# Deep Brain Stimulation in Neurological
and Psychiatric Disorders

# CURRENT CLINICAL NEUROLOGY

## Daniel Tarsy, MD, SERIES EDITOR

Deep Brain Stimulation in Neurological and Psychiatric Disorders, edited by Daniel Tarsy, Jerrold L. Vitek, Philip A. Starr, and Michael S. Okun, 2008
Stroke Recovery with Cellular Therapies, edited by Sean I. Savitz and Daniel M. Rosenbaum, 2008
Practicing Neurology: *What You Need to Know, What You Need to Do*, Second Edition, by Rahman Pourmand, 2007
Sleep Disorders in Women: *From Menarche Through Pregnancy to Menopause*, edited by Hrayr P. Attarian, 2006
Diagnostic Criteria in Neurology, edited by Alan J. Lerner, 2006
Psychiatry for Neurologists, edited by Dilip V. Jeste and Joseph H. Friedman, 2006
Status Epilepticus: *A Clinical Perspective*, edited by Frank W. Drislane, 2005
Thrombolytic Therapy for Acute Stroke, Second Edition, edited by Patrick D. Lyden, 2005
Parkinson's Disease and Nonmotor Dysfunction, edited by Ronald F. Pfeiffer and Ivan Bodis-Wollner, 2005
Movement Disorder Emergencies: *Diagnosis and Treatment*, edited by Steven J. Frucht and Stanley Fahn, 2005
Inflammatory Disorders of the Nervous System: *Pathogenesis, Immunology, and Clinical Management*, edited by Alireza Minagar and J. Steven Alexander, 2005
Neurological and Psychiatric Disorders: *From Bench to Bedside*, edited by Frank I. Tarazi and John A. Schetz, 2005
Multiple Sclerosis: Etiology, *Diagnosis, and New Treatment Strategies*, edited by Michael J. Olek, 2005
Seizures in Critical Care: *A Guide to Diagnosis and Therapeutics*, edited by Panayiotis N. Varelas, 2005
Vascular Dementia: *Cerebrovascular Mechanisms and Clinical Management*, edited by Robert H. Paul, Ronald Cohen, Brian R. Ott, Stephen Salloway, 2005
Atypical Parkinsonian Disorders: *Clinical and Research Aspects*, edited by Irene Litvan, 2005
Handbook of Neurocritical Care, edited by Anish Bhardwaj, Marek A. Mirski, and John A. Ulatowski, 2004
Handbook of Stroke Prevention in Clinical Practice, edited by Karen L. Furie and Peter J. Kelly, 2004
Clinical Handbook of Insomnia, edited by Hrayr P. Attarian, 2004
Critical Care Neurology and Neurosurgery, edited by Jose I. Suarez, 2004
Alzheimer's Disease: A *Physician's Guide to Practical Management*, edited by Ralph W. Richter and Brigitte Zoeller Richter, 2004
Field of Vision: *A Manual and Atlas of Perimetry*, edited by Jason J. S. Barton and Michael Benatar, 2003
Surgical Treatment of Parkinson's Disease and Other Movement Disorders, edited by Daniel Tarsy, Jerrold L. Vitek, and Andres M. Lozano, 2003
Myasthenia Gravis and Related Disorders, edited by Henry J. Kaminski, 2003
Seizures: *Medical Causes and Management*, edited by Norman Delanty, 2002
Clinical Evaluation and Management of Spasticity, edited by David A. Gelber and Douglas R. Jeffery, 2002
Early Diagnosis of Alzheimer's Disease, edited by Leonard F. M. Scinto and Kirk R. Daffner, 2000
Sexual and Reproductive Neurorehabilitation, edited by Mindy Aisen, 1997

# Deep Brain Stimulation in Neurological and Psychiatric Disorders

Edited by

**Daniel Tarsy, MD**
*Parkinson's Disease and Movement Disorders Center,
Department of Neurology,
Beth Israel Deaconess Medical Center,
Harvard Medical School,
Boston, MA*

**Jerrold L. Vitek, MD, PhD**
*Neuromodulation Research Center,
Lerner Research Institute,
The Cleveland Clinic Foundation,
Cleveland, OH*

**Philip A. Starr, MD, PhD**
*Department of Neurosurgery,
University of California,
San Francisco, CA*

**Michael S. Okun, MD**
*Departments of Neurology and Neurosurgery,
McKnight Brain Institute,
University of Florida,
Gainesville, FL*

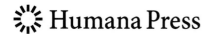

*Editors*
Daniel Tarsy
Beth Israel Deaconess Medical Center
Harvard Medical School
Boston, MA

Jerrold L. Vitek
The Cleveland Clinic Foundation
Cleveland, OH

Philip A. Starr
University of California
San Francisco, CA

Michael S. Okun
University of Florida
Gainesville, FL

*Series Editor*
Daniel Tarsy

ISBN: 978-1-58829-952-9     e-ISBN: 978-1-59745-360-8
DOI: 10.1008/978-1-59745-360-8

Library of Congress Control Number: 2007941161

© 2008 Humana Press, a part of Springer Science+Business Media, LLC
All rights reserved. This work may not be translated or copied in whole or in part without the written permission of the publisher (Humana Press, 999 Riverview Drive, Suite 208, Totowa, NJ 07512 USA), except for brief excerpts in connection with reviews or scholarly analysis. Use in connection with any form of information storage and retrieval, electronic adaptation, computer software, or by similar or dissimilar methodology now known or hereafter developed is forbidden.
The use in this publication of trade names, trademarks, service marks, and similar terms, even if they are not identified as such, is not to be taken as an expression of opinion as to whether or not they are subject to proprietary rights.
While the advice and information in this book are believed to be true and accurate at the date of going to press, neither the authors nor the editors nor the publisher can accept any legal responsibility for any errors or omissions that may be made. The publisher makes no warranty, express or implied, with respect to the material contained herein.

*Cover illustration:* Photo courtesy of Jeffrey T. Joseph, MD, PhD, Division of Neuropathology, Department of Neurology, Beth Israel Deaconess Medical Center, Boston, MA.

Printed on acid-free paper

9 8 7 6 5 4 3 2 1

springer.com

# Preface

Chronic deep brain stimulation (DBS) has been a rapidly evolving area of neurotherapeutics since its initial introduction for the treatment of Parkinson's disease and essential tremor in the 1990s. For these conditions, DBS is now considered accepted therapy for patients failing to adequately respond to medical treatment. Since the 1990s, new clinical indications, anatomic targets, and technologies have contributed to an expanding role for DBS in the treatment of other movement disorders such as dystonia and Tourette syndrome as well as for other neurologic disorders such as epilepsy and cluster headache. Early experience has also been reported for psychiatric syndromes, such as obsessive–compulsive disorder and depression. Experience with DBS in psychiatric disorders is very limited but is reviewed in this volume as neuropsychiatric indications are expected to grow in coming years.

Because of the rapidly increasing application of DBS for neurologic and psychiatric indications and the recruitment of increasing numbers of neurologic, neurosurgical, and psychiatric clinicians to the field, it is appropriate to provide a resource that updates the underlying scientific background, describes methodologies and standards of treatment, and provides information on new technologies essential for clinical success and to advance the field. *Deep Brain Stimulation in Neurological and Psychiatric Disorders* begins with reviews of the functional anatomy and physiology of motor and nonmotor aspects of the basal ganglia and their connections, which underlie the application of DBS to neurological and psychiatric disorders. This is followed by proposed mechanisms of action of DBS based on functional neuroimaging, molecular, modeling, and neurophysiologic studies in animals and man. Discussions of patient selection, preoperative assessment, operative complications, and brain targeting are followed by chapters concerning microelectrode mapping as well as new and emerging brain imaging alternatives for target localization inside the operating room.

DBS for movement disorders, which remains the most common indication, is reviewed in chapters on essential and other tremors, Parkinson's disease, atypical parkinsonism, dystonia, and Tourette syndrome. Postoperative management and treatment outcomes are reviewed in a series of chapters which address immediate and delayed complications, a particularly important chapter on programming. We have also included a discussion of DBS safety with regard to MRI and other electronic devices, neuropsychological sequelae, and quality of life. Finally, interesting new areas of DBS applications are addressed by experts with experience in epilepsy, obsessive–compulsive disorder, depression, and cluster headache.

We have gathered a group of experienced and recognized authors to review the current state of DBS in neurologic and psychiatric disorders. We thank them for providing a conservative and level-headed approach to the use of DBS with emphasis on objective assessment of clinical outcomes, particularly in the new and emerging applications. We greatly appreciate the efforts of Richard Lansing and Michele Seugling at Humana Press, who have helped to make this work a reality. We also wish to thank our understanding families, without whose love and support this book would not have been possible. Finally, we dedicate this book to our patients and their families, whose continued courage and cooperation in the face of great personal adversity have allowed this work to progress toward providing some measure of relief for their difficult conditions.

Daniel Tarsy, MD
Jerrold L. Vitek, MD, PhD
Philip A. Starr, MD, PhD
Michael S. Okun, MD

# Contents

Preface ................................................................................. v
Contributors ........................................................................ xi
List of Color Plates ............................................................ xv

**Part I.  Overview of Deep Brain Stimulation**

1. Functional Anatomy and Physiology of the Basal Ganglia:
   *Motor Functions* ............................................................. 3
   Yoland Smith and Thomas Wichmann

2. Functional Anatomy and Physiology of the Basal Ganglia:
   *Non-motor Functions* ..................................................... 33
   Suzanne N. Haber

3. History of the Therapeutic Use of Electricity on the Brain
   and the Development of Deep Brain Stimulation ............. 63
   Matthew A. Butler, Joshua M. Rosenow, and Michael S. Okun

4. Deep Brain Stimulation: *Patient Selection in Parkinson's Disease,
   Other Movement Disorders, and Neuropsychiatric Disorders.* ........ 83
   Mustafa Saad Siddiqui, Thomas Ellis, Stephen S. Tatter,
   Kelly D. Foote, and Michael S. Okun

5. Technical Alternatives in Performing Deep Brain
   Stimulator Implantation .................................................. 99
   Paul S. Larson

6. Intra-operative Microrecording and Stimulation ............. 111
   Frank Steigerwald and Jens Volkmann

7. Complication Avoidance and Management
   in Deep Brain Stimulation Surgery .................................. 135
   Philip A. Starr and Karl Sillay

8. Mechanisms of Deep Brain Stimulation ........................................... 151
   Svjetlana Miocinovic, Cameron C. McIntyre,
   Marc Savasta, and Jerrold L. Vitek

9. Functional Imaging of Deep Brain Stimulation:
   fMRI, SPECT, and PET ..................................................................... 179
   Robert Jech

**Part II.  Deep Brain Stimulation in Movement Disorders**

10. Thalamic Deep Brain Stimulation and Essential Tremor .............. 205
    Kelly E. Lyons and Rajesh Pahwa

11. Thalamic Deep Brain Stimulation for Other Tremors ................... 215
    Erwin B. Montgomery, Jr.

12. Thalamic Deep Brain Stimulation for Parkinson's
    Disease Tremor ................................................................................ 229
    Daniel Tarsy, Efstathios Papavassiliou, Kelly E. Lyons,
    and Rajesh Pahwa

13. Globus Pallidus Deep Brain Stimulation
    for Parkinson's Disease .................................................................... 243
    Frances Weaver, Kenneth Follett, and Matthew Stern

14. Deep Brain Stimulation of the Subthalamic Nucleus
    for the Treatment of Parkinson's Disease ....................................... 253
    Marcelo Merello

15. Deep Brain Stimulation of the Globus Pallidus
    Pars Interna and Subthalamic Nucleus in Parkinson's
    Disease: *Pros and Cons* .................................................................. 277
    Jorge Guridi, Maria C. Rodriguez-Oroz, and Jose A. Obeso

16. Deep Brain Stimulation in Atypical Parkinsonism ........................ 291
    Ludy Shih and Daniel Tarsy

17. Deep Brain Stimulation in Dystonia ............................................... 305
    Marie Vidailhet, David Grabli, and Emmanuel Roze

18. Deep Brain Stimulation in Tourette's Syndrome ........................... 321
    Linda Ackermans, Yasin Temel, and Veerle Visser-Vandewalle

19. The Role of Deep Brain Stimulation (DBS)
    in the Treatment of Postural Instability and Gait
    Disorders of Parkinson's Disease ..................................................... 333
    Helen Bronte-Stewart

## Part III.  Postoperative Management in Patients Undergoing Deep Brain Stimulation

20. Deep Brain Stimulation Programming for Movement Disorders ................................................................. 361
    *Ioannis U. Isaias and Michele Tagliati*

21. Neuropsychological Issues in Deep Brain Stimulation of Neurological and Psychiatric Disorders .................................... 399
    *Alexander I. Tröster, April B. McTaggart, and Ines A. Heber*

22. Deep Brain Stimulation Safety: *MRI and Other Electromagnetic Interactions* ............................................................ 453
    *Kenneth B. Baker and Michael D. Phillips*

23. Deep Brain Stimulation Fault Testing ............................................ 473
    *Jay L. Shils, Ron L. Alterman, and Jeffrey E. Arle*

24. Quality of Life and Cost Effectiveness of Deep Brain Stimulation in Movement Disorders .............................................. 495
    *Alan Diamond and Joseph Jankovic*

## Part IV.  Deep Brain Stimulation in Other Indications

25. Deep Brain Stimulation in Depression: *Background, Progress, and Key Issues* .......................................... 511
    *Benjamin D. Greenberg*

26. Deep Brain Stimulation in Obsessive–Compulsive Disorder ......... 531
    *Loes Gabriëls, Kris van Kuyck, Marleen Welkenhuyzen, Paul Cosyns, and Bart Nuttin*

27. Deep Brain Stimulation for Medically Intractable Cluster Headache ............................................................................ 547
    *Philip A. Starr and Andrew Ahn*

28. Deep Brain Stimulation in Epilepsy .............................................. 561
    *William J. Marks, Jr.*

29. The Future of Deep Brain Stimulation............................................ 571
    *Julie G. Pilitsis and Roy A.E. Bakay*

Index .................................................................................................... 593

# Contributors

Linda Ackermans, MD, Department of Neurosurgery, University Hospital Maastricht, Maastricht, The Netherlands

Andrew Ahn, MD, PhD, Department of Neurology, University of California, San Francisco, San Francisco, CA

Ron L. Alterman, MD, Department of Neurosurgery, Mount Sinai School of Medicine, New York, NY

Jeffrey E. Arle, MD, PhD, Lahey Clinic, Neurosurgery, Tufts University School of Medicine, Boston, MA

Roy A.E. Bakay, MD, Department of Neurosurgery, Rush University, Chicago, IL

Kenneth B. Baker, PhD, Department of Neurosciences, The Cleveland Clinic, Cleveland, OH

Helen Bronte-Stewart, MD, MSE, Departments of Neurology and Neurosciences and Neurosurgery, Stanford Movement Disorders Center, Stanford University, Stanford, CA

Matthew A. Butler, MD, Movement Disorders Center, University of Florida, Department of Neurology, McKnight Brain Institute, Gainesville, FL

Paul Cosyns, MD, PhD, Collaborative Antwerp Psychiatric Research Institute (CAPRI), University of Antwerp, Department of Psychiatry, University Hospital Antwerp, Antwerp, Belgium

Alan Diamond, DO, Colorado Neurological Institute, Englewood, CO

Thomas Ellis, MD, Departments of Neurology and Neurosurgery, Movement Disorders Program, Wake Forest University School of Medicine, Winston-Salem, NC

Kenneth Follett, MD, PhD, FACS, Department of Neurosurgery, University of Nebraska Medical Center, Omaha, NE

Kelly D. Foote, MD, Departments of Neurology and Neurosurgery, Movement Disorders Center, McKnight Brain Institute, University of Florida, Gainesville, FL

Loes Gabriëls, MD, MscEng, PhD, Collaborative Antwerp Psychiatric Research Institute (CAPRI), University of Antwerp, Antwerp, Belgium

David Grabli, MD, PhD, Department of Neurology, Salpêtrière Hospital, Paris, France

Benjamin D. Greenberg, MD, PhD, Butler Hospital, Department of Psychiatry and Human Behavior, Brown Medical School, Providence, RI

Jorge Guridi, MD, PhD, Neurological Surgery, Universidad de Navarra, Pamplona, Spain

Suzanne N. Haber, PhD, Department of Pharmacology and Physiology, University of Rochester School of Medicine, Rochester, NY

Ines A. Heber, DiplPsych, Department of Neurology, Rheinisch Westfälische Technische Hochschule, Aachen, Germany

Ioannis U. Isaias, MD, Department of Neurology, Mount Sinai School of Medicine, New York, NY

Joseph Jankovic, MD, Parkinson's Disease Center and Movement Disorders Clinic, Baylor College of Medicine, Houston, TX

Robert Jech, MD, PhD, Charles University, First Faculty of Medicine, Movement Disorders Center, Department of Neurology, Prague, Czech Republic

Paul S. Larson, MD, Department of Neurological Surgery, University of California, San Francisco, CA

Kelly E. Lyons, PhD, Department of Neurology, University of Kansas Medical Center, Kansas City, KS

William J. Marks, Jr., MD, Department of Neurology, University of California, San Francisco, CA

Cameron C. McIntyre, PhD, Department of Biomedical Engineering, The Cleveland Clinic Foundation, Cleveland, OH

April B. McTaggart, BS, Department of Neurology, University of North Carolina School of Medicine, Chapel Hill, NC

Marcelo Merello, MD, PhD, Raul Carrea Institute for Neurological Research (FLENI), Buenos Aires, Argentina

Svjetlana Miocinovic, PhD, Case Western Reserve University, School of Medicine, Cleveland, OH

Erwin B. Montgomery, Jr., MD, Department of Neurology, National Primate Research Center, Departments of Biomedical Engineering and Communicative Disorders, University of Wisconsin-Madison, Madison, WI

Bart Nuttin, MD, PhD, Department of Neurosurgery, University Hospital Gasthuisberg, Laboratory for Experimental Functional Neurosurgery, Katholieke Universiteit Leuven, Leuven, Belgium

Jose A. Obeso, MD, PhD, Neurological Department, Universidad de Navarra, Pamplona, Spain

Michael S. Okun, MD, Departments of Neurology and Neurosurgery, McKnight Brain Institute, University of Florida, Gainesville, FL

Rajesh Pahwa, MD, Department of Neurology, University of Kansas Medical Center, Kansas City, KS

Efstathios Papavassiliou, MD, Division of Neurosurgery, Beth Israel Deaconess Medical Center, Harvard Medical School, Boston, MA

Michael D. Phillips, MD, Department of Radiology, The Cleveland Clinic, Cleveland, OH

Julie G. Pilitsis, MD, PhD, Division of Neurosurgery, UMass Memorial Hospital Medical Center, Worcester, MA

Maria C. Rodriguez-Oroz, MD, PhD, Neurological Department, Universidad de Navarra, Pamplona, Spain

Joshua M. Rosenow, MD, Department of Neurosurgery, Feinberg School of Medicine, Northwestern University, Chicago, IL

Emmanuel Roze, MD, PhD, Department of Neurology, Salpêtrière Hospital and Pierre Marie Curie Paris 6 University, Paris, France

Mustafa Saad Siddiqui, MD, Departments of Neurology and Neurosurgery, Movement Disorders Program, Wake Forest University School of Medicine, Winston-Salem, NC

Marc Savasta, PhD, Grenoble Institut des Neurosciences, Université Joseph Fourier, UFR Biologie Bt B, Domaine Universitaire, Grenoble, France

Ludy Shih, MD, Department of Neurology, Beth Israel Deaconess Medical Center, Harvard Medical School, Boston, MA

Jay L. Shils, PhD, Lahey Clinic, Neurosurgery, Tufts University School of Medicine, Boston, MA

Karl Sillay, MD, Department of Neurosurgery, University of California, San Francisco, CA

Yoland Smith, PhD, Yerkes National Primate Center, Department of Neurology, Emory University, Atlanta, GA

Philip A. Starr, MD, PhD, Department of Neurosurgery, University of California, San Francisco, CA

Frank Steigerwald, MD, Department of Neurology, Christian-Albrechts-University, Kiel, Germany

Matthew Stern, MD, Department of Neurology, Philadelphia VAMC and University of Pennsylvania, Philadelphia, PA

Michele Tagliati, MD, Department of Neurology, Mount Sinai School of Medicine, New York, NY

Daniel Tarsy, MD, Parkinson's Disease and Movement Disorders Center, Department of Neurology, Beth Israel Deaconess Medical Center, Harvard Medical School, Boston, MA

Stephen S. Tatter, MD, PhD, Departments of Neurology and Neurosurgery, Movement Disorders Program, Wake Forest University School of Medicine, Winston-Salem, NC

Yasin Temel, MD, PhD, Department of Neurosurgery, University Hospital Maastricht, Maastricht, The Netherlands

Alexander I. Tröster, PhD, Department of Neurology, University of North Carolina School of Medicine, Chapel Hill, NC

Kris van Kuyck, PhD, Laboratory for Experimental Functional Neurosurgery, Katholieke Universiteit Leuven, Leuven, Belgium

Marie Vidailhet, MD, PhD, Department of Neurology, Salpêtrière Hospital, Paris, France

Veerle Visser-Vandewalle, MD, PhD, Department of Neurosurgery, University Hospital Maastricht, Maastricht, The Netherlands

Jerrold L. Vitek, MD, PhD, Neuromodulation Research Center, Lerner Research Institute, The Cleveland Clinic Foundation, Cleveland, OH

Jens Volkmann, MD, PhD, Department of Neurology, Christian-Albrechts-University, Kiel, Germany

Frances Weaver, PhD, Midwest Center for Health Services and Policy Research, Hines VAMC, Hines, IL

Thomas Wichmann, MD, Yerkes National Primate Center, Department of Neurology, Emory University, Atlanta, GA

Marleen Welkenhuyzen, MSc, Laboratory for Experimental Functional Neurosurgery, Katholieke Universiteit Leuven, Leuven, Belgium

# List of Color Plates

The images listed below appear in the color insert that follows page 304.

**Color Plate 1.** *Figure 1, Chapter 1:* Anatomical structure of the basal ganglia circuitry. Red arrows denote excitatory (glutamatergic) connections, black arrows indicate inhibitory (GABAergic) connections. (*See* complete caption on p. 4.)

**Color Plate 2.** *Figure 2, Chapter 1:* Intrinsic striatal circuitry. Red arrows denote excitatory (glutamatergic) connections, black arrows show inhibitory (GABAergic) projections, and green arrows symbolize cholinergic projections. (*See* complete caption on p. 6.)

**Color Plate 3.** *Figure 1, Chapter 9:* Manifestations of acute STN DBS in a 1.5 T fMRI scan of a PD patient (woman, 63 years, PD duration 12 years, UPDRS III: OFF = 53, ON = 30). (*See* complete caption on p. 182.)

**Color Plate 4.** *Figure 2, Chapter 9:* Effects of left-sided STN DBS on motion-related activity in eight patients with PD scanned with 1.5 T fMRI after overnight discontinuation of L-DOPA. (*See* complete caption on p. 186.)

**Color Plate 5.** *Figure 3, Chapter 9:* 1.5 T fMRI during acute VIM DBS in a patient with essential tremor (man, 58 years, tremor duration 20 years). (*See* complete caption on p. 191.)

**Color Plate 6.** *Figure 1, Chapter 18:* A schematic drawing of brain areas that have been targeted in surgery for Tourette's syndrome and other relevant neuroanatomical structures. (*See* complete caption on p. 323.)

**Color Plate 7.** *Figure 1, Chapter 20:* Strength-duration curve showing the inverse relationship between pulse width and voltage of stimulation. (*See* complete caption on p. 364.)

**Color Plate 8.** *Figure 7, Chapter 20:* Sagittal view of the thalamic and subthalamic area at 12 mm from the midline, illustrating the anatomical relationships of the subthalamic nucleus (STN). (*See* complete caption on p. 380.)

**Color Plate 9.** *Figure 8, Chapter 20:* Schematic representation of the 3387 DBS electrode placement in the subthalamic area, illustrating the approximate anatomical areas that can be stimulated by the four contacts. (*See* complete caption on p. 381.)

**Color Plate 10.** *Figure 8, Chapter 23:* Graphical representations of an analytic solution to the Voltage (A and C) and electric (B and D) fields generated by the Medtronic DBS lead. (*See* complete caption on p. 484.)

# Part I

# Overview of Deep Brain Stimulation

# Functional Anatomy and Physiology of the Basal Ganglia: Motor Functions

Yoland Smith and Thomas Wichmann

## Abstract

During the last few years, our understanding of basal ganglia anatomy and function has undergone major changes. It is now recognized that the basal ganglia participate in larger circuits that also involve regions of the cerebral cortex, thalamus, and brain stem. These circuits subserve motor and non-motor functions, and occupy separate territories within the basal ganglia. Specific abnormalities in the function of motor-related basal ganglia areas are thought to contribute to the signs and symptoms of movement disorders such as Parkinson's disease or dystonia, while abnormalities in non-motor circuits may be relevant for the pathophysiology of some of the neuropsychiatric disorders.

The insight that relatively local abnormalities in the basal ganglia may contribute to the pathophysiology of movement disorders has resulted in renewed interest in focal neurosurgical treatments for these conditions, such as deep brain stimulation, ablative techniques, or transplantation. This chapter discusses the results of anatomical and physiological studies that are relevant for our current understanding of the motor functions of the basal ganglia, and for the use of neurosurgical interventions in movement disorders.

**Keywords:** striatum, putamen, globus pallidus, subthalamic nucleus, substantia nigra, dopamine, Parkinson's disease, dystonia

## Introduction

In recent years, much progress has been made toward a better understanding of the pathophysiologic basis of movement disorders such as Parkinson's disease and dystonia. Besides opening the door to new pharmacologic therapies, this has resulted in renewed interest in neurosurgical techniques such as deep brain stimulation (DBS) to treat these diseases. DBS involves the continuous application of electrical stimulation pulses at high frequency to specific brain regions via chronically implanted electrodes. This technique makes it possible for the first time to reversibly alter the function of small and highly specific brain regions.

In most cases, movement disorders involve pathology in the basal ganglia or associated thalamocortical brain circuitry. This chapter discusses anatomical and physiological aspects of the basal ganglia–thalamocortical network of connections, which are important for the current use of DBS in these disorders. Specific information regarding the practical use of DBS to help patients with movement disorders is provided in other chapters of this book.

## General Structure of Basal Ganglia Circuits

As shown in Figure 1.1, the primate basal ganglia are a group of functionally related subcortical nuclei that include the dorsal striatum (comprised of the caudate nucleus and the putamen), the external globus pallidus (GPe); the internal globus pallidus (GPi); the substantia nigra, which comprises the dopaminergic neurons in the pars compacta (SNc) and the GABAergic neurons in the pars reticulata (SNr); and the subthalamic nucleus (STN). In rodents, the caudate nucleus and putamen are part of a single nucleus (the caudate–putamen complex). The rodent GP and the entopeduncular nucleus (EPN) are the functional homologues of the primate GPe and GPi, respectively.

Anatomically and physiologically, the basal ganglia structures are related to the thalamus and cerebral cortex. The striatum, and, to a lesser extent, the STN, are the main stations at which movement-related cortical information enters the basal ganglia circuitry, while GPi and SNr function as output nuclei, sending inhibitory (GABAergic) output to a variety of targets, including frontal areas of the cerebral cortex (via the ventral motor thalamic nuclei), as well as brainstem structures (superior colliculus, lateral habenular nucleus, pedunculopontine nucleus [PPN], parvicellular reticular formation). Basal ganglia outflow is also fed back into the basal ganglia via the thalamostriatal pathways.

All structures involved in the cortex-basal ganglia-thalamic-cortical circuits are topographically organized. Thus, each of the basal ganglia nuclei contains motor and non-motor areas. The motor circuit of the basal ganglia originates from frontal motor areas, and passes through the putamen (the motor portion of the striatum), as well as motor portions of GPe, STN, GPi, and SNr. GPi

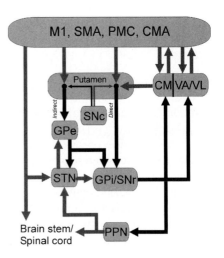

**Figure 1.1** Anatomical structure of the basal ganglia circuitry. Red arrows denote excitatory (glutamatergic) connections, black arrows indicate inhibitory (GABAergic) connections. Abbreviations: GPe, external pallidal segment; STN, subthalamic nucleus; GPi, internal pallidal segment; SNr, substantia nigra pars reticulata; SNc, substantia nigra pars compacta; PPN, pedunculopontine nucleus; CM, centromedian nucleus of the thalamus; VA/VL, ventral anterior and ventrolateral nucleus of the thalamus; M1, primary motor cortex; SMA, supple mentary motor area; PMC, premotor cortex; CMA, cingulate motor area. (To view this figure in color, see insert)

and SNr project to portions of the ventral anterior (VA) and ventrolateral (VL) nucleus of the thalamus, and from there, back to motor and pre-motor (PM) areas of frontal cortex.

It remains debated whether motor and non-motor basal ganglia-thalamocortical circuits are segregated throughout their entire course, or whether information from different domains converges at some levels of the circuitry. The anatomic concept of segregation is supported by evidence from electrophysiologic recording studies, which have shown that each basal ganglia region contains neurons that respond selectively to a narrow range of specific inputs or behaviors (at least within the experimental framework studied). For instance, the sensorimotor portion of the basal ganglia contains specific areas with neurons that are concerned with active or passive limb movements *(1–19)*. Furthermore, functional neurosurgical studies have demonstrated that lesions in the sensorimotor portion of the GPi alleviate the motor signs associated with parkinsonism without affecting cognitive functions, while lesions outside of this region do not improve motor function but may affect cognition (see, e.g., refs. *20* and *21*).

However, it is also clear that motor and non-motor circuits must converge to some extent, because the number of striatal neurons is much smaller than that of cortical neurons that project upon them, and much greater than the number of neurons in the nuclei that receive striatal inputs (see, e.g., refs. *22* and *23*). Communication between the basal ganglia-thalamocortical circuits may also occur through communication between cortical neurons *(24, 25)*. In addition, the spiral arrangement of the striato-nigro-striatal loops, which allows information to be channeled from limbic to cognitive to motor circuits provides another substrate for cross-talk between functionally segregated basal ganglia circuits (see refs. *26* and *27*).

The degree of interaction between neighboring circuits may also be dynamically regulated. Thus, release of dopamine or other neuromodulators may act to modulate synaptic collateral interactions, particularly in the striatum *(28–31)*. This could transiently affect the level of synchrony between neighboring basal ganglia neurons, for instance, during learning *(22, 23)*, or more permanently, in states of dopamine depletion, as is seen in parkinsonism, where a greater level of inter-neuronal synchrony is observed throughout the basal ganglia *(32–40)*.

## Intrinsic Neuronal Organization of Basal Ganglia Nuclei

Motor and non-motor areas of the basal ganglia differ mostly by their extrinsic connections, while the intrinsic organization and the connectivity within the basal ganglia is the same for all of these circuits. Most of the considerations in this section are therefore equally true for non-motor and motor circuits.

### Striatum

The intrinsic circuitry of the striatum and its relationship to cortical and striatal inputs is shown in Figure 1.2. The predominant neuronal cell type in the striatum is the spiny neuron (MSN), characterized by an abundance of dendritic spines. These GABAergic neurons are the output neurons of the

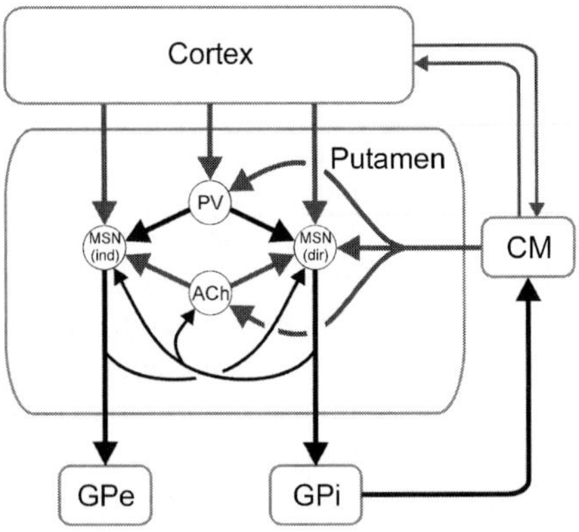

**Figure 1.2** Intrinsic striatal circuitry. Red arrows denote excitatory (glutamatergic) connections, black arrows show inhibitory (GABAergic) projections, and green arrows symbolize cholinergic projections. Abbreviations: Ach, striatal cholinergic interneurons; GPe, external pallidal segment; GPi, internal pallidal segment; CM, centromedian nucleus of the thalamus; MSN (ind), striatal GABAergic medium spiny neurons, projecting to GPe as part of the indirect pathway; MSN (dir), striatal GABAergic medium spiny neurons, projecting to GPi as part of the direct pathway; PV striatal GABAergic interneurons containing parvalbumin. (To view this figure in color, see insert)

striatum and can be further classified according to chemical and anatomical criteria. Neurons that contain enkephalin mRNA and express D2 dopamine receptors project preferentially to GPe as part of the so-called indirect pathway of the basal ganglia, while neurons that contain substance P and dynorphin and express D1 dopamine receptors project mainly to GPi and SNr *(41)*, constituting the direct pathway (see following paragraph).

Besides their classification as direct and indirect pathway neurons, MSNs can also be divided according to their association with the two distinct neurochemical striatal compartments, namely the patch (or striosome) and matrix compartment *(42, 43)*. Projections from sensorimotor cortices and most thalamic nuclei innervate preferentially the matrix *(43–50)*, while the patch compartment may be more closely associated with non-motor areas of the thalamus and cortex. The behavioral importance of the patch-matrix organization of the striatum is underscored by recent findings that a disturbance of the balance of activity between the patch and matrix compartments may lead to repetitive motor behaviors *(51–53)*, and that selective neurodegeneration of patches occurs in X-linked progressive dystonia-parkinsonism *(54)*. Another notable feature is that the dopaminergic innervation of patches seems to be more sensitive to the neurodegenerative processes underlying parkinsonism than the dopaminergic afferents to the matrix compartment *(55–57)*.

Aspiny striatal neurons are interneurons, and are less common than MSNs *(58, 59)*. Some of the anatomic connections of these interneurons are shown in Figure 1.2. A common aspiny interneuron type is cholinergic. These cells can be physiologically identified as tonically active neurons (see refs. *60* and *61*), and appear to play a role in reward-related learning and motivated behaviors *(62–64)*. These neurons receive excitatory input from the caudal intralaminar nuclei of the thalamus, and, at least in rats, inhibitory input from MSNs that project to GPi and SNr *(65, 66)*. Fifty percent of cholinergic interneurons co-express calretinin in the human striatum *(67)*. Other interneuron types are

GABAergic, but can be distinguished by their specific expression of neuropeptides or calcium-binding proteins. For instance, parvalbumin-containing cells correspond to the physiologic type of fast spiking interneurons that receive strong cortical inputs, and form axosomatic synapses on projection neurons. These neurons are connected to one another through gap junctions and provide fast feed-forward inhibition of striatal output neurons in response to cortical activation *(59, 68)*. Other types of GABAergic interneurons contain nitric oxide synthase, neuropeptide Y and somatostatin, or calretinin *(59, 67)*. An interesting population of tyrosine hydroxylase-immunoreactive interneurons has been identified in the striatum of animal models of parkinsonism and human patients with Parkinson's disease. These neurons are significantly increased in number in Parkinson's disease, are preferentially located in the associative striatum, receive very scarce extrinsic inputs and give rise to intrastriatal terminals that co-express tyrosine hydroxylase and GABA *(69–72)*. Striatal interneurons are selectively spared from the striatal degeneration which occurs in Huntington's disease *(73)*.

**Other Basal Ganglia Nuclei**

GPe and GPi are largely comprised of GABAergic projection neurons *(74–76)*. GPe projection neurons generate axon collaterals that may contribute to local inhibition in GPe, and may provide strong inhibitory influences to GPi and SNr *(77–79)*. Two populations of pallidal neurons have recently been identified in the rat GP (corresponding to the primate GPe), based on their location relative to the striatopallidal border (outer and inner neurons) and the number of intrinsic GABAergic terminals they give rise to *(80)*. Two types of projection neurons have also been identified in the monkey GPi *(81)*. The more common type consists of neurons that are located in the center of GPi and send projections to the ventral motor and caudal intralaminar nuclei of the thalamus, as well as the brainstem pedunculopontine region. Less numerous peripherally located neurons send axons to the lateral habenular nucleus *(81)*. Pallidothalamic axons travel through two main tracts to reach their targets, i.e., the ansa lenticularis and the lenticular fasciculus *(82)*. Of these, the lenticular fasciculus appears to contain most of the fibers that may carry movement-related information *(83)*.

Axon collaterals of SNr neurons innervate neighboring SNr neurons and dopaminergic SNc neurons in a highly organized and topographic manner, thereby contributing to an indirect route through which the striatum can upregulate its level of dopaminergic transmission via disinhibition of nigrostriatal neurons *(84, 85)*. The SNc also interacts with the SNr through dendritic release of dopamine (see below).

The STN mainly comprises glutamatergic projection neurons to GPe and GPi, but also includes a small population of GABAergic interneurons in humans *(78, 86, 87)*.

# Inputs to the Basal Ganglia

**Sensorimotor Corticostriatal Projections**

The corticostriatal projection terminates in a strict topographical organization *(88–91)*. In primates, the somatosensory, motor and PM cortices project in a somatotopically organized fashion to the post-commissural region of the putamen *(92–95)*. Projections from somatosensory and motor cortical areas related to the same body parts tightly overlap in the ipsilateral post-commissural putamen, while contralateral projections from the primary motor cortex (M1), except those from the face area, interdigitate with projections from the ipsilateral somatosensory and M1 cortices *(95)*.

The striatal neurons that give rise to either the direct or the indirect pathways may differ in the type of cortical inputs they receive. Thus, in rats, cortical intra-telencephalic (IT) neurons, which project to contralateral cortices and striatum, appear to target preferentially D1-containing direct striatofugal neurons, while pyramidal tract (PT) neurons, which project to the brainstem and spinal cord, innervate preferentially D2-containing indirect striatofugal neurons *(96)*. At the cortical level, corticostriatal IT neurons provide inputs to other IT neurons and PT neurons *(25)*, whereas PT neuron projections to IT neurons are far less common.

Other studies have also shown that the corticostriatal system differentially regulates the two main populations of striatofugal neurons. For instance, stimulation of sensorimotor cortices induces preferential immediate early gene expression in enkephalin-containing neurons in rats and monkeys *(97, 98)*, and injections of herpes simplex virus, used as a trans-neuronal anterograde tracer, into monkey M1 result in relatively selective virus accumulation in GPe neurons *(99)*. In monkeys, most data suggest that corticostriatal neurons are segregated from long-range corticospinal neurons *(100–102)*, but a recent single axon tracing study demonstrated that this segregation may not be as strict as previously thought *(103)*.

Dendritic spines of striatal output neurons are the main targets of corticostriatal afferents *(104)*, although the GABA/parvalbumin-containing interneurons also receive significant cortical inputs in rats and monkeys *(105)*. Recent *in vivo* electrophysiological data demonstrate that (spike) responses in these interneurons occur earlier and can be induced by a lower intensity of cortical stimulation than required for activation of MSNs *(68)*. In general, increased cortical activity facilitates responses in GABA/parvalbumin interneurons, while opposite effects are found in projection neurons, which indicates that feed-forward inhibition of GABA/parvalbumin interneurons filters cortical information transmitted to striatal output neurons *(59, 68)*. Cortical inputs to other interneuron populations are sparse and often located on distal dendrites *(106)*.

**Thalamostriatal Projections**

Most thalamic nuclei send topographically organized glutamatergic projections to the striatum *(48, 107–110)*. Projections from the caudal intralaminar nuclear group, the centromedian (CM) and the parafascicular (PF) nuclei are by far the most prominent among these inputs *(50, 104, 111, 112)*. We will focus here on a description of some of the properties of this projection. A comparison between these properties and those of other thalamostriatal projections is provided in Table 1.1. The CM/PF-striatal projection is also shown in Figure 1.2.

Compared to corticostriatal inputs, the CM/PF-striatal projections are more focused and give rise to a significantly larger number of terminals than individual corticostriatal axons *(103, 108–110, 113, 114)*. In rodents, the CM/PF projection arises from a common nucleus (the PF), while in primates, this projection originates in two separate nuclei (CM and PF), and terminates

**Table 1.1** Similarities and differences between thalamostriatal projections from CM/PF and from other thalamic nuclei.

| Projection from CM/PF | Projections from other thalamic nuclei |
|---|---|
| • Components of sub-cortical loops with basal ganglia and brainstem | • Components of basal ganglia-thalamocortico-thalamic loops |
| • Innervate preferentially the striatum with collaterals to cortex | • Innervate preferentially the cortex with collaterals to striatum |
| • Neurons have reticular dendrites | • Neurons have bushy dendrites |
| • Focal and highly convergent sites of termination in the striatum | • Diffuse and less convergent innervation of the striatum |
| • Form axo-dendritic synapses (75%) | • Form axo-spinous synapses (>95%) |
| • No relationships with dopaminergic afferents | • Converge with dopaminergic inputs onto common dendritic spines |
| • Discharge single spikes during cortical slow-wave activity | • Discharge low-threshold calcium bursts during cortical slow-wave activity |
| • Sensitive to attention-related multisensory information | • Respond to specific modalities (such as sensory, motor, or limbic signals) |
| • May provide the striatum with attention-related information from brainstem | • May convey context-dependent functionally specific cortical information |
| • Partly degenerate in Parkinson's disease | • Do not degenerate in Parkinson's disease |

in different functional territories of the striatum *(50, 115, 116)*. The medial portion of CM projects to the sensorimotor post-commissural putamen, whereas the lateral CM is reciprocally connected with the motor cortex and does not appear to contribute much to striatal innervation *(50, 107, 115–118)*. CM inputs innervate preferentially the dendritic shafts of striatal output neurons *(112, 117, 119, 120)*.

It is also well known that CM outputs affect striatal interneuron activity *(120, 121)*, which, in turn may affect striatal projection neurons. In monkeys, striatofugal neurons that project to GPi are more frequently contacted by CM inputs than striato-GPe neurons *(120)*, suggesting that CM may exert direct effects on the monosynaptic striato-GPi projection, while effects on GPe-projecting striatal neurons may be mediated via striatal interneurons. Surprisingly, a PF lesion prevents upregulation of enkephalin mRNA (marker of GPe-projecting neurons), but does not affect the downregulation of substance P mRNA (marker of GPi-projecting neurons) in 6-OHDA-treated rats *(122, 123)*.

The functional roles of the thalamostriatal system remain(s) poorly understood and likely differ between projections that arise from CM/PF and those arising from other thalamic nuclei *(107)*. Projections from CM/PF to the striatum are more focused, more massive and innervate preferentially the dendritic shafts of striatal projection neurons, whereas projections from other motor-related thalamic nuclei like VA/VL are more diffuse and target exclusively the spines of striatal output neurons *(107, 124, 125)*. CM and PF may provide feedback information to the basal ganglia. In addition, Kimura and colleagues have proposed that the CM and PF supply striatal neurons with information that have attentional values *(126–129)*. This is also supported by positron emission tomography (PET) studies in humans *(130)*. Another interesting hypothesis is that the thalamostriatal projections from intralaminar and non-intralaminar nuclei are part of parallel, functionally segregated subcortical loops *(131)*.

### Cortico- and Thalamo-Subthalamic Projections

The cortico-subthalamic projection is exclusively ipsilateral *(132, 133)*, and arises in large part from the primary motor cortex (M1), with lesser contributions from prefrontal cortex, premotor cortex (PMC), supplementary motor, area (SMA), and cingulate motor area *(CMA, 92, 132–135)*. M1-afferents are confined to the dorsolateral part of STN *(132, 134)*, while afferents from the other motor areas innervate mainly the medial third of the nucleus *(93, 132, 134–136)*. The M1-STN projection is somatotopically organized with the face area projecting laterally, the arm area centrally and the leg area medially *(7, 92, 132, 134, 137)*. A similar somatotopic organization has been reported in the STN of humans with Parkinson's disease undergoing microelectrode mapping during functional neurosurgical procedures *(138)*. Input from the supplementary motor area (SMA) to the STN shows a somatotopy which is reversed to the one from M1 *(134, 137)*. The cortico-striatal and cortico-subthalamic projections appear to originate from segregated populations of corticofugal neurons in monkeys *(103)*, whereas in rats and cats, the cortical input to the STN is a collateral of descending pathways to the brainstem and spinal cord *(139, 140)*.

A second source of excitatory inputs to the STN arises from CM/PF *(50, 141–143)*, although the relevance of this finding for primate anatomy remains disputed *(110)*. In the rat, the thalamo-subthalamic and thalamo-striatal projections arise largely from segregated sets of neurons (for a discussion of these findings, see refs. *109* and *142)*. Excitatory cortical and thalamic inputs to the STN may provide a faster route of transmission of cortical information to the basal ganglia output structures than that provided by the trans-striatal pathways *(137, 144–148)*.

## Intrinsic Basal Ganglia Connections

### Direct and Indirect Pathways

The topographical organization of the corticostriatal system and intrinsic basal ganglia connections provide the substrate for functionally segregated motor, limbic, associative, and oculomotor basal ganglia-thalamocortical loops *(88)*. Within the boundaries of each of these circuits, striatofugal pathways are divided into the so-called direct and indirect striatofugal projections, named after their presumed connection patterns to the basal ganglia output nuclei GPi and SNr *(149–151)*. The direct pathway arises from striatal MSNs that project directly to neurons of GPi and SNr. The indirect pathway involves a striatal projection to GPe *(41)*, and subsequent projections to GPi and SNr. In monkeys, GPe terminals account for more than 50% of the total number of terminals in contact with the perikarya of GPi neurons *(152–155)*. A portion of the indirect pathway passes through the intercalated STN *(154, 156–161)*. The STN also sends projections to GPe, the striatum *(115, 162, 163)* the SNc *(159, 164, 165)*, the pedunculopontine nucleus (PPN) *(163, 164, 166)*, and the spinal cord *(167)*. STN output is highly collateralized in the rat *(168, 169)*, but may be more specific in primates *(160, 163, 169–171)*.

The true extent of separation between direct and indirect pathways continues to be debated *(172–177)*. In favor of pathway segregation, findings in the recently developed EGFP-D1- and D2-transgenic mice have strongly supported the notion that D1 and D2 receptors are segregated in the striatum and along striatofugal projections to the GP and substantia nigra *(175, 176)*. However, single cell filling studies have reported a fairly high degree of axon collateralization of striatofugal neurons *(174, 177–179)*. In addition, striatal MSNs are known to form an extensive intrinsic axon collateral arbor that connects neighboring MSNs and interneurons. Although these connections were originally thought to be a substrate for lateral inhibition in the striatum *(152, 180, 181)*, electrophysiological and anatomical studies have demonstrated that these connections are weak and distal on the dendritic tree of striatal neurons so that their influence on neighboring neurons is likely to be subtle *(59, 182, 183)*.

**Dopaminergic Projections**

Dopamine is a key modulator of basal ganglia activity. The SNc (A9), ventral tegmental area (VTA, A10) and retrorubral field (RRF, A8) are the main sources of dopamine to the basal ganglia. The striatum is the main target of axons from neurons in these areas *(70)*. Both the caudate nucleus and putamen receive strong dopaminergic inputs from segregated populations of SNc and RRF neurons, while the VTA innervates mainly the ventral striatum *(41, 184, 185)*.

Most movement-related areas of the basal ganglia receive their dopaminergic inputs from the SNc. This nucleus contains two main populations of dopaminergic neurons that can be differentiated by their location and by the relative concentration of calbindin D28k and dopamine transporter *(186)*. The ventral tier of the SNc (SNc-v) comprises a densocellular part located dorsomedially and more ventrally located cell columns and clusters that interdigitate with the SNr. The sensorimotor striatum receives its main dopaminergic innervation from cell columns in the SNc-v. SNc-v neurons degenerate early in patients with Parkinson's disease and in animal models of parkinsonism. In contrast, calbindin-containing neurons in the dorsal tier of the SNc (SNc-d) and those of the VTA are relatively spared *(57, 187, 188)*. The two populations of dopaminergic SNc neurons provide specific patterns of innervation to the rat striatum *(189–191)*; SNc-v neurons innervate preferentially the patch compartment, whereas SNc-d neurons mainly project to the matrix *(189, 192)*. However, the relationships between nigrostriatal projections from subpopulations of SNc neurons and the regional or compartmental organization of the striatum appear to be more complex in primates *(27)*.

Dopaminergic inputs functionally regulate the activity of striatal MSNs through pre- and postsynaptic interactions with dopamine receptors belonging to the D1- and D2-family of receptors. Activation of D1-family receptors (which includes D1 and D5 receptors) exerts excitatory effects, while activation of D2-family receptors (D2, D3, and D4 receptors) is generally inhibitory towards striatofugal MSNs *(193, 194)*.

The distribution of dopaminergic receptors throughout the basal ganglia is shown in Table 1.2. In the striatum, postsynaptic D1 and D2 receptors are largely found in dendrites and spines of direct and indirect striatofugal neurons, respectively, where they may regulate corticostriatal transmission at dendritic spines, which receive glutamatergic terminals *(152, 195, 196)*. In addition, pre-synaptic

**Table 1.2** Distribution of dopamine receptors (D1–D5) in the basal ganglia and thalamus.

Striatum

- Presynaptic: D2 (on nigro- and corticostriatal projections)
- Postsynaptic:
  - Medium spiny neurons, direct pathway: D1 >> D2
  - Medium spiny neurons, indirect pathway: D2 >> D1
  - Cholinergic interneurons: D2, D5
  - Parvalbumin-positive interneurons: D5

GPe

- Presynaptic: D2 (striatal projection to GPe)
- Postsynaptic: D2, D3, D4, D5

GPi

- Presynaptic: D1 (striatal projection to GPi), D2 on SNc projection to GPi
- Postsynaptic: D3, D4, D5

STN

- Presynaptic: D1, D2 on glutamatergic inputs
- Postsynaptic: D1, D2, D3, D5

SNr

- Presynaptic: D1 (on striatal projection to SNr)
- Postsynaptic: D4, D5

Thalamus

- Presynaptic: D2 (on SNc projection to thalamus)
- Postsynaptic: D5

D2 receptors also play an important role in regulating corticostriatal glutamatergic activity. In rats, the dopamine regulation of glutamatergic inputs is highly specific and filters out selectively less active cortical inputs *(197, 198)*.

Another mechanism by which dopamine regulates intrinsic striatal activity is via dopamine receptors expressed in cholinergic interneurons. Most studies have focused on D2 receptors *(70)*, but D5 receptors may also be involved in the modulation of acetylcholine release *(199, 200)*. The dopaminergic regulation of striatal acetylcholine release is thought to play a role in the striatal processing of extrinsic inputs and learning *(194, 201, 202)*. The cholinergic interneurons also mediate some of the dopamine-regulated interactions between direct and indirect pathway neurons (see Figure 1.2). The cross-talk between cholinergic interneurons and MSNs is critical for the development of long-term synaptic plasticity in both populations of striatofugal neurons *(194, 202, 203)*.

In addition to its striatal actions, dopamine may also directly regulate pallidal, subthalamic and nigral activity (see Figure 1.3; refs. *70* and *204*). Dopamine is released from terminals of SNc projections to the rat GP and STN *(204, 205)*. In the SNr, dopamine is released from dendrites of SNc neurons that extend ventrally into the SNr *(70, 206)*. Neurons in these nuclei express pre- and post-synaptic D1- and D2-family dopamine receptors that may mediate the effects of dopaminergic ligands on GP, STN, and SNr neurons *(70, 207–213)*. Widespread dopamine innervation of the monkey thalamus has also been recently demonstrated *(214, 215)*. Albeit more modest than the massive nigrostriatal system, these extrastriatal dopaminergic projections may directly regulate basal ganglia outflow *(70)*.

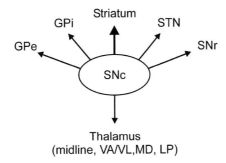

**Figure 1.3** Targets of dopaminergic projections arising in the substantia nigra pars compacta (SNc). The projection targeting the substantia nigra pars reticulata utilizes dendritic release of dopamine release. At all other projections sites, dopamine is released from axon terminals. Abbreviations: GPe, external segment of the globus pallidus; GPi, internal segment of the globus pallidus; LP, lateral posterior nucleus of the thalamus; MD, mediodorsal nucleus of the thalamus; STN, subthalamic nucleus; VA/VL, ventral anterior and ventrolateral nuclei of the thalamus

## Output Projections of the Basal Ganglia

### Nigrofugal Pathways

Based on the arrangement of striatal inputs and nigral outputs, the SNr in rats can be subdivided into a dorsolateral sensorimotor and a ventromedial associative territory (216). Recent single axon-tracing studies in rats and monkeys (84, 217–219) have shown that SNr neurons are highly heterogeneous in their degree of innervation and axonal collateralization to thalamic and other targets (217–219). Most SNr output to the thalamus appears to be related to non-motor functions. However, neurons in the lateral part of the SNr project preferentially to the lateral posterior region of the VAmc and to different parts of the mediodorsal nucleus (MD). These areas of the thalamus are predominately related to posterior regions of the frontal lobe including the frontal eye field and areas of the premotor cortex, respectively (220–222). In monkeys, the SNr also provides a projection to PF as part of an associative basal ganglia-thalamostriatal loop that involves the caudate nucleus (107, 118).

Other SNr projections reach the superior colliculus, PPN and the medullary reticular formation. Nigro-collicular fibers terminate mainly on tectospinal neurons in the intermediate layers of the superior colliculus (131, 223). The nigro-collicular system is thought to play a role in the regulation of visual saccades (131, 223). Nigro-tegmental projections terminate predominantly on noncholinergic neurons in the medial two-thirds of the PPN (224, 225), while the nigro-reticular projection terminates in the parvicellular reticular formation, which is directly connected with orofacial motor nuclei (226–228).

### Pallidofugal Pathways

The motor territory of the basal ganglia output nuclei is mostly contained within GPi. Sensorimotor information is conveyed almost exclusively to the posterior part of the ventrolateral nucleus (VLo in macaques; refs. 229–231). Via the thalamus, sensorimotor output from GPi is projected towards the SMA (232–235), M1 (234–241), and PM cortical area (237). Virus transport studies have suggested that the pallidal projections directed at cortical areas MI, PM, and SMA arise from segregated populations of GPi neurons in monkeys *(237, 242)*.

Most GPi neurons that project to VA/VLo also send axon collaterals to the caudal intralaminar nuclear group (CM/PF), which, in turn, projects predominately to the striatum (see previous paragraphs; ref. *229*). Neurons in the sensorimotor territory of GPi project exclusively to CM *(107, 118)*.

In monkeys, a large portion of GPi neurons that project to the VA/VLo also sends axon collaterals to the noncholinergic portion of the PPN *(243–247)*. This projection is than the GPi projections to the thalamus *(243)*. The PPN, in turn, gives rise to descending projections to the pons, medulla, and spinal cord as well as prominent ascending projections to the basal ganglia, the thalamus and the basal forebrain (see, e.g., refs. *248* and *249*).

## The Role of the Basal Ganglia in Motor Control

Voluntary movements are thought to be initiated at the cortical level of the motor circuit with simultaneous output to the brainstem and spinal cord, as well as to multiple subcortical targets, including the thalamus, putamen, and the STN. Insights into the anatomical organization of the basal ganglia have strongly influenced our view of the function of these circuits.

One line of reasoning has focused on the proposed dichotomy of direct and indirect pathways. It is thought that cortical movement-related inputs may activate striatal direct pathway neurons, resulting in inhibition of basal ganglia output, and subsequent disinhibition of thalamocortical neurons. In contrast, activation of indirect pathway neurons would result in activation of GPi output and inhibition of thalamocortical neurons. According to one hypothesis, interactions between the two pathways may be important for basal ganglia regulation of motor control. Cortical activity related to an intended movement may activate specific portions of the direct pathway, resulting in appropriate reduction of inhibitory basal ganglia output to the thalamus and facilitation of cortical activity related to the intended movement. Activation of the indirect pathway would have opposite effects, acting to suppress unintended movement *(137, 250–255)*. The most common change in GPi activity during movement is increased activity. Thus, suppression of unintended movements may be a particularly important role of the basal ganglia. Another possibility is that striatal output would first inhibit specific neuronal populations in GPi/SNr via the direct pathway, facilitating movement, followed after a delay by disinhibition of the same GPi/SNr neuron via inputs over the indirect pathway, leading to an inhibition of the ongoing movement. The resulting sequence of facilitation and inhibition would regulate the amplitude or velocity of individual movements *(256)*. Conceivably, neurons with short latency responses to movement could play such a role *(239, 257–265)*. Recent PET studies have reported that basal ganglia activity is modulated in relation to low-level parameters of movement, such as force or movement speed *(266, 267)*, thus supporting such a scaling function of the basal ganglia.

However, it is likely that interactions between basal ganglia circuits at a smaller scale strongly contribute to information processing in these circuits. For instance, transmission via local axon collaterals or interneurons may contribute to center-surround inhibition in the basal ganglia that are not accounted for in the simple direct/indirect pathway scheme mentioned previously. There is evidence for the existence of such collateral inhibition in the striatum. While some MSNs are directly activated by glutamatergic inputs from the cortex, neighboring neurons may be inhibited via axon collaterals of the activated neuron, or via intercalated fast-spiking interneurons *(68, 183, 268)*, thus favoring the (locally) strongest focus of corticostriatal stimulation, and reducing the excitability of neighboring areas of the striatum and related circuitry.

Other proposed motor functions of the basal ganglia include roles in internally generated movements, in motor learning and movement sequencing (e.g., refs. *24, 269–272*). For instance, both dopaminergic nigrostriatal neurons and tonically active neurons in the striatum develop transient responses to sensory conditioning stimuli during behavioral training in classical conditioning tasks *(270, 273–275)*. This supports a role of these cells, and of basal ganglia areas whose activity they influence, in motor learning. Shifts in the response properties of striatal output neurons during performance of a maze task that involved learning have been demonstrated in the rat *(276)*. In addition to these concepts, a number of other theories have gained varying degrees of popularity including concepts that the basal ganglia may globally act to extract cortical information through dimensionality reduction *(23)* or may assist in resource allocation *(131)*.

## Consequences of Abnormalities of Basal Ganglia Function

It is beyond the scope of this chapter to discuss disorders of basal ganglia function in detail. Thus, the spectrum of basal ganglia dysfunction is only briefly discussed, contrasting the effects of lesions of the basal ganglia output nuclei with those of alterations of the firing patterns in these structures.

### Lesions of the Basal Ganglia Output Nuclei

Perhaps surprisingly, complete cessation of basal ganglia output has few behavioral effects. Thus, in most studies, pallidal lesions in animals and humans produce either no or only short-latency effects on skilled fine movements or mild bradykinesia *(277–287)*. A notable exception is a study by Mink and Thach *(255, 288, 289)* in which co-contractions were observed after lesioning or inactivation of GPi, although this may have been due to inadvertent involvement of GPe in these experiments. While these studies could serve as evidence that the effects of the basal ganglia are only subtle or highly specialized, they most likely indicate that the motor system is, in fact, sufficiently redundant to be able to quickly compensate for complete loss of basal ganglia function. The fact that basal ganglia lesions appear to have few (negative) behavioral consequences has been exploited for decades in neurosurgical ablative treatments such as pallidotomy for Parkinson's disease or dystonia.

### Parkinson's Disease

Parkinsonism is the prototypical hypokinetic movement disorder. The primary movement abnormalities in Parkinson's disease or parkinsonism include bradykinesia (slowness of movement), tremor at rest, and muscular rigidity. It is thought that these signs are due to degeneration of dopaminergic neurons in the SNc and their projections to the striatum, which then results in striatal dopamine depletion, and subsequent activity changes in basal ganglia output, which are highly disruptive to movement. Recent evidence indicates that reduced dopaminergic inputs to basal ganglia regions other than the striatum (including GPi, SNr, and STN) may also play a role in the development of the motor signs of the disease. At least in the early stages of Parkinson's disease, the dopamine depletion preferentially affects the motor circuit, and the symptoms are often greatly ameliorated by administration of pharmacologic dopamine replacement therapy, such as levodopa or dopamine receptor agonists.

Although mechanistically not fully explained, dopamine depletion in the basal ganglia induces prominent changes in neuronal activity within the motor circuit. Thus, neuronal activity in GPi and STN is increased in parkinsonian animals and humans, and abnormal oscillatory activity and increased synchrony of neuronal discharge has been observed throughout all elements of the motor circuit (see example in Figure 1.4 and recent reviews *[290, 291]*). In addition to the frequently discussed abnormalities in the intrinsic basal ganglia circuitry, increased activity of the thalamo-subthalamic projection may also contribute to the increased (metabolic) activity of STN neurons in Parkinson's disease *(292)*.

While the link between specific basal ganglia discharge abnormalities and the behavioral manifestations of parkinsonism remains uncertain, it is likely that some or all signs of the disease arise from the fact that the abnormally patterned basal ganglia output functionally disables related thalamic and cortical areas. Functional imaging studies have demonstrated that changes in basal ganglia activity are associated with abnormal activation patterns in cortical motor (and other) areas both at rest and with movement. DBS within the motor portions of the STN or the GPi largely reverses these abnormalities. Curiously, DBS at these locations tends to treat specifically those parkinsonian signs that are also amenable to dopaminergic therapy, adding support to the notion that abnormalities in these dopamine-modulated circuits are at the core of the development of parkinsonian abnormalities.

DBS of other portions of the motor circuits in individuals affected by Parkinson's disease have also been described. For instance extradural motor cortex stimulation may have antiparkinsonian effects *(293, 294)*. Another target for DBS in Parkinson's disease is the PPN. Inactivation of the PPN induces akinesia in animals *(295)*, and low-frequency stimulation of the PPN may have antiparkinsonian efficacy, specifically against gait and balance problems *(296, 297)*.

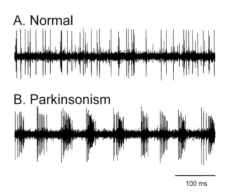

**Figure 1.4** Examples of traces of neuronal activity, recorded with standard extracellular electrophysiologic recording methods in a monkey before (A) and after (B) induction of parkinsonism with intracarotid injections of the dopaminergic neurotoxin 1-methyl-4-phenyl-1,2,3,6-tetrahydropyridine (MPTP). The traces neurons are each one second long

## Hemiballism

Hemiballism is a typical hyperkinetic disorder in which patients generate large-amplitude hemi-body limb movements. In humans, hemiballism results most often from lesions involving the STN, often due to discrete ischemic or hemorrhagic lesions of the nucleus (e.g., ref. *298*). Studies in monkeys have demonstrated that STN lesions that included at least 20% of the nucleus result in long-lasting, ballistic-appearing, choreiform movements *(299, 300)*. Similarly, small fiber-sparing lesions of the STN also result in dyskinesias of shorter duration *(301)*.

STN lesions interrupt the portion of the indirect pathway that traverses the STN. Metabolic and physiologic studies *(302, 303)* have demonstrated that STN lesions reduce neuronal activity in both GPe and GPi, and reduce the proportion of cells that respond to joint rotation with increases in discharge in GPe and GPi *(303)*. Thus, hemiballism is another disorder in which altered basal ganglia output appears to be highly disruptive to movement.

As is true for other movement disorders, changes in overall basal ganglia output are likely not the only reason for the development of hemiballism. Abnormally patterned activity may underlie the development of ballismus as well as other hyperkinetic disorders, and may, in fact, shape the specific features of the disorder in question.

## Dystonia

Dystonia is characterized by involuntary twisting movements, abnormal postures, muscular agonist/antagonist co-contraction, and muscle activation overflow phenomena. Dystonia is a highly heterogeneous condition. Neuroimaging studies in dystonic patients and other studies have demonstrated that portions of the motor circuit (cortical and subcortical) are often affected by dystonia *(304)*. Based on single cell recording studies in patients, it appears that at least some cases of dystonia are similar to Parkinson's disease with regard to the changes in the activity patterns of basal ganglia output, but that overall GPi activity is reduced in dystonia, while it is increased in Parkinson's disease *(305)*. In cases of focal dystonia, there is electrophysiologic evidence for reduced cortical inhibition, and aberrant organization of somatosensory cortical maps *(306)*. These findings, together with the delayed effects of surgery, support the concept that abnormal neuroplasticity may play a role in dystonia.

# Conclusions

There is a wealth of knowledge regarding the interactions between the basal ganglia, thalamus, cerebral cortex, and brainstem. Basal ganglia-thalamocortical circuitry is topographically organized into motor and non-motor portions. Given the anatomical and functional similarities between motor and non-motor circuits, information processing within these different circuits is likely similar. While it remains unclear which fundamental function(s) are carried out by this network of connections, testable hypotheses have been generated that will help us to elucidate this issue in the future. The role of the basal ganglia nuclei in movement disorders is more clearly defined than their normal functions. Neurosurgical interventions targeting individual portions of these circuits have become a highly efficacious method of treatment for Parkinson's disease and other conditions.

## References

1. DeLong MR (1971) Activity of pallidal neurons during movement. J Neurophysiol 34:414–427.
2. DeLong MR, Strick PL (1974) Relation of basal ganglia, cerebellum, and motor cortex units to ramp and ballistic limb movements. Brain Res 71:327–335.
3. DeLong MR, Crutcher MD, Georgopoulos AP (1983) Relations between movement and single cell discharge in the substantia nigra of the behaving monkey. J Neurosci 3:1599–1606.
4. Crutcher MD, DeLong MR (1984) Single cell studies of the primate putamen. I. Functional organization. Exp Brain Res 53:233–243.
5. Crutcher MD, DeLong MR (1984) Single cell studies of the primate putamen. II. Relations to direction of movement and pattern of muscular activity. Exp Brain Res 53:244–258.
6. DeLong MR, Crutcher MD, Georgopoulos AP (1985) Primate globus pallidus and subthalamic nucleus: functional organization. J Neurophysiol 53:530–543.
7. Wichmann T, Bergman H, DeLong MR (1994) The primate subthalamic nucleus. I. Functional properties in intact animals. J Neurophysiol 72:494–506.
8. Magarinos-Ascone C, Buno W, Garcia-Austt E (1992) Activity in monkey substantial nigra neurons related to a simple learned movement. Exp Brain Res 88:283–291.
9. Allum JHJ, Anner-Baratti REC, Hepp-Raymond MC (1983) Activity of neurons in the motor thalamus and globus pallidus during the control of isometric finger force in the monkey. In: Paillard MJ, Schultz W, Wiesendanger M, eds. Neural Coding of Motor Performance Exp Brain Res Suppl 7. New York: Springer, pp. 194–203.
10. Apicella P, Scarnati E, Ljungberg T, Schultz W (1992) Neuronal activity in monkey striatum related to the expectation of predictable environmental events. J Neurophysiol 68:945–960.
11. Schultz W (1986) Activity of pars reticulata neurons of monkey substantia nigra in relation to motor, sensory, and complex events. J Neurophysiol 4:660–677.
12. Ashe J, Georgopoulos AP (1994) Movement parameters and neural activity in motor cortex and area 5. Cerebr Cortex 4(6):590–600.
13. Bauswein E, Fromm C, Werner W, Ziemann U (1991) Phasic and tonic responses of premotor and primary motor cortex neurons to torque changes. Exp Brain Res 86:303–310.
14. Crutcher MD, Alexander GE (1990) Movement-related neuronal activity selectively coding either direction or muscle pattern in three motor areas of the monkey. J Neurophysiol 64:151–163.
15. Fu QG, Suarez JI, Ebner TJ (1993) Neuronal specification of direction and distance during reaching movements in the superior precentral premotor area and primary motor cortex of monkeys. J Neurophysiol 70(5):2097–2116.
16. Hepp-Reymond MC, Husler EJ, Maier MA, Ql HX (1994) Force-related neuronal activity in two regions of the primate ventral premotor cortex. Can J Physiol Pharmacol 72:571–579.
17. Kurata K (1993) Premotor cortex of monkeys: set- and movement-related activity reflecting amplitude and direction of wrist movements. J Neurophysiol 69(1):187–200.
18. Smith AM (1979) The activity of supplementary motor area neurons during a maintained precision grip. Brain Res 172:315–327.
19. Werner W, Bauswein E, Fromm C (1991) Static firing rates of premotor and primary motor cortical neurons associated with torque and joint position. Exp Brain Res 86(2):293–302.
20. Vitek JL, Hashimoto T, Baron MS, et al (1994) Lesion location related to outcome in microelectrode-guided pallidotomy. American Neurological Association.

21. Gross RE, Lombardi WD, Hutchison WD, et al (1998) Lesion location and outcome following pallidotomy: support for multiple output channels in the human pallidum. Movement Disorders 13(Suppl 2):262.
22. Bar-Gad I, Bergman H (2001) Stepping out of the box: information processing in the neural networks of the basal ganglia. Curr Opinion Neurobiol 11(6):689–695.
23. Bar-Gad I, Morris G, Bergman H (2003) Information processing, dimensionality reduction and reinforcement learning in the basal ganglia. Prog Neurobiol 71(6):439–473.
24. Joel D, Weiner I (1994) The organization of the basal ganglia-thalamocortical circuits: open interconnected rather than closed segregated. Neuroscience 63(2):363–379.
25. Morishima M, Kawaguchi Y (2006) Recurrent connection patterns of corticostriatal pyramidal cells in frontal cortex. J Neurosci 26(16):4394–4405.
26. Haber SN, Fudge JL, McFarland NR (2000) Striatonigrostriatal pathways in primates form an ascending spiral from the shell to the dorsolateral striatum. J Neurosci 20(6):2369–2382.
27. Joel D, Weiner I (2000) The connections of the dopaminergic system with the striatum in rats and primates: an analysis with respect to the functional and compartmental organization of the striatum. Neuroscience 96(3):451–474.
28. Guzman JN, Hernandez A, Galarraga E, et al (2003) Dopaminergic modulation of axon collaterals interconnecting spiny neurons of the rat striatum. J Neurosci 23(26):8931–8940.
29. Onn SP, Grace AA (1995) Repeated treatment with haloperidol and clozapine exerts differential effects on dye coupling between neurons in subregions of striatum and nucleus accumbens. J Neurosci 15(11):7024–7036.
30. Onn SP, Grace AA (1994) Dye coupling between rat striatal neurons recorded in vivo: compartmental organization and modulation by dopamine. J Neurophysiol 71(5):1917–1934.
31. O'Donnell P, Grace AA (1995) Different effects of subchronic clozapine and haloperidol on dye-coupling between neurons in the rat striatal complex. Neuroscience 66(4):763–767.
32. Filion M, Tremblay L, Bedard PJ (1988) Abnormal influences of passive limb movement on the activity of globus pallidus neurons in parkinsonian monkeys. Brain Res 444:165–176.
33. Miller WC, DeLong MR (1987) Altered tonic activity of neurons in the globus pallidus and subthalamic nucleus in the primate MPTP model of parkinsonism. In: Carpenter MB, Jayaraman A, eds. The Basal Ganglia II. New York: Plenum Press, pp. 415–427.
34. Bergman H, Wichmann T, Karmon B, DeLong MR (1994) The primate subthalamic nucleus. II. Neuronal activity in the MPTP model of parkinsonism. J Neurophysiol 72:507–520.
35. Nini A, Feingold A, Slovin H, Bergman H (1995) Neurons in the globus pallidus do not show correlated activity in the normal monkey, but phase-locked oscillations appear in the MPTP model of parkinsonism. J Neurophysiol 74(4):1800–1805.
36. Raz A, Feingold A, Zelanskaya V, et al (1996) Neuronal synchronization of tonically active neurons in the striatum of normal and parkinsonian primates. J Neurophysiol 76(3):2083–2088.
37. Filion M, Tremblay L (1991) Abnormal spontaneous activity of globus-pallidus neurons in monkeys with Mptp-induced parkinsonism. Brain Res 547(1):142–151.
38. Tremblay L, Filion M, Bedard PJ (1989) Responses of pallidal neurons to striatal stimulation in monkeys with MPTP-induced parkinsonism. Brain Res 498:17–33.
39. Williams D, Kuhn A, Kupsch A, et al (2005) The relationship between oscillatory activity and motor reaction time in the parkinsonian subthalamic nucleus. Eur J Neurosci 21(1):249–258.
40. Brown P (2003) Oscillatory nature of human basal ganglia activity: relationship to the pathophysiology of Parkinson's disease. Mov Dis 18(4):357–363.

41. Gerfen CR, Wilson CJ (1996) The basal ganglia. In: Björklund A, Hökfeld T, Swanson L, eds. Handbook of Chemical Neuroanatomy, Integrated Systems of the CNS, Part III. Amsterdam: Elsevier, p. 369.
42. Graybiel AM, Ragsdale CW Jr, Yoneoka ES, Elde RP (1981) An immunohistochemical study of enkephalins and other neuropeptides in the striatum of the cat with evidence that the opiate peptides are arranged to form mosaic patterns in register with the striosomal compartments visible by acetylcholinesterase staining. Neuroscience 6(3):377–397.
43. Herkenham M, Pert C (1981) Mosaic distribution of opiate receptors, parafascicular projections and acetylcholinesterase in rat striatum. Nature London 291:415–417.
44. Ragsdale CW Jr, Graybiel AM (1981) The fronto-striatal projection in the cat and monkey and its relationship to inhomogeneities established by acetylcholinesterase histochemistry. Brain Res 208:259–266.
45. Gerfen CR (1989) The neostriatal mosaic: striatal patch-matrix organization is related to cortical lamination. Science 246:385–388.
46. Gerfen CR (1992) The neostriatal mosaic: multiple levels of compartmental organization. Trends Neurosci 14:133–139.
47. Gerfen CR (1984) The neostriatal mosaic: compartmentalization of corticostriatal input and striatonigral output systems. Nature 311(5985):461–464.
48. Berendse HW, Groenewegen HJ (1990) Organization of the thalamostriatal projections in the rat, with special emphasis on the ventral striatum. J Comp Neurol 299(2):187–228.
49. Ragsdale CW Jr, Graybiel AM (1991) Compartmental organization of the thalamostriatal connection in the cat. J Comp Neurol 311(1):134–167.
50. Sadikot AF, Parent A, Smith Y, Bolam JP (1992) Efferent connections of the centromedian and parafascicular thalamic nuclei in the squirrel monkey: a light and electron microscopic study of the thalamostriatal projection in relation to striatal heterogeneity. J Comp Neurol 320(2):228–242.
51. Graybiel AM, Canales JJ, Capper-Loup C (2000) Levodopa-induced dyskinesias and dopamine-dependent stereotypies: a new hypothesis. Trends Neurosci 23(10 Suppl):S71–S77.
52. Canales JJ, Capper-Loup C, Hu D, et al (2002) Shifts in striatal responsivity evoked by chronic stimulation of dopamine and glutamate systems. Brain 125(Pt 10):2353–2363.
53. Graybiel AM, Canales JJ (2001) The neurobiology of repetitive behaviors: clues to the neurobiology of Tourette syndrome. Adv Neurol 85:123–131.
54. Goto S, Lee LV, Munoz EL, et al (2005) Functional anatomy of the basal ganglia in X-linked recessive dystonia-parkinsonism. Ann Neurol 58(1):7–17.
55. Kish SJ, Shannak K, Hornykiewicz O (1988) Uneven pattern of dopamine loss in the striatum of patients with idiopathic Parkinson's disease. New Engl J Med 318:876–880.
56. Moratalla R, Quinn B, DeLanney LE, et al (1992) Differential vulnerability of primate caudate-putamen and striosome-matrix dopamine systems to the neurotoxic effects of 1-methyl-4-phenyl-1,2,3,6-tetrahydropyridine. Proc Natl Acad Sci USA 89(9):3859–3863.
57. Iravani MM, Syed E, Jackson MJ, et al (2005) A modified MPTP treatment regime produces reproducible partial nigrostriatal lesions in common marmosets. Eur J Neurosci 21(4):841–854.
58. Graveland GA, Difiglia M (1985) The frequency and distribution of medium-sized neurons with indented nuclei in the primate and rodent neostriatum. Brain Res 327:307–311.
59. Tepper JM, Bolam JP (2004) Functional diversity and specificity of neostriatal interneurons. Curr Opin Neurobiol 14(6):685–692.
60. Kawaguchi Y, Wilson CJ, Augood SJ, Emson PC (1995) Striatal interneurones: chemical, physiological and morphological characterization. Trends Neurosci 18(12):527–535.

61. Bennett BD, Wilson CJ (1999) Spontaneous activity of neostriatal cholinergic interneurons in vitro. J Neurosci 19(13):5586–5596.
62. Aosaki T, Tsubokawa H, Ishida A, et al (1994) Responses of tonically active neurons in the primate's striatum undergo systematic changes during behavioral sensorimotor conditioning. J Neurosci 14(6):3969–3984.
63. Yamada H, Matsumoto N, Kimura M (2004) Tonically active neurons in the primate caudate nucleus and putamen differentially encode instructed motivational outcomes of action. J Neurosci 3500–3510.
64. Shimo Y, Hikosaka O (2001) Role of tonically active neurons in primate caudate in reward-oriented saccadic eye movement. J Neurosci 21(19):7804–7814.
65. Martone ME, Armstrong DM, Young SJ, Groves PM (1992) Ultrastructural examination of enkephalin and substance P input to cholinergic neurons within the rat neostriatum. Brain Res 594(2):253–262.
66. Bolam JP, Ingham CA, Izzo PN, et al (1986) Substance P-containing terminals in synaptic contact with cholinergic neurons in the neostriatum and basal forebrain: a double immunocytochemical study in the rat. Brain Res 397(2):279–289.
67. Cicchetti F, Beach TG, Parent A (1998) Chemical phenotype of calretinin interneurons in the human striatum. Synapse 30(3):284–297.
68. Mallet N, Le Moine C, Charpier S, Gonon F (2005) Feedforward inhibition of projection neurons by fast-spiking GABA interneurons in the rat striatum in vivo. J Neurosci 25(15):3857–3869.
69. Betarbet R, Turner R, Chockkan V, et al (1997) Dopaminergic neurons intrinsic to the primate striatum. J Neurosci 17(17):6761–6768.
70. Smith Y, Kieval JZ (2000) Anatomy of the dopamine system in the basal ganglia. Trends Neurosci 23(10 Suppl):S28–S33.
71. Cossette M, Levesque D, Parent A (2005) Neurochemical characterization of dopaminergic neurons in human striatum. Parkinsonism Relat Disord 11(5):277–286.
72. Mazloom M, Smith Y (2006) Synaptic microcircuitry of tyrosine hydroxylase-containing neurons and terminals in the striatum of 1-methyl-4-phenyl-1,2,3,6-tetrahydropyridine-treated monkeys. J Comp Neurol 495(4):453–469.
73. Vonsattel JP, DiFiglia M (1998) Huntington disease. J Neuropathol Exp Neurol 57(5):369–384.
74. Difiglia M, Pasik P, Pasik T (1982) A golgi and ultrastructural study of the monkey globus pallidus. J Comp Neurol 212:53–75.
75. Francois C, Percheron G, Yelnik J, Heyner S (1984) A Golgi analysis of the primate globus pallidus. I. Inconstant processes of large neurons, other neuronal types, and afferent axons. J Comp Neurol 227(2):182–199.
76. Hassler R, Chung YW (1984) Identification of eight types of synapses in the pallidum externum and internum in squirrel monkey (Saimiri sciureus). Acta Anat (Basel) 118(2):65–81.
77. Kita H, Kitai ST (1994) The morphology of globus pallidus projection neurons in the rat: an intracellular staining study. Brain Res 636(2):308–319.
78. Sato F, Parent M, Levesque M, Parent A (2000) Axonal branching pattern of neurons of the subthalamic nucleus in primates. J Comp Neurol 424(1):142–152.
79. Smith Y, Shink E, Sidibe M (1998) Neuronal circuitry and synaptic connectivity of the basal ganglia. Neurosurg Clin N Am 9(2):203–222.
80. Sadek AR, Magill PJ, Bolam JP (2007) A single-cell analysis of intrinsic connectivity in the rat globus pallidus. J Neurosci 27(24):6352–6362.
81. Parent M, Levesque M, Parent A (2001) Two types of projection neurons in the internal pallidum of primates: single-axon tracing and three-dimensional reconstruction. J Comp Neurol 439(2):162–175.
82. Kuo JS, Carpenter MB (1973) Organization of pallidothalamic projections in the rhesus monkey. J Comp Neurol 151:201–236.
83. Baron MS, Sidibe M, DeLong MR, Smith Y (2001) Course of motor and associative pallidothalamic projections in monkeys. J Comp Neurol 429(3):490–501.

84. Mailly P, Charpier S, Menetrey A, Deniau JM (2003) Three-dimensional organization of the recurrent axon collateral network of the substantia nigra pars reticulata neurons in the rat. J Neurosci 23(12):5247–5257.
85. Tepper JM, Lee CR (2007) GABAergic control of substantia nigra dopaminergic neurons. Prog Brain Res 160:189–208.
86. Yelnik J, Percheron G (1979) Subthalamic neurons in primates: a quantitative and comparative analysis. Neuroscience 4(11):1717–1743.
87. Levesque JC, Parent A (2005) GABAergic interneurons in human subthalamic nucleus. Mov Disord 20(5):574–584.
88. Alexander GE, DeLong MR, Strick PL (1986) Parallel organization of functionally segregated circuits linking basal ganglia and cortex. Ann Rev Neurosci 9:357–381.
89. Alexander GE, Crutcher MD, DeLong MR (1990) Basal ganglia-thalamocortical circuits: parallel substrates for motor, oculomotor, 'prefrontal' and 'limbic' functions. Prog Brain Res 85:119–146.
90. Parent A (1990) Extrinsic connections of the basal ganglia. Trends Neurosci 13: 254–258.
91. Romanelli P, Esposito V, Schaal DW, Heit G (2005) Somatotopy in the basal ganglia: experimental and clinical evidence for segregated sensorimotor channels. Brain Res Brain Res Rev 48(1):112–128.
92. Kunzle H (1975) Bilateral projections from precentral motor cortex to the putamen and other parts of the basal ganglia. An autoradiographic study in macaca fascicularis. Brain Res 88:195–209.
93. Kunzle H (1978) An autoradiographic analysis of the efferent connections from premotor and adjacent prefrontal regions (areas 6 and 9) in macaca fascicularis. Brain Behav Evol 15:185–234.
94. Flaherty AW, Graybiel AM (1991) Corticostriatal transformations in the primate somatosensory sstem. Projections from physiologically mapped body-part representations. J Neurophysiol 66:1249–1263.
95. Flaherty AW, Graybiel AM (1993) Two input systems for body representations in the primate striatal matrix: Experimental evidence in the squirrel monkey. J Neurosci 13:1120–1137.
96. Lei W, Jiao Y, Del Mar N, Reiner A (2004) Evidence for differential cortical input to direct pathway versus indirect pathway striatal projection neurons in rats. J Neurosci 24(38):8289–8299.
97. Berretta S, Parthasarathy HB, Graybiel AM (1997) Local release of GABAergic inhibition in the motor cortex induces immediate-early gene expression in indirect pathway neurons of the striatum. J Neurosci 17(12):4752–4763.
98. Parthasarathy HB, Graybiel AM (1997) Cortically driven immediate-early gene expression reflects modular influence of sensorimotor cortex on identified striatal neurons in the squirrel monkey. J Neurosci 17(7):2477–2491.
99. Zemanick MC, Strick PL, Dix RD (1991) Direction of transneuronal transport of herpes simplex virus 1 in the primate motor system is strain-dependent. Proc Natl Acad Sci USA 88(18):8048–8051.
100. Jones EG, Coulter JD, Burton H, Porter R (1977) Cells of origin and terminal distribution of corticostriatal fibers arising in the sensory-motor cortex of monkeys. J Comp Neurol 173:53–80.
101. Turner RS, DeLong MR (2000) Corticostriatal activity in primary motor cortex of the macaque. J Neurosci 20(18):7096–7108.
102. Bauswein E, Fromm C, Preuss A (1989) Corticostriatal cells in comparison with pyramidal tract neurons: contrasting properties in the behaving monkey. Brain Res 493(1):198–203.
103. Parent M, Parent A (2006) Single-axon tracing study of corticostriatal projections arising from primary motor cortex in primates. J Comp Neurol 496(2):202–213.

104. Kemp JM, Powell TPS (1971) The connections of the striatum and globus pallidus: synthesis and speculation. Phil Trans R Soc Lond 262:441–457.
105. Lapper SR, Smith Y, Sadikot AF, et al (1992) Cortical input to parvalbumin-immunoreactive neurones in the putamen of the squirrel monkey. Brain Res 580(1–2):215–224.
106. Thomas TM, Smith Y, Levey AI, Hersch SM (2000) Cortical inputs to m2-immunoreactive striatal interneurons in rat and monkey. Synapse 37(4):252–261.
107. Smith Y, Raju DV, Pare JF, Sidibe M (2004) The thalamostriatal system: a highly specific network of the basal ganglia circuitry. Trends Neurosci 27(9):520–527.
108. Deschenes M, Bourassa J, Parent A (1996) Striatal and cortical projections of single neurons from the central lateral thalamic nucleus in the rat. Neuroscience 72:679–687.
109. Deschenes M, Bourassa J, Doan VD, Parent A (1996) A single-cell study of the axonal projections arising from the posterior intralaminar thalamic nuclei in the rat. Eur J Neurosci 8:329–343.
110. Parent M, Parent A (2005) Single-axon tracing and three-dimensional reconstruction of centre median-parafascicular thalamic neurons in primates. J Comp Neurol 481(1):127–144.
111. Wilson CJ, Chang HT, Kitai ST (1983) Origins of post synaptic potentials evoked in spiny neostriatal projection neurons by thalamic stimulation in the rat. Exp Brain Res 51:217–226.
112. Dube L, Smith AD, Bolam JP (1988) Identification of synaptic terminals of thalamic or cortical origin in contact with distinct medium-size spiny neurons in the rat neostriatum. J Comp Neurol 267:455–471.
113. Cowan RL, Wilson CJ (1994) Spontaneous firing patterns and axonal projections of single corticostriatal neurons in the rat medial agranular cortex. J Neurosci 71:17–32.
114. Levesque M, Parent A (1998) Axonal arborization of corticostriatal and corticothalamic fibers arising from prelimbic cortex in the rat. Cereb Cortex 8(7):602–613.
115. Smith Y, Parent A (1986) Differential connections of caudate nucleus and putamen in the squirrel monkey (Saimiri sciureus). Neuroscience 18(2):347–371.
116. Nakano K, Hasegawa Y, Tokushige A, et al (1990) Topographical projections from the thalamus, subthalamic nucleus and pedunculopontine tegmental nucleus to the striatum in the Japanese monkey, Macaca fuscata. Brain Res 537(1–2):54–68.
117. Sadikot AF, Parent A, Francois C (1992) Efferent connections of the centromedian and parafascicular thalamic nuclei in the squirrel monkey: a PHA-L study of subcortical projections. J Comp Neurol 315(2):137–159.
118. Sidibe M, Pare JF, Smith Y (2002) Nigral and pallidal inputs to functionally segregated thalamostriatal neurons in the centromedian/parafascicular intralaminar nuclear complex in monkey. J Comp Neurol 447(3):286–299.
119. Smith Y, Bennett BD, Bolam JP, et al (1994) Synaptic relationships between dopaminergic afferents and cortical or thalamic input in the sensorimotor territory of the striatum in monkey. J Comp Neurol 344:1–19.
120. Sidibe M, Smith Y (1996) Differential synaptic innervation of striatofugal neurones projecting to the internal or external segments of the globus pallidus by thalamic afferents in the squirrel monkey. J Comp Neurol 365(3):445–465.
121. Zackheim J, Abercrombie ED (2005) Thalamic regulation of striatal acetylcholine efflux is both direct and indirect and qualitatively altered in the dopamine-depleted striatum. Neuroscience 131(2):423–436.
122. Salin P, Kachidian P (1998) Thalamo-striatal deafferentation affects preproenkephalin but not preprotachykinin gene expression in the rat striatum. Brain Res Mol Brain Res 57(2):257–265.
123. Bacci JJ, Kachidian P, Kerkerian-Le Goff L, Salin P (2004) Intralaminar thalamic nuclei lesions: widespread impact on dopamine denervation-mediated cellular defects in the rat basal ganglia. J Neuropathol Exp Neurol 63(1):20–31.

124. McFarland NR, Haber SN (2000) Convergent inputs from thalamic motor nuclei and frontal cortical areas to the dorsal striatum in the primate. J Neurosci 20(10):3798–3813.
125. Raju DV, Shah DJ, Wright TM, et al (2006) Differential synaptology of vGluT2-containing thalamostriatal afferents between the patch and matrix compartments in rats. J Comp Neurol 499(2):231–243.
126. Matsumoto N, Minamimoto T, Graybiel AM, Kimura M (2001) Neurons in the thalamic CM-Pf complex supply striatal neurons with information about behaviorally significant sensory events. J Neurophysiol 85(2):960–976.
127. Minamimoto T, Kimura M (2002) Participation of the thalamic CM-Pf complex in attentional orienting. J Neurophysiol 87(6):3090–3101.
128. Kimura M, Minamimoto T, Matsumoto N, Hori Y (2004) Monitoring and switching of cortico-basal ganglia loop functions by the thalamo-striatal system. Neurosci Res 48(4):355–360.
129. Minamimoto T, Hori Y, Kimura M (2005) Complementary process to response bias in the centromedian nucleus of the thalamus. Science 308(5729):1798–1801.
130. Kinomura S, Larsson J, Gulyas B, Roland PE (1996) Activation by attention of the human reticular formation and thalamic intralaminar nuclei. Science 271(5248):512–515.
131. McHaffie JG, Stanford TR, Stein BE, et al (2005) Subcortical loops through the basal ganglia. Trends Neurosci 28(8):401–407.
132. Hartmann-von Monakow K, Akert K, Kunzle H (1978) Projections of the precentral motor cortex and other cortical areas of the frontal lobe to the subthalamic nucleus in the monkey. Exp Brain Res 33:395–403.
133. Afsharpour S (1985) Topographical projections of the cerebral cortex to the subthalamic nucleus. J Comp Neurol 236(1):14–28.
134. Nambu A, Takada M, Inase M, Tokuno H (1996) Dual somatotopical representations in the primate subthalamic nucleus: evidence for ordered but reversed body-map transformations from the primary motor cortex and the supplementary motor area. J Neurosci 16(8):2671–2683.
135. Takada M, Tokuno H, Hamada I, et al (2001) Organization of inputs from cingulate motor areas to basal ganglia in macaque monkey. Eur J Neurosci 14(10):1633–1650.
136. Nambu A, Tokuno H, Inase M, Takada M (1997) Corticosubthalamic input zones from forelimb representations of the dorsal and ventral divisions of the premotor cortex in the macaque monkey: comparison with the input zones from the primary motor cortex and the supplementary motor area. Neurosci Lett 239(1):13–16.
137. Nambu A, Tokuno H, Takada M (2002) Functional significance of the cortico-subthalamo-pallidal 'hyperdirect' pathway. Neurosci Res 43(2):111–117.
138. Rodriguez-Oroz MC, Rodriguez M, Guridi J, et al (2001) The subthalamic nucleus in Parkinson's disease: somatotopic organization and physiological characteristics. Brain 124(Pt 9):1777–1790.
139. Kitai ST, Deniau JM (1981) Cortical inputs to the subthalamus: intracellular analysis. Brain Res 214(2):411–415.
140. Giuffrida R, Li Volsi G, Maugeri G, Perciavalle V (1985) Influences of pyramidal tract on the subthalamic nucleus in the cat. Neurosci Lett 54(2–3):231–235.
141. Sugimoto T, Hattori T, Mizuno N, et al (1983) Direct projections from the centre median-parafascicular complex to the subthalamic nucleus in the cat and rat. J Comp Neurol 214:209–216.
142. Feger J, Bevan M, Crossman AR (1994) The projections from the parafascicular thalamic nucleus to the subthalamic nucleus and the striatum arise from separate neuronal populations: a comparison with the corticostriatal and corticosubthalamic efferents in a retrograde double-labelling study. Neuroscience 60(1):125–132.
143. Lanciego JL, Gonzalo N, Castle M, et al (2004) Thalamic innervation of striatal and subthalamic neurons projecting to the rat entopeduncular nucleus. Eur J Neurosci 19(5):1267–1277.

144. Ryan LJ, Clark KB (1991) The role of the subthalamic nucleus in the response of globus pallidus neurons to stimulation of the prelimbic and agranular frontal cortices in rats. Exp Brain Res 86(3):641–651.
145. Kita H (1994) Physiology of two disynaptic pathways from the sensorimotor cortex to the basal ganglia output nuclei. In: Percheron G, McKenzie JS, Feger J, eds. The Basal Gnaglia IV New ideas and data on structure and function. New York and London: Plenum Press, p. 263–276.
146. Maurice N, Deniau JM, Glowinski J, Thierry AM (1998) Relationships between the prefrontal cortex and the basal ganglia in the rat: physiology of the corticosubthalamic circuits. J Neurosci 18(22):9539–9546.
147. Maurice N, Deniau JM, Glowinski J, Thierry AM (1999) Relationships between the prefrontal cortex and the basal ganglia in the rat: physiology of the corticonigral circuits. J Neurosci 19(11):4674–4681.
148. Kolomiets BP, Deniau JM, Glowinski J, Thierry AM (2003) Basal ganglia and processing of cortical information: functional interactions between trans-striatal and trans-subthalamic circuits in the substantia nigra pars reticulata. Neuroscience 117(4):931–938.
149. Albin RL, Young AB, Penney JB (1989) The functional anatomy of basal ganglia disorders. Trends Neurosci 12:366–375.
150. Alexander GE, Crutcher MD (1990) Functional architecture of basal ganglia circuits: neural substrates of parallel processing. Trends Neurosci 13:266–271.
151. Bergman H, Wichmann T, DeLong MR (1990) Amelioration of Parkinsonian symptoms by inactivation of the subthalamic nucleus (STN) in MPTP treated green monkeys. Mov Dis 5(Suppl 1):79.
152. Smith AD, Bolam JP (1990) The neural network of the basal ganglia as revealed by the study of synaptic connections of identified neurones. Trends Neurosci 13(7):259–265.
153. Smith Y, Bolam JP (1991) Convergence of synaptic inputs from the striatum and the globus pallidus onto identified nigrocollicular cells in the rat: a double anterograde labelling study. Neuroscience 44(1):45–73.
154. Shink E, Smith Y (1995) Differential synaptic innervation of neurons in the internal and external segments of the globus pallidus by the GABA- and glutamate-containing terminals in the squirrel monkey. J Comp Neurol 358(1):119–141.
155. Smith Y, Bevan MD, Shink E, Bolam JP (1998) Microcircuitry of the direct and indirect pathways of the basal ganglia. Neuroscience 86(2):353–387.
156. Nauta HJ, Cole M (1978) Efferent projections of the subthalamic nucleus: an autoradiographic study in monkey and cat. J Comp Neurol 180(1):1–16.
157. Carpenter MB, Batton RRI, Carleton SC, Keller JT (1981) Interconnections and organization of pallidal and subthalamic nucleus neurons in the monkey. J Comp Neurol 197:579–603.
158. Moriizumi T, Nakamura Y, Kitao Y, Kudo M (1987) Ultrastructural analyses of afferent terminals in the subthalamic nucleus of the cat with a combined degeneration and horseradish peroxidase tracing method. J Comp Neurol 265(2):159–174.
159. Smith Y, Hazrati LN, Parent A (1990) Efferent projections of the subthalamic nucleus in the squirrel monkey as studied by PHA-L anterograde tracing method. J Comp Neurol 294:306–323.
160. Shink E, Bevan MD, Bolam JP, Smith Y (1996) The subthalamic nucleus and the external pallidum: two tightly interconnected structures that control the output of the basal ganglia in the monkey. Neuroscience 73(2):335–357.
161. Bevan MD, Clarke NP, Bolam JP (1997) Synaptic integration of functionally diverse pallidal information in the entopeduncular nucleus and subthalamic nucleus in the rat. J Neurosci 17(1):308–324.
162. Beckstead RM (1983) A reciprocal axonal connection between the subthalamic nucleus and the neostriatum in the cat. Brain Res 275(1):137–142.
163. Parent A, Smith Y (1987) Organization of efferent projections of the subthalamic nucleus in the squirrel monkey as revealed by retrograde labeling methods. Brain Res 436:296–310.

164. Kita H, Kitai ST (1987) Efferent projections of the subthalamic nucleus in the rat: light and electron microscope analysis with the PHA-L method. J Comp Neurol 260:435–452.
165. Smith ID, Grace AA (1992) Role of the subthalamic nucleus in the regulation of nigral dopamine neuron activity. Synapse 12(4):287–303.
166. Hammond C, Rouzaire-Dubois B, Feger J, et al (1983) Anatomical and electrophysiological studies on the reciprocal projections between the subthalamic nucleus and nucleus tegmenti pedunculopontinus in the rat. Neuroscience 9(1):41–52.
167. Takada M, Li ZK, Hattori T (1987) Long descending direct projection from the basal ganglia to the spinal cord: a revival of the extrapyramidal concept. Brain Res 436(1):129–135.
168. Deniau JM, Hammond C, Riszk A, Feger J (1978) Electrophysiological properties of identified output neurons of the rat substantia nigra (pars compacta and pars reticulata): evidences for the existence of branched neurons. Exp Brain Res 32(3):409–422.
169. Van Der Kooy D, Hattori T (1980) Single subthalamic nucleus neurons project to both the globus pallidus and substantia nigra in rat. J Comp Neurol 192(4):751–768.
170. Berendse HW, Groenewegen HJ (1989) The connections of the medial part of the subthalamic nucleus in the rat. Evidence for a parallel organization. In: Bernardi G, Carpenter MB, Di Chiara G, et al., eds. The Basal Ganglia II. New York: Plenum Press, pp. 89–98.
171. Haber SN, Lynd-Balta E, Mitchell SJ (1993) The organization of the descending ventral pallidal projections in the monkey. J Comp Neurol 329:111–128.
172. Surmeier DJ, Song WJ, Yan Z (1996) Coordinated expression of dopamine receptors in neostriatal medium spiny neurons. J Neurosci 16(20):6579–6591.
173. Aizman O, Brismar H, Uhlen P, et al (2000) Anatomical and physiological evidence for D1 and D2 dopamine receptor colocalization in neostriatal neurons. Nature Neuroscience 3(3):226–230.
174. Parent A, Sato F, Wu Y, et al (2000) Organization of the basal ganglia: the importance of axonal collateralization. Trends Neurosci 23(10 Suppl):S20–S27.
175. Day M, Wang Z, Ding J, et al (2006) Selective elimination of glutamatergic synapses on striatopallidal neurons in Parkinson disease models. Nat Neurosci 9(2):251–259.
176. Gerfen CR (2006) Indirect-pathway neurons lose their spines in Parkinson disease. Nat Neurosci 9(2):157–158.
177. Nadjar A, Brotchie JM, Guigoni C, et al (2006) Phenotype of striatofugal medium spiny neurons in parkinsonian and dyskinetic nonhuman primates: a call for a reappraisal of the functional organization of the basal ganglia. J Neurosci 26(34):8653–8661.
178. Kawaguchi Y, Wilson CJ, Emson PC (1990) Projection subtypes of rat neostriatal matrix cells revealed by intracellular injection of biocytin. J Neurosci 10(10):3421–3438.
179. Levesque M, Parent A (2005) The striatofugal fiber system in primates: a reevaluation of its organization based on single-axon tracing studies. Proc Natl Acad Sci USA 102(33):11888–11893.
180. Wilson CJ, Groves PM (1980) Fine structure and synaptic connections of the common spiny neuron of the rat neostriatum: a study employing intracellular inject of horseradish peroxidase. J Comp Neurol 194(3):599–615.
181. Bishop GA, Chang HT, Kitai ST (1982) Morphological and physiological properties of neostriatal neurons: an intracellular horseradish peroxidase study in the rat. Neuroscience 7(1):179–191.
182. Jaeger D, Kita H, Wilson CJ (1994) Surround inhibition among projection neurons is weak or nonexistent in the rat neostriatum. J Neurophysiol 72(5):2555–2558.
183. Koos T, Tepper JM, Wilson CJ (2004) Comparison of IPSCs evoked by spiny and fast-spiking neurons in the neostriatum. J Neurosci 24(36):7916–7922.

184. Parent A, Hazrati LN (1995) Functional anatomy of the basal ganglia. I. The cortico-basal ganglia-thalamo-cortical loop. Brain Res Brain Res Rev 20(1):91–127.
185. Parent A, Hazrati L-N (1995) Functional anatomy of the basal ganglia. II. The place of subthalamic nucleus and external pallidum in basal ganglia circuitry. Brain Res Rev 20:128–154.
186. Gerfen CR, Baimbridge KG, Miller JJ (1985) The neostriatal mosaic: compartmental distribution of calcium-binding protein and parvalbumin in the basal ganglia of the rat and monkey. Proc Natl Acad Sci USA 82:8780–8784.
187. Iacopino A, Christakos S, German D, et al (1992) Calbindin-D28K-containing neurons in animal models of neurodegeneration: possible protection from excitotoxicity. Brain Res Mol Brain Res 13(3):251–261.
188. Haber SN, Ryoo H, Cox C, Lu W (1995) Subsets of midbrain dopaminergic neurons in monkeys are distinguished by different levels of mRNA for the dopamine transporter: comparison with the mRNA for the D2 receptor, tyrosine hydroxylase and calbindin immunoreactivity. J Comp Neurol 362(3):400–410.
189. Gerfen CR, Herkenham M, Thibault J (1987) The neostriatal mosaic: II. Patch- and matrix-directed mesostriatal dopaminergic and non-dopaminergic systems. J Neurosci 7(12):3915–3934.
190. Lynd-Balta E, Haber SN (1994) Primate striatonigral projections: a comparison of the sensorimotor-related striatum and the ventral striatum. J Comp Neurol 345(4):562–578.
191. Lynd-Balta E, Haber SN (1994) The organization of midbrain projections to the ventral striatum in the primate. Neuroscience 59(3):609–623.
192. Prensa L, Parent A (2001) The nigrostriatal pathway in the rat: A single-axon study of the relationship between dorsal and ventral tier nigral neurons and the striosome/matrix striatal compartments. J Neurosci 21(18):7247–7260.
193. Nicola SM, Surmeier J, Malenka RC (2000) Dopaminergic modulation of neuronal excitability in the striatum and nucleus accumbens. Annu Rev Neurosci 23:185–215.
194. Surmeier DJ, Ding J, Day M, et al (2007) D1 and D2 dopamine-receptor modulation of striatal glutamatergic signaling in striatal medium spiny neurons. Trends Neurosci 30(5):228–235.
195. Bouyer JJ, Park DH, Joh TH, Pickel VM (1984) Chemical and structural analysis of the relation between cortical inputs and tyrosine hydroxylase-containing terminalsin rat neostriatum. Brain Res 302:267–275.
196. Freund TF, Powell JF, Smith AD (1984) Tyrosine hydroxylase-immunoreactive boutons in synaptic contact with identified striatonigral neurons, with particular reference to dendritic spines. Neuroscience 13(4):1189–1215.
197. Bamford NS, Zhang H, Schmitz Y, et al (2004) Heterosynaptic dopamine neurotransmission selects sets of corticostriatal terminals. Neuron 42(4):653–663.
198. Dani JA, Zhou FM (2004) Selective dopamine filter of glutamate striatal afferents. Neuron 42(4):522–524.
199. Hersi AI, Kitaichi K, Srivastava LK, et al (2000) Dopamine D-5 receptor modulates hippocampal acetylcholine release. Brain Res Mol Brain Res 76(2):336–340.
200. Suzuki T, Miura M, Nishimura K, Aosaki T (2001) Dopamine-dependent synaptic plasticity in the striatal cholinergic interneurons. J Neurosci 21(17):6492–6501.
201. Graybiel AM, Aosaki T, Flaherty AW, Kimura M (1994) The basal ganglia and adaptive motor control. Science 265(5180):1826–1831.
202. Wang Z, Kai L, Day M, et al (2006) Dopaminergic control of corticostriatal long-term synaptic depression in medium spiny neurons is mediated by cholinergic interneurons. Neuron 50(3):443–452.
203. Wilson CJ (2006) Striatal D2 receptors and LTD: yes, but not where you thought they were. Neuron 50(3):347–348.
204. Cragg SJ (2005) Singing to the tune of dopamine. Focus on "Properties of dopamine release and uptake in the songbird basal ganglia." J Neurophysiol 93(4):1827–1828.

205. Fuchs H, Nagel J, Hauber W (2005) Effects of physiological and pharmacological stimuli on dopamine release in the rat globus pallidus. Neurochem Int 47(7):474–481.
206. Cheramy A, Leviel V, Glowinski J (1981) Dendritic release of dopamine in the substantia nigra. Nature 289:537–542.
207. Waszczak BL (1990) Differential effects of D1 and D2 dopamine receptor agonists on substantia nigra pars reticulata neurons. Brain Res 513(1):125–135.
208. Hoover BR, Marshall JF (2002) Further characterization of preproenkephalin mRNA-containing cells in the rodent globus pallidus. Neuroscience 111(1):111–125.
209. Billings LM, Marshall JF (2003) D2 antagonist-induced c-fos in an identified subpopulation of globus pallidus neurons by a direct intrapallidal action. Brain Res 964(2):237–243.
210. Galvan A, Kliem MA, Smith Y, Wichmann T (2005) GABAergic and dopaminergic modulation of basal ganglia output in primates. In: Bolam JP, Ingham CA, Magill PJ, eds. The Basal Ganglia VIII. New York: Springer, pp. 575–584.
211. Kliem MA, Maidment NT, Ackerson LC, et al (2007) Activation of nigral and pallidal dopamine D1-like receptors modulates basal ganglia outflow in monkeys. J Neurophysiol 98:1489–1500.
212. Baufreton J, Atherton JF, Surmeier DJ, Bevan MD (2005) Enhancement of excitatory synaptic integration by GABAergic inhibition in the subthalamic nucleus. J Neurosci 25(37):8505–8517.
213. Cragg SJ, Baufreton J, Xue Y, et al (2004) Synaptic release of dopamine in the subthalamic nucleus. Eur J Neurosci 20(7):1788–1802.
214. Freeman A, Ciliax B, Bakay R, et al (2001) Nigrostriatal collaterals to thalamus degenerate in parkinsonian animal models. Ann Neurol 50(3):321–329.
215. Sanchez-Gonzalez MA, Garcia-Cabezas MA, Rico B, Cavada C (2005) The primate thalamus is a key target for brain dopamine. J Neurosci 25(26):6076–6083.
216. Deniau JM, Thierry AM (1997) Anatomical segregation of information processing in the rat substantia nigra pars reticulata. Adv Neurol 74:83–96.
217. Kha HT, Finkelstein DI, Tomas D, et al (2001) Projections from the substantia nigra pars reticulata to the motor thalamus of the rat: single axon reconstructions and immunohistochemical study. J Comp Neurol 440(1):20–30.
218. Francois C, Tande D, Yelnik J, Hirsch EC (2002) Distribution and morphology of nigral axons projecting to the thalamus in primates. J Comp Neurol 447(3):249–260.
219. Cebrian C, Parent A, Prensa L (2005) Patterns of axonal branching of neurons of the substantia nigra pars reticulata and pars lateralis in the rat. J Comp Neurol 492(3):349–369.
220. Ilinsky IA, Jouandet ML, Goldman-Rakic PS (1985) Organization of the nigrothalamocortical system in the rhesus monkey. J Comp Neurol 236:315–330.
221. Middleton FA, Strick PL (2000) Basal ganglia and cerebellar loops: motor and cognitive circuits. Brain Res Brain Res Rev 31(2–3):236–250.
222. Clower DM, Dum RP, Strick PL (2005) Basal ganglia and cerebellar inputs to 'AIP.' Cereb Cortex 15(7):913–920.
223. Wurtz RH, Hikosaka O (1986) Role of the basal ganglia in the initiation of saccadic eye movements. Prog Brain Res 64:175–190.
224. Spann BM, Grofova I (1989) Origin of ascending and spinal pathways from the nucleus tegmenti pedunculopontinus in the rat. J Comp Neurol 283(1):13–27.
225. Grofova I, Zhou M (1998) Nigral innervation of cholinergic and glutamatergic cells in the rat mesopontine tegmentum: light and electron microscopic anterograde tracing and immunohistochemical studies. J Comp Neurol 395(3):359–379.
226. Chandler SH, Turman J Jr, Salem L, Goldberg LJ (1990) The effects of nanoliter ejections of lidocaine into the pontomedullary reticular formation on cortically induced rhythmical jaw movements in the guinea pig. Brain Res 526(1):54–64.
227. von Krosigk M, Smith Y, Bolam JP, Smith AD (1993) Synaptic organization of gabaergic inputs from the striatum and the globus pallidus onto neurons in the substantia nigra and retrorubral field which project to the medullary reticular formation. Neuroscience 50:531–549.

228. Mogoseanu D, Smith AD, Bolam JP (1994) Monosynaptic innervation of facial motoneurones by neurones of the parvicellular reticular formation. Exp Brain Res 101(3):427–438.
229. Sidibe M, Bevan MD, Bolam JP, Smith Y (1997) Efferent connections of the internal globus pallidus in the squirrel monkey: I. Topography and synaptic organization of the pallidothalamic projection. J Comp Neurol 382(3):323–347.
230. Kim R, Nakano K, Jayaraman A, Carpenter MB (1976) Projections of the globus pallidus and adjacent structures: an autoradiographic study in the monkey. J Comp Neurol 169(3):263–290.
231. DeVito JL, Anderson ME (1982) An autoradiographic study of efferent connections of the globus pallidus in Macaca mulatta. Exp Brain Res 46(1):107–117.
232. Schell GR, Strick PL (1984) The origin of thalamic inputs to the arcuate premotor and supplementary motor areas. J Neurosci 4(2):539–560.
233. Strick PL (1985) How do the basal ganglia and cerebellum gain access to the cortical motor areas? Behav Brain Res 18(2):107–123.
234. Inase M, Tanji J (1995) Thalamic distribution of projection neurons to the primary motor cortex relative to afferent terminal fields from the globus pallidus in the macaque monkey. J Comp Neurol 353(3):415–426.
235. Sakai ST, Inase M, Tanji J (2002) The relationship between MI and SMA afferents and cerebellar and pallidal efferents in the macaque monkey. Somatosens Motor Res 19(2):139–148.
236. Nambu A, Yoshida S, Jinnai K (1988) Projection on the motor cortex of thalamic neurons with pallidal input in the monkey. Exp Brain Res 71:658–662.
237. Hoover JE, Strick PL (1993) Multiple output channels in the basal ganglia. Science 259:819–821.
238. Hoover JE, Strick PL (1999) The organization of cerebellar and basal ganglia outputs to primary motor cortex as revealed by retrograde transneuronal transport of herpes simplex virus type 1. J Neurosci 19(4):1446–1463.
239. Jinnai K, Nambu A, Yoshida S, Tanibuchi I (1993) The two separate neuron circuits through the basal ganglia concerning the preparatory or execution processes of motor control. In: Mamo N, Hamada I, DeLong MR, eds. Role of the Cerebellum and Basal Ganglia in Voluntary Movement. Elsevier Science, pp. 153–161.
240. Rouiller EM, Liang F, Babalian A, et al (1994) Cerebellothalamocortical and pallidothalamocortical projections to the primary and supplementary motor cortical areas: a multiple tracing study in macaque monkeys. J Comp Neurol 345(2):185–213.
241. Kayahara T, Nakano K (1996) Pallido-thalamo-motor cortical connections: an electron microscopic study in the macaque monkey. Brain Res 706(2):337–342.
242. Middleton FA, Strick PL (2000) Basal ganglia output and cognition: evidence from anatomical, behavioral, and clinical studies. Brain Cogn 42(2):183–200.
243. Shink E, Sidibe M, Smith Y (1997) Efferent connections of the internal globus pallidus in the squirrel monkey: II. Topography and synaptic organization of pallidal efferents to the pedunculopontine nucleus. J Comp Neurol 382(3):348–363.
244. Harnois C, Filion M (1982) Pallidofugal projections to thalamus and midbrain: a quantitative antidromic activation study in monkeys and cats. Exp Brain Res 47(2):277–285.
245. Parent A, DeBellefeuille L (1982) Organization of efferent projections from the internal segment of globus pallidus in primate as revealed by fluorescence retrograde labeling method. Brain Res 245:201–213.
246. Rye DB, Lee HJ, Saper CB, Wainer BH (1988) Medullary and spinal efferents of the pedunculopontine tegmental nucleus and adjacent mesopontine tegmentum in the rat. J Comp Neurol 269(3):315–341.
247. Steininger TL, Rye DB, Wainer BH (1992) Afferent projections to the cholinergic pedunculopontine tegmental nucleus and adjacent midbrain extrapyramidal area in the albino rat. I. Retrograde tracing studies. J Comp Neurol 321(4):515–543.
248. Inglis WL, Winn P (1995) The pedunculopontine tegmental nucleus: where the striatum meets the reticular formation. Prog Neurobiol 47:1–29.

249. Mena-Segovia J, Bolam JP, Magill PJ (2004) Pedunculopontine nucleus and basal ganglia: distant relatives or part of the same family? Trends Neurosci 27(10):585–588.
250. Kaji R (2001) Basal ganglia as a sensory gating devise for motor control. J Med Invest 48(3–4):142–146.
251. Nambu A (2005) A new approach to understand the pathophysiology of Parkinson's disease. J Neurol 252(Suppl 4):iv1–iv4.
252. Kita H, Tachibana Y, Nambu A, Chiken S (2005) Balance of monosynaptic excitatory and disynaptic inhibitory responses of the globus pallidus induced after stimulation of the subthalamic nucleus in the monkey. J Neurosci 25(38):8611–8619.
253. Nambu A, Tokuno H, Hamada I, et al (2000) Excitatory cortical inputs to pallidal neurons via the subthalamic nucleus in the monkey. J Neurophysiol 84(1):289–300.
254. Boraud T, Bezard E, Bioulac B, Gross CE (2000) Ratio of inhibited-to-activated pallidal neurons decreases dramatically during passive limb movement in the MPTP-treated monkey. J Neurophysiol 83(3):1760–1763.
255. Mink JW (1996) The basal ganglia: focused selection and inhibition of competing motor programs. Prog Neurobiol 50(4):381–425.
256. Georgopoulos AP, DeLong MR, Crutcher MD (1983) Relations between parameters of step-tracking movements and single cell discharge in the globus pallidus and subthalamic nucleus of the behaving monkey. J Neurosci 3:1586–1598.
257. Jaeger D, Gilman S, Aldridge JW (1993) Primate basal ganglia activity in a pre-cued reaching task: preparation for movement. Exp Brain Res 95:51–64.
258. Alexander GE, Crutcher MD (1987) Preparatory activity in primate motor cortex and putamen coded in spatial rather than limb coordinates. Soc Neurosci Abstr 13:245.
259. Alexander GE, Crutcher MD (1989) Coding in spatial rather than joint coordinates of putamen and motor cortex preparatory activity preceding planned limb movements. In: Sambrook MA, Crossman AR, eds. Neural Mechanisms in Disorders of Movement. London: Blackwell, pp. 55–62.
260. Anderson M, Inase M, Buford J, Turner R (1992) Movement and preparatory activity of neurons in pallidal-receiving areas of the monkey thalamus. In: Mano N, Hamada I, DeLong MR, eds. Role of Cerebellum and Basal Ganglia in Voluntary Movement. Amsterdam: Elsevier, pp. 163–170.
261. Apicella P, Scarnati E, Schultz W (1991) Tonically discharging neurons of monkey striatum respond to preparatory and rewarding stimuli. Exp Brain Res 84:672–675.
262. Boussaoud D, Kermadi I (1997) The primate striatum: neuronal activity in relation to spatial attention versus motor preparation. Eur J Neurosci 9(10):2152–2168.
263. Crutcher MD, Alexander GE (1988) Supplementary motor area (SMA): Coding of both preparatory and movement-related neural activity in spatial rather than joint coordinates. Soc Neurosci Abstr 14:342.
264. Kubota K, Hamada I (1979) Preparatory activity of monkey pyramidal tract neurons related to quick movement onset during visual tracking performance. Brain Res 168:435–439.
265. Schultz W, Romo R (1992) Role of primate basal ganglia and frontal cortex in the internal generation of movement. I. Preparatory activity in the anterior striatum. Exp Brain Res 91:363–384.
266. Dettmers C, Fink GR, Lemon RN, et al (1995) Relation between cerebral activity and force in the motor areas of the human brain. J Neurophysiol 74(2):802–815.
267. Turner RS, Grafton ST, Votaw JR, et al (1998) Motor subcircuits mediating the control of movement velocity: a PET study. J Neurophysiol 80(4):2162–2176.
268. Tepper JM, Koos T, Wilson CJ (2004) GABAergic microcircuits in the neostriatum. Trends Neurosci 27(11):662–669.
269. Marsden CD, Obeso JA (1994) The functions of the basal ganglia and the paradox of stereotaxic surgery in Parkinson's disease. Brain 117:877–897.
270. Graybiel AM (1995) Building action repertoires: memory and learning functions of the basal ganglia. Curr Opinion Neurobiol 5:733–741.

271. Beiser DG, Hua SE, Houk JC (1997) Network models of the basal ganglia. Curr Opinion Neurobiol 7(2):185–190.
272. Beiser DG, Houk JC (1998) Model of cortical-basal ganglionic processing: encoding the serial order of sensory events. J Neurophysiol 79(6):3168–3188.
273. Schultz W (1998) The phasic reward signal of primate dopamine neurons. Advance Pharmacol 42:686–690.
274. Aosaki T, Kimura M, Graybiel AM (1995) Temporal and spatial characteristics of tonically active neurons of the primate striatum. J Neurophysiol 73:1234–1252.
275. Aosaki T, Tsubokawa H, Watanabe K, et al (1994) Responses of tonically active neurons in the primate's striatum undergo systematic changes during behavioral sensory-motor conditioning. J Neurosci 14:3969–3984.
276. Jog MS, Kubota Y, Connolly CI, et al (1999) Building neural representations of habits. Science 286(5445):1745–1749.
277. Hore J, Villis T (1980) Arm movement performance during reversible basal ganglia lesions in the monkey. Exp Brain Res 39:217–228.
278. Inase M, Buford JA, Anderson ME (1996) Changes in the control of arm position, movement, and thalamic discharge during local inactivation in the globus pallidus of the monkey. J Neurophysiol 75(3):1087–1104.
279. Kato M, Kimura M (1992) Effects of reversible blockade of basal ganglia on a voluntary arm movement. J Neurophysiol 68(5):1516–1534.
280. Horak FB, Anderson ME (1984) Influence of globus pallidus on arm movements in monkeys. II. Effects of stimulation. J Neurophysiol 52:305–322.
281. Horak FB, Anderson ME (1984) Influence of globus pallidus on arm movements in monkeys. I. Effects of kainic-induced lesions. J Neurophysiol 52:290–304.
282. Alamy M, Pons JC, Gambarelli D, Trouche E (1995) A defective control of small-amplitude movements in monkeys with globus pallidus lesions: an experimental study on one component of pallidal bradykinesia. Behav Brain Res 72(1–2):57–62.
283. Alamy M, Trouche E, Nieoullon A, Legallet E (1994) Globus pallidus and motor initiation: the bilateral effects of unilateral quisqualic acid-induced lesion on reaction times in monkeys. Exp Brain Res 99(2):247–258.
284. DeLong MR, Georgopoulos AP (1981) Motor functions of the basal ganglia. In: Brookhart JM, Mountcastle VB, Brooks VB, Geiger SR, eds. Handbook of Physiology The Nervous System Motor Control Sect 1, Vol II, Pt 2. Bethesda: American Physiological Society, pp. 1017–1061.
285. Laitinen LV (1995) Pallidotomy for Parkinson's diesease. Neurosurg Clin N Am 6:105–112.
286. Baron MS, Vitek JL, Bakay RAE, et al (1996) Treatment of advanced Parkinson's disease by GPi pallidotomy: 1 year pilot-study results. Ann Neurol 40:355–366.
287. Lozano AM, Lang AE, Galvez-Jimenez N, et al (1995) Effect of GPi pallidotomy on motor function in Parkinson's disease. Lancet 346(8987):1383–1387.
288. Mink JW, Thach WT (1991) Basal ganglia motor control. III. Pallidal ablation: normal reaction time, muscle cocontraction, and slow movement. J Neurophysiol 65:330–351.
289. Mink JW, Thach WT (1993) Basal ganglia intrinsic circuits and their role in behavior. Curr Opinion Neurobiol 3(6):950–957.
290. Gatev P, Darbin O, Wichmann T (2006) Oscillations in the basal ganglia under normal conditions and in movement disorders. Mov Disord 21(10):1566–1577.
291. Hammond C, Bergman H, Brown P (2007) Pathological synchronization in Parkinson's disease: networks, models and treatments. Trends Neurosci 30(7):357–364.
292. Hirsch EC, Perier C, Orieux G, et al (2000) Metabolic effects of nigrostriatal denervation in basal ganglia. Trends Neurosci 23(10 Suppl):S78–S85.
293. Drouot X, Oshino S, Jarraya B, et al (2004) Functional recovery in a primate model of Parkinson's disease following motor cortex stimulation. Neuron 44(5):769–778.

294. Pagni CA, Altibrandi MG, Bentivoglio A, et al (2005) Extradural motor cortex stimulation (EMCS) for Parkinson's disease. History and first results by the study group of the Italian neurosurgical society. Acta Neurochir Suppl 93:113–119.
295. Kojima J, Yamaji Y, Matsumura M, et al (1997) Excitotoxic lesions of the pedunculopontine tegmental nucleus produce contralateral hemiparkinsonism in the monkey. Neurosci Lett 226(2):111–114.
296. Nandi D, Liu X, Winter JL, et al (2002) Deep brain stimulation of the pedunculopontine region in the normal non-human primate. J Clin Neurosci 9(2):170–174.
297. Plaha P, Gill SS (2005) Bilateral deep brain stimulation of the pedunculopontine nucleus for Parkinson's disease. Neuroreport 16(17):1883–1887.
298. Provenzale JM, Glass JP (1995) Hemiballismus: CT and MR findings. J Comput Assist Tomogr 19(4):537–540.
299. Carpenter MB, Whittier JR, Mettler FA (1950) Analysis of choreoid hyperkinesia in the rhesus monkey: surgical and pharmacological analysis of hyperkinesia resulting from lesions in the subthalamic nucleus of Luys. J Comp Neurol 92:293–332.
300. Whittier JR, Mettler FA (1949) Studies of the subthalamus of the rhesus monkey. II. Hyperkinesia and other physiologic effects of subthalamic lesions with special references to the subthalamic nucleus of Luys. J Comp Neurol 90:319–372.
301. Hamada I, DeLong MR (1992) Excitotoxic acid lesions of the primate subthalamic nucleus result in transient dyskinesias of the contralateral limbs. J Neurophysiol 68:1850–1858.
302. Mitchell IJ, Sambrook MA, Crossman AR (1985) Subcortical changes in the regional uptake of [3H]-2-deoxyglucose in the brain of the monkey during experimental choreiform dyskinesia elicited by injection of a gamma-aminobutyric acid antagonist into the subthalamic nucleus. Brain 108(Pt 2):405–422.
303. Hamada I, DeLong MR (1992) Excitotoxic acid lesions of the primate subthalamic nucleus result in reduced pallidal neuronal activity during active holding. J Neurophysiol 68:1859–1866.
304. Carbon M, Trost M, Ghilardi MF, Eidelberg D (2004) Abnormal brain networks in primary torsion dystonia. Adv Neurol 94:155–161.
305. Starr PA, Rau GM, Davis V, et al (2005) Spontaneous pallidal neuronal activity in human dystonia: comparison with Parkinson's disease and normal macaque. J Neurophysiol 93(6):3165–3176.
306. Hallett M (2004) Dystonia: abnormal movements result from loss of inhibition. Adv Neurol 94:1–9.

# 2
# Functional Anatomy and Physiology of the Basal Ganglia: Non-motor Functions

Suzanne N. Haber

## Abstract

While typically associated with motor control, the basal ganglia are also involved in reward-based learning, decision making, and habit formation. The cortico-basal ganglia circuitry constitutes a system in which frontal cortex exploits the basal ganglia for additional processing of reward and cognition to effectively modulate learning that leads to the development of action plans and motor behaviors. This chapter first addresses basic basal ganglia anatomy and circuitry. Second, it focuses on the non-motor pathways associated with prefrontal cortex, in both limbic and cognitive areas. While each basal ganglia structure can generally be divided along limbic, cognitive, and motor pathways, recent evidence supports the hypothesis that complex interactions may occur between these functional systems. This chapter discusses the potential routes by which information can cross functional (limbic, cognitive, and motor control) domains thereby providing a network that supports both parallel and integrative function across motor and nonmotor circuits.

**Keywords:** ventral striatum, dorsal striatum, ventral pallidum, dorso-lateral prefrontal cortex, orbital cortex, cingulate cortex, dopamine, reward, cognition, motor control

## Introduction

The basal ganglia (BG) and cortex work in concert to orchestrate and execute planned behaviors. While the BG are best known for their motor functions, they also play an equally important role in motivation and cognition. Indeed, the role of the BG in cognitive and emotional behaviors is now well accepted. Areas within each of the BG nuclei are associated with limbic and cognitive aspects of behavior in addition to motor control regions. The dorsolateral striatum is the area generally associated with motor control (for review, see refs. *1* and *2*). Central BG areas are involved in cognitive functions such as procedural learning and working memory tasks (*3–6*). The ventro-medial regions play a key role

From: *Current Clinical Neurology: Deep Brain Stimulation in Neurological and Psychiatric Disorders*
Edited by: D. Tarsy, J.L. Vitek, P.A. Starr, and M.S. Okun © Humana Press, Totowa, NJ

in reward and reinforcement *(7–10)* and are important in the development of addictive behaviors and habit formation *(11–13)*. Diseases affecting motor control as well as mental health, including schizophrenia, drug addiction, and obsessive–compulsive disorder, are all linked to pathology in the BG *(13–17)*. The association of different BG regions with specific functions has lead to the concept of parallel and separate processing of functional information (motor, cognitive, and emotional) via segregated channels *(18)*. A major drawback of completely separate functional pathways is that most actions do not occur in isolation of motivation and cognition, but rather are the result of a combination of these behaviors requiring complex information processing. The development and execution of appropriate responses to environmental stimuli require continual updating and learning to adjust the response. A segregated system would create a system without sufficient temporal flexibility to change behaviors under different conditions. Indeed, the emerging consensus is that BG also plays a key role not only in the execution of behaviors, but also in the learning process and the development of action plans.

Recent physiological and imaging data show changes during learning which occur not only in cortex, but also within the BG. These studies show BG involvement in set shifting, response learning, and the development of behavioral guiding rules, and habit formation *(19–25)*. Indeed, there are a growing number of anatomical studies that clearly demonstrate a complex pattern of cortico-BG connections, providing an anatomical substrate for integrative processing across functional domains. This chapter first reviews basic BG anatomy and circuitry. Second, it discusses the non-motor pathways and addresses the evidence for integration across the functional domains of frontal cortical BG circuits.

## Basal Ganglia Structures and Connectivity

The primary structures of the BG are the striatum (the caudate nucleus, putamen, and n. accumbens), the globus pallidus, substantia nigra (SN), and the subthalamic nucleus (STN; Figure 2.1). The BG are divided into dorsal and ventral systems, associated with motor and cognitive functions (dorsal striatum) and motivational functions (ventral striatum), respectively. The concept of the ventral system was introduced with the recognition that medial and ventral portions of BG structures are connected to cortical and subcortical areas mediating emotion and motivation *(26, 27)*. The ventral system includes the ventral striatum (the n. accumbens, the ventromedial parts of the rostral caudate, and putamen), the ventral pallidum, the ventral tegmental area (VTA) and the medial region of the STN. The pallidal complex is comprised of the external (GPe) and internal segments (GPi) of the globus pallidus (the dorsal pallidum) and the ventral pallidum (specifically connected to the ventral striatum). The GPe and GPi, along with the putamen, form the lentiform nucleus. The ventral pallidum is that part of the pallidal complex that receives input from the ventral striatum. The ventral pallidum is located ventral to the anterior commissure and extends rostrally where it invades parts of the ventral striatum (Figure 2.1B). Caudally it occupies the ventral and medial extremes of the external and internal pallidal segments. The SN is divided into two parts, the pars compacta (SNc), and the pars reticulata (SNr); *(1, 28,* and *29)*.

The basic cortical-BG pathway flows from the cortex through BG structures, to the thalamus and back to cortex. This basic pathway is further divided

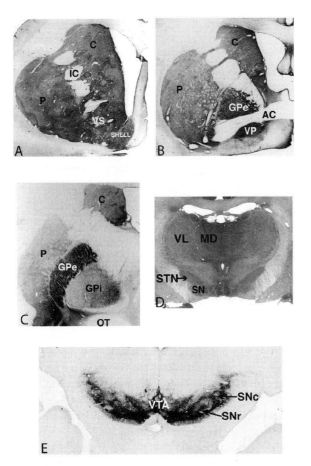

**Figure 2.1** Photomicrographs at coronal levels using different markers to illustrate specific basal ganglia structures in the non-human primate brain (A–C stained for enkephalin immunoreactivity, D stained for Nissl, E stained for tyrosine hydroxylase immunoreactivity). (A) the rostral striatum; (B) at the level of the anterior commissure; (C) at the level of both the internal and external segments of the globus pallidus; (D) at the level of the thalamus and subthalamic nucleus; (E) at the level of the substantia nigra. AC, anterior commissure; C, caudate nucleus; GPe, globus pallidus external segment; GPi, globus pallidus internal segment; IC, internal capsule; MD, mediolateral nucleus of the thalamus, P, putamen; OT, optic tract; SNc, substantia nigra, pars compacta; SNr, substantia nigra, pars reticulata; STN, subthalamic nucleus; VL, ventral lateral nucleus of the thalamus; VP, ventral pallidum; VS, ventral striatum; VTA, ventral tegmental area

into two circuits: (1) A direct circuit in which the striatum projects to the GPi/SNr and back to cortex via the thalamus; and (2) an indirect circuit via the GPe which projects to the STN, then from the STN to the GPi/SNr and back to cortex via the thalamus (Figure 2.2).

## The Striatum

### *Afferent Connections*
The striatum is the main input structure of the BG. Its afferent projections are derived from three major sources: *(1)* it receives a massive and topographic

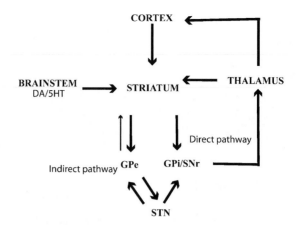

**Figure 2.2** Diagram demonstrating the connections of the basal ganglia, including the direct and indirect pathways. 5HT, serotonin; DA, dopamine; GPe, globus pallidus external segment; GPi, globus pallidus internal segment; SNr, substantia nigra, pars reticulata; STN, subthalamic nucleus

input from all of cerebral cortex; (2) the second largest input is derived from the thalamus; and (3) the third major input is from the brainstem, primarily from the dopaminergic cells of the midbrain (Figure 2.2). Afferent projections to the striatum terminate in a general topographic manner, such that the dorsolateral striatum receives cortical input from sensory-motor areas, the central striatum receives input from associative cortical areas, and the ventromedial striatum receives input from limbic areas. Within this organization, afferent projections terminate in a dense and patchy manner *(30)*. In addition to the dense, or focal projections, each cortical area sends axons that travel long distances to innervate a broad striatal region *(31)*. Indeed, intracellular tracer injections of single cortical neurons show that these cortico-striatal axons can innervate up to 14% of the striatum *(32)*. These projections (referred to as diffuse projections), not only expand the borders of the focal projections, but also extend into striatal territories, which are innervated by focal projections derived from other function regions of cortex.

Thalamo-striatal inputs are also topographically organized. The midline and intralaminar nuclei are the source of the most widely reported thalamo-striatal projections *(33–40)*. However, there is an equally large projection to the striatum from the BG relay thalamic nuclei, including, the mediodorsal (MD), ventral anterior (VA) and ventral lateral (VL) nuclei in primates *(38, 40–42)*. These thalamic nuclei are associated with limbic, association, and motor systems, respectively, by virtue of their connectivity with cortical and subcortical regions *(43–46)*.

The ascending midbrain dopaminergic striatal afferents terminate on the spines of the medium spiny projection neurons, in close apposition to cortical synapses, and are in a position to influence cortical input *(47)*. In this way, a relatively smaller midbrain projection to the striatum has a large impact on modulation of the larger cortical projection. This dopamine (DA) projection has a mediolateral topographic arrangement as well as an inverse dorsoventral topography. The ventral SNc neurons project to the dorsal striatum and the dorsally located DA neurons project to the ventral striatum *(48)*. Medium spiny neurons (MSNs) are divided into two groups based on DA receptor distributions. Those that contain high mRNA expression levels for the $D_1$ receptors also co-contain substance P (SP) and those that contain high mRNA expression levels for the $D_2$ receptor subtype also co-contain enkephalin (ENK) *(49)*. Inputs to the striatum also include projections from the dorsal and median raphe nuclei and from other components of the BG including the external globus pallidus (and comparable regions of the ventral pallidum. In addition to the extrinsic inputs, the projection neurons also receive input from interneurons and from local collaterals of other medium spiny cells *(50–53)*.

*Intrinsic Cells of the Striatum*

The striatum contains two general cell groups: projection neurons and interneurons. Projection neurons are the most common cell type and are referred to as MSNs or the principal neurons of the striatum (Figure 2.3). In non-primate species, they account for more than 90% of the cells. They account for about 70% of cells in primates *(54–56)*. These medium-sized cells (14–20 μm) have four to seven radiating dendrites that are densely covered with spines. This dendritic arbor extends in all directions with a radius of up to 0.5 mm. Extracellular physiological recordings in awake, behaving monkeys show that the MSNs are phasically active neurons (PANs), with a low spontaneous discharge rate (0.5–1 spike/s), but a relatively high firing rate associated with behavior, including the performance of learned tasks *(5, 57, 58)*. PANs are activated antidromically from either GPe or GPi, thus identifying them as the projection neurons. MSNs are bistable, shifting between two membrane states: an upstate and a downstate *(59, 60)*. In the downstate, the membranes are hyperpolarized and cannot generate action potentials. In the upstate, the membranes are relatively depolarized and close to threshold for spike generation. Movement from a downstate to an upstate occurs in response to the combined

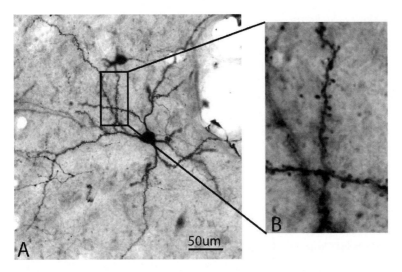

**Figure 2.3** (A) Photomicrograph of a medium spiny neuron (MSN) filled with Lucifer Yellow. (B) Enlargement of the dendritic tree shown (framed in A), demonstrating the dense spines

effects of temporally coherent and convergent excitatory input from cortex and/or thalamus. Neurons in the upstate are primed to fire in response to further depolarization. However, in the absence of the coherent excitatory input, the membrane returns to the downstate. Therefore, it is generally believed that a relatively large (temporally and spatially coordinated) excitatory input is required to move the MNS from the downstate to the upstate in order to result in activation. Both cortical and thalamic fibers provide this input via their dense, focal projections that terminate primarily on the dendritic spines of the MSN. These terminals form asymmetric, glutamatergic synapses *(61, 62)*.

There are four classes of aspiny interneurons *(63, 64)*. Cholinergic cells comprise the largest striatal cells (30–40 μm) and represent approximately 1% of the population, both receiving input from and projecting to the MSN. A central role for the functional balance between dopaminergic/cholinergic populations is well documented in both Parkinson's disease and in experimental animal models *(65, 66)*. The cholinergic interneurons are spontaneously active and referred to as tonically active neurons (TANS). In contrast to the membrane properties responsible for the physiological (up and down) states of the MSNs that are controlled by extrinsic connections, the TANS spontaneous firing patterns are a function of their intrinsic membrane properties *(67)*. TANs are involved in the detection of stimuli that have inherent motivational significance and are associated with the delivery of primary rewards throughout the striatum, including the dorsal region *(68–70)*. A second population of interneurons co-contains the calcium binding protein, parvalbumin. These cells are fast spiking neurons that receive a powerful input from cortex. Their response to cortical activation is faster and earlier than the response of the MSNs to cortical input. Moreover, they appear to have an inhibitory affect on MSNs, as their firing is associated with a decrease in MSN activity *(71, 72)*. There are two additional interneuron types: a GABA-containing interneurons that stain positively for the neuropeptides somatostatin and neuropeptide Y, and co-contain nitric oxide synthase (NOS); and GABA-containing cells that co-contain calretinin, a calcium-binding protein *(50, 73)*.

### *The Ventral Striatum*

While the ventral striatum is similar to the dorsal striatum in most respects, nonetheless, there are some unique features *(27)*. The ventral striatum contains a subterritory, called the shell (Figure 2.1A; ref. *74*). Experiments show that this area plays a particularly important role in the circuitry underlying goal-directed behaviors, behavioral sensitization, and changes in affective states *(75–79)*. While several transmitter and receptor distribution patterns distinguish the shell, lack of calbindin-positive staining is the most consistent marker *(80)*. Embedded within the ventral striatum are the islands of Calleja. Finally, while the basic cortical BG loop is similar in all BG circuits, the ventral striatum alone receives an additional subcortical input from the amygdala and from the hippocampus, for which there is no comparable input to the other BG territories *(82, 83)*.

## The Pallidal Complex and the SN, SNr

The main output from the striatum is to the GP and the SNr. Based on histochemical localization of neuropeptides, there are two general types of medium spiny cells: one that co-contains SP and GABA; and one that co-contains

ENK and GABA. SP-containing MSNs project primarily to the GPi/SNr, while the ENK-containing cells project primarily to the GPe *(84)*. The dorsal globus pallidus is divided by the internal medullary lamina into the external (GPe) and internal (GPi) pallidal segments. The ventral pallidum (VP) extends ventrally, below the anterior commissure and rostrally to invade the rostral and ventral portions of the ventral striatum, sending finger-like extensions into the anterior perforated space *(84)*. The pallidal complex is primarily made of large cells (20–60 μm) that give rise to thick, long, dendrites *(85–87)*. These dendrites are densely ensheathed with synapses originating primarily from the striatum and STN. All pallidal neurons use GABA as their transmitter *(88)*. While the projections of the two dorsal pallidal segments GPe and GPi (and comparable parts of the ventral pallidum) differ, their main input is from the striatum. ENK/D2R-positive MSNs project primarily to GPe and parts of the VP. In contrast, the SP/D1R-postive MSNs send fibers to the GPi and parts of the VP (Figure 2.4). In addition to this GABAergic striatal input, there is the well-characterized glutamatergic input from the STN nucleus to all pallidal components *(89, 90)*. Terminals from STN intermingle with the much larger GABAergic innervation from the striatum *(91)*. Both the GPi and GPe also receive input from the midbrain DA cells *(92)*.

The GPi (and parts of the VP) project directly to the thalamus and brainstem (Figure 2.4). These projection fibers are divided into three bundles, the ansa lenticularis, the lenticular fasciculus, and the pallidotegmental fibers *(93, 94)*. Fibers in the ansa lenticularis arise from the outer portion of the GPi, forming a clearly defined bundle that sweeps ventromedially and rostrally, around the internal capsule and continuing caudally to merge with Forel's field H. Fibers of the lenticular fasciculus arise from the medial portion of the GPi, traverse the internal capsule, and form a discrete bundle, ventral to the zona incerta. This

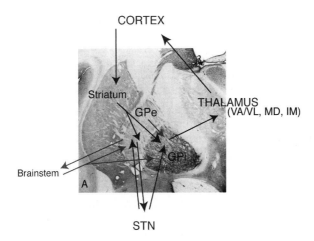

**Figure 2.4** Diagram demonstrating the connections of the two segments of the globus pallidus. The tissue is processed for SP immunoreactivity to highlight the internal pallidal segment. The main connections (black lines) and less prominent connections (gray lines) are indicated. GPe, globus pallidus external segment; GPi, globus pallidus internal segment; IM, intralaminar nuclei of the thalamus; MD, mediodorsal nucleus of the thalamus; STN, subthalamic nucleus, VA/VL, ventral anterior/ventral lateral nuclei of the thalamus

bundle joins the ansa lenticularis in Forel's field H and both fiber groups then become part of the thalamic fasciculus to terminate in different thalamic nuclei *(95, 96)*. GPi fibers projecting to the thalamic relay nuclei also give off collaterals that terminate in the centromedian and parafasicular intralaminar nuclei *(96–98)*. The third fiber bundle arising from the GPi, the pallidotegmental fibers, terminates in the pedunculopontine n *(99)*. While projections from the GPi to the ventral tier nuclear group of the thalamus have been considered to be segregated from cerebellar inputs to the thalamus, recent evidence suggests that there may be some overlap between them *(100–102)*. The GPe projects primarily to the STN, via the subthalamic fasciculus. It also projects to the striatum, to the internal pallidal segment, and to the midbrain. Neurons in the GPe segment have been further classified according to their projection targets: those that target the STN and SNr; those that target the internal segment and STN; and those that target the striatum *(103)*. Although the GPe and GPi have different firing patterns, they are both tonically active and change their firing in relationship to behavioral activity *(104, 105)*. These changes are presumably due to a combination of excitatory, glutamatergic inputs from STN and/or inhibitory, GABAergic inputs from the striatum *(106, 107)*.

The SNr cells of the SN, are GABAergic and, like the pallidum, are primarily large neurons with long, thick dendrites, which are almost completely ensheathed with synaptic contacts with dense SP-positive striatal fibers *(84, 86)*. However, it is important to point out that in primates, a clear demarcation between the SNc and the SNr is often difficult to visualize, particularly in caudal regions, due to the invasion into the SNr by DA neurons and their dendritic arborizations (see Figure 2.1E). The connections of the SNr are also similar to those of the GPi. Moreover, changes in firing patterns in association with behavioral activity are consistent with those seen with cells of the GP *(108)*. However, the SNr also receives a major serotonergic input from the dorsal raphe nucleus *(109, 110)*. In addition, the SNr projects to the superior colliculus, a pathway which arises primarily from the lateral SNr and is important in the control of eye movements associated with specific behavioral tasks *(111)*.

**The STN**

The STN is a well-defined compact oval structure, located medial to the peduncular portion of the internal capsule at its rostral level, which extends caudally to overlie the rostral part of the SN (see Figure 2.1E). The principal neurons in the STN nucleus are medium to large cells (25–40 µm) and are pyramidal, or round in shape and give rise to dendritic trees, which branch extensively to cover a large area of the nucleus *(112)*. STN neurons are glutamatergic and project to all pallidal components (Figure 2.5; ref. *113*). The external segment of the globus pallidus and parts of the ventral pallidum provide one of its most massive afferent projections *(93, 114)*. Connections of the STN include inputs not only from the pallidum, but also from the brainstem, including the midbrain DA cells *(92, 115)*. Interest in the direct DA innervation of the STN has increased recently due to the recognition of its hyperactivity in Parkinson's disease and the fact that at least a subpopulation of the DA cells that project to the STN are vulnerable to degeneration in Parkinson's disease and in animal models of PD *(116, 117)*. Additional brainstem inputs to the STN are derived from cholinergic cells of the pedunculopontine region, more medially placed cells that are noncholinergic, and cells from the laterodorsal tegmental nucleus *(118, 119)*.

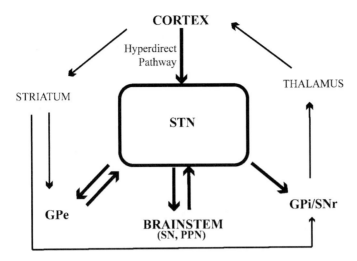

**Figure 2.5** Diagram demonstrating the connections of the subthalamic nucleus (STN). Direct afferent and efferent projections of the STN are shown in thick lines. Connections between the other basal ganglia nuclei are indicated with thin lines. GPe, globus pallidus external segment; GPi, globus pallidus internal segment; PPN, pedunculopontine nucleus; SNr, substantia nigra, pars reticulata

In addition to input from the pallidum and brainstem, the STN receives a direct afferent projection from cortex. This pathway is referred to as the hyperdirect pathway *(120)*. Through this connection, information from cortex reaches the STN prior to that from the GPe whose signal first must pass through the striatum. The STN projects to all pallidal regions including the GPe, GPi, and VP, and SN, primarily terminating in the SNr. These target structures receive input from collateral axons. One population of STN cells project to all three target regions, the GPi, GPe, and SN; a second population, the largest, sends axons to the GPi and GPe; a third group of cells innervates only the GPe *(121)*. In addition, the STN also projects back to the pedunculopontine tegmentum *(118)*.

### The SN, SNc and VTA

*Organization and Connections of the Midbrain DA Cells*
The midbrain DA neurons are divided into the SN, SNc, and the VTA (Figure 2.6). The SNc is further divided into three groups: a dorsal group; a main, densocellular region; and a ventral group, or the cell columns *(122, 123)*. The dorsal group of neurons is composed of loosely, horizontally oriented cells, which extend dorsolaterally and circumvent the ventral and lateral superior cerebellar peduncle and the red nucleus. These cells merge with the immediately adjacent DA neurons of the VTA and form a continuous mediodorsal band of cells. Calbindin (CaBP), a calcium-binding protein, is a marker for both the VTA and the dorsal SNc, but not for the ventral cell groups (the densocellular group and the cell columns), which are calbindin negative *(123, 124)*. The dendritic arborizations of the ventral cell groups are oriented ventrally and occupy the major portion of the SNr in primates. The densocellular group and the cell

columns, in addition to being calbindin-negative, have high expression levels for DA transporter (DAT) and for the D2 receptor mRNAs. Based on the phenotypic characteristics of the DA neurons, they are divided into two tiers: a dorsal tier (calbindin-positive) and a ventral tier (Figure 2.6A; ref. *123*). The ventral tier cells are more vulnerable to degeneration in Parkinson's disease and to N-methyl-4-phenyl-1,2,3,6-tetrahydropyridine (MPTP)-induced toxicity, while the calbindin-positive dorsal tier cells are selectively spared in these disorders *(125, 126)*.

Input to the midbrain DA neurons is from the striatum, from both the external segment of the globus pallidus and the ventral pallidum, and from the pedunculopontine nucleus (Figure 2.6B). In addition, there are projections to the VTA and the dorsomedial SNc from the bed nucleus of the stria terminalis, from the sublenticular substantia innominata and the extended amygdala *(114, 127–131)*. These DA cells project massively to the striatum. The dorsal tier cells also project widely throughout cortex. The DA innervation of primate cortex is more extensive than in rats and found not only in granular areas but also in agranular frontal regions, parietal cortex, temporal cortex, and albeit sparsely, in occipital cortex *(132–134)*. The majority of DA cortical projections are from the parabrachial pigmented nucleus of the VTA and the dorsal SNc *(135, 136)*. The ventral tier does not project extensively to cortex.

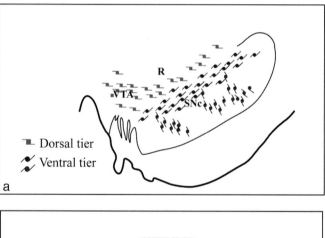

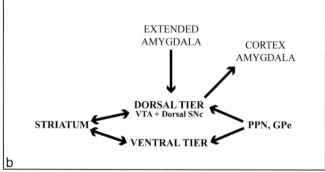

**Figure 2.6** (A) Midbrain dopamine cell groups, dorsal tier, cells = light gray; ventral tier cells, dark gray. (B) Diagram demonstrating the connections of the dorsal and ventral tiers of midbrain dopamine neurons. GPe, globus pallidus external segment; PPN, pedunculopontine nucleus; R, red nucleus; SNc, substantia nigra, pars compacta; VTA, ventral tegmental area

In addition, DA cells from the VTA and the adjoining dorsal SNc innervate the amygdala (Figure 2.6; refs. *137–139*).

*Functional Correlates of the DA Cells*

The midbrain DA neurons play a unique role in BG and cortical circuits in modulating a broad range of behaviors including reward, learning, and "working memory" to motor control. In fact, while the subpopulations of DA neurons have been associated with these different functions based on the connections to the striatum, physiological studies suggest their primary function is to focus attention on significant and rewarding or salient stimuli *(140, 141)*. DA cells fire tonically at about 5 spikes/s but are activated when a rewarding or salient stimuli is not expected. However, when the animal expects the reward, cells no longer respond to the reward, but rather respond to the signal that indicates the beginning of a trial that might result in a reward *(140)*. Moreover, DA neurons pause if a predicted reward fails to occur *(142;* see also ref. *143)*. These and other experiments clearly show that it is not the movement but the relevance of the stimulus that is important *(144)*. Thus, unlike other major inputs to the striatum, the DA cells are more difficult to categorize based on their association with different cortical functions. Rather, as a group, they appear to mediate aspects of the reward or salient response. In this respect the DA system has been an intense focus of productive research in the development of reward-based learning, drug addiction, and plasticity *(145–149)*.

## Integration Across Cortico-BG Circuits

The BG are tightly linked to frontal cortex both anatomically and physiologically and, as indicated above, are involved not only in motor control, but also in the learning process and habit formation. The components of the frontal cortex that mediate behaviors, including motivation and emotional drive, coupled with planning and cognitive components to plan actions, and finally, the movement itself, are reflected in the organization, physiology, and connections between areas of frontal cortex and the striatum. While the functional topography of these inputs has been extensively studied (for review, see refs. *1* and *2*), recent experiments demonstrate that convergence between functional regions also occurs. Anatomical studies show that cortico-striatal inputs from different functional regions are not strictly segregated *(31)*, rather there are clear areas of convergence between cortico-striatal dense terminal fields (or focal projections) from different functional regions of cortex. Moreover, in addition to these well-described focal projections, there are the diffuse cortical projections that invade regions which receive focal projections from other functional cortical areas. Additional potential interactions between functional circuits are again seen at the level of the GP/SNr and its outputs *(150–152)*. Finally, there are connections between limbic, cognitive, and motor regions of the striatum via non-reciprocal networks in the midbrain DA cells and thalamo-cortical pathways *(101, 153, 154)*.

**Functional Organization of Frontal Cortical Striatal Projections**

The main input to the striatum is from cortex. The BG project back primarily to the frontal cortex. The frontal cortex is often considered the cortex of action and divided into regions that mediate motivation and emotion, cognition, and motor control. The anterior cingulate cortex (ACC) and orbital frontal cortex (OFC) are involved in different aspects of emotional expression, reward-based behaviors, error prediction and the choice between short and long-term gains *(155–158)*. The OFC and ACC project primarily to the rostral and ventral striatum (the medial caudate N., the medial and ventral rostral putamen, and the nucleus accumben), including both the shell and the core *[159, 160]*. The shell receives the densest innervation from medial areas 25, 14, and 32 and from agranular insular cortex, areas involved in monitoring the internal milieu. The entire reward-related striatum, as defined by ACC/OFC inputs, occupies a large rostral region and encompasses at least 22% of the entire striatum. This region is not limited to the ventral striatum at rostral levels, but extends into a large medial and central area, occupying much of the rostral pole before tapering off caudally. Diffuse projections from these areas extend the projection influence of the ACC/OFC, by invading other functional domains of the striatum *(31)*. Moreover, consistent with the anatomical distribution of OFC and dACC focal and diffuse projections, reward-responsive activation is not limited to the ventral striatum, but rather found throughout a large dorsal-ventral striatal region (Figure 2.7; refs. *161–166*).

The dorsolateral prefrontal cortex (DLPFC) plays an important role in executive functions *(167–170)*. The DLPFC projects primarily to the rostral central region of the caudate N. and extends from the rostral pole of the striatum through its caudal extent *(171, 172)*. Consistent with input from this cortical area, cells in the head of the caudate nucleus discharge during the delayed portion of the task resembling activity observed in the DLPFC *(3, 173, 174)*. Furthermore, imaging studies support the idea that the head of the caudate is instrumental in delayed tasks, particularly in specific working memory tasks *(175–178)*. Taken together, a particularly large part of the head of the caudate nucleus N, is involved in working memory and strategic

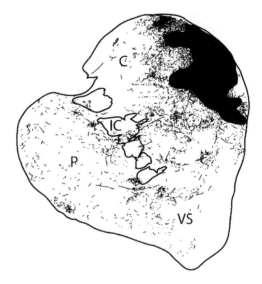

**Figure 2.7** Diagram illustrating focal projections (black filled area) and diffuse projections (line drawings) following an injection of an anterograde tracer into the dorsolateral prefrontal cortex

planning processes. Importantly innervation from the DLPFC interfaces with inputs from several other cortical areas, including those from both the ACC and OFC *(31)*. Although each cortical projection (limbic and cognitive) does occupy its own territory to some extent, projections from all prefrontal cortical areas converge in a central, rostral region, with each cortical projection extending into non-overlapping zones. As with limbic projections, the diffuse cortical fibers from the DLPFC extend deeper into other functional territories (Figure 2.7). Convergence between these projection fields is less prominent caudally, and there is almost a complete separation of DLPFC and ACC/OFC focal projections just rostral to the anterior commissure *(31)*. However, at the level of the anterior commissure, there is convergence between DLPFC fibers and rostral motor control areas. Thus, there is convergence between terminals from the DLPFC with those from limbic cortical regions in rostral striatal areas and with motor control cortical regions more caudally.

The dorsolateral putamen and caudate nucleus form the striatal area associated with motor control. This region receives input from the motor, premotor, supplementary motor, and cingulate motor cortices (for review, see refs. *1* and *2*). Moreover, physiological and imaging studies support its involvement in motor control and motor planning *(57, 179–182)*. Taken together, the motor and premotor areas (including the frontal eye fields) mediate different aspects of motor behavior. However, as indicated above, there are specific areas within the striatum that receive a convergent input from motor control areas, specifically rostral areas, and the DLPFC. These regions are likely to play a specific role in planning and learning and action.

Some convergence between focal projections from different functional domains appears to be a consistent rule in fronto-striatal circuitry. Indeed, EM studies show that cortico-striatal terminals from the sensory and motor systems converge in the striatum where they synapse onto the same parvalbumin interneuron. These fast spiking GABAergic interneurons, as mentioned previously, are more responsive to cortical input than the medium spiny cells *(72, 183–186)*. Because MSNs have a large dendritic field, regions of convergence between the focal terminal fields from different functional cortical areas are likely to be larger than can be determined by the area of each focal projection. These regions of converging terminals may represent hot spots of plasticity required for updating an action plan. Given that behavioral guiding rules are developed from different aspects of reward-related information, cognition, and motor control, regions of converging inputs may be particularly critical for the coordination of these processes.

In addition to its focal projection, each cortical area sends terminal fibers that extend outside of the dense, focal projection field. This diffuse projection invades striatal regions that receive their focal input from other cortical areas (Figure 2.7; ref. *31*). The distribution and extent of these fiber clusters is consistent with the distance a single cortical axon travels within the striatum *(32)*. As mentioned previously, activation of MSNs requires a large coordinated glutamatergic input, and therefore little attention has been paid to these fibers. Nonetheless, they are a prominent feature of all frontal projections. While their numbers may not be sufficient to activate MSNs in a given region, they may serve a separate function from the denser, focal projection fields. First, taken together, diffuse projections from widespread cortical areas collectively represent a large population of axons invading each focal projection field.

Under certain conditions, if these axons were activated as a group, they could provide the recruitment strength necessary to modulate the incoming focal signal. Second, these invading clusters of axons might target a different population of striatal cells, such as the tonically active cholinergic interneurons, a subpopulation of interneurons that are specifically activated by motivationally salient stimuli and found throughout the striatum *(187, 188)*. Alternatively, clusters of cortical axons that invade other functional territories may interact more specifically with thalamic glutamatergic input, providing a small, but potentially significant and functionally diverse signal. While a specific role for the diffuse projections is unclear, it likely serves to broadly disseminate cortical activity to a wide striatal region.

**Pathways of the GP/SNr**

The pathways that flow from the striatum and back to cortex via the GP/SNr and thalamus, are also somewhat topographically organized (for review, see refs. *1* and *2*). Despite the general topographic arrangement of these pathways, anatomical studies also demonstrate some integration between functional systems in the GP/SN connections that may underlie meditation of complex behaviors. The dendrites of both the GP and SNr are long and stretch across multiple functional regions *(85, 150, 189)*. The distal regions of these dendrites therefore receive input from several functional regions via their striatal projections. Indeed, while physiological studies demonstrate the continuity of striatal functional areas in the pallidal complex, particularly in motor control function *(104, 190–192)*, these studies do not support the role of GP neurons in the initial activation of muscles, but rather in the coordination of voluntary actions. Consistent with an integrative role for these pathways, a growing body of evidence suggests that GPi neurons are selectively modulated during movement behaviors performed in different behavioral contexts, including learning paradigms *(193)*. Moreover, descending projections from different functional regions of the GP converge within their hypothalamic and brainstem targets. In particular, those from the GPe that project to the STN converge with those from the VP that project to the medial STN at the border with the lateral hypothalamic nucleus. These convergent regions may account for the fact that, functional segregation is only partially maintained in the STN, following activation of different cortical regions *(151, 152, 194)*.

**The Striato-Nigro-Striatal Network**

While behavioral and pharmacological studies of DA pathways have lead to the association of the mesolimbic pathway and nigrostriatal pathway with reward and motor activity, respectively, more recently both of these cell groups have been associated with the development of reward-based learning, the acquisition of newly acquired behaviors, and plasticity *(142, 149, 195–199)*. As described previously, while the midbrain DA cells project to the striatum, the striatum is also a main input to the DA cells. There is an inverse dorsal-ventral topographic organization to this reciprocal projection system. Thus, the dorsal aspects of the striatum terminate in the ventral regions of the midbrain, while the ventral areas terminate dorsally *(48, 131, 154, 200–202)*. In addition to the inverse topography, there is also a differential ratio of DA projections to the different striatal areas. The DA input to the ventral striatum is derived from the most limited midbrain region, while the input to the dorsolateral striatum is derived from the largest midbrain area. In contrast, projections from the ventromedial striatum to the midbrain are the most extensive projecting to a wide mediolateral range of dopaminergic cells including much of the densocellular SNc. The dorsolateral striatal projection to the DA cells is the most limited and terminates in a relatively confined ventrolateral region of the SNr and the dopaminergic cell columns that extend into this region.

Thus, when considered separately, each limb of the system (striato-nigral or nigro-striatal pathway) creates a loose topographic organization indicating that the VTA and medial SN are associated with the limbic system, and the lateral and ventral SN are related to the associative and motor striatal regions (Figure 2.8). However, the ascending and descending limb for each functional area of the striatum differs in their proportional projections. The ventral striatum influences a wide range of DA neurons, but is itself influenced by

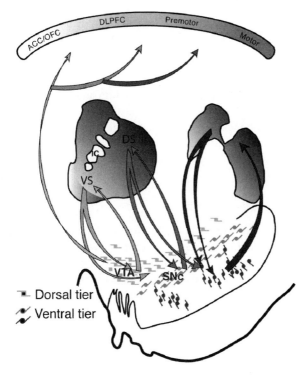

**Figure 2.8** Diagram of the organization of striato-nigro-striatal (SNS) projections *(156)*. The gray scale gradient illustrates the organization of functional corticostriatal projections. Light gray, input from limbic cortical areas; medium gray, input from association cortical areas; dark gray, input from motor control cortical areas. Midbrain projections from the ventral striatum target both the VTA and ventromedial SNc. Midbrain projections from the VTA to the ventral striatum forms a "closed," reciprocal SNS loop (light gray arrows). Projections from the medial SN feed-forward to the dorsal striatum forming the first part of a spiral (medium gray arrow). The spiral continues through the SNS projections (medium and dark gray arrows), projecting more dorsally (dark gray arrows). In this way, ventral striatal regions influence more dorsal striatal regions via spiraling SNS projections. DLPFC, dorsal lateral prefrontal cortex; ACC, anterior cingulate cortex; DS, dorsal striatum; OFC, orbital frontal cortex; SNc, substantia nigra, pars compacta; VS, ventral striatum; VTA, ventral tegmental area

a relatively limited group of DA cells. In contrast, the dorsolateral striatum influences a limited midbrain region, but is affected by a relatively large midbrain region. Moreover, for each striatal region there is one reciprocal and two non-reciprocal connections with the midbrain. Dorsal to the reciprocal connection lies a group of cells that project to the striatal region, but does not receive projections from it. Ventral to the reciprocal component lie efferent terminals without an ascending reciprocal connection. Finally, these three components for each SNS projection system occupy a different position within the midbrain. The ventral striatum system lies dorsomedially, the dorsolateral striatum system lies ventrolaterally, and the central striatum system is positioned between the two (156).

With this arrangement, information from the limbic system can reach the motor system through a series of connections. For example, the ventral striatum, which receives input from the limbic cortical areas, sends an efferent projection to the midbrain that extends beyond its reciprocal connection, terminating lateral and ventral to it. This terminal region projects to the central (or associative) striatum. The central striatum is reciprocally connected to the densocellular region but also projects ventrally and thus in a position to interact with cells projecting to the dorsolateral (or motor) striatum. Taken together, the interface between different striatal regions via the midbrain DA cells is organized in an ascending spiral which interconnects different functional regions of the striatum and creates a feed-forward organization (Figure 2.8). Information can thus be channeled from limbic to cognitive to motor circuits. Pharmacological, physiological and functional imaging data support this flow of information and the recruitment of the dorsal striatum following activation of the ventral striatum and limbic circuits (21, 203, 204).

**Thalamo-Cortico-Thalamic Interface**

The thalamic-cortical pathway is the last link in the cortico-BG circuit and is often treated as a simple relay back to cortex. However this pathway does not transfer information passively but rather plays a key role in regulating cortical ensembles of neurons through its projections to different cortical layers (205–208). Moreover, the emphasis on the thalamic link in cortico-BG processing is placed on the thalamocortical projection. However, the most massive input to thalamus, including the BG relay nuclei, is from the cortex, not from the GP/SNr. The cortical connection to the VA/VL and MD is far more extensive than its reciprocal thalamocortical projection, a concept that is seen in other corticothalamocortical systems (205, 206, 209–212). Of particular importance here is that the cortical innervation of the BG relay nuclei of the thalamus will activate these cell groups prior to information that flows via the striatum and GP/SNr to the thalamus thereby priming the thalamus for BG input, before sending those signals back to cortex. Furthermore, in addition to the reciprocal connection, there is a non-reciprocal cortico-thalamic connection, such that, projections to the VA/VL/MD are derived from cortical areas not innervated by the same thalamic region. For example, the central MD has reciprocal connections with the lateral and orbital prefrontal areas and also a non-reciprocal input from medial prefrontal areas; VA has reciprocal connections with dorsal premotor areas, and caudal area DLPFC and also a non-reciprocal connection from medial prefrontal areas; and VL has reciprocal connections with caudal motor areas along with a non-reciprocal connection from rostral motor regions *(205)*. The potential for relaying information between circuits through thalamic connections, therefore, can be accomplished through these non-reciprocal cortico-thalamic pathways (Figure 2.9). Therefore, like the striato-nigro-striatal system described previously, the cortico-thalamo-cortical system is in a critical position for integrating information across functional circuits.

**A Role for Both Parallel Circuit and Integrative Networks**

The BG serves, in part, as a throughput system back to cortex that allows smooth execution of action plans that can be maintained and reproduced over time. Consistent with this important function, there are cortico-BG-thalamic connections that link regions of these structures that are associated with similar functions (maintaining parallel networks). However, the cortex and the BG must also work together in the learning process, to acquire new behaviors, and for the modification of those behaviors *(20, 58, 144, 168, 196, 213–220)*. For this to occur, integration between circuits is critical. Thus, a key component of BG function must also be a mechanism for integration across functional domains. Information must to be channeled through limbic, to cognitive, to motor circuits, allowing the animal to respond appropriately to environmental cues. Parallel and integrative circuits must therefore both be present for coordinated behaviors to be maintained and focused (via parallel networks),

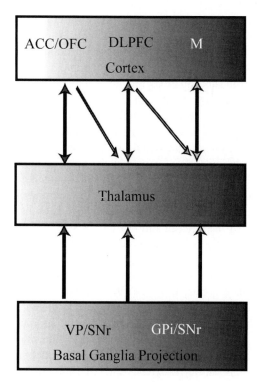

**Figure 2.9** Diagram of potential information transfer through functional circuits via a non-reciprocal connection to the thalamic relay nuclei. ACC, anterior cingulate cortex; GPi, globus pallidus internal segment; M, motor control areas of cortex; OFC, orbital frontal cortex; SNr, substantia nigra, pars reticulata; VP, ventral pallidum

but also to be modified and changed according the appropriate external and internal stimuli (via integrative networks). Indeed, the inability to maintain and focus in the execution of specific behaviors, as well as the inability to adapt appropriately to external and internal cues, are key deficits in all diseases affecting the BG.

## Neurocircuitry of Obsessive–Compulsive Disorder (OCD) and Depression

While the pathophysiology of OCD and depression remain incompletely understood, converging lines of evidence point to abnormalities in the medial and orbital frontal–BG circuit for these disorders *(221, 222)*. The structures associated with this network are: the ACC, the OFC, the striatum, the thalamus, and the amygdala and hippocampus. For example, in OCD, there are subtle differences in OFC, striatal and thalamic volumes in subjects with OCD vs. controls *(223–227)* and functional neuroimaging studies show hyperactivity at rest in this circuit when comparing OCD subjects to controls. This regional hyperactivity is accentuated during provocation of the OCD symptomatic state versus control states *(16, 221)*. Conversely, there is a reduction in activity in these regions following successful treatment of OCD including pharmacological, behavioral, and neurosurgical therapies *(228–231)* Pretreatment regional activity within OFC predicts subsequent response to treatment with medication or behavior therapy *(232–234)*. Moreover, effective treatments for OCD are obtained by modulating the activity in this circuitry *(235)*.

Significant subpopulations of OCD and depressive patients are refractory to available psychological and pharmacological treatments *(236)*. Stereotactic neurosurgical lesions in the anterior limb of the internal capsule, the anterior cingulate, and/or the subcaudate region, all of which interrupt the medial and orbital frontal descending circuits, are effective in the treatment of refractory OCD and depression *(237)*. The development of implantable, programmable chronic stimulating devices and improved stereotactic MRI localization has revolutionized the field of functional neurosurgery over the last 15 years. Deep brain stimulation (DBS), a proven therapy for intractable tremor in Parkinson's disease, is now being actively investigated for mental health disorders including OCD and depression, with encouraging initial clinical results *(238–240)*. The most effective targets have been either: *(1)* centered down the middle of the anterior limb of the capsule with extension into the caudal nucleus accumbens, at the border of the anterior commissure in the coronal plane; or *(2)* in the white matter bundle adjacent to area 25 in the ventral, medial prefrontal cortex. Connections between the ACC/OFC and subcortical regions are carried, in part through the ventral internal capsule. The most ventral region of ventral internal capsule breaks up into relatively small bundles that are imbedded within the ventral striatum. These bundles merge rostrally with the underlying subcaudate white matter. The subcaudate white matter lies immediately ventral to the caudate nucleus rostral to the nucleus accumbens. As it extends laterally, circumventing the caudate nucleus, it divides into the external and extreme capsules. Cortico-cortical and descending fibers from the OFC/ACC, along with ascending fibers to these cortical regions, enter either the internal capsule, remain in the subcaudate white matter, or pass through the ventral striatum. Importantly, fibers passing through this region include not only cortico-striatal and thalamic bundles, but also connections with the amygdala, whose role in fear conditioning is now well established *(241)*, and the hippocampus. The demonstration of effective DBS targets for depression and OCD along the trajectories of these white matter tracts is consistent with current hypotheses of pathophysiology underlying these mental health disorders.

*Acknowledgements*: This work was supported by NIH grants NS22311 and MH45573.

## References

1. Haber SN, Gdowski MJ (2004) The Basal Ganglia. In: Paxinos G, Mai JK, eds. The Human Nervous System, second edition. Academic Press, pp. 677–738.
2. Parent A, Hazrati LN (1995) Functional anatomy of the basal ganglia. I. The cortico-basal ganglia-thalamo-cortical loop. Brain Res Rev 20(1):91–127.
3. Levy R, Friedman HR, Davachi L, Goldman-Rakic PS (1997) Differential activation of the caudate nucleus in primates performing spatial and nonspatial working memory tasks. J Neurosci 17.
4. Hikosaka O, Rand MK, Miyachi S, Miyashita K (1995) Procedural learning in the monkey. In: Kimura M, Graybiel, A.M., ed. Functions of the Cortico-Basal Ganglia Loop. New York: Springer-Verlag, pp. 18–30.
5. Pasupathy A, Miller EK (2005) Different time courses of learning-related activity in the prefrontal cortex and striatum. Nature 433(7028):873–876.
6. Tricomi EM, Delgado MR, Fiez JA (2004) Modulation of caudate activity by action contingency. Neuron 41(2):281–292.
7. Robbins TW, Everitt BJ (1999) Motivation and reward. In: IV Sensory Systems. Academic Press.
8. Rolls ET (2000) The orbitofrontal cortex and reward. Cerebral Cortex 10(3):284–294.
9. Christakou A, Robbins TW, Everitt BJ (2004) Prefrontal cortical-ventral striatal interactions involved in affective modulation of attentional performance: implications for corticostriatal circuit function. J Neurosci 24(4):773–780.
10. Knutson B, Adams CM, Fong GW, Hommer D (2001) Anticipation of increasing monetary reward selectively recruits nucleus accumbens. J Neurosci 21(16):RC159.
11. Koob (1999) Drug Reward and Addiction. In: Fundamental Neuroscience. Academic Press, pp. 1261–1279.
12. Nestler EJ, Hope BT, Widnell KL (1993) Drug addiction: a model for the molecular basis of neural plasticity. Neuron 11:995–1006.
13. Kalivas PW, Volkow ND (2005) The neural basis of addiction: a pathology of motivation and choice. Am J Psychiatry 162(8):1403–1413.
14. Rauch SL, Savage CR, Alpert NM, et al (1997) Probing striatal function in obsessive-compulsive disorder: a PET study of implicit sequence learning. J Neuropsychiatry Clin Neurosci 9(4):568–573.
15. Breiter HC, Rauch SL, Kwong KK, et al (1996) Functional magnetic resonance imaging of symptom provocation in obsessive-compulsive disorder. Arch Gen Psych 53:595–606.
16. McGuire PK, Bench CJ, Frith CD, Marks IM, Frackowiak RS, Dolan RJ (1994) Functional anatomy of obsessive-compulsive phenomena. Brit J Psych 164:459–468.
17. Pantelis C, Barnes TR, Nelson HE, et al (1997) Frontal-striatal cognitive deficits in patients with chronic schizophrenia. Brain 120(Pt 10):1823–1843.
18. Alexander GE, DeLong MR, Strick PL (1986) Parallel organization of functionally segregated circuits linking basal ganglia and cortex. Ann Rev Neurosci 9:357–381.

19. Elliott R, Newman JL, Longe OA, Deakin JF (2003) Differential response patterns in the striatum and orbitofrontal cortex to financial reward in humans: a parametric functional magnetic resonance imaging study. J Neurosci 23(1):303–307.
20. Wise SP, Murray EA, Gerfen CR (1996) The frontal cortex-basal ganglia system in primates. Crit Rev Neurobiol 10:317–356.
21. Everitt BJ, Robbins TW (2005) Neural systems of reinforcement for drug addiction: from actions to habits to compulsion. Nat Neurosci 8(11):1481–1489.
22. Brasted PJ, Wise SP (2004) Comparison of learning-related neuronal activity in the dorsal premotor cortex and striatum. Eur J Neurosci 19(3):721–740.
23. Schultz W, Tremblay L, Hollerman JR (2003) Changes in behavior-related neuronal activity in the striatum during learning. Trends Neurosci 26(6):321–328.
24. Graybiel AM (2005) The basal ganglia: learning new tricks and loving it. Curr Opin Neurobiol 15(6):638–644.
25. Berns GS, Sejnowski TJ (1996) How the basal ganglia make decisions. In: Damasio A, Damasio H, Christen Y, eds. The Neurobiology of Decision Making. Berlin: Springer-Verlag, pp. 101–114.
26. Heimer L, Alheid GF, Zahm DS (1994) Basal forebrain organization: An anatomical framework for motor aspects of drive and motivation. In: Kalivas PW, Barnes CD, eds. Limbic Motor Circuits and Neuropsychiatry. Boca Raton, Florida: CRC Press, Inc.
27. Haber SN, McFarland NR (1999) The concept of the ventral striatum in nonhuman primates. In: McGinty JF, ed. Advancing from the ventral striatum to the extended amygdala. New York: The New York Academy of Sciences, pp. 33–48.
28. Parent A (1986) Comparative Neurobiology of the Basal Ganglia. New York: John Wiley and Sons.
29. Olszewski, J., Baxter, D., (1982) Cytoarchitecture of the human brain stem. Basal: S. Rarger
30. Graybiel AM (1995) The basal ganglia. Trends Neurosci 18(2):60–62.
31. Haber SN, Kim KS, Mailly P, Calzavara R (2006) Reward-related cortical inputs define a large striatal region in primates that interface with associative cortical inputs, providing a substrate for incentive-based learning. J Neurosci 26(32):8368–8376.
32. Zheng T, Wilson CJ (2002) Corticostriatal combinatorics: the implications of corticostriatal axonal arborizations. J Neurophysiol 87(2):1007–1017.
33. Sadikot AF, Parent A, Francois C (1990) The centre median and parafascicular thalamic nuclei project respectively to the sensorimotor and associative-limbic striatal territories in the squirrel monkey. Brain Res 510:161–165.
34. Francois C, Percheron G, Parent A, Sadikot AF, Fenelon G, Yelnik J (1991) Topography of the projection from the central complex of the thalamus to the sensorimotor striatal territory in monkeys. J Comp Neurol 305:17–34.
35. Giménez-Amaya JM, McFarland NR, de las Heras S, Haber SN (1995) Organization of thalamic projections to the ventral striatum in the primate. J Comp Neurol 354:127–149.
36. Fenelon G, Francois C, Percheron G, Yelnik J (1991) Topographic distribution of the neurons of the central complex (Centre median-parafascicular complex) and of other thalamic neurons projecting to the striatum in macaques. Neuroscience 45(2):495–510.
37. Smith Y, Bennett BD, Bolam JP, Parent A, Sadikot AF (1994) Synaptic relationships between dopaminergic afferents and cortical or thalamic input in the sensorimotor territory of the striatum in monkey. J Comp Neurol 344:1–19.
38. Nakano K, Hasegawa Y, Tokushige A, Nakagawa S, Kayahara T, Mizuno N (1990) Topographical projections from the thalamus, subthalamic nucleus and pedunculopontine tegmental nucleus to the striatum in the Japanese monkey, Macaca fuscata. Brain Res 537:54–68.

39. Nakano K, Kayahara T, Chiba T (1999) Afferent connections to the ventral striatum from the medial prefrontal cortex (area 25) and the thalamic nuclei in the macaque monkey. Ann NY Acad Sci 877:667–670.
40. McFarland NR, Haber SN (2000) Convergent inputs from thalamic motor nuclei and frontal cortical areas to the dorsal striatum in the primate. J Neurosci 20(10):3798–3813.
41. McFarland NR, Haber SN (2001) Organization of thalamostriatal terminals from the ventral motor nuclei in the macaque. J Comp Neurol 429:321–336.
42. Druga R, Rokyta R, Benes V (1991) Thalamocaudate projections in the macaque monkey (a horseradish peroxidase study). J Hirnforsch 6:765–774.
43. Schell GR, Strick PL (1984) The origin of thalamic inputs to the arcuate premotor and supplementary motor areas. J Neurosci 4:539–560.
44. Rouiller EM, Liang F, Babalian A, Moret V, Wiesendanger M (1994) Cerebellothalamocortical and pallidothalamocortical projections to the primary and supplementary motor cortical areas: A multiple tracing study in macaque monkeys. J Comp Neurol 345:185–213.
45. Matelli M, Luppino G (1996) Thalamic input to mesial and superior area 6 in the Macaque monkey. J Comp Neurol 372:59–87.
46. Akert K, Hartmann-von Monakow K (1980) Relationships of precentral, premotor and prefrontal cortex to the mediodorsal and intralaminar nuclei of the monkey thalamus. Acta Neurobiol Exp 40:7–25.
47. Bouyer JJ, Joh TH, Pickel VM (1984) Ultrastructural localization of tyrosine hydroxylase in rat nucleus accumbens. J Comp Neurol 227(1):92–103.
48. Lynd-Balta E, Haber SN (1994) The organization of midbrain projections to the striatum in the primate: Sensorimotor-related striatum versus ventral striatum. Neuroscience 59:625–640.
49. Gerfen CR, Engber TM, Mahan LC, et al (1990) D1 and D2 dopamine receptor-regulated gene expression of striatonigral and striatopallidal neurons. Science 250:1429–1432.
50. Takagi H, Somogyi P, Somogyi J, Smith AD (1983) Fine structural studies on a type of somatostatin-immunoreactive neuron and its synaptic connections in the rat neostriatum: A correlated light and electron microscopic study. J Comp Neurol 214:1–16.
51. Izzo PN, Bolam JP (1988) Cholinergic synaptic input to different parts of spiny stratonigral neurons in the rat. J Comp Neurol 269:219–236.
52. Spooren WPJM, Lynd-Balta E, Mitchell S, Haber SN (1996) Ventral pallidostriatal pathway in the monkey: Evidence for modulation of basal ganglia circuits. J Comp Neurol 370(3):295–312.
53. Smith Y, Bevan MD, Shink E, Bolam JP (1998) Microcircuitry of the direct and indirect pathways of the basal ganglia. Neuroscience 86:353–387.
54. DiFiglia M, Pasik P, Pasik T (1976) A Golgi study of neuronal types in the neostriatum of monkeys. Brain Res 114:245–256.
55. Graveland GA, DiFiglia M (1985) The frequency and distribution of medium-sized neurons with indented nuclei in the primate and rodent neostriatum. Brain Res 327(1–2):307–311.
56. Fox CA, Andrade AN, Hillman DE, Schwyn RC (1971) The spiny neurons in the primate striatum: a Golgi and electron microscopic study. J Hirnforschung 13(3):181–201.
57. Kimura M (1990) Behaviorally contingent property of movement-related activity of the primate putamen. J Neurophysiol 63:1277–1296.
58. Jog MS, Kubota Y, Connolly CI, Hillegaart V, Graybiel AM (1999) Building neural representations of habits. Science 286(26):1745–1749.
59. Wilson CJ (2004) The basal ganglia. In: Shepherd GM, ed. Synaptic Organization of the Brain, fifth ed. New York, NY: Oxford University Press, pp. 361–413.

60. Plenz D, Kitai ST (1998) Up and down states in striatal medium spiny neurons simultaneously recorded with spontaneous activity in fast-spiking interneurons studied in cortex-striatum-substantia nigra organotypic cultures. J Neurosci 18:266–283.
61. Kemp JM, Powell TP (1971) The termination of fibres from the cerebral cortex and thalamus upon dendritic spines in the caudate nucleus: a study with the Golgi method. Philos Trans R Soc Lond B Biol Sci 262(845):429–439.
62. Dubé L, Smith AD, Bolam JP (1988) Identification of synaptic terminals of thalamic or cortical origin in contact with distinct medium-size spiny neurons in the rat neurostriatum. J Comp Neurol 267:455–471.
63. Fox CA, Andrade AN, Schwyn RC, Rafols JA (1971) The aspiny neurons and the glia in the primate striatum: a golgi and electron microscopic study. J Hirnforschung 13(4):341–362.
64. Kawaguchi Y, Wilson CJ, Augood SJ, Emson PC (1995) Striatal interneurones: chemical, physiological and morphological characterization. Trends Neurosci 18(12):527–535.
65. Lehmann J, Langer SZ (1983) The striatal cholinergic interneuron: synaptic target of dopaminergic terminals? Neuroscience 10(4):1105–1120.
66. Kubota Y, Inagaki S, Shimada S, Kito S, Eckenstein F, Tohyama M (1987) Neostriatal cholinergic neurons receive direct synaptic inputs from dopaminergic axons. Brain Res 413(1):179–184.
67. Bennett BD, Callaway JC, Wilson CJ (2000) Intrinsic membrane properties underlying spontaneous tonic firing in neostriatal cholinergic interneurons. J Neurosci 20(22):8493–8503.
68. Ravel S, Sardo P, Legallet E, Apicella P (2001) Reward unpredictability inside and outside of a task context as a determinant of the responses of tonically active neurons in the monkey striatum. J Neurosci 21(15):5730–5739.
69. Kimura M, Rajkowski J, Evarts E (1984) Tonically discharging putamen neurons exhibit set-dependent responses. Proc Natl Acad Sci USA 81:4998–5001.
70. Apicella P, Legallet E, Trouche E (1997) Responses of tonically discharging neurons in the monkey striatum to primary rewards delivered during different behavioral states. Exp Brain Res 116(3):456–466.
71. Lapper SR, Smith Y, Sadikot AF, Parent A, Bolam JP (1992) Cortical input to parvalbumin-immunoreactive neurones in the putamen of the squirrel monkey. Brain Res 580:215–224.
72. Mallet N, Le Moine C, Charpier S, Gonon F (2005) Feedforward inhibition of projection neurons by fast-spiking GABA interneurons in the rat striatum in vivo. J Neurosci 25(15):3857–3869.
73. Vuillet J, Kerkerian L, Salin P, Nieoullon A (1989) Ultrastructural features of NPY-containing neurons in the rat striatum. Brain Res 477(1–2):241–251.
74. Zaborszky L, Alheid GF, Beinfeld MC, Eiden LE, Heimer L, Palkovits M (1985) Cholecystokinin innervation of the ventral striatum: A morphological and radioimmunological study. Neuroscience 14(2):427–453.
75. Pecina S, Berridge KC (2005) Hedonic hot spot in nucleus accumbens shell: where do mu-opioids cause increased hedonic impact of sweetness? J Neurosci 25(50):11777–11786.
76. Bassareo V, De Luca MA, Di Chiara G (2002) Differential expression of motivational stimulus properties by dopamine in nucleus accumbens shell versus core and prefrontal cortex. J Neurosci 22(11):4709–4719.
77. Ito R, Dalley JW, Howes SR, Robbins TW, Everitt BJ (2000) Dissociation in conditioned dopamine release in the nucleus accumbens core and shell in response to cocaine cues and during cocaine-seeking behavior in rats. J Neurosci 20(19):7489–7495.
78. Corbit LH, Muir JL, Balleine BW (2001) The role of the nucleus accumbens in instrumental conditioning: evidence of a functional dissociation between accumbens core and shell. J Neurosci 21(9):3251–3260.

79. Parkinson JA, Olmstead MC, Burns LH, Robbins TW, Everitt BJ (1999) Dissociation in effects of lesions of the nucleus accumbens core and shell on appetitive pavlovian approach behavior and the potentiation of conditioned reinforcement and locomotor activity by D-amphetamine. J Neurosci 19(6):2401–2411.
80. Meredith GE, Pattiselanno A, Groenewegen HJ, Haber SN (1996) Shell and core in monkey and human nucleus accumbens identified with antibodies to calbindin-D28k. J Comp Neurol 365:628–639.
81. Chronister RB, Sikes RW, Trow TW, DeFrance JF (1981) The organization of the nucleus accumbens. In: Chronister RB, DeFrance JF, eds. The Neurobiology of the Nucleus Accumbens. Brunswick, ME: Haer Institute, pp. 97–146.
82. Russchen FT, Bakst I, Amaral DG, Price JL (1985) The amygdalostriatal projections in the monkey. An anterograde tracing study. Brain Res 329:241–257.
83. Fudge JL, Kunishio K, Walsh C, Richard D, Haber SN (2002) Amygdaloid projections to ventromedial striatal subterritories in the primate. Neuroscience 110:257–275.
84. Haber SN (1986) Neurotransmitters in the human and nonhuman primate basal ganglia. Human Neurobiology 5:159–168.
85. Yelnik J, Percheron G, Francois C (1984) A golgi analysis of the primate globus pallidus. II. Quantitative morphology and spatial orientation of dendritic arborizations. J Comp Neurol 227:200–213.
86. Fox CH, Andrade HN, Du Qui IJ, Rafols JA (1974) The primate globus pallidus. A Golgi and electron microscope study. J R Hirnforschung 15:75–93.
87. Francois C, Percheron G, Yelnik J, Heyner S (1984) A golgi analysis of the primate globus pallidus. I. Inconstant processes of large neurons, other neuronal types, and afferent axons. J Comp Neurol 227:182–199.
88. Smith Y, Parent A, Seguela P, Descarries L (1987) Distribution of GABA-immunoreactive neurons in the basal ganglia of the squirrel monkey (saimiri sciureus). J Comp Neurol 259:50–64.
89. Carpenter MB, Baton RRd, Carleton SC, Keller JT (1981) Interconnections and organization of pallidal and subthalamic nucleus neurons in the monkey. J Comp Neurol 197(4):579–603.
90. Nauta HJW, Cole M (1978) Efferent projections of the subthalamic nucleus: An autoradiographic study in monkey and cat. J Comp Neurol 180:1–16.
91. Shink E, Smith Y (1995) Differential synaptic innervation of neurons in the internal and external segments of the globus pallidus by the GABA- and glutamate-containing terminals in the squirrel monkey. J Comp Neurol 358:119–141.
92. Hedreen JC (1999) Tyrosine hydroxylase-immunoreactive elements in the human globus pallidus and subthalamic nucleus. J Comp Neurol 409(3):400–410.
93. Nauta WJ, Mehler WR (1966) Projections of the lentiform nucleus in the monkey. Brain Res 1(1):3–42.
94. DeVito JL, Anderson ME (1982) An autoradiographic study of efferent connections of the globus pallidus in *Macaca mulatta*. Exp Brain Res 46:107–117.
95. Carpenter MB (1976) Anatomical organization of the corpus striatum and related nuclei. In: Yahr MD, ed. The Basal Ganglia. New York: Raven Press, pp. 1–36.
96. Kuo J, Carpenter MB (1973) Organization of pallidothalamic projections in the rhesus monkey. J Comp Neurol 151:201–236.
97. Kim R, Nakano K, Jayaraman A, Carpenter MB (1976) Projections of the globus pallidus and adjacent structures: an autoradiographic study in the monkey. J Comp Neurol 169(3):263–290.
98. Parent M, Levesque M, Parent A (2001) Two types of projection neurons in the internal pallidum of primates: single-axon tracing and three-dimensional reconstruction. J Comp Neurol 439(2):162–175.
99. Shink E, Sidibé M, Smith Y (1997) Efferent connections of the internal globus pallidus in the squirrel monkey: II. Topography and synaptic organization of pallidal efferents to the penduclulopontine nucleus. J Comp Neurol 382:348–363.

100. Sakai ST, Inase M, Tanji J (1996) Comparison of cerebellothalamic and pallidothalamic projections in the monkey (Macaca fuscata): a double anterograde labeling study. J Comp Neurol 368(2):215–228.
101. McFarland NR, Haber SN (2002) Thalamic connections with cortex from the basal ganglia relay nuclei provide a mechanism for integration across multiple cortical areas. J Neurosci in press.
102. Hoshi E, Tremblay L, Feger J, Carras PL, Strick PL (2005) The cerebellum communicates with the basal ganglia. Nat Neurosci 8(11):1491–1493.
103. Sato F, Lavallee P, Levesque M, Parent A (2000) Single-axon tracing study of neurons of the external segment of the globus pallidus in primate. J Comp Neurol 417(1):17–31.
104. Mink JW, Thach WT (1991) Basal ganglia motor control. I. Nonexclusive relation of pallidal discharge to five movement modes. J Neurophysiol 65(2):273–300.
105. Raz A, Vaadia E, Bergman H (2000) Firing patterns and correlations of spontaneous discharge of pallidal neurons in the normal and the tremulous 1-methyl-4-phenyl-1,2,3,6-tetrahydropyridine vervet model of parkinsonism. J Neurosci 20(22):8559–8571.
106. Mink JW (1996) The basal ganglia: focused selection and inhibition of competing motor programs. Prog Neurobiol 50(4):381–425.
107. Nambu A, Tokuno H, Hamada I, et al (2000) Excitatory cortical inputs to pallidal neurons via the subthalamic nucleus in the monkey. J Neurophysiol 84(1):289–300.
108. Basso MA, Wurtz RH (2002) Neuronal activity in substantia nigra pars reticulata during target selection. J Nuerosci 22(5):1883–1894.
109. Lavoie B, Parent A (1990) Immunohistochemical study of the serotoninergic innervation of the basal ganglia in the squirrel monkey. J Comp Neurol 299:1–16.
110. Moukhles H, Bosler O, Bolam JP, et al (1997) Quantitative and morphometric data indicate precise cellular interactions between serotonin terminals nd postsynaptic targets in rat substantia nigra. Neuroscience 76:1159–1171.
111. Hikosaka O, Wurtz RH (1983) Visual and oculomotor functions of monkey substantia nigra pars reticulata. IV. Relation of substantia nigra to superior colliculus. J Neurophysiol 49(5):1285–1301.
112. Rafols JA, Fox CA (1976) The neurons in the primate subthalamic nucleus: a Golgi and electron microscopic study. J Comp Neurol 168(1):75–111.
113. Smith Y, Shink E, Sidibe M (1998) Neuronal circuitry and synaptic connectivity of the basal ganglia. Neurosurg Clin North Am 9(2):203–222.
114. Haber SN, Lynd-Balta E, Mitchell SJ (1993) The organization of the descending ventral pallidal projections in the monkey. J Comp Neurol 329(1):111–129.
115. Hassani OK, Francois C, Yelnik J, Feger J (1997) Evidence for a dopaminergic innervation of the subthalamic nucleus in the rat. Brain Res 749(1):88–94.
116. Bergman H, Wichmann T, DeLong MR (1990) Reversal of experimental Parkinsonism by lesions of the subthalamic nucleus. Science 249:1436–1438.
117. Francois C, Savy C, Jan C, Tande D, Hirsch EC, Yelnik J (2000) Dopaminergic innervation of the subthalamic nucleus in the normal state, in MPTP-treated monkeys, and in Parkinson's disease patients. J Comp Neurol 425(1):121–129.
118. Rye DB, Saper CB, Lee HJ, Wainer BH (1987) Pedunculopontine tegmental nucleus of the rat: cytoarchitecture, cytochemistry, and some extrapyramidal connections of the mesopontine tegmentum. J Comp Neurol 259:483–528.
119. Bevan MD, Bolam JP (1995) Cholinergic, GABAergic, and glutamate-enriched inputs from the mesopontine tegmentum to the subthalamic nucleus in the rat. J Neurosci 15:7105–7120.
120. Nambu A, Tokuno H, Takada M (2002) Functional significance of the cortico-subthalamo-pallidal 'hyperdirect' pathway. Neurosci Res 43(2):111–117.

121. Sato F, Parent M, Levesque M, Parent A (2000) Axonal branching pattern of neurons of the subthalamic nucleus in primates. J Comp Neurol 424(1):142–152.
122. Olszewski J, Baxter D (1982) Cytoarchitecture of the Human Brain Stem, second ed. Basel: S. Karger.
123. Haber SN, Ryoo H, Cox C, Lu W (1995) Subsets of midbrain dopaminergic neurons in monkeys are distinguished by different levels of mRNA for the dopamine transporter: Comparison with the mRNA for the D2 receptor, tyrosine hydroxylase and calbindin immunoreactivity. J Comp Neurol 362:400–410.
124. McRitchie DA, Halliday GM (1995) Calbindin D28K-containing neurons are restricted to the medial substantia nigra in humans. Neuroscience 65:87–91.
125. Parent A, Lavoie B (1993) The heterogeneity of the mesostriatal dopaminergic system as revealed in normal and Parkinsonian monkeys. Adv Neurol 60:25–30.
126. Pifl C, Schingnitz G, Hornykiewicz O (1991) Effect of 1-methyl-4-phenyl-1,2,3,6-tetrahydropyridine on the regional distribution of brain monoamines in the rhesus monkey. Neuroscience 44(3):591–605.
127. Fudge JL, Haber SN (2000) The central nucleus of the amygdala projection to dopamine subpopulations in primates. Neuroscience 97(3):479–494.
128. Parent A, DeBellefeuille L (1983) The pallidointralaminar and pallidonigral projections in primate as studied by retrograde double-labeling method. Brain Res 278:11–27.
129. Lavoie B, Parent A (1994) Pedunculopontine nucleus in the squirrel monkey: Projections to the basal ganglia as revealed by anterograde tract-tracing methods. J Comp Neurol 344:210–231.
130. Fudge JL, Haber SN (2001) Bed nucleus of the stria terminalis and extended amygdala inputs to dopamine subpopulations in primates. Neuroscience 104(3):807–827.
131. Lynd-Balta E, Haber SN (1994) Primate striatonigral projections: A comparison of the sensorimotor-related striatum and the ventral striatum. J Comp Neurol 345(4):562–578.
132. Gaspar P, Berger B, Febvret A, Vigny A, Henry JP (1989) Catecholamine innervation of the human cerebral cortex as revealed by comparative immunohistochemistry of tyrosine hydroxylase and dopamine-beta-hydroxylase. J Comp Neurol 279:249–271.
133. Lewis DA, Campbell MJ, Foote SL, Goldstein M, Morrison JH (1987) The distribution of tyrosine hydroxylase-immunoreactive fibers in primate neocortex is widespread but regionally specific. J Neurosci 7(1):279–290.
134. Lidow MS, Goldman-Rakic PS, Gallager DW, Rakic P (1991) Distribution of dopaminergic receptors in the primate cerebral cortex: quantitative autoradiographic analysis using [3H] raclopride, [3H] spiperone and [3H]sch23390. Neuroscience 40(3):657–671.
135. Gaspar P, Stepneiwska I, Kaas JH (1992) Topography and collateralization of the dopaminergic projections to motor and lateral prefrontal cortex in owl monkeys. J Comp Neurol 325:1–21.
136. Porrino LJ, Goldman-Rakic PS (1982) Brainstem innervation of prefrontal and anterior cingulate cortex in the rhesus monkey revealed by retrograde transport of HRP. J Comp Neurol 205:63–76.
137. Mehler WR (1980) Subcortical afferent connections of the amygdala in the monkey. J Comp Neurol 190:733–762.
138. Norita M, Kawamura K (1980) Subcortical afferents to the monkey amygdala: an HRP study. Brain Res 190:225–230.
139. Aggleton JP, Burton MJ, Passingham RE (1980) Cortical and subcortical afferents to the amygdala of the rhesus monkey (Macaca mulatta). Brain Res 190:347–368.
140. Schultz W, Dayan P, Montague PR (1997) A neural substrate of prediction and reward. Science 275:1593–1599.

141. Dommett E, Coizet V, Blaha CD, et al (2005) How visual stimuli activate dopaminergic neurons at short latency. Science 307(5714):1476–1479.
142. Schultz W (1998) Predictive reward signal of dopamine neurons. J Neurophysiol 80(1):1–27.
143. Schultz W, Tremblay L, Hollerman JR (2000) Reward processing in primate orbitofrontal cortex and basal ganglia. Cerebral Cortex 10(3):272–284.
144. Morris G, Nevet A, Arkadir D, Vaadia E, Bergman H (2006) Midbrain dopamine neurons encode decisions for future action. Nat Neurosci 9(8):1057–1063.
145. Wise RA (2004) Dopamine, learning and motivation. Nat Rev Neurosci 5(6):483–494.
146. Arbuthnott GW, Ingham CA, Wickens JR (2000) Dopamine and synaptic plasticity in the neostriatum. J Anat 196(Pt 4):587–596.
147. Centonze D, Grande C, Saulle E, et al (2003) Distinct roles of D1 and D5 dopamine receptors in motor activity and striatal synaptic plasticity. J Neurosci 23(24):8506–8512.
148. Kawagoe R, Takikawa Y, Hikosaka O (2004) Reward-predicting activity of dopamine and caudate neurons—a possible mechanism of motivational control of saccadic eye movement. J Neurophysiol 91(2):1013–1024.
149. Berke JD, Hyman SE (2000) Addiction, dopamine, and the molecular mechanisms of memory. Neuron 25(3):515–532.
150. Percheron G, Filion M (1991) Parallel processing in the basal ganglia: Up to a point. Trends Neurosci 14:55–59.
151. Bevan MD, Clarke NP, Bolam JP (1997) Synaptic integration of functionally diverse pallidal information in the entopeduncular nucleus and subthalamic nucleus in the rat. J Neurosci 17:308–324.
152. Bevan MD, Smith AD, Bolam JP (1996) The substantia nigra as a site of synaptic integration of functionally diverse information arising from the ventral pallidum and the globus pallidus in the rat. Neuroscience 75:5–12.
153. Somogyi P, Bolam JP, Totterdell S, Smith AD (1981) Monosynaptic input from the nucleus accumbens-ventral striatum region to retrogradely labelled nigrostriatal neurones. Brain Res 217:245–263.
154. Haber SN, Fudge JL, McFarland NR (2000) Striatonigrostriatal pathways in primates form an ascending spiral from the shell to the dorsolateral striatum. J Neurosci 20(6):2369–2382.
155. Hadland KA, Rushworth MF, Gaffan D, Passingham RE (2003) The anterior cingulate and reward-guided selection of actions. J Neurophysiol 89(2):1161–1164.
156. Walton ME, Devlin JT, Rushworth MF (2004) Interactions between decision making and performance monitoring within prefrontal cortex. Nat Neurosci 7(11):1259–1265.
157. Fellows LK, Farah MJ (2005) Different underlying impairments in decision-making following ventromedial and dorsolateral frontal lobe damage in humans. Cereb Cortex 15(1):58–63.
158. Elliott R, Dolan RJ, Frith CD (2000) Dissociable functions in the medial and lateral orbitofrontal cortex: evidence from human neuroimaging studies. Cereb Cortex 10(3):308–317.
159. Haber SN, Kunishio K, Mizobuchi M, Lynd-Balta E (1995) The orbital and medial prefrontal circuit through the primate basal ganglia. J Neurosci 15:4851–4867.
160. Freedman LJ, Insel TR, Smith Y (2000) Subcortical projections of area 25 (subgenual cortex) of the macaque monkey. Jour of Comp Neur 421(2):172–188.
161. Hassani OK, Cromwell HC, Schultz W (2001) Influence of expectation of different rewards on behavior-related neuronal activity in the striatum. J Neurophysiol 85(6):2477–2489.

162. Takikawa Y, Kawagoe R, Hikosaka O (2002) Reward-dependent spatial selectivity of anticipatory activity in monkey caudate neurons. J Neurophysiol 87(1):508–515.
163. Tanaka SC, Doya K, Okada G, Ueda K, Okamoto Y, Yamawaki S (2004) Prediction of immediate and future rewards differentially recruits cortico-basal ganglia loops. Nat Neurosci 7(8):887–893.
164. Watanabe K, Hikosaka O (2005) Immediate changes in anticipatory activity of caudate neurons associated with reversal of position-reward contingency. J Neurophysiol 94(3):1879–1887.
165. Apicella P, Ljungberg T, Scarnati E, Schultz W (1991) Responses to reward in monkey dorsal and ventral striatum. Exp Brain Res 85:491–500.
166. Nakamura K, Hikosaka O (2006) Role of dopamine in the primate caudate nucleus in reward modulation of saccades. J Neurosci 26(20):5360–5369.
167. Goldman-Rakic PS (1987) Circuitry of the frontal association cortex and its relevance to dementia. Arch Gerontol Geriatr 6:299–309.
168. Fuster JM (2000) Prefrontal neurons in networks of executive memory. Brain Res Bull 52(5):331–336.
169. Jonides J, Smith EE, Koeppe RA, Awh E, Minoshima S, Mintun MA (1993) Spatial working memory in humans as revealed by PET. Nature 363(6430):623–625.
170. Smith EE, Jonides J (1997) Working memory: a view from neuroimaging. Cog Psychol 33(1):5–42.
171. Selemon LD, Goldman-Rakic PS (1985) Longitudinal topography and interdigitation of corticostriatal projections in the rhesus monkey. J Neurosci 5:776–794.
172. Arikuni T, Kubota K (1986) The organization of prefrontocaudate projections and their laminar origin in the macaque monkey: A retrograde study using HRP-gel. J Comp Neurol 244:492–510.
173. Apicella P, Scarnati E, Ljungberg T, Schultz W (1992) Neuronal activity in monkey striatum related to the expectation of predictable environmental events. J Neurophysiol 68(3):1–16.
174. Hikosaka O, Sakamoto M, Usui S (1989) Functional properties of monkey caudate neurons. III. Activities related to expectation of target and reward. J Neurophysiol 61(4):814–832.
175. Elliott R, Dolan RJ (1999) Differential neural responses during performance of matching and nonmatching to sample tasks at two delay intervals. J Neurosci 19(12):5066–5073.
176. Battig K, Rosvold HE, Mishkin M (1960) Comparison of the effect of frontal and caudate lesions on delayed response and alternation in monkeys. J Comp Physiol Psychol 53:400–404.
177. Butters N, Rosvold HE (1968) Effect of caudate and septal nuclei lesions on resistance to extinction and delayed-alternation. J Comp Physiol Psychol 65(3):397–403.
178. Partiot A, Verin M, Pillon B, Teixeira-Ferreira C, Agid Y, Dubois B (1996) Delayed response tasks in basal ganglia lesions in man: further evidence for a striato-frontal cooperation in behavioural adaptation. Neuropsychologia 34(7):709–721.
179. Miyachi S, Hikosaka O, Miyashita K, Karadi Z, Rand MK (1997) Differential roles of monkey striatum in learning of sequential hand movement. Exper Brain Res 115(1):1–5.
180. Boecker H, Dagher A, Ceballos-Baumann AO, et al (1998) Role of the human rostral supplementary motor area and the basal ganglia in motor sequence control: investigations with H2 15O PET. J Neurophysiol 79(2):1070–1080.
181. Hikosaka O, Sakai K, Miyauchi S, Takino R, Sasaki Y, Putz B (1996) Activation of human presupplementary motor area in learning of sequential procedures: a functional MRI study. J Neurophysiol 76:617–621.
182. Aldridge JW, Anderson RJ, Murphy JT (1980) Sensory-motor processing in the caudate nucleus and globus pallidus: a single-unit study in behaving primates. Can J Physiol Pharmacol 58(10):1192–1201.

183. Flaherty AW, Graybiel AM (1993) Two input systems for body representations in the primate striatal matrix: experimental evidence in the squirrel monkey. J Neurosci 13(3):1120–1137.
184. Takada M, Tokuno H, Nambu A, Inase M (1998) Corticostriatal input zones from the supplementary motor area overlap those from the contra rather than ipsilateral primary motor cortex. Brain Res 791(1–2):335–340.
185. Ramanathan S, Hanley JJ, Deniau JM, Bolam JP (2002) Synaptic convergence of motor and somatosensory cortical afferents onto GABAergic interneurons in the rat striatum. J Neurosci 22:8158–8169.
186. Charpier S, Mahon S, Deniau JM (1999) In vivo induction of striatal long-term potentiation by low-frequency stimulation of the cerebral cortex. Neuroscience 91(4):1209–1222.
187. Yamada H, Matsumoto N, Kimura M (2004) Tonically active neurons in the primate caudate nucleus and putamen differentially encode instructed motivational outcomes of action. J Neurosci 24(14):3500–3510.
188. Apicella P (2002) Tonically active neurons in the primate striatum and their role in the processing of information about motivationally relevant events. Eur J Neurosci 16(11):2017–2026.
189. Percheron G, Yelnik J, Francois C (1984) The primate striato-pallido-nigral system: An integrative system for cortical information. In: McKenzie JS, Kemm RE, Wilcock LN, eds. The Basal Ganglia: Structure and Function. London: Plenum Press, pp. 87–105.
190. Anderson ME, Turner RS (1991) A quantitative analysis of pallidal discharge during targeted reaching movement in the monkey. Exp Brain Res 86(3):623–632.
191. Brotchie P, Iansek R, Horne M (1991) A neural network model of neural activity in the monkey globus pallidus. Neurosci Lett 131(1):33–36.
192. Aldridge JW, Anderson RJ, Murphy JT (1980) The role of the basal ganglia in controlling a movement initiated by a visually presented cue. Brain Res 192:3–16.
193. Inase M, Li BM, Takashima I, Iijima T (2001) Pallidal activity is involved in visuomotor association learning in monkeys. Eur J Neurosci 14(5):897–901.
194. Kolomiets BP, Deniau JM, Mailly P, Menetrey A, Glowinski J, Thierry AM (2001) Segregation and convergence of information flow through the cortico-subthalamic pathways. J Neurosci 21(15):5764–5772.
195. Bonci A, Malenka RC (1999) Properties and plasticity of excitatory synapses on dopaminergic and GABAergic cells in the ventral tegmental area. J Neurosci 19(10):3723–3730.
196. Matsumoto N, Hanakawa T, Maki S, Graybiel AM, Kimura M (1999) Nigrostriatal dopamine system in learning to perform sequential motor tasks in a predictive manner. J Neurophysiol 82(2):978–998.
197. Hollerman JR, Schultz W (1998) Dopamine neurons report an error in the temporal prediction of reward during learning. Nat Neurosci 1(4):304–309.
198. Anglade P, Blanchard V, Raisman-Vozari R, et al (1996) Is dopaminergic cell death accompanied by concomitant nerve plasticity? In: Battistin L, Scarlato G, Caraceni T, Ruggieri S, eds. Parkinson's Disease. Philadelphia: Lippincott-Raven Publishers, pp. 195–208.
199. Ljungberg T, Apicella P, Schultz W (1991) Responses of monkey midbrain dopamine neurons during delayed alternation performance. Brain Res 567:337–341.
200. Hedreen JC, DeLong MR (1991) Organization of striatopallidal, striatonigral, and nigrostriatal projections in the Macaque. J Comp Neurol 304:569–595.
201. Haber SN, Lynd E, Klein C, Groenewegen HJ (1990) Topographic organization of the ventral striatal efferent projections in the rhesus monkey: An anterograde tracing study. J Comp Neurol 293:282–298.
202. Szabo J (1979) Strionigral and nigrostriatal connections. Anatomical studies. Appl Neurophysiol 42(1–2):9–12.

203. Porrino LJ, Lyons D, Smith HR, Daunais JB, Nader MA (2004) Cocaine self-administration produces a progressive involvement of limbic, association, and sensorimotor striatal domains. J Neurosci 24(14):3554–3562.
204. Martinez D, Slifstein M, Broft A, et al (2003) Imaging human mesolimbic dopamine transmission with positron emission tomography. Part II: amphetamine-induced dopamine release in the functional subdivisions of the striatum. J Cereb Blood Flow Metab 23(3):285–300.
205. McFarland NR, Haber SN (2002) Thalamic relay nuclei of the basal ganglia form both reciprocal and nonreciprocal cortical connections, linking multiple frontal cortical areas. J Neurosci 22(18):8117–8132.
206. Sherman SM, Guillery RW (1996) Functional organization of thalamocortical relays. J Neurophysiol 76(3):1367–1395.
207. Castro-Alamancos MA, Connors BW (1997) Thalamocortical synapses. Prog Neurobiol 51(6):581–606.
208. Jones EG (1985) The Thalamus. New York: Plenum Press.
209. Murphy PC, Duckett SG, Sillito AM (1999) Feedback connections to the lateral geniculate nucleus and cortical response properties. Science 286(5444):1552–1554.
210. Deschenes M, Veinante P, Zhang ZW (1998) The organization of corticothalamic projections: reciprocity versus parity. Brain Res Rev 28(3):286–308.
211. Darian-Smith C, Tan A, Edwards S (1999) Comparing thalamocortical and corticothalamic microstructure and spatial reciprocity in the macaque ventral posterolateral nucleus (VPLc) and medial pulvinar. J Comp Neurol 410(2):211–234.
212. Jones EG (1998) The thalamus of primates. In: Bloom FE, Björklund A, Hökfelt T, eds. The Primate Nervous System, Part II. Amsterdam: Elsevier Science, pp. 1–298.
213. Owen AM, Roberts AC, Hodges JR, Summers BA, Polkey CE, Robbins TW (1993) Contrasting mechanisms of impaired attentional set-shifting in patients with frontal lobe damage or Parkinson's disease. Brain 116:1159–1175.
214. Passingham RE (1995) The Frontal Lobes and Voluntary Action. Oxford: OUP.
215. Grafton ST, Hazeltine E (1995) Functional mapping of sequence learning in normal humans. J Cog Neurosci 7:497–510.
216. Hikosaka O, Miyashita K, Miyachi S, Sakai K, Lu X (1998) Differential roles of the frontal cortex, basal ganglia, and cerebellum in visuomotor sequence learning. Neurobiol Learn Mem 70(1–2):137–149.
217. Doyon J, Gaudreau D, Laforce R Jr, et al (1997) Role of the striatum, cerebellum, and frontal lobes in the learning of a visuomotor sequence. Brain Cogn 34(2):218–245.
218. Jaeger D, Gilman S, Aldridge JW (1995) Neuronal activity in the striatum and pallidum of primates related to the execution of externally cued reaching movements. Brain Res 694(1–2):111–127.
219. Aosaki T, Graybiel AM, Kimura M (1994) Effect of the nigrostriatal dopamine system on acquired neural responses in the striatum of behaving monkeys. Science 265:412–410.
220. Schultz W (1997) Dopamine neurons and their role in reward mechanisms. Curr Opin Neurobiol 7:191–197.
221. Rauch SL, Jenike MA, et al (1994) Regional cerebral blood flow measured during symptom provocation in obsessive-compulsive disorder using oxygen 15-labeled carbon dioxide and positron emission tomography. Arch Gen Psychiatry 51(1):62–70.
222. Mayberg HS, Brannan SK, et al (2000) Regional metabolic effects of fluoxetine in major depression: serial changes and relationship to clinical response. Bio Psych 48(8):830–843.
223. Szeszko PR, Robinson D, et al (1999) Orbital frontal and amygdala volume reductions in obsessive-compulsive disorder. Arch Gen Psych 56(10):913–919.

224. Gilbert AR, Moore GJ, et al (2000) Decrease in thalamic volumes of pediatric patients with obsessive-compulsive disorder who are taking paroxetine. Arch Gen Psych 57(5):449–456.
225. Scarone S, Colombo C, et al (1992) Increased right caudate nucleus size in obsessive-compulsive disorder: detection with magnetic resonance imaging. Psychiatry Res 45(2):115–121.
226. Robinson D, Wu H, et al (1995) Reduced caudate nucleus volume in obsessive-compulsive disorder. Arch Gen Psych 52:393–398.
227. Jenike MA, Breiter HC, et al (1996) Cerebral structural abnormalities in obsessive-compulsive disorder. A quantitative morphometric magnetic resonance imaging study. Arch Gen Psych 53(7):625–632.
228. Schwartz JM, Stoessel PW, et al (1996) Systematic changes in cerebral glucose metabolic rate after successful behavior modification treatment of obsessive-compulsive disorder. Arch Gen Psych 53:109–113.
229. Mindus P, Bergstrom K, et al (1986) Magnetic resonance imaging of stereotactic radiosurgical lesions in the internal capsule. Acta Radiol Suppl 369:614–617.
230. Baxter LR Jr, Schwartz JM, et al (1992) Caudate glucose metabolic rate changes with both drug and behavior therapy for obsessive-compulsive disorder. Arch Gen Psych 49(9):681–689.
231. Swedo SE, Pietrini P, et al (1992) Cerebral glucose metabolism in childhood-onset obsessive-compulsive disorder. Revisualization during pharmacotherapy. Arch Gen Psych 49(9):690–694.
232. Brody AL, Saxena S, et al (1998) FDG-PET predictors of response to behavioral therapy and pharmacotherapy in obsessive compulsive disorder. Psychiatry Res 84(1):1–6.
233. Saxena S, Brody AL, et al (1999) Localized orbitofrontal and subcortical metabolic changes and predictors of response to paroxetine treatment in obsessive-compulsive disorder. Neuropsychopharmacology 21(6):683–693.
234. Rauch SL, Shin LM, et al (2002) Predictors of fluvoxamine response in contamination-related obsessive compulsive disorder: a PET symptom provocation study. Neuropsychopharmacology 27(5):782–791.
235. Rauch SL, Dougherty DD, et al (2006) A functional neuroimaging investigation of deep brain stimulation in patients with obsessive-compulsive disorder. J Neurosurg 104(4):558–565.
236. Rasmussen SA, Eisen JL (1997) Treatment strategies for chronic and refractory obsessive-compulsive disorder. J Clin Psychiatry 58(Suppl 13):9–13.
237. Greenberg BD, Price LH, et al (2003) Neurosurgery for intractable obsessive-compulsive disorder and depression: Critical issues. Neurosurg Clin North Am 14(2):199–212.
238. Greenberg BD (2004) Deep brain stimulation: Clinical findings in intractable OCD and depression. Bio Psych 55(Suppl 1):197S.
239. Nuttin BJ, Gabriels LA, et al (2003) Long-term electrical capsular stimulation in patients with obsessive-compulsive disorder. Neurosurgery 52(6):1263–1272; discussion 1272–1274.
240. Mayberg HS, Lozano AM, et al (2005) Deep brain stimulation for treatment-resistant depression. Neuron 45(5):651–660.
241. Corcoran KA, Quirk GJ (2007) Activity in prelimbic cortex is necessary for the expression of learned, but not innate, fears. J Neurosci 27(4):840–844.

# 3
# History of the Therapeutic Use of Electricity on the Brain and the Development of Deep Brain Stimulation

Matthew A. Butler, Joshua M. Rosenow, and Michael S. Okun

## Abstract

Neuroscientists have long attempted to use external electrical signals to modulate brain function. Brain stimulation has evolved from the early application of torpedo fish to the use of modern anatomic and functional imaging methods to implant chronic stimulating electrodes into deep centers of the brain for a variety of neurologic and psychiatric disorders, many of which are reviewed in this volume. With the future evolution of technology and neurophysiology, applications of this technique will likely continue to increase.

**Keywords:** deep brain stimulation, electricity, Parkinson's disease, dystonia

## Electrical Stimulation Up to 1700

The human fascination with electricity has been well documented and spans many centuries. The ancient Greeks believed that Zeus' main weapon, a lightning strike, was "sacred." Temples were commonly built at the sites of lightening strikes in an effort to allay the anger of the gods. Although the Greeks were not aware that lightning possessed the properties of electricity, they appreciated some of its electrical properties. The word "electricity," first coined by William Gilbert (1544–1603) in 1600, was derived from the Greek word for amber *(1)*. However, the actual discovery of electricity was credited to the ancient Greek scholar Thales of Miletus *(2)*. His writings from approximately 600 B.C. detailed the attraction of straw particles to fur rubbed with amber. This phenomenon, known as static electricity, was the result of the generation of a charge on the surface of the fur. Centuries later Benjamin Franklin (1706–1790) discovered the electrical properties of lightning with his famous kite experiment *(1)*.

The first medical use of electricity is credited to the Roman physician Scribbonius Largus, who used the electric torpedo fish to treat ailments such as headache and gouty arthritis. Largus' text, *Compositiones Medicae*, outlined a number of remedies using these special fish, and many of his works were later incorporated into those of Galen. The fish discharged an electrical shock when laid across the forehead of headache sufferers. Alternatively, this effect was used to treat conditions such as gout by placing the fish under the feet. Moreover, numbing effects of the electrical discharge were used to transiently relieve musculoskeletal pain. For several centuries the electric torpedo fish and electric eel represented the only harnessed sources of therapeutic electricity *(3)*.

## Electrical Stimulation of the Nervous System, 1700–1900 (Table 3.1)

By the late 1600s, it was more fully appreciated that electricity could be generated via mechanical means, allowing physicians and scientists to embark on important experiments. The era of electrical stimulation in medicine exploded in 1745 when Pieter von Musschebroek (1692–1761) revealed that an electrical charge could be stored in a Leyden jar and could later be discharged *(4)*. This observation impacted and influenced Galvani's later description of the theory of animal electricity. Galen, the great Roman physician, had posited that the central nervous system was a large secretory center supplying spirits or humors. The spirit was conducted through the nerves, which were believed to serve as simple hollow tubes for transport. Galen's theory remained widely accepted until 1791 when Luigi Galvani (1737–1798) published his theory of animal electricity. His work was based on an ability to stimulate a frog's legs with sparks of electricity. He stated that the brain secreted animal electricity, and he believed this electricity was stored in muscles and then carried by nerves *(5)*. Galvani's staunchest opponent, Allesandro Volta (1745–1827), developed the "voltaic" pile in 1800, which led to the widespread availability of more powerful electric currents for experimentation and therapeutic application *(6)*. Volta's pile was later used in experiments whose results supported Galvani's theory, rather than his own *(7)*.

Over the next 75 years, other scientists, including Galvani's nephew, Giovanni Aldini (1762–1834) conducted experiments and public displays of the effects of electricity on nervous system tissue *(8)*. Aldini and others stimulated the exposed brains of oxen and the spinal cords of decapitated criminals,

**Table 3.1** Early Advances in Neurostimulation.

| Year/Person | Event | Reference |
|---|---|---|
| 600 B.C./Thales of Miletus | Discovers electricity | 2 |
| 47 A.D./Scribbonius Largus | Electric fish used to treat human disease | 3 |
| 1600/William Gilbert | Coins the term "electricity" | 1 |
| 1874/Roberts Bartholow | Stimulates the cortex of human brain | 13 |
| 1948/J Lawrence Pool | Implants human electric stimulators | 15 |
| 1950/Robert G Heath | Uses a stereotactic apparatus to implant electrodes in a human | 16 |
| 1960/Rolf Hassler | Describes the effect of stimulation on tremor | 17 |

causing visible contractions of the extremities, thus proving that electricity could be applied centrally with peripheral effects. This was an advance over the work of Galvani, who had excited only peripheral nerves.

The career of Karl Weinhold (1782–1829) provides an extreme example of a scientist's fascination with animal electricity *(9)*. Weinhold claimed to have removed the brain and spinal cord of a cat and replaced it with a crude zinc and silver battery. His published report in 1817 *(9)* argued that the nervous system was similar to a galvanic cell. The cat survived his experiment for an unspecified time period. This story, as well as others like it, influenced Mary Shelley's famous horror novel, *Frankenstein*, which was authored in the same historical period.

Roberts Bartholow (1831–1904) is credited as the first person to electrically stimulate the human brain *(10–12)*. In 1874, he supplied an electric current to the cortex and dura of Mary Rafferty in Cincinnati *(13)*. Rafferty was described as a "feeble-minded servant girl" who presented with a cancerous ulceration on her scalp. This ulceration extended through the cranium and eroded into the dura, thus allowing easy access to the cerebral cortex. Bartholow used faradic current to electrically stimulate the exposed cortex. He described the production of muscle contractions in the right arm and leg when conducting wires were inserted into the left pre-central gyrus. Similarly, the left side began to spasm when the right parietal lobe was stimulated. When the wire was further inserted on the left, the patient experienced a tingling sensation on the right side of the body. When the electrical current was increased she had a generalized seizure and then slipped into a coma. Two days later, Rafferty developed a right hemiparesis and expired on the third day of the experiment. Although Barthelow claimed to have received consent from the patient for these experiments, he was ostracized by the Medical College of Ohio and was forced to move to Philadelphia where he continued his work at Thomas Jefferson Hospital *(14)*.

## Electrical Stimulation of the Brain, 1900–1987 (Table 3.2)

As neurosurgery blossomed during the early part of the 20th century and came into its own as a surgical specialty, greater strides were made in applying electricity to the study of the brain. One of the great pioneers in the field was Wilder Penfield (1891–1976) who stimulated a variety of cortical regions *(18, 19)* in patients undergoing epilepsy surgery at the Montreal Neurological Institute (the so-called "Montreal procedure") *(20)*. With these investigations, he was able to construct a map correlating cerebral architecture with function. His 1937 landmark paper introduced his seminal map of the sensorimotor

Table 3.2 Early Applications of Deep Brain Stimulation for Pain.

| Year/Person | Target | Reference |
|---|---|---|
| 1952/Heath | Limbic system | *34* |
| 1962/Mazars | Hypothalamus | *36* |
| 1967/Shealy | Dorsal columns | *37* |
| 1973/Hosobuchi | Thalamus | *38* |

cortex that is now referred to as "the homunculus" *(21)*. The promulgation of this map and others like it involving the thalamus and other brain regions served as the starting point for further acquisition of knowledge about cerebral centers involved in complex neurological functions such as movement, sensation, and memory.

During the first half of the 20th century, a primary therapeutic use of brain surgery was in the performance of ablative procedures for psychiatric disorders. Early operations were largely based on observations that ablating areas of the cortex in monkeys, dogs, and other experimental animals changed or improved behavior *(22)*. In the 1930s prefrontal lobotomy and prefrontal topectomies emerged as a treatment for institutionalized mentally ill patients *(23)*.

J. Lawrence Pool (1906–2004), working at Columbia University in New York, was an advocate of such operations *(24–27)*. Influenced by early lesioning and resective procedures, Pool took the next major step by exploring electrical stimulation of the brain for psychiatric disease. In 1948, he attempted to treat an elderly woman's anorexia and depression by implanting a stimulation electrode in the patient's caudate nucleus. Pool performed a traditional craniotomy and implanted the electrodes (Figure 3.1). The stimulator was used daily for a period of 8 weeks with favorable results, according to Pool, until one of the wires was found to be fractured. Pool's patient may have been the first example of a permanently implanted stimulation system used on the human brain *(15)*.

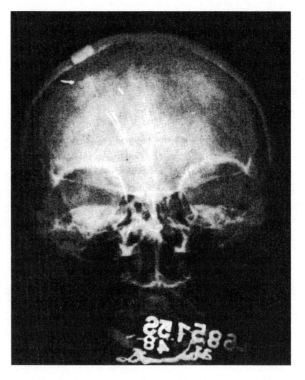

**Figure 3.1** Electrodes implanted by Dr. Pool in 1948 into the caudate nucleus *(15)*

The procedure for implantation of deep electrodes would not have been widely accepted without the subsequent development of the stereotactic frame, which greatly improved targeting accuracy. In 1947, Ernest Spiegel (1895–1985), an Austrian trained neurologist who fled from Vienna during World War II, along with his student Henry Wycis (1911–1971), developed the first stereotactic frame for use on humans at Temple University in Philadelphia *(28, 29)*. This new method employed an apparatus similar to a prototype first introduced by Clarke and Horsely in 1906 and was based on intracerebral landmarks such as the pineal body *(30)*. The Spiegel-Wycis device, introduced in 1947 for human use, was a ring that was fixed to the skull and stabilized by a custom plaster casting of the patient's head (Figure 3.2). A frame was attached to the ring and coordinates were determined using radiographic landmarks, such as the pineal body. Spiegel and Wycis subsequently published the first atlas for stereotactic surgery in 1952 *(31)*. These advances were critical for the future of stereotactic approaches in implanting neurostimulators *(32)*.

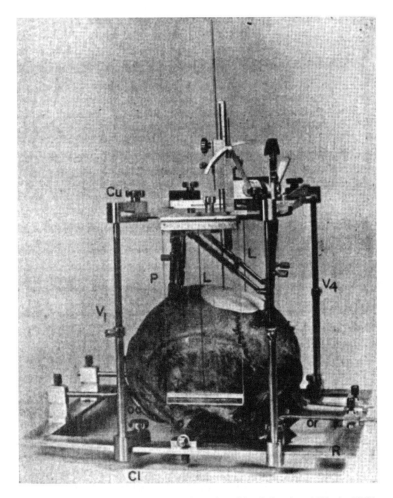

**Figure 3.2** An example of the apparatus introduced by Spiegel and Wycis *(178)*

In 1954, Robert Heath (1915–1999), a neurosurgeon at Tulane University in New Orleans and Pool's former pupil, published the first account of an electrical stimulator implanted utilizing stereotactic techniques *(16)*. Many of Heath's studies had bizarre underpinnings and some were controversial and ethically questionable. His studies centered on the limbic system, and he stimulated the human brain with the goal of elucidating emotional responses. For example, Heath stimulated the septal region and other reward areas of the brain in homosexual men with an ultimate goal of converting the men from homosexual to heterosexual *(33)*. These experiments were precursors of later efforts at treatment of pain with brain stimulation *(34)*.

During the 1960s and 1970s the most common therapeutic application of chronic brain stimulation was to treat intractable pain (Table 3.2). In 1960, Mazars reported a series of 14 patients treated with intermittent hypothalamic stimulation for painful syndromes that he believed resulted from "lack of proprioceptive information" *(35)*. Mazars reported that the pain was completely resolved in 13 of these cases. Another series of patients categorized by Mazars as having pain with "excessive nociceptive stimuli" such as neoplastic pain were not helped by this therapy *(36)*. In 1967, Norman Shealy implanted neurostimulators in the dorsal columns to treat intractable pain *(37)*. In 1973, Hosobuchi reported five patients with anesthesia dolorosa resulting from rhizotomy who were treated successfully with chronic thalamic stimulation *(38)*. Four of the patients had favorable relief of facial pain. Mundinger also reported the use of thalamic stimulation for chronic pain *(39–42)*.

During the 1950s and 1960s, two ablative procedures, pallidotomy and thalamotomy, were introduced for the relief of symptoms associated with movement disorders such as Parkinson's disease (PD; refs. *43–50*). In the course of localizing the region to be ablated, it was routine to perform stimulation within the basal ganglia and other areas of interest prior to performing definitive coagulation. Spiegel and Wycis reported that, at low frequencies, pallidal stimulation before pallidotomy could elicit tremor and even unmask anesthetic-induced suppression of tremor *(51)*.

Importantly, this led to the awareness that deep brain stimulation (DBS) could suppress tremor. Having published the first report of the effects of thalamotomy on movement disorders *(52)*, Rolf Hassler published a paper describing the relief of extrapyramidal motor symptoms during intraoperative stimulation *(17)*. He found that low stimulation frequencies 60Hz exacerbated tremor and >100Hz reduced it, but that a suppressive effect could be observed with high frequency stimulation.

The discovery, in the late 1960s, of the effectiveness of levodopa for the treatment of PD *(53–60)*, along with the complications of ablative surgery *(61–64)*, led to a great decrease in the volume of ablative surgery for movement disorders. The use of brain stimulation continued for treatment of chronic pain, and was later applied to other neurological disorders such as spasticity, epilepsy, and blindness *(65)*.

In 1973, Irving Cooper reported the results of stimulating the anterior surface of the cerebellum for spasticity and epilepsy *(66)*. Three patients with spasticity were treated with high frequency stimulation, which decreased their rigidity and spasticity. Four other patients were successfully treated with low frequency cerebellar stimulation for convulsive disorders. Cooper conducted many significant studies of cerebral stimulation (both cortical and DBS) from the late 1960s through the 1980s *(67)*. He treated numerous patients with spasticity, dystonia, and epilepsy with cerebellar cortical stimulation *(68, 69)*. Avery Laboratories (Farmingdale, NY) manufactured the first generation of stimulators Cooper implanted. These stimulators were radio receivers activated by an external battery-powered transmitter. Patients wore a battery pack on their belts and the transmitter was taped to the chest over the implanted receiver. The pulse amplitude dial on these transmitters was labeled with a simple 0 to 10 scale, which had no direct relationship to the current delivered, thus necessitating calibration by the investigators. A later generation of fully implantable stimulators (neurolith 601) was manufactured by Pacemaker Systems-Neurodyne Corporation (Sylmar, CA) and used after 1979 by investigators other than Cooper *(70)*.

Despite Cooper's optimistic publications documenting significant clinical improvements, further trials in the 1980s cast doubt on his methodologies and results, leading to the essential cessation of this technique *(67)*. However, in 1980, Schvarcz *(71)* implanted electrodes into the dentate nucleus of a 25-year-old patient with spastic cerebral palsy, reporting that stimulation at 100 Hz and 2 V produced marked improvement in speech quality and spasticity in the ipsilateral body.

In January 1979, Cooper *(72)* implanted Medtronic quadripolar electrodes in the left pulvinar and posterior internal capsule of a 34-year-old male with chronic lower extremity pain and spasticity. The patient experienced pain relief after 15 minutes of stimulation as well as decreased spasticity. Cooper subsequently implanted electrodes in the thalamus or internal capsule of five other patients with tremor, spasticity, dystonia, dysarthria, and torticollis. Five of these initial six patients obtained sustained relief from their symptoms. Several of these patients had already undergone cerebellar stimulation or cryogenic thalamic lesioning. Optimal results were achieved with stimulation at 4–7 V, 0.3 millisecond pulse duration, and a frequency of 50–75 Hz.

In his 1980 report, Cooper *(72)* most often selected the ventrolateral nucleus as his thalamic site because of its importance in the extrapyramidal motor system loop and its role as a target for dentatorubrothalamic projections. He believed that motor symptoms may reflect a "net loss of excitation" and that DBS would "provide sufficient background excitation to the motor cortex such that otherwise intact motor programmes may become operational once more."

Emboldened by these positive results, Cooper expanded his work in this field. In 1981, he presented the results from the treatment of his first 49 patients in Zurich at the 8th Meeting of the World Society of Stereotactic and Functional Neurosurgery *(73)*. Approximately half (27 of 49) of these patients improved with DBS. The procedure was a failure for patients with dystonia of unspecified etiology, as five of six did not improve. Even though the procedure was not uniformly successful, Cooper stated that it would be useful in patients who already had a contralateral cryothalamectomy. In a prescient move, he speculated in this paper that the reversible nature of chronic stimulation would avoid the complications of bilateral thalamic lesions *(73)*.

Noting that the anterior nucleus of the thalamus serves as a vital relay in Papez's classic circuit, Cooper hypothesized that this region could serve as a key location to disrupt limbic seizures. Six patients underwent implantation of bilateral thalamic electrodes into the anterior nucleus between 1979 and 1982. These were coupled to external RF transmitters similar to the early cerebellar stimulators. The findings from this small group of patients were presented at several scientific meetings and formed the basis for several publications *(74, 75)*.

More detailed physiological and imaging results were published on the final two patients to undergo the procedure *(76, 77)*. Both individuals experienced improved mood, affect, and reaction time during stimulation. "Obsessional thinking" and "viscosity of thought" decreased over the same time period. PET studies performed with the stimulators off revealed bilateral temporal hypometabolism that normalized with initiation of stimulation. These scans were repeated multiple times over 2 years in these patients with identical results. While no complications were reported, some patients experienced euphoria. Patients first noted this sensation in association with the mild increase in voltage that accompanies the insertion of a new battery. However, when patients began increasing their stimulation voltage on their own to obtain a high, Cooper was forced to place a locking device on the external stimulator controls.

During the 1970s and 1980s scattered reports of DBS for tremor and for other movement disorders began to appear. One of the first reports was by Bechtereva in Leningrad, USSR during the early 1970s *(78)*. Bechtereva reported promising results, although her data on specific disorders and the total number of patients treated was not well documented. In the United States, Brice described five patients with intention tremor secondary to multiple sclerosis who were treated with some success by stimulating areas in the midbrain and basal ganglia *(79)*.

## The Modern Era of DBS: 1987 to the Present (Table 3.3)

The modern era of DBS began in 1987 when Alim Benabid published his landmark paper reporting the use of ventral intermediate nucleus (Vim) stimulation for PD *(80)*. He reported the positive effects of Vim stimulation in patients who had previous contralateral thalamotomy, and in whom he did not wish to

**Table 3.3** Recent History of DBS.

| Year/Person | Target | Disorder | Reference |
|---|---|---|---|
| 1975/Bechtereva | Basal ganglia | Movement disorders | 78 |
| 1979/Cooper | Anterior thalamus | Epilepsy | 72 |
| 1987/Benabid | Vim thalamus | Tremor | 80 |
| 1994/Benabid | Subthalamic nucleus | Parkinson's disease | 94 |
| 1994/Siegfried | Internal pallidum | Parkinson's disease | 100 |
| 1999/Nuttin | Internal capsule | Obsessive–compulsive disorder | 157 |
| 1999/Vandewalle | Thalamus | Tourette's syndrome | 173 |
| 2003/Broggi | Hypothalamus | Cluster headache | 141 |
| 2005/Mayberg | Brodmann area 25 | Depression | 170 |

perform a second lesion because of fear of causing pseudobulbar symptoms *(80)*. In a subsequent paper, Benabid *(81)* reported on 26 patients with parkinsonian tremor all treated with chronic Vim stimulation, who all experienced remarkable benefits. Benabid's findings were quickly reproduced *(81)*. Since that time, the era of DBS for PD and other movement disorders has flourished and become a highly efficacious treatment, mainly as a result of target flexibility, device "programmability," and safety.

Reports of thalamic DBS for tremor subsequently appeared, confirming the beneficial effects of this modality *(82–90)*. Lyons et al. *(83)* confirmed that the suppressive effect of Vim DBS on Parkinsonian tremor was long lasting and noted that tolerance was minimal, with no adjustment in stimulation parameters required for most patients after 3 months postoperatively. Hariz *(84)* noted that while DBS was effective, some tolerance did develop among the patients in his series. In the 22 PD patients, mean voltage increased almost 50% from 1 week to 1 year postoperatively. In addition, the percentage of patients who were tremor free fell from 90 to 70%. Hubble et al. *(85)* analyzed various subtypes of tremor and stated that both proximal and distal postural tremor, resting tremor, and intention tremor all improved significantly with thalamic DBS. Tasker's *(86)* comparison of thalamotomy and thalamic stimulation demonstrated that chronic stimulation was associated with a lower incidence of ataxia and dysarthria (common complications of bilateral thalamotomy). When these problems occurred in the DBS group, adjusting stimulation parameters served to abolish them. Importantly, 15% of thalamotomy patients required a repeat procedure due to recurrence of tremor. Schuurman et al. *(87)* reported the results of a randomized trial of thalamotomy versus thalamic DBS. Even though both techniques were effective at suppressing tremor, only DBS was associated with significantly improved functional status and was associated with significantly fewer adverse events than thalamotomy.

Prior to the advent of subthalamic and pallidal DBS for PD, several investigators utilized thalamic stimulation for symptomatic relief in these patients. An important observation made by Kumar et al. *(88)* was that, while tremor was significantly reduced with Vim stimulation, dopaminergic medication was unchanged. Ondo et al. *(89)* analyzed 19 PD patients with thalamic stimulators and verified that while writing and subjective functional measures improved in these patients, overall activities of daily living (ADL) scores did not improve due to a lack of effect of stimulation on other aspects of the disease besides tremor. The European multicenter study *(90)* noted a 10% improvement in rigidity and 35% improvement in akinesia, both of which were significant. However, given that stimulation of either the subthalamic nucleus (STN) or the globus pallidus interna (GPi) provided relief of tremor as well as the other cardinal symptoms of PD (as discussed later), the role for Vim stimulation for PD appeared limited at best.

The rapid ascendance of STN DBS for PD was a notable change in the field, given the traditional view that STN lesions cause hemiballismus. However, after primate models of PD demonstrated that STN lesions could alleviate motor symptoms of parkinsonism *(91–93)*, human trials followed. The Grenoble group led the way in performing chronic electrical stimulation the STN *(94, 95)*. The ADL and motor score portions of the Unified Parkinson's Disease Rating Scale (UPDRS) improved more than 50%. Some transient, stimulation-induced hemiballismus occurred but was controlled by adjusting the stimulation parameters. One-year *(96)* follow-up studies of 24 patients with bilateral STN stimulators demonstrated that UPDRS ADL and motor scores improved by 60% in the off-medication state. The UPDRS subscores for akinesia (56%), tremor (80%), rigidity (68%), and gait (55%) also improved, in contrast to results seen with Vim stimulation. However, the effect in the on-medication state was not as pronounced, with only a 10% improvement in motor scores. While recent studies have attested to the long-term durability of STN stimulation for PD *(97)*, no change in disease progression had been noted.

After Laitinen revived pallidotomy as a method of addressing all the cardinal features of PD *(98, 99)*, chronic GPi stimulation for PD was reported in 1994. Siegfried and Lippitz *(100)* described their results in three patients who underwent implantation of bilateral GPi DBS systems using Leksell's target. All three achieved significant reduction in medication-induced side effects and on–off fluctuations. Bradykinesia, freezing, and speech also improved.

Reports concerning patients undergoing pallidal DBS have proliferated. Loher's *(101)* 1-year results in 16 patients showed a 38% improvement in medication-off UPDRS motor scores and a 33% improvement in ADL score in those patients receiving unilateral stimulation. Bilateral stimulation led to a slight improvement in these results. It was shown in a larger series of 36 patients *(102)* that bilateral pallidal stimulation results in a median motor improvement of 37% and an increase from 28 to 64% of the day spent without disabling involuntary movements. Kumar et al. *(103)* reported 6-month follow-up data on 22 patients (17 implanted bilaterally). Their total UPDRS motor score improved 31% and the ADL score improved 39%. Medication-induced dyskinesias decreased by two-thirds. Subsequent reports have confirmed the beneficial effects of GPi DBS on dyskinesia, motor fluctuations, and tremor *(104–109)*.

Chronic pallidal stimulation has also been validated in the setting of prior pallidotomy *(104)*. In 4 patients who underwent GPi stimulation contralateral to a prior pallidotomy, motor scores improved by almost 50% while bradykinesia was decreased by 37% and tremor by 93% without serious adverse cognitive or motor effects. While bilateral pallidotomy has been avoided due to concern for cognitive impairment, this has been shown to be relatively well preserved during bilateral GPi stimulation *(110–113)*. Patients who do experience cognitive decline after pallidal stimulation have tended to be elderly and taking large doses of dopaminergic medication *(113)*.

A handful of direct comparisons beteen GPi and STN DBS for PD have been published *(102, 114–116)*. A large multicenter study *(102)* found that STN stimulation was significantly more efficacious and enabled patients to reduce their medication while GPi stimulation did not. The series published by Krause et al. *(114)* and Krack et al. *(115)* also gave the edge to the STN as the target of choice. Burchiel et al. *(117)* conducted a randomized trial of pallidal versus STN stimulation. While the results off medication were similar for the 2 groups (44% with STN stimulation and 39% with GPi), pallidal, but not subthalamic, stimulation improved parkinson motor symptoms while patients were in the medication-on state. While both targets provided equal improvements in rigidity (37–47%), bradykinesia (25%), and tremor (74%), axial symptomatology was relieved only by GPi stimulation. However, only

STN stimulation allowed patients to reduce their medication dosage. Using the results of their comparison between the two targets, Volkman et al. *(118)* argued that there exists a tradeoff between STN and pallidal DBS. STN stimulation allowed patients to reduce their medication by 63% while using one-third of the power required for effective GPi stimulation. The incidence of stimulation-induced side effects such as dysarthria, hypophonia, and eyelid opening apraxia was greater with STN than GPi DBS. The results from currently ongoing randomized trials of GPi versus STN stimulation in PD are eagerly awaited.

Dystonia has a long history of neurosurgical treatment, and reports have emerged describing the use of DBS in dystonia with a variety of subcortical targets. However, the disorder is heterogenous, with a wide clinical spectrum and multiple etiologies, making the assembly of large patient populations problematic *(120–127)*.

In reviewing their experience with Vim DBS, the Grenoble group found that results in their five patients with dystonia were unimpressive *(119)*. However, pallidal stimulation has become increasingly utilized for this purpose. Multiple small series have been published documenting improvement in the Burke-Fahn-Marsden (BFM) score. In addition, GPi stimulation has been found to maintain a robust effect 4 years after implantation *(129)*. Best results have been in patients with idiopathic generalized dystonia, either DYT1 gene positive or negative *(128, 130, 131)*. Phasic or mobile dystonia appears to respond better than more fixed dystonia.

The last several years have been characterized by many emerging indications and new intracranial targets for DBS. These include new targets for PD such as the posterior subthalamic region *(132, 133)* and the pedunculopontine nucleus *(134–137)*. It is hoped that stimulation in these areas will address some aspects of advanced PD that are not improved by STN or GPi DBS, such as gait difficulties and postural instability. With the advent of functional imaging has come the introduction of rationally derived targets, such as the use of hypothalamic stimulation for the treatment of intractable cluster headache *(138–141)*, This area was targeted after hypothalamic hyperactivity was observed on functional imaging during cluster attacks *(142)*.

Cooper's early work with DBS for epilepsy has attracted renewed interest. Several groups have shown that anterior thalamic stimulation is effective at reducing seizure frequency in animal models of epilepsy *(143, 144)*. This spurred new human trials *(145–147)*, albeit with more rigorous patient selection, better surgical techniques, and better outcomes evaluation than in Cooper's series.

Velasco and colleagues *(148–150)* have actively explored stimulation of the centromedian nucleus of the thalamus for treatment of medically refractory epilepsy. They and others *(145, 148)* have also stimulated the hippocampus for treatment of refractory seizures, although this has not been consistently effective in blinded trials *(151)*. There has also been interest in targeting the STN for seizure suppression *(152–155)* but this remains unproven as a consistently successful therapy.

Probably the most closely watched area of expansion for DBS is behavioral and psychiatric disorders, including Tourette's syndrome, major depression, and obsessive–compulsive disorder (OCD). Initial attempts at DBS for OCD utilized the same anterior internal capsule target as that of radiofrequency and radiosurgical capsulotomy *(156)*. Nuttin and colleagues have demonstrated short and longer term benefit in uncontrolled trials of DBS in anterior limb of internal capsule *(157, 158)*. Additional reports of DBS for OCD have appeared *(159–166)*.

Functional imaging of patients with major depression has shown localized metabolic changes in cingulate gyrus during depressive episodes *(167–169)*. This led Mayberg et al. *(170)* to conduct a trial of DBS in the subgenual cingulate region (Brodmann area 25), in six patients with major depression. Chronic stimulation was associated with significant remission of depression in four of the six patients *(170)*. Moreover, PET scans revealed that the antidepressant effects of stimulation were associated with a marked reduction in local cerebral blood flow as well as changes in downstream limbic and cortical sites.

Tourette syndrome has also attracted interest for treatment with DBS *(171)*. Using the region of the anterior and intralaminar thalamus which had been lesioned by Hassler *(172)*, Vandewalle *(173)* reported nearly complete resolution of tics in patients undergoing chronic stimulation *(173, 174)*. Other targets have also been utilized, including the anterior internal capsule *(175)*, globus pallidum *(176, 177)*, and centromedian-parafascicular complex (Ce-Pf) of the thalamus *(177)*.

## Conclusion

As reviewed in this chapter, neuroscientists have long attempted to use external electrical signals to modulate brain function. Brain stimulation has evolved from the application of torpedo fish to the use of modern anatomic and functional imaging methods to implant chronic stimulating electrodes into deep centers of the brain for a variety of neurologic and psychiatric disorders many of which are reviewed in this volume. With the future evolution of technology and neurophysiology, applications of this technique will likely continue to increase.

## References

1. Gilbert W (1991) De Magnete. New York, NY: Dover Books.
2. Lloyd G (1970) Early Greek Science: Thales to Aristotle. New York, NY: WW Norton and Company.
3. Largus S (1529) De Compositionibus Medicamentorum. Paris, France: Wechel.
4. Musschenbroek Pv. Essai de Physique…Avec une Description de nouvelles sortes de Machines pneumatiques, et un Recueil d'Expériences.
5. Foley M (1953) Lugi Galvani: Commentary on the effects of electricity on muscular motion. Norwalk, CT: Burndy Library.
6. Pancaldi G (2003) Volta: Science and Culture in the Age of Enlightenment. Princeton, NJ: Princeton University Press.
7. Licht S (1967) Therapeutic Electricity and Ultraviolet Radiation. Baltimore, MD: Weaverly Press.
8. Parent A (2004) Giovanni Aldini: from animal electricity to human brain stimulation. Can J Neurol Sci 31:576–584.
9. Weinholdt K (1817) Versuche Uber das Leben und seine, Grudkafte auf dem wege derr experimental-physiologie. Magdeburg: Creutz.
10. Morgan JP (1982) The first reported case of electrical stimulation of the human brain. J Hist Med Allied Sci 37:51–64.

11. Thomas RK, Young CD (1993) A note on the early history of electrical stimulation of the human brain. J Gen Psychol 120:73–81.
12. Zimmermann M (1982) Electrical stimulation of the human brain. Hum Neurobiol 1:227–229.
13. Bartholow R (1874) Experimental investigations into the functions of the human brain. Am J Med Sci 67:305–313.
14. Walker AE (1957) Stimulation and ablation; their role in the history of cerebral physiology. J Neurophysiol 20:435–449.
15. Pool JL (1954) Psychosurgery in older people. J Am Geriat Soc 2:456–465.
16. Heath R (1954) Studies in schizophrenia: a multidisciplinary approach to mind-brain relationships. Cambridge, MA: Harvard University Press.
17. Hassler R, Riechert T, Mundinger F, Umbach W, Ganglberger JA (1960) Physiological observations in stereotaxic operations in extrapyramidal motor disturbances. Brain 83:337–350.
18. Penfield W (1972) The electrode, the brain and the mind. Z Neurol 201:297–309.
19. Penfield W, Welch K (1949) Instability of response to stimulation of the sensorimotor cortex of man. J Physiol 109:358–365, illust.
20. Preul MC, Feindel W (1991) Origins of Wilder Penfield's surgical technique. The role of the "Cushing ritual" and influences from the European experience. J Neurosurg 75:812–820.
21. Penfield W (1937) Somatic motor and sensory representation in the cerebral cortex of man as studied by electrical stimulation. Brain 60:389–443.
22. Goltz F (1888) Uber dieVerrichtungen des Grosshirins. Pflug er's Archiv fur die gesammte Physiologie 42:419–467.
23. Finger S (1994) Origins of neuroscience: a history of explorations into brain function. New York: Oxford University Press.
24. Glusman M, Ransohoff J, Pool JL, Grundfest H, Mettler FA (1952) Electrical excitability of the human motor cortex. I. The parameters of the electrical stimulus. J Neurosurg 9:461–471.
25. Glusman M, Ransohoff J, Pool JL, Sloan N (1953) Electrical excitability of human uncus. J Neurophysiol 16:528–536.
26. Pool JL, Langford W, Glaser GH (1951) Treatment of psychomotor syndromes by operations on the temporal lobe. AMA Arch Neurol Psychiatry 65:538–541.
27. Pool JL, Ransohoff J (1949) Autonomic effects on stimulating rostral portion of cingulate gyri in man. J Neurophysiol 12:385–392.
28. Gildenberg PL (2001) Spiegel and Wycis—the early years. Stereotact Funct Neurosurg 77:11–16.
29. Spiegel EA, Wycis HT, Marks M, Lee AJ (1947) Stereotaxic apparatus for operations on the human brain. Science 106:349–350.
30. Clark RH, Horsley VA (1906) On a method of investigating the deep ganglia and tracts of the central nervous system (cerebellum). BMJ 2:1799–1800.
31. Spiegel EA, Wycis HT (1952) Stereoencephalotomy: thalamotomy and related procedures. New York: Grune and Stratton.
32. Spiegel EA, Wycis HT (1961) Chronic implantation of intracerebral electrodes in humans. In: Sheer DE, ed. Electrical Stimulation of the Brain. Austin, TX: University of Texas Press, pp. 37–44.
33. Moan CE, Heath RG (1972) Septal stimulation for the initiation of heterosexual activity in a homosexual male. J Behav Ther Exper Psych 3:23–30.
34. Heath RG (1963) Electrical self-stimulation of the brain in man. Am J Psychiatry 120:571–577.
35. Mazars G, Roge R, Mazars Y (1960) [Results of the stimulation of the spinothalamic fasciculus and their bearing on the physiopathology of pain.]. Rev Prat 103:136–138.
36. Mazars G (1973) Stimulations thalaiques intermittentes Antalgiques. Rev Neurol 128:273–279.

37. Shealy CN, Mortimer JT, Reswick JB (1967) Electrical inhibition of pain by stimulation of the dorsal columns: preliminary clinical report. Anesthetic Analgesia 46:489–491.
38. Hosobuchi Y, Adams JE, Rutkin B (1973) Chronic thalamic stimulation for the control of facial anesthesia dolorosa. Arch Neurol 29:158–161.
39. Mundinger F, Neumuller H (1982) Programmed stimulation for control of chronic pain and motor diseases. Appl Neurophysiol 45:102–111.
40. Mundinger F, Salomao JF (1980) Deep brain stimulation in mesencephalic lemniscus medialis for chronic pain. Acta Neurochir Suppl (Wien) 30:245–258.
41. Mundinger F (1977) [Treatment of chronic pain with intracerebral stimulators]. Dtsch Med Wochenschr 102:1724–1729.
42. Strassburg HM, Thoden U, Mundinger F (1979) Mesencephalic chronic electrodes in pain patients. An electrophysiological study. Appl Neurophysiol 42:284–293.
43. Gillingham J (2000) Forty-five years of stereotactic surgery for Parkinson's disease: a review. Stereotact Funct Neurosurg 74:95–98.
44. Guridi J, Lozano AM (1997) A brief history of pallidotomy. Neurosurgery 41:1169–1180; discussion 1180–1163.
45. Hornyak M, Rovit RL, Simon AS, Couldwell WT (2001) Irving S. Cooper and the early surgical management of movement disorders. Video history. Neurosurg Focus 11:E6.
46. Redfern RM (1989) History of stereotactic surgery for Parkinson's disease. Br J Neurosurg 3:271–304.
47. Zesiewicz TA, Hauser RA (2001) Neurosurgery for Parkinson's disease. Semin Neurol 21:91–101.
48. Narabayashi H (1962) Neurophysiological ideas on pallidotomy and ventrolateral thalamotomy for hyperkinesis. Confin Neurol 22:291–303.
49. Narabayashi H (1998) Stereotactic surgery and Parkinson's disease. Stereotact Funct Neurosurg 70:114–121.
50. Svennilson E, Torvik A, Lowe R, Leksell L (1960) Treatment of parkinsonism by stereotatic thermolesions in the pallidal region. A clinical evaluation of 81 cases. Acta Psychiatr Scand 35:358–377.
51. Spiegel EA, Wycis HT, Baird HW, Szekely EG (1960) Physiopathologic observations on the basal ganglia. In: Ramey E, O'Doherty DS, eds. Electrical Studies on the Unanesthetized Brain. New York: Harper & Brothers, pp. 192–213.
52. Hassler R, Riechert T (1954) Indikationen and Lokalizationensmethode der Hirnoperationen. Nervenarzt 25:441–447.
53. Cotzias GC (1968) L-Dopa for Parkinsonism. N Engl J Med 278:630.
54. Cotzias GC, Papavasiliou PS, Fehling C, Kaufman B, Mena I (1970) Similarities between neurologic effects of L-dipa and of apomorphine. N Engl J Med 282:31–33.
55. Cotzias GC, Papavasiliou PS, Gellene R (1968) Experimental treatment of parkinsonism with L-Dopa. Neurology 18:276–277.
56. Cotzias GC, Papavasiliou PS, Gellene R (1969) L-dopa in parkinson's syndrome. N Engl J Med 281:272.
57. Cotzias GC, Papavasiliou PS, Gellene R (1969) Modification of Parkinsonism—chronic treatment with L-dopa. N Engl J Med 280:337–345.
58. Cotzias GC, Papavasiliou PS, Gellene R, Aronson RB (1968) Parkinsonism and DOPA. Trans Assoc Am Physicians 81:171–183.
59. Cotzias GC, Papavasiliou PS, Steck A, Duby S (1971) Parkinsonism and levodopa. Clin Pharmacol Ther 12:319–322.
60. Cotzias GC, Van Woert MH, Schiffer LM (1967) Aromatic amino acids and modification of parkinsonism. N Engl J Med 276:374–379.
61. Gildenberg PL (1984) The present role of stereotactic surgery in the management of Parkinson's disease. Adv Neurol 40:447–452.

62. Gildenberg PL (1987) Whatever happened to stereotactic surgery? Neurosurgery 20:983–987.
63. Gildenberg PL (1990) The history of stereotactic neurosurgery. Neurosurg Clin N Am 1:765–780.
64. Gildenberg PL (1998) The history of surgery for movement disorders. Neurosurg Clin N Am 9:283–294.
65. Brindley GS (1970) Sensations produced by electrical stimulation of the occipital poles of the cerebral hemispheres, and their use in constructing visual prostheses. Ann R Coll Surg Engl 47:106–108.
66. Cooper IS (1973) Effect of chronic stimulation of anterior cerebellum on neurological disease. Lancet 1:206.
67. Rosenow J, Das K, Rovit RL, Couldwell WT, Irving S (2002) Cooper and his role in intracranial stimulation for movement disorders and epilepsy. Stereotact Funct Neurosurg 78:95–112.
68. Cooper IS, Amin I (1973) The effect of chronic cerebellar stimulation upon epilepsy in man. Trans Am Neurol Assoc 98:192–196.
69. Cooper IS, Amin I (1976) Chronic cerebellar stimulation in epilepsy. Clinical and anatomic studies. Arch Neurol 33:558–570.
70. Davis R, Emmonds SE (1992) Cerebellar stimulation for seizure control: 17-year study. Stereotact Funct Neurosurg 58:200–208.
71. Schvarcz JR, Sica RE, Morita E (1980) Chronic self-stimulation of the dentate nucleus for the relief of spasticity. Acta Neurochir Suppl (Wien) 30:351–359.
72. Cooper IS, Upton AR, Amin I (1980) Reversibility of chronic neurologic deficits. Some effects of electrical stimulation of the thalamus and internal capsule in man. Appl Neurophysiol 43:244–258.
73. Cooper IS, Upton AR, Amin I (1982) Chronic cerebellar stimulation (CCS) and deep brain stimulation (DBS) in involuntary movement disorders. Appl Neurophysiol 45:209–217.
74. Cooper IS, Upton AR (1985) Therapeutic implications of modulation of metabolism and functional activity of cerebral cortex by chronic stimulation of cerebellum and thalamus. Biol Psychiatry 20:811–813.
75. Upton AR, Cooper IS, Springman M, Amin I (1985) Suppression of seizures and psychosis of limbic system origin by chronic stimulation of anterior nucleus of the thalamus. Int J Neurol 19–20:223–230.
76. Cooper IS, Upton ARM (1985) Therapeutic implications of modulation of metabolism and functional activity of cerebral cortex by chronic stimulation of cerebellum and thalamus. Biol Psych 20:811–813.
77. Upton ARM, Amin I, Garnett S, Springman M, Nahmias C, Cooper IS (1987) Evoked metabolic responses in the limbic-striate system produced by stimulation of anterior thalamic nucleus in man. Pace 10:217–225.
78. Bechtereva NP, Bondartchuk AN, Smirnov VM, Meliutcheva LA, Shandurina AN (1975) Method of electrostimulation of the deep brain structures in treatment of some chronic diseases. Confin Neurol 37:136–140.
79. Brice J, McLellan L (1980) Suppression of intention tremor by contingent deep-brain stimulation. Lancet 1:1221–1222.
80. Benabid AL, Pollak P, Louveau A, Henry S, de Rougemont J (1987) Combined (thalamotomy and stimulation) stereotactic surgery of the VIM thalamic nucleus for bilateral Parkinson disease. Appl Neurophysiol 50:344–346.
81. Benabid AL, Pollak P, Gervason C, et al (1991) Long-term suppression of tremor by chronic stimulation of the ventral intermediate thalamic nucleus. Lancet 337:403–406.
82. Koller W, Pahwa R, Busenbark K, et al (1997) High-frequency unilateral thalamic stimulation in the treatment of essential and parkinsonian tremor. Ann Neurol 42:292–299.

83. Lyons KE, Koller WC, Wilkinson SB, Pahwa R (2001) Long term safety and efficacy of unilateral deep brain stimulation of the thalamus for parkinsonian tremor. J Neurol Neurosurg Psych 71:682–684.
84. Hariz MI, Shamsgovara P, Johansson F, Hariz G, Fodstad H (1999) Tolerance and tremor rebound following long-term chronic thalamic stimulation for Parkinsonian and essential tremor. Stereotact Funct Neurosurg 72:208–218.
85. Hubble JP, Busenbark KL, Wilkinson S, et al (1997) Effects of thalamic deep brain stimulation based on tremor type and diagnosis. Mov Disord 12:337–341.
86. Tasker RR (1998) Deep brain stimulation is preferable to thalamotomy for tremor suppression. Surg Neurol 49:145–153; discussion 153–144.
87. Schuurman PR, Bosch DA, Bossuyt PM, et al (2000) A comparison of continuous thalamic stimulation and thalamotomy for suppression of severe tremor. N Engl J Med 342:461–468.
88. Kumar K, Kelly M, Toth C (1999) Deep brain stimulation of the ventral intermediate nucleus of the thalamus for control of tremors in Parkinson's disease and essential tremor. Stereotact Funct Neurosurg 72:47–61.
89. Ondo W, Jankovic J, Schwartz K, Almaguer M, Simpson RK (1998) Unilateral thalamic deep brain stimulation for refractory essential tremor and Parkinson's disease tremor. Neurology 51:1063–1069.
90. Limousin P, Speelman JD, Gielen F, Janssens M (1999) Multicentre European study of thalamic stimulation in parkinsonian and essential tremor. J Neurol Neurosurg Psych 66:289–296.
91. Aziz TZ, Peggs D, Agarwal E, Sambrook MA, Crossman AR (1992) Subthalamic nucleotomy alleviates parkinsonism in the 1-methyl-4-phenyl-1,2,3,6-tetrahydropyridine (MPTP)-exposed primate. Br J Neurosurg 6:575–582.
92. Aziz TZ, Peggs D, Sambrook MA, Crossman AR (1991) Lesion of the subthalamic nucleus for the alleviation of 1-methyl-4-phenyl-1,2,3,6-tetrahydropyridine (MPTP)-induced parkinsonism in the primate. Mov Disord 6:288–292.
93. Bergman H, Wichmann T, DeLong MR (1990) Reversal of experimental parkinsonism by lesions of the subthalamic nucleus. Science 249:1436–1438.
94. Benabid AL, Pollak P, Gross C, et al (1994) Acute and long-term effects of subthalamic nucleus stimulation in Parkinson's disease. Stereotact Funct Neurosurg 62:76–84.
95. Limousin P, Pollak P, Benazzouz A, et al (1995) Effect of parkinsonian signs and symptoms of bilateral subthalamic nucleus stimulation. Lancet 345:91–95.
96. Limousin P, Pollak P, Benazzouz A, et al (1995) Bilateral subthalamic nucleus stimulation for severe Parkinson's disease. Mov Disord 10:672–674.
97. Krack P, Batir A, Van Blercom N, et al (2003) Five-year follow-up of bilateral stimulation of the subthalamic nucleus in advanced Parkinson's disease. N Engl J Med 349:1925–1934.
98. Laitinen LV, Bergenheim AT, Hariz MI (1992) Leksell's posteroventral pallidotomy in the treatment of Parkinson's disease. J Neurosurg 76:53–61.
99. Laitinen LV, Bergenheim AT, Hariz MI (1992) Ventroposterolateral pallidotomy can abolish all parkinsonian symptoms. Stereotact Funct Neurosurg 58:14–21.
100. Siegfried J, Lippitz B (1994) Bilateral chronic electrostimulation of ventroposterolateral pallidum: a new therapeutic approach for alleviating all parkinsonian symptoms. Neurosurgery 35:1126–1129; discussion 1129–1130.
101. Loher TJ, Burgunder JM, Pohle T, Weber S, Sommerhalder R, Krauss JK (2002) Long-term pallidal deep brain stimulation in patients with advanced Parkinson disease: 1-year follow-up study. J Neurosurg 96:844–853.
102. [No authors listed] (2001) Bilateral deep brain stimulation (DBS) of the subthalamic nucleus (STN) or the globus pallidus interna (GPi) for treatment of advanced Parkinson's disease. Tecnologica MAP Suppl 1–8.
103. Kumar R, Lang AE, Rodriguez-Oroz MC, et al (2000) Deep brain stimulation of the globus pallidus pars interna in advanced Parkinson's disease. Neurology 55: S34–S39.

104. Galvez-Jimenez N, Lozano A, Tasker R, Duff J, Hutchison W, Lang AE (1998) Pallidal stimulation in Parkinson's disease patients with a prior unilateral pallidotomy. Can J Neurolog Sci 25:300–305.
105. Ghika J, Villemure JG, Fankhauser H, Favre J, Assal G, Ghika-Schmid F (1998) Efficiency and safety of bilateral contemporaneous pallidal stimulation (deep brain stimulation) in levodopa-responsive patients with Parkinson's disease with severe motor fluctuations: a 2-year follow-up review. J Neurosurg 89:713–718.
106. Gross C, Rougier A, Guehl D, Boraud T, Julien J, Bioulac B (1997) High-frequency stimulation of the globus pallidus internalis in Parkinson's disease: a study of seven cases. J Neurosurg 87:491–498.
107. Pahwa R, Wilkinson S, Smith D, Lyons K, Miyawaki E, Koller WC (1997) High-frequency stimulation of the globus pallidus for the treatment of Parkinson's disease. Neurology 49:249–253.
108. Peppe A, Pierantozzi M, Bassi A, et al (2004) Stimulation of the subthalamic nucleus compared with the globus pallidus internus in patients with Parkinson disease. J Neurosurg 101:195–200.
109. Volkmann J, Sturm V, Weiss P, et al (1998) Bilateral high-frequency stimulation of the internal globus pallidus in advanced Parkinson's disease. Ann Neurol 44:953–961.
110. Pillon B, Ardouin C, Damier P, et al (2000) Neuropsychological changes between "off" and "on" STN or GPi stimulation in Parkinson's disease. Neurology 55:411–418.
111. Troster AI, Fields JA, Wilkinson SB, et al (1997) Unilateral pallidal stimulation for Parkinson's disease: neurobehavioral functioning before and 3 months after electrode implantation. Neurology 49:1078–1083.
112. Vingerhoets G, Lannoo E, van der Linden C, et al (1999) Changes in quality of life following unilateral pallidal stimulation in Parkinson's disease. J Psychosomat Res 46:247–255.
113. Vingerhoets G, van der Linden C, Lannoo E, et al (1999) Cognitive outcome after unilateral pallidal stimulation in Parkinson's disease. J Neurol Neurosurg Psych 66:297–304.
114. Krause M, Fogel W, Heck A, et al (2001) Deep brain stimulation for the treatment of Parkinson's disease: subthalamic nucleus versus globus pallidus internus. J Neurol Neurosurg Psych 70:464–470.
115. Krack P, Pollak P, Limousin P, et al (1998) Subthalamic nucleus or internal pallidal stimulation in young onset Parkinson's disease. Brain 121:451–457.
116. Burchiel KJ, Anderson VC, Favre J, Hammerstad JP (1999) Comparison of pallidal and subthalamic nucleus deep brain stimulation for advanced Parkinson's disease: results of a randomized, blinded pilot study. Neurosurg 45:1375–1382; discussion 1382–1374.
117. Krack P, Poepping M, Weinert D, Schrader B, Deuschl G (2000) Thalamic, pallidal, or subthalamic surgery for Parkinson's disease? J Neurol 247:II122–134.
118. Volkmann J, Allert N, Voges J, Weiss PH, Freund HJ, Sturm V (2001) Safety and efficacy of pallidal or subthalamic nucleus stimulation in advanced PD. Neurology 56:548–551.
119. Benabid AL, Pollak P, Gao D, et al (1996) Chronic electrical stimulation of the ventralis intermedius nucleus of the thalamus as a treatment of movement disorders. J Neurosurg 84:203–214.
120. Bereznai B, Steude U, Seelos K, Botzel K (2002) Chronic high-frequency globus pallidus internus stimulation in different types of dystonia: a clinical, video, and MRI report of six patients presenting with segmental, cervical, and generalized dystonia. Mov Disord 17:138–144.
121. Coubes P, Roubertie A, Vayssiere N, Hemm S, Echenne B (2000) Treatment of DYT1-generalised dystonia by stimulation of the internal globus pallidus. Lancet 355:2220–2221.

122. Islekel S, Zileli M, Zileli B (1999) Unilateral pallidal stimulation in cervical dystonia. Stereotact Funct Neurosurg 72:248–252.
123. Krauss JK, Loher TJ, Pohle T, et al (2002) Pallidal deep brain stimulation in patients with cervical dystonia and severe cervical dyskinesias with cervical myelopathy. J Neurol Neurosurg Psych 72:249–256.
124. Krauss JK, Pohle T, Weber S, Ozdoba C, Burgunder JM (1999) Bilateral stimulation of globus pallidus internus for treatment of cervical dystonia. Lancet 354:837–838.
125. Kumar R, Dagher A, Hutchison WD, Lang AE, Lozano AM (1999) Globus pallidus deep brain stimulation for generalized dystonia: clinical and PET investigation. Neurology 53:871–874.
126. Tronnier VM, Fogel W (2000) Pallidal stimulation for generalized dystonia. Report of three cases. J Neurosurg 92:453–456.
127. Vayssiere N, Hemm S, Zanca M, et al (2000) Magnetic resonance imaging stereotactic target localization for deep brain stimulation in dystonic children. J Neurosurg 93:784–790.
128. Vesper J, Klostermann F, Funk T, Stockhammer F, Brock M (2002) Deep brain stimulation of the globus pallidus internus (GPI) for torsion dystonia—a report of two cases. Acta Neurochir Suppl 79:83–88.
129. Loher TJ, Hasdemir MG, Burgunder JM, Krauss JK (2000) Long-term follow-up study of chronic globus pallidus internus stimulation for posttraumatic hemidystonia. J Neurosurg 92:457–460.
130. Krack P, Vercueil L (2001) Review of the functional surgical treatment of dystonia. Eur J Neurol 8:389–399.
131. Vercueil L, Krack P, Pollak P (2002) Results of deep brain stimulation for dystonia: a critical reappraisal. Mov Disord 17(Suppl 3):S89–S93.
132. Plaha P, Ben-Shlomo Y, Patel NK, Gill SS (2006) Stimulation of the caudal zona incerta is superior to stimulation of the subthalamic nucleus in improving contralateral parkinsonism. Brain 129:1732–1747.
133. Plaha P, Patel NK, Gill SS (2004) Stimulation of the subthalamic region for essential tremor. J Neurosurg 101:48–54.
134. Bastian AJ, Kelly VE, Revilla FJ, Perlmutter JS, Mink JW (2003) Different effects of unilateral versus bilateral subthalamic nucleus stimulation on walking and reaching in Parkinson's disease. Mov Disord 18:1000–1007.
135. Plaha P, Gill SS (2005) Bilateral deep brain stimulation of the pedunculopontine nucleus for Parkinson's disease. Neuroreport 16:1883–1887.
136. Mazzone P, Lozano A, Stanzione P, et al (2005) Implantation of human pedunculopontine nucleus: a safe and clinically relevant target in Parkinson's disease. Neuroreport 16:1877–1881.
137. Jenkinson N, Nandi D, Aziz TZ, Stein JF (2005) Pedunculopontine nucleus: a new target for deep brain stimulation for akinesia. Neuroreport 16:1875–1876.
138. Leone M, Franzini A, Felisati G, et al (2005) Deep brain stimulation and cluster headache. Neurol Sci 26(Suppl 2):s138–s139.
139. Schoenen J, Di Clemente L, Vandenheede M, et al (2005) Hypothalamic stimulation in chronic cluster headache: a pilot study of efficacy and mode of action. Brain 128:940–947.
140. Leone M, Franzini A, Broggi G, Bussone G (2003) Hypothalamic deep brain stimulation for intractable chronic cluster headache: a 3-year follow-up. Neurol Sci 24(Suppl 2):S143–S145.
141. Franzini A, Ferroli P, Leone M, Broggi G (2003) Stimulation of the posterior hypothalamus for treatment of chronic intractable cluster headaches: first reported series. Neurosurgery 52:1095–1099; discussion 1099–1101.
142. Sprenger T, Boecker H, Tolle TR, Bussone G, May A, Leone M (2004) Specific hypothalamic activation during a spontaneous cluster headache attack. Neurology 62:516–517.

143. Shi LH, Luo F, Woodward D, Chang JY (2006) Deep brain stimulation of the substantia nigra pars reticulata exerts long lasting suppression of amygdala-kindled seizures. Brain Res 1090:202–207.
144. Usui N, Maesawa S, Kajita Y, Endo O, Takebayashi S, Yoshida J (2005) Suppression of secondary generalization of limbic seizures by stimulation of subthalamic nucleus in rats. J Neurosurg 102:1122–1129.
145. Vonck K, Boon P, Claeys P, Dedeurwaerdere S, Achten R, Van Roost D (2005) Long-term deep brain stimulation for refractory temporal lobe epilepsy. Epilepsia 46(Suppl 5):98–99.
146. Graves NM, Fisher RS (2005) Neurostimulation for epilepsy, including a pilot study of anterior nucleus stimulation. Clin Neurosurg 52:127–134.
147. Hodaie M, Wennberg RA, Dostrovsky JO, Lozano AM (2002) Chronic anterior thalamus stimulation for intractable epilepsy. Epilepsia 43:603–608.
148. Velasco AL, Velasco M, Velasco F, et al (2000) Subacute and chronic electrical stimulation of the hippocampus on intractable temporal lobe seizures: preliminary report. Arch Med Res 31:316–328.
149. Velasco F, Velasco M, Jimenez F, et al (2000) Predictors in the treatment of difficult-to-control seizures by electrical stimulation of the centromedian thalamic nucleus. Neurosurgery 47:295–305.
150. Velasco M, Velasco F, Velasco AL, Jimenez F, Brito F, Marquez I (2000) Acute and chronic electrical stimulation of the centromedian thalamic nucleus: modulation of reticulo-cortical systems and predictor factors for generalized seizure control. Arch Med Res 31:304–315.
151. Tellez-Zenteno JF, McLachlan RS, Parrent A, Kubu CS, Wiebe S (2006) Hippocampal electrical stimulation in mesial temporal lobe epilepsy. Neurology 66:1490–1494.
152. Benabid AL, Koudsie A, Benazzouz A, et al (2001) Deep brain stimulation of the corpus luysi (subthalamic nucleus) and other targets in Parkinson's disease. Extension to new indications such as dystonia and epilepsy. J Neurol 248:III37–III47.
153. Benabid AL, Minotti L, Koudsie A, De Saint Martin A, Hirsch E (2002) Antiepileptic effect of high-frequency stimulation of the subthalamic nucleus (corpus luysi) in a case of medically intractable epilepsy caused by focal dysplasia: a 30-month follow-up: technical case report. Neurosurgery 50:1385–1392.
154. Shon YM, Lee KJ, Kim HJ, et al (2005) Effect of chronic deep brain stimulation of the subthalamic nucleus for frontal lobe epilepsy: subtraction SPECT analysis. Stereotact Funct Neurosurg 83:84–90.
155. Vercueil L, Benazzouz A, Deransart C, et al (1998) High-frequency stimulation of the subthalamic nucleus suppresses absence seizures in the rat: comparison with neurotoxic lesions. Epilepsy Res 31:39–46.
156. Nuttin BJ, Gabriels L, van Kuyck K, Cosyns P (2003) Electrical stimulation of the anterior limbs of the internal capsules in patients with severe obsessive-compulsive disorder: anecdotal reports. Neurosurg Clin N Am 14:267–274.
157. Nuttin B, Cosyns P, Demeulemeester H, Gybels J, Meyerson B (1999) Electrical stimulation in anterior limbs of internal capsules in patients with obsessive-compulsive disorder. Lancet 354:1526.
158. Nuttin BJ, Gabriels LA, Cosyns PR, et al (2003) Long-term electrical capsular stimulation in patients with obsessive-compulsive disorder. Neurosurgery 52:1263–1272; discussion 1272–1264.
159. Abelson JL, Curtis GC, Sagher O, et al (2005) Deep brain stimulation for refractory obsessive-compulsive disorder. Biol Psychiatry 57:510–516.
160. Aouizerate B, Cuny E, Martin-Guehl C, et al (2004) Deep brain stimulation of the ventral caudate nucleus in the treatment of obsessive-compulsive disorder and major depression. Case report. J Neurosurg 101:682–686.
161. Canterbury RJ (2003) Deep brain stimulation for obsessive-compulsive disorder. J Neurosurg 98:941–942; discussion 942.

162. Greenberg BD, Malone DA, Friehs GM, et al (2006) Three-year outcomes in deep brain stimulation for highly resistant obsessive-compulsive disorder. Neuropsychopharmacology 31(11):2384–2393.
163. Greenberg BD, Price LH, Rauch SL, et al (2003) Neurosurgery for intractable obsessive-compulsive disorder and depression: critical issues. Neurosurg Clin N Am 14:199–212.
164. Sturm V, Lenartz D, Koulousakis A, et al (2003) The nucleus accumbens: a target for deep brain stimulation in obsessive-compulsive- and anxiety-disorders. J Chem Neuroanat 26:293–299.
165. Tass PA, Klosterkotter J, Schneider F, Lenartz D, Koulousakis A, Sturm V (2003) Obsessive-compulsive disorder: development of demand-controlled deep brain stimulation with methods from stochastic phase resetting. Neuropsychopharmacology 28(Suppl 1):S27–S34.
166. Van Laere K, Nuttin B, Gabriels L, et al (2006) Metabolic imaging of anterior capsular stimulation in refractory obsessive-compulsive disorder: a key role for the subgenual anterior cingulate and ventral striatum. J Nucl Med 47:740–747.
167. Mayberg H (2002) Depression, II: localization of pathophysiology. Am J Psychiatry 159:1979.
168. Mayberg HS (2002) Modulating limbic-cortical circuits in depression: targets of antidepressant treatments. Semin Clin Neuropsychiatry 7:255–268.
169. Mayberg HS, Liotti M, Brannan SK, et al (1999) Reciprocal limbic-cortical function and negative mood: converging PET findings in depression and normal sadness. Am J Psychiatry 156:675–682.
170. Mayberg HS, Lozano AM, Voon V, et al (2005) Deep brain stimulation for treatment-resistant depression. Neuron 45:651–660.
171. Temel Y, Visser-Vandewalle V (2004) Surgery in Tourette syndrome. Mov Disord 19:3–14.
172. Hassler R, Dieckmann G (1970) [Stereotaxic treatment of tics and inarticulate cries or coprolalia considered as motor obsessional phenomena in Gilles de la Tourette's disease]. Rev Neurol (Paris) 123:89–100.
173. Vandewalle V, van der Linden C, Groenewegen HJ, Caemaert J (1999) Stereotactic treatment of Gilles de la Tourette syndrome by high frequency stimulation of thalamus. Lancet 353:724.
174. Visser-Vandewalle V, Temel Y, Boon P, et al (2003) Chronic bilateral thalamic stimulation: a new therapeutic approach in intractable Tourette syndrome. Report of three cases. J Neurosurg 99:1094–1100.
175. Flaherty AW, Williams ZM, Amirnovin R, et al (2005) Deep brain stimulation of the anterior internal capsule for the treatment of Tourette syndrome: technical case report. Neurosurgery 57:E403; discussion E403.
176. Diederich NJ, Kalteis K, Stamenkovic M, Pieri V, Alesch F (2005) Efficient internal pallidal stimulation in Gilles de la Tourette syndrome: a case report. Mov Disord 20:1496–1499.
177. Houeto JL, Karachi C, Mallet L, et al (2005) Tourette's syndrome and deep brain stimulation. J Neurol Neurosurg Psychiatry 76:992–995.
178. Sheer D (1961) Electrical stimulation of the brain: An interdisciplinary survey of neurobehavioral sciences. Austin, TX: University of Texas Press.

# 4

# Deep Brain Stimulation: Patient Selection in Parkinson's Disease, Other Movement Disorders, and Neuropsychiatric Disorders

Mustafa Saad Siddiqui, Thomas Ellis, Stephen S. Tatter, Kelly D. Foote, and Michael S. Okun

## Abstract

Selecting the appropriate candidate for deep brain stimulation (DBS) may be the most important factor to determine the success of surgery *(1–4)*. The process of patient selection appears to vary widely among DBS centers in different regions of the world. The majority of large centers prefer a multidisciplinary approach involving a neurologist, a neurosurgeon, a psychologist, a psychiatrist, and a nurse specialist *(5)*. This chapter focuses on reviewing the factors involved in selecting appropriate DBS candidates for Parkinson's disease (PD) as well as other movement and neuropsychiatric disorders.

**Keywords:** deep brain stimulation, patient selection, Parkinson's disease, movement disorders, multidisciplinary assessment

## The Importance of Multidisciplinary Assessment Prior to DBS Surgery

A complete multidisciplinary assessment (neurologist, neurosurgeon, neuropsychologist, and psychiatrist) should be performed prior to consideration of DBS surgery *(6, 7)*. We usually recommend that the assessments are performed by experienced DBS teams and that the results of individual evaluations are discussed in a multidisciplinary team meeting prior to proceeding with surgery.

## Patient Selection for DBS in PD (Algorithm)

### Role of the Neurologist

*Confirmation of Diagnosis and Evaluation of Severity of Symptoms*

A neurologist plays a central role in the candidate selection process by confirming the PD diagnosis, assessing the severity of symptoms and disability, verifying responsiveness to levodopa and adjunctive medications using objective scales such as the UPDRS, and instilling realistic patient expectations.

The first step in this process is confirming the idiopathic PD diagnosis (6). The clinical evaluation of a PD patient should be focused on uncovering the presence of atypical features, which could indicate atypical parkinsonism (multiple system atrophy, progressive supranuclear palsy, corticobasal degeneration, dementia with diffuse Lewy bodies, vascular, and drug-induced parkinsonism). Possible "red flags" that should indicate atypical parkinsonism include gait ataxia, early appearance of hallucinations and dementia, early autonomic involvement, early and severe postural instability and gait abnormality, vertical gaze palsy, cortical deficits such as agraphaesthesia and apraxia, history of neuroleptic use, and a poor and unsustained response to levodopa.

In general, levodopa-responsive symptoms will improve with DBS (3, 8). An exception to this rule is tremor. Documented accounts of symptom improvement with medications are essential in rendering a PD diagnosis as subjective descriptions by patients of their treatment response can often be misleading (9). It is therefore recommended that objective assessment for levodopa responsiveness be performed by utilizing validated tools such as the motor portion of the Unified Parkinson's Disease Rating Scale (UPDRS) and CAPSIT criteria (6). A minimum 30% improvement in UPDRS motor scores following a levodopa challenge is usually required to justify the risks and benefits of a surgical approach to treatment (6, 10). When judging responsiveness to therapy it is useful to use a supratherapeutic dose during a levodopa challenge (1.5 to 2 times the patient's current dose), and patients should be tested during their best on state condition. The levodopa challenge should occur following a scale performed in a practically defined off state (off medications overnight or for 12 hours).

Once the objective idiopathic PD confirmation has been made, the severity and medical refractoriness of symptoms should be determined. Apart from tremor in some cases, PD symptoms can usually be satisfactorily managed with dopaminergic medications during the initial five years of treatment. Following five or more years of dopaminergic therapy patients typically begin to experience motor fluctuations. Many types of motor fluctuations have been described. Two of the earliest symptoms to appear are dyskinesias (involuntary choreiform/hyperkinetic movements in an on-state) and wearing off (predictable worsening of parkinsonism prior to the next medication dose). These may be present in up to 40% of patients following 4 to 6 years of levodopa therapy (11). As the disease continues to advance, the off states may become less predictable and shorter dose intervals and other medication adjustments may be necessary.

Other types of motor fluctuations may include "delay to on" (the period between ingesting the dose of levodopa and the onset of effect), dose failures

**Algorithm: Suggested Scheme for a Multidisciplinary Approach to Patient Selection for DBS in PD**

---
**Neurologist**
- Confirm diagnosis
- Levodopa challenge and UPDRS motor scoring (preferably video taped)
- Confirm medical refractoriness of symptoms. Possible medication trial
- Address patient expectations from DBS

---

| **Neurosurgeon** | **Psychiatrist** | **Neuropsychologist** |
|---|---|---|
| • Evaluate risks/benefits for DBS.<br>• Explain the operative process | Identify and treat any psychiatric problems | Cognitive and behavioral testing using standardized tests |

---

**Multidisciplinary Clinical Conference**
- Final selection is made based on evaluations by each discipline

---

(when a dose of levodopa fails to produce any effect), on-off state yo-yo-ing (rapid fluctuations between the on and off states), or sudden offs (an unpredictable off state that may be unrelated to the timing of the levodopa dose). In advanced PD, patients spend a considerable amount of time in an off state, and their on states are often complicated by disabling dyskinesias *(11)*. In the hands of an experienced clinician, many medication strategies are available to manage motor fluctuations. When a reasonable number of medication strategies fail to provide satisfactory alleviation of motor symptoms, DBS may be considered. Triage tools such as FLASQ-PD, which has been developed and validated for identification of appropriate DBS surgical candidates, can be utilized in patient selection prior to multidisciplinary screening *(12)*.

*Setting Realistic Patient Expectations*

The importance of instilling realistic patient expectations before surgery cannot be over-emphasized *(2, 13)*. What is perceived as a success by the clinician can be judged as a failure by the patient, especially if patients are not adequately educated on what to expect following surgery. As noted earlier, DBS can improve only those PD symptoms that are demonstrably improved during the best levodopa on state *(3)*. The degree of levodopa responsiveness of the motor symptoms seems to be the best known predictor of the extent of benefit following surgery *(3, 14–16)*. It is important to understand that if on- medication UPDRS scores remain in the moderate to severe PD range, even with a greater than 30% improvement in off scores, the degree of improvement following surgery, may be insufficient for the patient to gain functional independence. As previously mentioned, an exception to this rule is medically refractory tremor where a 30% improvement in UPDRS motor scores does not predict a lack of response to surgery and is therefore not required for DBS candidacy. Typical motor symptoms which respond to DBS include tremor, rigidity, bradykinesia, off state painful dystonia, dyskinesias, and gait dysfunction (Table 4.1). The total amount of daily off time may be considerably reduced as a result of DBS *(15–17)*. "Freezing" usually improves only if it has been proven to be levodopa responsive *(14)*. However, gait and balance changes following surgery are among the least predictable symptoms. Other symptoms which fail to improve with medications will not improve with DBS. Speech, autonomic, cognitive, and behavioral symptoms are not expected to improve with DBS (Table 4.1). It is useful for patients to enumerate and rank their most disabling symptoms and even assign a priority order. Each symptom and the possibility of its improvement should be individually addressed, and this discussion should be documented. DBS has been shown to improve disability and quality of life scores *(18)*.

Although medication dose reduction may be expected with subthalamic nucleus (STN) DBS *(17)*, it should not be included as a patient expectation, but rather should be discussed as a possibility. Patients should understand the significant time commitment required for successful postoperative management. Multiple postoperative visits are needed for treatment optimization (both with medications and stimulation). A useful mnemonic device to improve patient expectations for PD DBS is included in Table 4.2 *(19)*.

### *Role of the Neuropsychologist*

Patients with PD suffer various levels of cognitive deficit. These include deficits in executive functioning *(20)*, problem solving, concept formation, verbal fluency *(21)*, visuospatial function *(22)*, memory *(23)*, attention *(24)*, and set shifting *(25)*. Frank dementia may be present in up to 40% of patients with PD *(26, 27)*. Most groups have been reluctant to perform DBS in patients with significant cognitive impairment *(1)*. However, defining the level of impairment which should preclude surgery has resulted in some controversy. A minimal level of cognitive ability is required to tolerate and cooperate with awake surgery, to accurately articulate symptoms during follow-up visits, and to perform lifestyle modifications and care required following surgery *(6)*.

Table 4.1 Responsiveness of PD Symptoms with DBS.

| PD Symptoms Known to Respond to DBS | PD Symptoms That Do Not Respond Consistency to DBS |
| --- | --- |
| • Motor symptoms, which respond to the best on medication state | • Speech (may worsen) |
| • Rigidity | • Cognition |
| • Tremor | • Gait and postural instability (if not levodopa responsive) |
| • Bradykinesia | • Autonomic symptoms |
| • Dyskinesias, dystonia (if not fixed) | • Mood and behavior |
| • Motor fluctuations | |
| • Gait and postural instability, if levodopa responsive | |
| • Pain as a result of PD sometimes responds to surgery | |
| • Some sleep disorders | |

**Table 4.2** Mnemonic: DBS in PD *(19)*.

**D**oes not cure.

**B**ilateral DBS is often required to improve gait, although sometimes unilateral DBS has a marked effect on walking.

**S**mooths out on/off fluctuations.

**I**mproves tremor, stiffness (rigidity), bradykinesia, and dyskinesia in most cases, but may not completely eliminate them.

**N**ever improves symptoms that are unresponsive to your best "on." For example, if gait or balance do not improve with best medication response, it is very unlikely to improve with surgery.

**P**rogramming visits are likely to occur many times during the first 6 months, and then follow-up visits as frequently as every 6 months. There will be multiple adjustments in the stimulator and in the medications.

**D**ecreases medications in many, but not all patients.

---

There is no consistent evidence that DBS alters or hastens the cognitive decline in PD patients *(28)*, although at least one study did show that STN DBS may adversely affect cognition *(25)*. Decreases in verbal fluency are the most frequently reported cognitive symptom following bilateral STN stimulation *(29, 30)*.

Neuropsychological testing is helpful in excluding patients with dementia. In addition it can also be helpful for separating medication induced encephalopathy from true dementia *(31)*. Commonly used tests for evaluating cognition in PD patients pre- and postsurgery are listed in Table 4.3. Many clinicians use Mattis Dementia Rating Scale (MDRS) scores of <130 *(6)* or mini-mental status scores (MMSE) of <24 *(32)* as cut offs for candidacy for DBS. However, we advise a complete interview and examination of neurocognitive features prior to surgical consideration.

**Role of the Psychiatrist**

The principal role of the psychiatrist is to identify and treat patients with underlying psychiatric conditions, especially those that may be worsened by DBS. Only a minority of centers screen patients psychiatrically but we recommend psychiatric screening as an important safety measure. Suicide (0.5–2.9%) has been reported in patients following bilateral STN DBS *(17, 33–35)*, however the specific relationship of suicide to DBS or surgery has been uncertain *(36)*. Postoperative symptoms of depression, mania, anxiety, panic, and apathy have been described *(30, 33, 34, 37)*. A list of neuropsychiatric side effects from DBS is shown in Table 4.4. However, a cause–effect relationship between DBS and these symptoms has not been definitively established as many of these symptoms may be due to PD. A number of validated tools have been utilized for screening patients with depression. The structured clinical interview (SCID; ref. *38*) is perhaps the most important screening test as this may uncover underlying psychiatric disease, substance abuse, and propensity for future difficulties following the stress of surgery *(39)*. Among the most commonly used tools are the Beck Depression "self-report" Inventory, the Hamilton Depression Rating Scale *(40)*, the Montgomery Asberg Depression Rating Scale *(41)*, the Young Mania scale *(42)*, and the Hamilton

**Table 4.3** Commonly Used Tools for Cognitive Testing *(1)*.

| | |
|---|---|
| Overall cognitive function | Mattis Dementia Rating Scale *(99)* |
| | Mini Mental Status Examination *(100)* |
| Abstraction/reasoning/planning | Wisconsin Card Sorting Test *(101)* |
| | Delis-Kaplan Executive Function System (D-KEFS; ref. *102*) |
| | Matrix Reasoning (Raven's matrices; Wechsler Adult Intelligence Scales Matrix Reasoning; refs. *103* and *104*) |
| | Tower Tests (D-KEFS, Tower of London, Tower of Toronto; refs. *102* and *105*) |
| Attention/working memory | Digit Span *(106)* |
| | Spatial Span *(106)* |
| | Symbol Search *(106)* |
| | Trailmaking *(107)* |
| | Stroop *(108)* |
| | Digit Symbol/Symbol Digit *(104)* |
| | Letter Number Sequencing *(104)* |
| Visuoperceptual | Hooper Visual Organization Test |
| | Judgement of Line Orientation *(109)* |
| | Block Design *(104)* |
| Memory | Prose (Logical Memory; ref. *106*) |
| | List learning (Hopkins Verbal Learning Test, California Verbal Learning Test, Auditory Verbal Learning Test [after Rey]; Selective Reminding Test [after Buschke]; ref. *107*) |
| | Wechsler Memory Scale III *(106)* |
| | Facial Recognition *(106)* |
| | Benton Visual Memory Test Recognition *(110)* |
| | Brief Visual Memory Test Revised *(111)* |
| Language | Letter and category fluency *(107)* |
| | Boston Naming Test *(112)* |
| | Multilingual Aphasia Examination *(113)* |
| | Complex Ideational Material *(114)* |

List of validated and non-validated tests commonly used in cognitive testing in patients with Parkinson's disease *(1)*.

Anxiety Rating Scale *(43)*. DBS should be deferred in patients with active psychiatric issues, and should be closely monitored following surgery in patients with treated psychiatric co-morbidity.

**Role of the Neurosurgeon**

The neurosurgeon and the neurologist should work closely to evaluate the benefits and risks of DBS. Together they share the responsibility for evaluating the degree of disability as well as discussing patient expectations. Evaluating the surgical risks and carefully explaining all details of the procedure to the patient and family is usually performed by the neurosurgeon. Possible complications related to the surgical procedure, the implanted device, and the stimulation conditions are listed in Table 4.4.

**Table 4.4** Possible Complications of DBS *(15, 17, 18, 25, 33, 46, 72, 115–121)*.

| Surgery-related | Hardware-related | Stimulation-related |
|---|---|---|
| Seizure: <1 to 3% | Device malfunction | Paresthesias |
| Hemorrhage: 2–3% | Lead fracture | Muscle contractions |
| Fatal cerebral hemorrhage: <1% | Lead migration | Dysarthria |
| Infection: 2–25% (vast majority are superficial) | Lead disconnection | Diplopia |
| Permanent neurologic deficit: 0–0.6% | Skin erosion | Cognitive changes |
| Misplaced leads: 0–12.5% |  | Depression |
| Venous air embolism |  | Mania |
|  |  | Suicide |
|  |  | Pseudobulbar affect |
|  |  | Obsessive/compulsive thoughts |
|  |  | Anxiety/panic attacks |
|  |  | Aggressive behavior |

# Risk factors for DBS

### Age

Although there is an impression that younger patients have less surgical risk, no well defined upper age limit has been set for DBS surgery *(1)*. The majority of centers have arbitrarily utilized an upper age limit of 75 years but there is no consensus on what a safe upper age limit should be for DBS surgery. Older age is associated with a higher prevalence of medical comorbidities such as amyloid angiopathy *(44)* and cognitive impairment *(45)*. Some but not all reports indicate lower rates of efficacy in DBS in older patients when compared to younger patients *(3, 8)*, but these differences may ultimately fail to be significant and remain to be better elucidated by future studies *(46)*. Transient postoperative confusion sometimes occurs following DBS *(47)* and patients should be warned of this possibility. It is recommended that patients older than 75 should be evaluated on a case-by-case basis and consideration for the level of disability, degree of expected improvement, presence of medical comorbidities, life expectancy, cognition, and the ability to satisfactorily meet the operative and postoperative requirement of surgery should all be weighed rather than age alone.

### Imaging

MRI is recommended as part of the pre-surgical evaluation for DBS[1]. MRI helps to exclude patients with atypical parkinsonism, moderate to severe cortical atrophy, significant vascular white matter changes, and structural lesions. One report found that significant white matter changes were associated with a suboptimal outcome *(48)*. Mild cortical atrophy is frequently present in PD. Safety and efficacy of DBS in patients with severe cortical atrophy has not been carefully studied but many surgeons will exclude these patients because of subdural bleeding risk, less certain target localization, and co-morbid cognitive dysfunction. MRI is not necessarily required for DBS. Some groups effectively use ventriculography *(17, 49, 50)*. Other groups use CT scanning. Each DBS team should employ the technique they are most comfortable with and refine their targets with microelectrode recording *(50, 51)*.

### Medical Co-morbidities

The role of individual co-morbidities such as diabetes, heart disease, pulmonary dysfunction and hypertension in predicting the outcome of DBS has not been specifically studied. Uncontrolled hypertension poses an increased risk of bleeding, and has been associated with increased frequency of hemorrhage following microelectrode recording *(52, 53)*. Uncontrolled diabetes can result in increased risk of infection and possibly delayed healing. Because of safety concerns, patients who are expected to require frequent body MRI due to a medical condition may not be appropriate for DBS.

### Patients with Prior Ablative Surgery

DBS can be safely performed in patients who have had prior ablative surgery for PD *(54–56)*. Studies have reported varying degrees of success with bilateral STN DBS in patients with previous unilateral pallidotomy *(54, 56)* and thalamotomy *(57)*. Bilateral STN DBS in patients with bilateral pallidotomy has not been uniformly successful unless the previous ablative lesions were misplaced or too small *(58)*. Similarly, PD patients who have had unilateral STN DBS contralateral to a previous pallidotomy may experience some problems in the adjustment of medications *(59)*. Ipsilateral DBS on the same side as a lesion but in a different target has also been performed in a small number of cases *(57)* and results, although less robust, may be meaningful in individual patients. The most important factors to consider in patients with previous ablative surgery are the size of the previous lesion, lesion location, and responsiveness of symptoms to a levodopa challenge.

## Patient Selection for DBS in Dystonia

A humanitarian device exemption was issued by the U.S. Food and Drug Administration for the treatment of medically refractory symptoms of generalized dystonia. DBS has recently also been reported to be effective in cervical dystonia *(60)* and tardive dystonia *(61)*. DBS may be the best available treatment for disabling symptoms of generalized, cervical, tardive and other dystonias which are medically refractory, and have not developed fixed muscle contractures. Open-label *(62)* and double-blind trials *(63)* of bilateral globus pallidus interna (GPi) DBS have shown an approximate 50 to 80% improvement in 12-month motor scores in patients with both DYT-1 and non-DYT-1 generalized dystonia. Bilateral GPi DBS in patients with cervical dystonia has shown 64% improvement in the Toronto Western Spasmodic Torticollis Rating Scale (TWSTRS), 60% improvement in disability scores, and 60% improvement in pain relief *(64)*. There may be less interpatient variability in response to DBS in patients with cervical dystonia when compared to other dystonias, but this remains to be confirmed *(65)*. The response to DBS in secondary dystonias and hemi-dystonias is less predictable and has ranged from no response *(66, 67)* to significant improvement in functional benefit and pain *(68, 69)*. DBS has shown promising results in some patients with primary segmental dystonias including Meige syndrome *(65)*. Although there are only a few uncontrolled trials of DBS in tardive dystonia, rapid and sustained relief of symptoms has been observed with bilateral pallidal DBS *(61)*.

In evaluating a dystonic patient for DBS, the history and examination should focus on the identification of secondary causes of dystonia. Birth, developmental, medication, toxin, family and traumatic histories are important to identify. Brain imaging may be required to exclude secondary causes of dystonia. Metabolic disorders which produce dystonia such as glutaric acidemia, pantothenate kinase deficiciency, and Wilson's disease should be excluded (although in select cases DBS may also help with these disorders). If the dystonia is generalized and onset has occurred before age 26 patients should be tested for the DYT 1 gene *(70)*.

Examination should include careful characterization of the dystonia and evaluation for reducibility of potential contractures. Exclusion of contractures may in some cases require anaesthesia. Contractures that fail to reduce are not expected to respond to DBS. Mobile and phasic dystonic movements appear to be more responsive to DBS than more fixed dystonic postures *(63)*. Patients selected for surgical intervention should have failed trials of levodopa to exclude dopa-responsive dystonia and have experienced suboptimal responses to anticholinergic drugs, baclofen and, in some cases, tetrabenazine. In cases of cervical and other focal dystonias, an adequate trial of botulinum toxin treatment should be administered. Patients need to be educated that unlike PD and essential tremor (ET), dystonia symptoms frequently show delayed improvement and require repeated programming sessions *(63)*. A complete multidisciplinary assessment (neurologist, neurosurgeon, neuropsychologist, and psychiatrist) should be performed prior to consideration of DBS surgery for dystonia.

## Patient Selection for DBS in ET

DBS of the ventral intermediate (VIM) nucleus of the thalamus has proven to be a very effective and safe treatment in patients with medically refractory ET *(71–74)*. Appropriate surgical candidates have experienced postural and action tremors that significantly impair their ability to perform simple everyday tasks *(75)*. ET candidates should have failed medication trials with primidone, a beta blocker, a benzodiazepine, and in some cases more novel anticonvulsant medications. The typical candidate has medication refractory symptoms that affect quality of life and ability to work *(75)*. Medical co-morbidities, imaging, and a complete neurological, neurosurgical, psychological, and psychiatric evaluation should be reviewed prior to consideration of DBS. Formal neuropsychological testing is not usually required in patients with ET. Although mild cognitive abnormalities have been identified in patients with ET *(76–78)*, these are not usually clinically significant unless a coincidental underlying dementia is also present.

Patients may undergo unilateral or bilateral VIM DBS. Unilateral stimulation reliably results in marked improvement of contralateral action, postural and resting tremor and in some cases may also produce a mild ipsilateral effect *(79–81)*. Unilateral VIM stimulation does not reliably improve voice tremor *(74, 82, 83)*. Voice tremor, therefore, should not be a primary indication for DBS. Head tremor has been shown to improve following unilateral VIM DBS *(71, 84, 85)* and to show an even greater sustained response following bilateral stimulation.

Many patients elect bilateral stimulation for ET. Patients should be counseled that dysarthria and gait dysequilibrium are more common with bilateral DBS *(86, 87)*. One approach is to stage the operations and perform the first procedure for either the dominant hand or the more affected side. A decision can then be made later as to the need for contralateral surgery.

## Patient Selection for DBS in Neuropsychiatric Disorders

DBS is in very early experimental stages for patients with medication refractory depression, Tourette's syndrome (TS), and obsessive–compulsive disorder (OCD). It may eventually be applied to other disorders. DBS applied in these targets should be performed only under the guidance of institutional review and ethics board approval.

The criteria for using DBS in depression have yet to be fully developed, but a similar multidisciplinary screening including failure of an adequate number of antidepressants of different classes and also electroconvulsive therapy will likely be required. Further, it is unknown which patients with major depression will benefit from this procedure. Targets currently under study include white matter tracts adjacent to the subgenual region of the cingulate gyrus, and the nucleus accumbens region *(88, 89)*.

Currently studied targets for motor symptoms of TS include the centromedian-parafascicular complex of the thalamus, the anterior limb of the internal capsule, and the ventral and postero-ventral GPi *(90–94)*. The Tourette's Syndrome Association published guidelines for appropriate patient selection criteria and appropriate conduct of TS trials *(95)*. A full multidisciplinary evaluation must be performed and patients must meet standards for age (past the age where tics wane) and disability and have had documented unsuccessful medication trials in the hands of experts before consideration of DBS. Early results have been promising for motor tics, but the extent to which behavioral features have responded remains unclear *(90, 92, 93)*.

DBS for OCD has been performed using several targets including the anterior limb of the internal capsule/nucleus accumbens, the STN, and the striatum *(91, 96, 97)*. The best target is unknown but preliminary studies of the anterior limb of the internal capsule and nucleus accumbens have been promising *(97, 98)*. The selection criteria for patients in these studies have been previously discussed *(95)*, but must include a full multidisciplinary evaluation and medication refractoriness. A psychiatrist is a crucial member of the team in addressing any of the neuropsychiatric indications for DBS.

## Conclusion

In summary, DBS can be an effective surgical treatment for PD, ET, and dystonia and has the potential to expand into new targets for the treatment of neuropsychiatric disorders. The most important step in successful DBS remains attention to selecting the appropriate candidate. A multi-disciplinary approach is the best and safest method for selecting DBS patients.

## References

1. Lang AE, Houeto JL, Krack P, et al (2006) Deep brain stimulation: preoperative issues. Mov Disord 21(Suppl 14):S171–S196.
2. Okun MS, Tagliati M, Pourfar M, et al (2005) Management of referred deep brain stimulation failures: a retrospective analysis from 2 movement disorders centers. Arch Neurol 62(8):1250–125.
3. Charles PD, Van Blercom N, Krack P, et al (2002) Predictors of effective bilateral subthalamic nucleus stimulation for PD. Neurology 59(6):932–934.
4. Lang AE, Widner H (2002) Deep brain stimulation for Parkinson's disease: patient selection and evaluation. Mov Disord 17(Suppl 3):S94–S101.
5. Ondo WG, Bronte-Stewart H (2005) The North American survey of placement and adjustment strategies for deep brain stimulation. Stereotact Funct Neurosurg 83(4):142–147.
6. Defer GL, Widner H, Marie RM, Remy P, Levivier M (1999) Core assessment program for surgical interventional therapies in Parkinson's disease (CAPSIT-PD). Mov Disord 14(4):572–584.
7. Houeto JL, Damier P, Bejjani PB, et al (2000) Subthalamic stimulation in Parkinson disease: a multidisciplinary approach. Arch Neurol 57(4):461–465.
8. Welter ML, Houeto JL, Tezenas du Montcel S, et al (2002) Clinical predictive factors of subthalamic stimulation in Parkinson's disease. Brain 125(Pt 3): 575–583.
9. Cubo E, Rojo A, Ramos S, et al (2002) The importance of educational and psychological factors in Parkinson's disease quality of life. Eur J Neurol 9(6):589–593.
10. Lopiano L, Rizzone M, Bergamasco B, et al (2002) Deep brain stimulation of the subthalamic nucleus in PD: an analysis of the exclusion causes. J Neurolog Sci 195(2):167–170.
11. Ahlskog JE, Muenter MD (2001) Frequency of levodopa-related dyskinesias and motor fluctuations as estimated from the cumulative literature. Mov Disord 16(3):448–458.
12. Okun MS, Fernandez HH, Pedraza O, et al (2004) Development and initial validation of a screening tool for Parkinson disease surgical candidates. Neurology 63(1):161–163.
13. Hariz MI (2005) What is deep brain stimulation "failure" and how do we manage our own failures? Arch Neurol 62(12):1938; author reply 9.
14. Bejjani BP, Gervais D, Arnulf I, et al (2000) Axial parkinsonian symptoms can be improved: the role of levodopa and bilateral subthalamic stimulation. J Neurol Neurosurg Psychiatry 68(5):595–600.
15. Benabid AL, Benazzouz A, Hoffmann D, Limousin P, Krack P, Pollak P (1998) Long-term electrical inhibition of deep brain targets in movement disorders. Mov Disord 13(Suppl 3):119–125.
16. Krack P, Pollak P, Limousin P, et al (1998) Subthalamic nucleus or internal pallidal stimulation in young onset Parkinson's disease. Brain 121(Pt 3):451–457.

17. Krack P, Batir A, Van Blercom N, et al (2003) Five-year follow-up of bilateral stimulation of the subthalamic nucleus in advanced Parkinson's disease. N Engl J Med 349(20):1925–1934.
18. Deuschl G, Schade-Brittinger C, Krack P, et al (2006) A randomized trial of deep-brain stimulation for Parkinson's disease. N Engl J Med 355(9):896–908.
19. Okun MS, Foote KD (2004) A mnemonic for Parkinson disease patients considering DBS: a tool to improve perceived outcome of surgery. Neurologist 10(5):290.
20. Pillon BFB, Levy R, Dubois B (2001) Cognitive deficits and dementia in Parkinson's disease. In: F Boller and S Cappa, eds. Handbook of Neuropsychology, second edition. Amsterdam: Elsevier Science, pp. 311–371.
21. Stern Y, Richards M, Sano M, Mayeux R (1993) Comparison of cognitive changes in patients with Alzheimer's and Parkinson's disease. Arch Neurol 50(10):1040–1045.
22. Levin BE, Llabre MM, Reisman S, et al (1991) Visuospatial impairment in Parkinson's disease. Neurology 41(3):365–369.
23. Helkala EL, Laulumaa V, Soininen H, Riekkinen PJ (1989) Different error pattern of episodic and semantic memory in Alzheimer's disease and Parkinson's disease with dementia. Neuropsychologia 27(10):1241–1248.
24. Litvan I, Mohr E, Williams J, Gomez C, Chase TN (1991) Differential memory and executive functions in demented patients with Parkinson's and Alzheimer's disease. J Neurol Neurosurg Psychiatry 54(1):25–29.
25. Saint-Cyr JA, Trepanier LL, Kumar R, Lozano AM, Lang AE (2000) Neuropsychological consequences of chronic bilateral stimulation of the subthalamic nucleus in Parkinson's disease. Brain 123(Pt 10):2091–2108.
26. Emre M (2003) Dementia associated with Parkinson's disease. Lancet Neurol 2(4):229–237.
27. Cummings JL (1988) Intellectual impairment in Parkinson's disease: clinical, pathologic, and biochemical correlates. J Geriatr Psychiatry Neurol 1(1):24–36.
28. Ardouin C, Pillon B, Peiffer E, et al (1999) Bilateral subthalamic or pallidal stimulation for Parkinson's disease affects neither memory nor executive functions: a consecutive series of 62 patients. Ann Neurol 46(2):217–223.
29. Alegret M, Junque C, Valldeoriola F, et al (2001) Effects of bilateral subthalamic stimulation on cognitive function in Parkinson disease. Arch Neurol 58(8):1223–1227.
30. Rodriguez RL, Miller K, Bowers D, et al (2005) Mood and cognitive changes with deep brain stimulation. What we know and where we should go. Minerva Medica 96(3):125–144.
31. Saint-Cyr JA, Taylor AE, Lang AE (1993) Neuropsychological and psychiatric side effects in the treatment of Parkinson's disease. Neurology 43(12 Suppl 6):S47–S52.
32. Pollak P (2000) Deep Brain Stimulation. Annual Course of the American Academy of Neurology.
33. Houeto JL, Mesnage V, Mallet L, et al (2002) Behavioural disorders, Parkinson's disease and subthalamic stimulation. J Neurol Neurosurg Psychiatry 72(6):701–707.
34. Voon V, Moro E, Saint-Cyr JA, Lozano AM, Lang AE (2005) Psychiatric symptoms following surgery for Parkinson's disease with an emphasis on subthalamic stimulation. Advances Neurol 96:130–147.
35. Voon VPK, Lang A, Lozano AM, Dujardin K, Tamma F, Thobois S, Schupbach M, Herzog J, Samanta J, Kubu C, Poon YY, Ardouin C, Rossignol H, Saint Cyr J, Moro E (2006) Frequency and risk factors for suicidal outcomes following subthalamic deep brain stimulation for Parkinson's disease: A multicenter retrospective survey. 58th Annual Meeting of American Academy of Neurology, San Diego, CA.
36. Voon VKP, Lang A, et al (2006) Frequency and risk factors for suicidal outcomes following subthalamic deep brain stimulation for Parkinson's disease: a multicenter retrospective study. Neurology 66(suppl 2):A195.

37. Takeshita S, Kurisu K, Trop L, Arita K, Akimitsu T, Verhoeff NP (2005) Effect of subthalamic stimulation on mood state in Parkinson's disease: evaluation of previous facts and problems. Neurosurg Rev 28(3):179–186; discussion 87.
38. Spitzer RL, Williams JB, Gibbon M, First MB (1992) The Structured Clinical Interview for DSM-III-R (SCID). I: History, rationale, and description. Arch Gen Psychiatry 49(8):624–629.
39. Voon V, Kubu C, Krack P, Houeto JL, Troster AI (2006) Deep brain stimulation: neuropsychological and neuropsychiatric issues. Mov Disord 21(Suppl 14): S305–S327.
40. Leentjens AF, Verhey FR, Lousberg R, Spitsbergen H, Wilmink FW (2000) The validity of the Hamilton and Montgomery-Asberg depression rating scales as screening and diagnostic tools for depression in Parkinson's disease. Int J Geriatr Psychiatry 15(7):644–649.
41. Montgomery SA, Asberg M (1979) A new depression scale designed to be sensitive to change. Br J Psychiatry 134:382–389.
42. Young RC, Biggs JT, Ziegler VE, Meyer DA (1978) A rating scale for mania: reliability, validity and sensitivity. Br J Psychiatry 133:429–435.
43. Guy W (1976) 048 HAMA Hamilton Anxiety Scale: ECDEU assessment manual. Bethesda, MD: Department of Health and Human Services, Public Health Service, Alcohol, Drug Abuse and Mental Health Administration, pp. 194–198.
44. Vinters HV (1987) Cerebral amyloid angiopathy. A critical review. Stroke 18(2):311–324.
45. Ritchie K, Touchon J (2000) Mild cognitive impairment: conceptual basis and current nosological status. Lancet 355(9199):225–228.
46. Kleiner-Fisman G, Fisman DN, Sime E, Saint-Cyr JA, Lozano AM, Lang AE (2003) Long-term follow up of bilateral deep brain stimulation of the subthalamic nucleus in patients with advanced Parkinson disease. J Neurosurg 99(3):489–495.
47. Hariz MI (2002) Complications of deep brain stimulation surgery. Mov Disord 17(Suppl 3):S162–S166.
48. Broggi G, Franzini A, Ferroli P, et al (2001) Effect of bilateral subthalamic electrical stimulation in Parkinson's disease. Surg Neurol 56(2):89–94; discussion 6.
49. Benabid AL, Krack PP, Benazzouz A, Limousin P, Koudsie A, Pollak P (2000) Deep brain stimulation of the subthalamic nucleus for Parkinson's disease: methodologic aspects and clinical criteria. Neurology 55(12 Suppl 6):S40–S44.
50. Starr PA, Christine CW, Theodosopoulos PV, et al (2002) Implantation of deep brain stimulators into the subthalamic nucleus: technical approach and magnetic resonance imaging-verified lead locations. J Neurosurg 97(2):370–387.
51. Bejjani BP, Dormont D, Pidoux B, et al (2000) Bilateral subthalamic stimulation for Parkinson's disease by using three-dimensional stereotactic magnetic resonance imaging and electrophysiological guidance. J Neurosurg 92(4):615–625.
52. Binder DK, Rau GM, Starr PA (2005) Risk factors for hemorrhage during microelectrode-guided deep brain stimulator implantation for movement disorders. Neurosurgery 56(4):722–732; discussion 32.
53. Binder DK, Rau G, Starr PA (2003) Hemorrhagic complications of microelectrode-guided deep brain stimulation. Stereotact Funct Neurosurg 80(1–4):28–31.
54. Moro E, Esselink RA, Van Blercom N, et al (2000) Bilateral subthalamic nucleus stimulation in a parkinsonian patient with previous unilateral pallidotomy and thalamotomy. Mov Disord 15(4):753–755.
55. Mogilner AY, Sterio D, Rezai AR, Zonenshayn M, Kelly PJ, Beric A (2002) Subthalamic nucleus stimulation in patients with a prior pallidotomy. J Neurosurg 96(4):660–665.
56. Kleiner-Fisman G, Fisman DN, Zamir O, et al (2004) Subthalamic nucleus deep brain stimulation for parkinson's disease after successful pallidotomy: clinical and electrophysiological observations. Mov Disord 19(10):1209–1214.

57. Goto S, Yamada K, Ushio Y (2004) Subthalamic nucleus stimulation in a parkinsonian patient with previous bilateral thalamotomy. J Neurol Neurosur Psychiatry 75(1):164–165.
58. Samii A, Giroux ML, Slimp JC, Goodkin R (2003) Bilateral subthalamic nucleus stimulation after bilateral pallidotomies in a patient with advanced Parkinson's disease. Parkinsonism Related Disord 9(3):159–162.
59. Merello M (1999) Subthalamic stimulation contralateral to a previous pallidotomy: an erroneous indication? Mov Disord 14(5):890.
60. Krauss JK, Loher TJ, Pohle T, et al (2002) Pallidal deep brain stimulation in patients with cervical dystonia and severe cervical dyskinesias with cervical myelopathy. J Neurol Neurosurg Psychiatry 72(2):249–256.
61. Trottenberg T, Volkmann J, Deuschl G, et al (2005) Treatment of severe tardive dystonia with pallidal deep brain stimulation. Neurology 64(2):344–346.
62. Coubes P, Cif L, El Fertit H, et al (2004) Electrical stimulation of the globus pallidus internus in patients with primary generalized dystonia: long-term results. J Neurosurg 101(2):189–194.
63. Vidailhet M, Vercueil L, Houeto JL, et al (2005) Bilateral deep-brain stimulation of the globus pallidus in primary generalized dystonia. N Engl J Med 352(5):459–467.
64. Yianni J, Bain P, Giladi N, et al (2003) Globus pallidus internus deep brain stimulation for dystonic conditions: a prospective audit. Mov Disord 18(4):436–442.
65. Krauss JK, Yianni J, Loher TJ, Aziz TZ (2004) Deep brain stimulation for dystonia. J Clin Neurophysiol 21(1):18–30.
66. Krauss JK, Jankovic J (2002) Head injury and posttraumatic movement disorders. Neurosurgery 50(5):927–939; discussion 39–40.
67. Yianni J, Bain PG, Gregory RP, et al (2003) Post-operative progress of dystonia patients following globus pallidus internus deep brain stimulation. Eur J Neurol 10(3):239–247.
68. Loher TJ, Hasdemir MG, Burgunder JM, Krauss JK (2000) Long-term follow-up study of chronic globus pallidus internus stimulation for posttraumatic hemidystonia. J Neurosurg 92(3):457–460.
69. Vercueil L, Pollak P, Fraix V, et al (2001) Deep brain stimulation in the treatment of severe dystonia. J Neurol 248(8):695–700.
70. Ozelius L, Kramer PL, Moskowitz CB, et al (1989) Human gene for torsion dystonia located on chromosome 9q32–q34. Neuron 2(5):1427–1434.
71. Koller WC, Lyons KE, Wilkinson SB, Troster AI, Pahwa R (2001) Long-term safety and efficacy of unilateral deep brain stimulation of the thalamus in essential tremor. Mov Disord 16(3):464–468.
72. Limousin P, Speelman JD, Gielen F, Janssens M (1999) Multicentre European study of thalamic stimulation in parkinsonian and essential tremor. J Neurol Neurosurg Psychiatry 66(3):289–296.
73. Rehncrona S, Johnels B, Widner H, Tornqvist AL, Hariz M, Sydow O (2003) Long-term efficacy of thalamic deep brain stimulation for tremor: double-blind assessments. Mov Disord 18(2):163–170.
74. Sydow O, Thobois S, Alesch F, Speelman JD (2003) Multicentre European study of thalamic stimulation in essential tremor: a six year follow up. J Neurol Neurosurg Psychiatry 74(10):1387–1391.
75. Lyons KE, Pahwa R (2004) Deep brain stimulation and essential tremor. J Clin Neurophysiol 21(1):2–5.
76. Lombardi WJ, Woolston DJ, Roberts JW, Gross RE (2001) Cognitive deficits in patients with essential tremor. Neurology 57(5):785–790.
77. Gasparini M, Bonifati V, Fabrizio E, et al (2001) Frontal lobe dysfunction in essential tremor: a preliminary study. J Neurol 248(5):399–402.
78. Lacritz LH, Dewey R Jr, Giller C, Cullum CM (2002) Cognitive functioning in individuals with "benign" essential tremor. J Int Neuropsychol Soc 8(1):125–129.

79. Troster AI, Fields JA, Pahwa R, et al (1999) Neuropsychological and quality of life outcome after thalamic stimulation for essential tremor. Neurology 53(8):1774–1780.
80. Kumar R, Lozano AM, Sime E, Halket E, Lang AE (1999) Comparative effects of unilateral and bilateral subthalamic nucleus deep brain stimulation. Neurology 53(3):561–566.
81. Kumar K, Kelly M, Toth C (1999) Deep brain stimulation of the ventral intermediate nucleus of the thalamus for control of tremors in Parkinson's disease and essential tremor. Stereotact Funct Neurosurg 72(1):47–61.
82. Carpenter MA, Pahwa R, Miyawaki KL, Wilkinson SB, Searl JP, Koller WC (1998) Reduction in voice tremor under thalamic stimulation. Neurology 50(3):796–798.
83. Obwegeser AA, Uitti RJ, Turk MF, Strongosky AJ, Wharen RE (2000) Thalamic stimulation for the treatment of midline tremors in essential tremor patients. Neurology 54(12):2342–2344.
84. Koller WC, Lyons KE, Wilkinson SB, Pahwa R (1999) Efficacy of unilateral deep brain stimulation of the VIM nucleus of the thalamus for essential head tremor. Mov Disord 14(5):847–850.
85. Ondo W, Jankovic J, Schwartz K, Almaguer M, Simpson RK (1998) Unilateral thalamic deep brain stimulation for refractory essential tremor and Parkinson's disease tremor. Neurology 51(4):1063–1069.
86. Ondo W, Almaguer M, Jankovic J, Simpson RK (2001) Thalamic deep brain stimulation: comparison between unilateral and bilateral placement. Arch Neurol 58(2):218–222.
87. Putzke JD, Uitti RJ, Obwegeser AA, Wszolek ZK, Wharen RE (2005) Bilateral thalamic deep brain stimulation: midline tremor control. J Neurol Neurosurg Psychiatry 76(5):684–690.
88. Mayberg HS, Lozano AM, Voon V, et al (2005) Deep brain stimulation for treatment-resistant depression. Neuron 45(5):651–660.
89. Greenberg BD, Price LH, Rauch SL, et al (2003) Neurosurgery for intractable obsessive-compulsive disorder and depression: critical issues. Neurosurg Clin North Am 14(2):199–212.
90. Houeto JL, Karachi C, Mallet L, et al (2005) Tourette's syndrome and deep brain stimulation. J Neurol Neurosurg Psychiatry 76(7):992–995.
91. Visser-Vandewalle V, Temel Y, Boon P, et al (2003) Chronic bilateral thalamic stimulation: a new therapeutic approach in intractable Tourette syndrome. Report of three cases. J Neurosurg 99(6):1094–1100.
92. Visser-Vandewalle V, Ackermans L, van der Linden C, et al (2006) Deep brain stimulation in Gilles de la Tourette's syndrome. Neurosurgery 58(3):E590.
93. Ackermans L, Temel Y, Cath D, et al (2006) Deep brain stimulation in Tourette's syndrome: two targets? Mov Disord 21(5):709–713.
94. Flaherty AW, Williams ZM, Amirnovin R, et al (2005) Deep brain stimulation of the anterior internal capsule for the treatment of Tourette syndrome: technical case report. Neurosurgery 57(4 Suppl):E403; discussion E.
95. Mink JW, Walkup J, Frey KA, Como P, Cath D, DeLong MR, Erenberg G, Jankovic J, Juncos J, Leckman JF, Swerdlow N, Visser-Vandewalle V, Vitek JL, Tourette Syndrome Association, Inc (2006) Patient selection and assessment recommendations for deep brain stimulation in Tourette syndrome. Mov Disord 99:89–98.
96. Gabriels L, Cosyns P, Nuttin B, Demeulemeester H, Gybels J (2003) Deep brain stimulation for treatment-refractory obsessive-compulsive disorder: psychopathological and neuropsychological outcome in three cases. Acta psychiatrica Scandinavica 107(4):275–282.
97. Nuttin B, Cosyns P, Demeulemeester H, Gybels J, Meyerson B (1999) Electrical stimulation in anterior limbs of internal capsules in patients with obsessive-compulsive disorder. Lancet 354(9189):1526.

98. Sturm V, Lenartz D, Koulousakis A, et al (2003) The nucleus accumbens: a target for deep brain stimulation in obsessive-compulsive- and anxiety-disorders. J Chem Neuroanat 26(4):293–299.
99. Jurica PJ LC, Mattis S (2001) Dementia Rating Scale-2. Lutz, FL: Psychological Assessment Resources.
100. Folstein MF, Folstein SE, McHugh PR (1975) "Mini-mental state." A practical method for grading the cognitive state of patients for the clinician. J Psychiatric Res 12(3):189–198.
101. Heaton RK CG, Talley JL, et al (1993) Wisconsin Card Sorting Test: manual revised and expanded. Odessa, FL: Psychological Assessment Resources.
102. Delis DKE, Kramer J (2001) Delis-Kaplan Executive Function Scale. San Antonio, TX: Psychological Corporation.
103. Raven J SB, Birchfield M, et al (1990) Manual for Raven's Progressive Matrices and Vocabulary Scales: research supplement 3 - a compendium of North American normative and validity studies. Oxford: Oxford Psychologists Press.
104. Wechsler D. Wechsler Adult Intelligence Scale-III. San Antonio TPC.
105. Lezak MDHD, Loring DW (2004) Neuropsychological Assessment, fourth edition. New York: Oxford University Press.
106. Wechsler D (1997) Wechsler Memory Scale. San Antonio, TX: Psychological Corporation.
107. Spreen OSE (1998) A compendium of neuropsychological tests: administration, norms, and commentary, second edition. New York: Oxford University Press.
108. Golden C (1978) Stroop Color and Word Test. Stoelting, Chicago.
109. Benton ALSA, Hamsher K, Varney NR, Spreen O (1994) Contributions to Neuropsychological Assessment, A Clinical Manual, second edition. New York: Oxford University Press.
110. Benton AL Revised Visual Retention Test teNYPC.
111. Benedict RHB Brief Visuospatial Memory Test-Revised. Odessa FPAR.
112. Kaplan EF GH, Weintraub S (1983) The Boston Naming Test. Philadelphia, PA: Lea and Febiger.
113. Benton ALHK, Sivan AB (1994) Multilingual Aphasia Examination, third edition. San Antonio, TX: Psychological Corporation.
114. Goodglass H, Kaplan E (1987) Boston Diagnostic Aphasia Examination (BDAE), 2nd ed. Philadelphia, PA: Lea and Febiger.
115. Lyons KE, Wilkinson SB, Overman J, Pahwa R (2004) Surgical and hardware complications of subthalamic stimulation: a series of 160 procedures. Neurology 63(4):612–616.
116. Oh MY, Abosch A, Kim SH, Lang AE, Lozano AM (2002) Long-term hardware-related complications of deep brain stimulation. Neurosurgery 50(6):1268–1274; discussion 74–76.
117. (2001) Deep-brain stimulation of the subthalamic nucleus or the pars interna of the globus pallidus in Parkinson's disease. N Engl J Med 345(13):956–963.
118. Kulisevsky J, Berthier ML, Gironell A, Pascual-Sedano B, Molet J, Pares P (2002) Mania following deep brain stimulation for Parkinson's disease. Neurology 59(9):1421–1424.
119. Bejjani BP, Houeto JL, Hariz M, et al (2002) Aggressive behavior induced by intraoperative stimulation in the triangle of Sano. Neurology 59(9):1425–1427.
120. Deogaonkar A, Avitsian R, Henderson JM, Schubert A (2005) Venous air embolism during deep brain stimulation surgery in an awake supine patient. Stereotact Funct Neurosurg 83(1):32–35.
121. Goodman RR, Kim B, McClelland S 3rd, et al (2006) Operative techniques and morbidity with subthalamic nucleus deep brain stimulation in 100 consecutive patients with advanced Parkinson's disease. J Neurol Neurosurg Psychiatry 77(1):12–17.

# 5
# Technical Alternatives in Performing Deep Brain Stimulator Implantation

Paul S. Larson

## Abstract

Traditional methods of deep brain stimulator (DBS) implantation utilize a rigid, head mounted stereotactic frame to deliver electrodes to the intended brain target. New surgical navigation systems have provided the substrate for the development of frameless DBS delivery techniques that now provide a viable alternative to frame-based implantations, and may have advantages for both the surgical team and the patient. Intraoperative MR imaging and purely image-guided implantation may represent the next generation of implantation strategies.

**Keywords:** deep brain stimulator (DBS), stereotactic surgery, surgical navigation, frameless DBS, NexFrame™, StarFix™, intraoperative MRI, interventional MRI

## Introduction

The word stereotactic literally means to touch in three dimensions. From the earliest days of stereotactic surgery, the traditional method of "touching" targets within the brain has been through the use of a stereotactic frame. In the early 1900s, Horsley and Clarke were the first to describe the use of a stereotactic frame and atlas in animals. In the 1940s, Spiegel and Wycis were the first to routinely employ the use of frames in human stereotactic procedures. Their work and that of others provided the foundation for many stereotactic systems that followed, including the popular Leksell (Elekta, Stockholm, Sweden) and CRW (Integra Radionics, Burlington, MA) frames that are widely used today by centers performing DBS surgery.

Traditional stereotactic systems rely on an external frame of reference of known dimensions that is rigidly attached to the patient's head. Some form of imaging is then used to identify internal landmarks, such as the anterior commissure (AC) and posterior commissure (PC), as well as a number of fiducial markers attached to the frame. Measurements are made relative to the AC-PC plane to determine the specific location of a target of interest, and that target is then spatially related to the fiducials to determine its coordinates in frame space. A historical alternative to frame-based systems were the so-called burr hole-mounted systems, such as the one developed by Professor Sano in Tokyo, which were aiming devices mounted on the skull directly over the burr hole. These systems did not gain widespread acceptance with many stereotactic surgeons, in large part because tedious mathematical calculations were required and small inaccuracies at the level of the device translated to large angular errors at the target.

In addition to the use of stereotactic or anatomical targeting, modern era practitioners of DBS surgery also often employ physiological targeting. The most common form of physiological targeting is microelectrode recording (MER), although the specific techniques of physiological targeting that are used vary greatly among centers. These include single cell or multicellular recordings, field potential recordings, measurement of tissue impedance changes, microstimulation, macrostimulation, or a combination of these techniques. Regardless of the methods used, the goal is to map the intended target, usually a deep nucleus, by determining its physiologic characteristics, mapping its borders, and/or identifying adjacent structures. Physiological mapping provides further target refinement and can overcome errors in anatomical targeting, although its utility may vary depending on the target being implanted and the disease being treated.

## Modern Surgical Navigation

The advent of surgical navigation systems over the last decade, based on optical tracking, such as the StealthStation® (Medtronic, Minneapolis, MN), VectorVision® (BrainLAB, Heimstetten, Germany), and Stryker® Navigation System (Stryker Leibinger, Freiburg, Germany), has provided the substrate for a revolution in the field of stereotaxy. These systems allow surgeons to fuse different pre-operative imaging modalities such as CT and MR and view them in multiple planes simultaneously while using high-speed image reconstruction. Surgeons can use these systems to improve targeting with a traditional stereotactic frame or alternatively can now perform frameless DBS implantation utilizing several techniques. These navigation systems use a camera system to optically track fiducial markers and a stationary reference frame as well as specific instruments within the surgical field. In a typical neurosurgical procedure, the use of skin mounted fiducials and freehand tools provides accuracy in the submillimeter to less than 2 mm range. Such accuracy is satisfactory for many surgical applications, but DBS requires a system that can consistently deliver an accuracy of less than 1 mm.

Two more recent developments have provided the consistent submillimetric accuracy necessary for frameless DBS placement. First is the use of bone implanted fiducials, which provide a much more stable marker than their more mobile skin mounted counterparts. Several types of fiducials have been developed, but all have a base with a self-tapping screw that secures to the bone and some sort of sphere, visible on CT or MR imaging, that sits at or just above the level of the scalp. The second innovation is the development of skull mounted aiming devices that provide the stability and accuracy needed to perform physiological mapping and DBS implantation. The two most widely used frameless DBS systems are the NexFrame™ (Medtronic, Minneapolis, MN) and the StarFix™ micro Targeting® Platform (FHC, Bowdoinham, ME). Both systems meet accuracy demands which are required for DBS, although they accomplish this in very different ways. The NexFrame uses optical tracking and an adjustable aiming device to acquire the desired target. The StarFix uses pre-operative planning to create a customized aiming platform that is "pre-set" to the desired target. Both systems have matured through several generations of refinements, and have been in routine clinical use for several years *(1, 2)*.

## Medtronic NexFrame

The NexFrame is a plastic, burr hole-mounted aiming device that has two degrees of freedom. It has two main components, the base ring and the socket assembly. The base ring is a shallow, funnel-shaped base that attaches to the skull over the burr hole with three self-tapping screws. The socket assembly is an inverted, bowl-shaped component that sits on top of the base ring. The socket assembly rotates freely on the fixed base, providing one degree of freedom; it has a platform that slides linearly in a limited arc along its curved surface, providing the second degree of freedom. These two degrees of freedom allow the device to aim electrodes within a 50-degree cone with its apex at the burr hole. The platform itself has an electrode holder with five holes in the shape of a cross, 2 mm apart, which allows it to interface with most micropositioners. The socket assembly has a cutout window in it so the surgeon can see the burr hole and manipulate the guide tubes and DBS lead during surgery.

The NexFrame technique utilizes five to six bone-implanted fiducials and an optically tracked reference arc attached to the base ring to register the patient using a surgical navigation system. The fiducials are placed with local anesthetic using small stab incisions and are often placed several days before surgery (Figure 5.1). In this manner, imaging and targeting can be decoupled from the day of surgery if desired, allowing the actual surgical procedure to start at a predictable time and earlier in the day. This can prove beneficial for Parkinson's patients, who must be off their medications on the day of surgery for proper MER and often do not tolerate being off medications for an extended time. It also provides more efficient use of operating room (OR) time and more predictable scheduling for members of the DBS team and allows the surgeon to perform targeting prior to the day of surgery. Fiducial placement and imaging may also be done the morning of surgery if desired.

Most centers obtain a high-resolution, volumetric outpatient MR scan and then a thin-cut CT scan after the fiducials have been placed within a few days of surgery. The two imaging volumes are fused on a surgical planning workstation to perform targeting and trajectory planning. The geometric center of the fiducial spheres is identified on the planning workstation, in a similar manner to marking the fiducials in a frame-based system. Once in the OR, the fiducials are included in the sterile field to allow registration to occur. Registration is the process by which the patient's anatomy in "imaging space" (in the computer) is matched with the actual patient's head in "physical space"

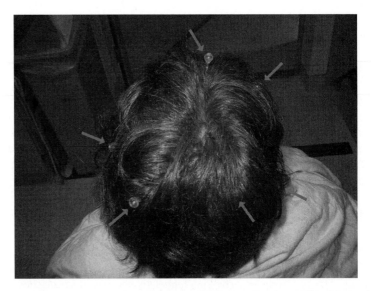

**Figure 5.1** View of the top of a patient's head with bone implanted fiducials in place. Arrows point to CT and MR visible spheres that temporarily snap into the base of this particular type of fiducial for imaging

(in the OR). Four things make this possible: (1) the planning workstation's optical camera system, which uses two or more cameras to spatially resolve objects; (2) the bone implanted fiducials; (3) the reference arc, a small metal device that holds four reflective spheres in a unique geometry that can be tracked by the computer's optical camera system; and (4) a handheld probe, also with four reflective spheres in a different unique geometry and a known distance between the spheres and the probe tip. The probe is used to "teach" the computer the position of the reference arc and the fiducials in real space, and the computer then relates that data to the patient's anatomy in imaging space. One distinct advantage of this technique is that, because the reference arc and fiducials are all rigidly mounted to the skull and move as one when the skull moves, the patient's head does not have to be fixed during the procedure. Some surgeons who regularly use the NexFrame feel that the patient's ability to adjust their position during surgery has advantages in terms of patient comfort and tolerability of the procedure while others have not noted such an advantage (Larson, personal communication).

Once registration is completed, the process of alignment takes place. This involves moving the socket assembly of the NexFrame along its two degrees of freedom until the platform is aligned with the target trajectory. The position of the NexFrame is optically tracked in real time, and the computer workstation provides the surgeon with visual feedback to indicate when the NexFrame is aligned (Figure 5.2). One of the disadvantages of the NexFrame compared to an arc-centered system like the Leksell is a relatively limited ability to alter the entry point in the cortex in order to miss undesirable features on the cortical surface such as sulci or vessels. There is an offset adapter that does allow the entry point to be offset by several millimeters, which provides some flexibility, but not as much as a Leksell frame provides. Once aligned, the surgeon may proceed with MER and DBS lead placement in the usual manner (Figure 5.3).

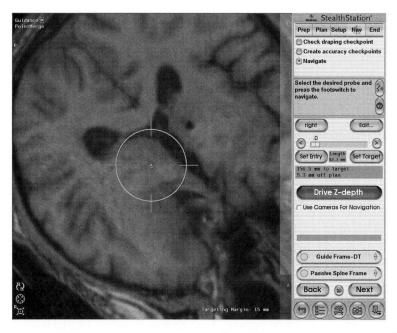

**Figure 5.2** Screen shot from a StealthStation® during alignment in a NexFrame™ frameless case. The surgeon manipulates the NexFrame until the small dot is inside the small inner circle, indicating that the device is properly aligned with the target. A contralateral lead has already been implanted

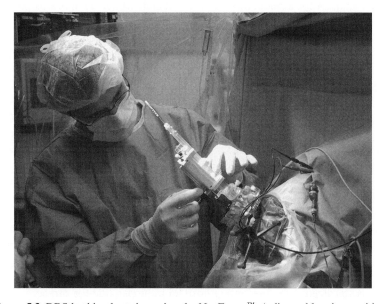

**Figure 5.3** DBS lead implantation using the NexFrame™. A disposable micropositioner is mounted on the NexFrame and is being used to lower the electrode to the target

Medtronic makes a disposable micropositioner specifically for the NexFrame, or a third-party drive can be used. The base ring is designed to integrate with the Medtronic StimLock™ lead anchoring device to secure the DBS electrode following implantation.

## FHC StarFix

The StarFix micro Targeting Platform (FHC, Bowdoinham, ME) replaces the traditional stereotactic frame with a different variation of a skull mounted system. In essence, the micro Targeting Platform (MTP) is a custom-designed, skull-mounted aiming device that is specifically manufactured for each patient based on a pre-operative plan created by the surgeon days before the procedure. In essence, the MTP is a device that comes out of the box pre-set to the chosen target, with parallel channels for MER that are also pre-set to be aligned to the AC-PC plane. No optical tracking system is used in the OR, and there is no registration or alignment process required. Unlike the NexFrame device, which is fairly compact and mounted directly around the burr hole, the MTP is an open tripod design with legs that reach out to secure to skull mounted anchors. This system also gives the surgeon the ability to decouple the imaging and targeting from the day of surgery. In the case of the MTP, however, the separation of imaging from the day of surgery is mandatory, as the device is manufactured based on pre-operative CT scans and the manufacturing process takes several days to complete.

The first stage of the procedure takes place in an outpatient setting approximately one week before surgery. The surgeon identifies a roughly 50-mm diameter region as the intended entry area, and percutaneously implants three anchors into the bone, spaced about 120 degrees apart in a 50- to 80-mm radius from the center of the intended entry area. These anchors sit below the level of the scalp, and can stay in place for up to 28 days. The head of each anchor can accept a temporary locator fiducial, which is placed to provide accurate localization of the anchors on imaging. The patient is sent for high-resolution CT and MR imaging, after which the locator fiducials are removed and the patient is sent home with the anchors left in place.

The surgeon then loads the CT and MR images onto the MTP Planning and Design Workstation. The system provides the ability to fuse CT and MR volumes and, based on the CT scan, creates a detailed 3D model of the skull surface and implanted anchors, which will be used to create the MTP. The target or targets are selected, and entry point and trajectory planning is performed with multiplanar views available. Once the target and entry point are selected, the system will build a virtual MTP that is of appropriate geometry to be centered over the entry point with legs that will attach to the bone implanted anchors (Figure 5.4). For bilateral simultaneous implants, a combination of two separate platforms can be used, or the computer can create one complex platform that attaches to four anchors spanning the top of the head. Once the surgeon is satisfied with the surgical plan, the platform planning files are transmitted to the manufacturer who uses rapid prototyping technology to make the actual MTP and ships it to the surgeon within 24 to 72 hours. The MTP is sterilized at the implanting hospital in preparation for surgery.

On the day of surgery, the patient is taken directly to the OR at the desired time. Because the MTP is skull mounted, no rigid fixation of the patient's head is required. Once in the OR, the anchors are exposed so the platform can be attached. The MTP can be readily attached and removed as many times as needed. It is usually temporarily placed to mark the skin incision and then again to mark the appropriate position for the burr hole. Once the dura is open and the team is ready to perform MER or DBS lead placement, the MTP is again

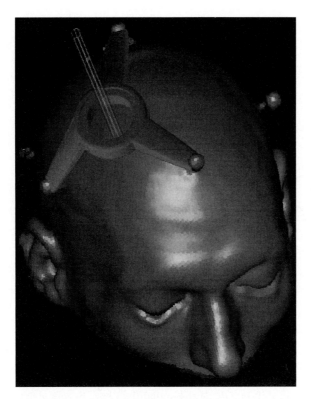

**Figure 5.4** Computer model of a virtual StarFix™ MTP created by the MTP Planning and Design Workstation during pre-operative targeting. This model will be transferred to the manufacturing facility, which will use it to create the actual MTP using rapid prototyping technology

secured into position and a metallic ring is placed in the hole of the platform to provide a stable base for the micropositioner (Figure 5.5). Again, an offset device is available if there is a sulcus or vessel that the surgeon feels is in the way of the initially planned trajectory, but the exact entry point options within the exposed burr hole are somewhat limited compared to an arc-centered frame like the Leksell. At this point, the surgeon can perform DBS implantation using standard techniques including MER. One unique advantage of the StarFix system is the ability to perform bilateral simultaneous MER if desired. Another advantage of this system is its simplicity and non-reliance on an optical tracking system or need for alignment in the OR. However, this simplicity comes at a potential price, as any error in pre-operative targeting or MTP manufacturing could result in an improper trajectory and a misplaced electrode.

## Localization Using Peri-operative and Intra-operative Imaging

Although image guidance systems have proven their value in DBS surgery, they do have shortcomings. The images used for registration and navigation are obtained pre-operatively with the patient in a supine position. When the patient is taken to the OR and has a burr hole placed (typically in a semi-sitting

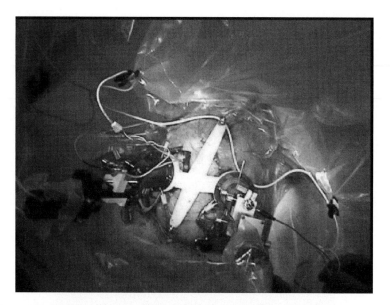

**Figure 5.5** Intraoperative photograph showing one MTP platform being used for a bilateral simultaneous implantation. Note that two micropositioners are in use at once, providing the capacity for simultaneous bilateral MER

position), brain shift due to cerebrospinal fluid loss, pneumocephalus, and the effects of gravity can occur, altering the accuracy of the planned cortical entry point, trajectory and even the target *(3)*. Errors in registration or alignment can result in poor lead placement. Many surgeons have come to rely heavily on brain atlases that are provided with the stereotactic planning software. However, these atlases are simple, minimally deformable to individual patient anatomy, and are frequently a poor representation of the anatomy in the target region. Finally, the only true measure of anatomically successful electrode placement is postoperative imaging with either CT or MRI. Any cases of errant electrode placement with suboptimal benefit that cannot be overcome with programming of the DBS device often require a second procedure to surgically reposition the electrode.

For these reasons and others, some centers have turned to intra-operative imaging as a means of confirming electrode placement. The imaging modalities used have included CT as well as MRI of varying field strengths. Surgeons that employ this technique use standard frame-based or frameless methods to determine the target coordinates and then use MER or purely anatomical targeting to place the DBS electrode. They then move the patient into a scanner, ideally located within the operating suite or immediately adjacent to it, for confirmation of acceptable lead location. If the lead is suboptimally positioned, a correction can be made before the patient leaves the operating theater. An advantage of this technique is that the surgeon can continue to use the implantation tools (frame, physiologic mapping methods, etc.) that he or she is familiar with, while gaining the advantage of immediate feedback with regard to lead location.

While helpful, the use of imaging in this context is somewhat limited. First, if CT is used as the imaging modality, the direct visualization of the lead relative to the actual target is essentially non-existent due to the poor tissue discrimination inherent with CT. The lead location can be inferred by taking measurements of the center of the lead artifact relative to the AC-PC plane, and/or fusing postoperative images with pre-operative MR studies. If MRI is used, there are considerations related to the field strength of the magnet. Lower-field MRI can allow the surgical team to use the usual surgical equipment at some minimum distance from the magnet, however low field MRI generally does not allow adequate visualization of the target. High-field MRI (1.5T) often provides good target visualization, but precludes the use of much of the usual DBS instrumentation, such as MER equipment, at least within some distance from the magnet. Finally, most centers using intra-operative imaging in this setting are not really utilizing real-time imaging to its fullest potential. Rather, they are performing a standard, frame-based implantation and using "immediate postoperative imaging" to detect complications before leaving the OR.

## Interventional MRI

On an investigational basis, our center has started using high field interventional MRI to place DBS electrodes into the subthalamic nucleus (STN) to treat Parkinson's disease using real-time imaging as the only method of targeting *(4)*. The idea for this technique came in part from prior experience with intra-operative MR-guided brain biopsies *(5)*. The other catalyst was our observation that patients with postoperative MRI who showed lead locations in the dorsolateral motor subterritory of the STN, centered within the nucleus in the mediolateral dimension and equal to or just behind the anterior border of the red nucleus in the anteroposterior dimension, experienced a good clinical outcome *(6)*. At our center, the goal of MER and macrostimulation is to localize this region of the STN. Because the STN is visible at 1.5T using optimized MR sequences, a logical extension of this observation was to use real-time imaging instead of physiological mapping to place electrodes into the dorsolateral STN. No stereotactic frame or fiducial markers are required, no pre-operative targeting is performed, and no physiological mapping of any kind is undertaken.

This technique, referred to as iMRI DBS implantation, takes place with the patient entirely within the bore of a 1.5T Philips Intera MRI (Philips, Best, The Netherlands). The scanner is located in radiology, not in an OR, hence the use of the term interventional MRI as opposed to intra-operative MRI. The procedure requires the use of MR compatible titanium instruments and a custom MR compatible drill (The Anspach Effort, Inc., Palm Beach Gardens, FL). Unilateral or simultaneous bilateral implantations can be performed. The patient is first placed under general anesthesia. Once asleep, the head is fixed to the MR gantry using a carbon fiber head holder and flexible loop MR coils are positioned on either side of the head. The implantation technique requires that the patient not move between the time the final target is selected and the point at which the lead is implanted, so secure fixation of the head is required. The patient is then placed into the imaging center (isocenter) of the magnet bore, and a series of brief scans are obtained to choose an appropriate entry point and trajectory to the target region. Once the entry points are selected, the patient's head is moved from isocenter to the far edge of the bore, where the scalp is prepared in the usual manner. A custom sterile drape sticks to the top of the head and extends outward to attach to the far end of the magnet, providing a sterile field that moves with the head as it moves from the bore edge to isocenter during the procedure. An incision or incisions are made over the entry points, burr holes are created, and NexFrame towers are mounted over the burr holes. Bilateral simultaneous implants are performed with two separate NexFrame towers mounted at the same time. The dura is opened early in the procedure so that any early brain shift that may occur happens prior to target selection.

Once the NexFrames are mounted, an aiming device called an alignment stem is placed into the socket assembly. The saline-filled alignment stem has a sphere at the end closest to the brain and is engineered such that the center of the sphere sits at the "pivot point" of the NexFrame system, meaning that the sphere remains stationary regardless of where the NexFrame and upper portion of the alignment stem are aimed. When the patient is moved back to isocenter for high-resolution imaging, definitive target selection, and implantation, the 3D coordinates for the center of the pivot point can be determined in MR space, which remains constant provided the patient is not moved. When the target is selected and its coordinates in MR space are also determined, the target and pivot point define a linear path, which is the trajectory to the target. It is then a simple matter of manipulating the alignment stem until it is in line with this trajectory. This is accomplished by using a rapid fluoroscopic MR acquisition through the distal portion of the alignment stem, perpendicular to the intended trajectory. The fluoroscopic sequence acquires images at several frames per second, allowing the surgeon to reach into the bore of the magnet and align the stem with the target while watching real-time images (Figure 5.6). The surgeon sees the actual position of the alignment stem and a mathematically calculated annotation of the target trajectory on a monitor in the MR suite and manipulates the NexFrame until the two are aligned.

Once aligned, the NexFrame is locked into position and a stylet with a plastic peel away sheath is passed to the target. Rapid MR sequences at right angles to the trajectory are obtained to confirm proper trajectory (Figure 5.7). Once the target has been reached, a high-resolution scan is used to confirm proper placement in the desired portion of the STN. In the vast majority of cases, only a single pass is required (4). Once proper placement is confirmed, the stylet is removed, leaving the peel away sheath in place. A 28-cm Medtronic DBS lead with a custom titanium stylet is then passed down the peel away sheath to the target, and the peel away is removed. A final confirmation scan is obtained, and the lead is anchored using the StimLock device. The end of the DBS lead is tucked underneath the scalp and the incision is closed. Pulse generator implantation takes place approximately 2 weeks later as an outpatient procedure.

The iMRI technique appears to have several advantages. It is time efficient in that no fiducials are placed, no pre-operative studies are required, and the overall time of the procedure is significantly shorter than a standard implantation. The patients do not have to be awake and Parkinson's disease patients do not need to be off medications. The implantation can be done with one penetration of the brain, which may translate into a lower risk of hemorrhage although this remains to be seen. Finally, there is a high degree of confidence that the lead is placed in a favorable position at the end of the procedure. The disadvantages are that the technique requires facilities that allow interventional procedures to be done in a MR scanner and, at the present

5 Technical Alternatives in DBS    109

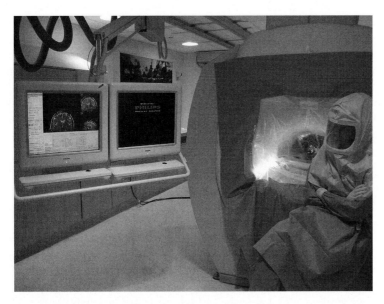

**Figure 5.6** A view of the iMRI DBS suite from the far end of the bore. The NexFrame™ mounted on the top of the patient's head is visible inside the bore of the magnet. During alignment, the surgeon reaches into the bore to aim the device while watching real-time images on the monitors to the left. A sterile hood is worn to maintain sterility of the bore drape while reaching into the magnet

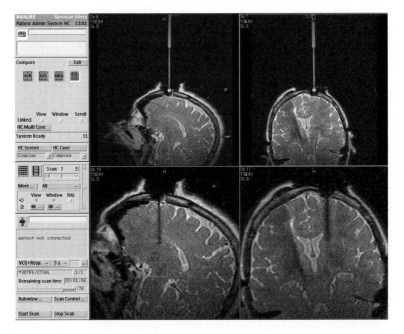

**Figure 5.7** Screen shot from the iMRI console after alignment showing rapidly acquired, low-resolution images. The upper row of images show the saline-filled alignment stem with the pivot point in the burr hole. The NexFrame™ holding the alignment stem is plastic and not visible on MRI. The lower row of images show the stylet and peel away partially advanced toward the target; the patient has already had a contralateral lead placed

time, requires a significant amount of technical expertise from a MR physicist. It also requires a strong institutional commitment and radiology, anesthesia and OR personnel that are willing to work in a unique and sometimes adverse working environment. This technique has recently been adapted to implantation of the globus pallidus for the treatment of dystonia, and is currently being expanded to a second hospital using a different MR platform. In the STN DBS patients, a comparison of clinical outcomes to those following frame-based, microelectrode recorded implantations is currently underway.

## Conclusions

In summary, viable alternatives to traditional frame-based DBS implantation now exist. While each technique has its advantages and disadvantages, all of these techniques appear to be safe and accurate. Frame-based implantations have an extensive track record and are a familiar and comfortable technique for many surgeons. The newer frameless techniques may be more time efficient for many centers and may provide some increased comfort for patients. Frameless systems also lower the upfront costs for hospitals starting new DBS programs, as most of the components are disposable and inexpensive compared to the purchase of a stereotactic frame and other associated components. Teams performing DBS implantation would be well served to explore these various options and employ whichever technique provides the greatest efficiency, consistency and comfort level for their particular team.

*Acknowledgments*: The author would like to thank Dr. Peter Konrad from Vanderbilt University and Keith Sootsman from Medtronic/IGN for providing some of the figures used in this chapter.

## References

1. Holloway KL, Gaede SE, Starr PA, Rosenow JM, Ramakrishnan, Henderson JM (2005) Frameless stereotaxy using bone fiducial markers for deep brain stimulation. J Neurosurg 103:404–413.
2. Fitzpatrick JM, Konrad PE, Nickele C, Cetinkaya E, Kao C (2005) Accuracy of customized miniature stereotactic platforms. Stereotact Funct Neurosurg 83:25–31.
3. Ivan ME, Martin AJ, Starr PA, Sootsman K, Larson PS (2006) Brain shift analysis during burr hole based procedures using interventional MRI. Presented at the Annual Meeting of the American Association of Neurological Surgeons, San Francisco, CA.
4. Martin AJ, Larson PS, Ostrem JL, Keith Sootsman W, Talke P, Weber OM, Levesque N, Meyers J, Starr PA (2005) Placement of deep brain stimulator electrodes using real-time high-field interventional magnetic resonance imaging. Magn Reson Med 54(5):1107–1114.
5. Moriarty TM, Quinones-Hinojosa A, Larson PS, Alexander E III, Gleason PL, Schwartz RB, Jolesz FA, Black PM (2000) Frameless stereotactic neurosurgery using intraoperative magnetic resonance imaging: stereotactic brain biopsy. Neurosurgery 47(5):1138–1145.
6. Starr PA, Christine CW, Theodosopoulos PV, Lindsey N, Byrd D, Mosley A, Marks WJ (2002) Implantation of deep brain stimulators into the subthalamic nucleus: technical approach and magnetic resonance imaging-verified lead locations. J Neurosurg 97:370–387.

# 6
# Intra-operative Microrecording and Stimulation

Frank Steigerwald and Jens Volkmann

## Abstract

Electrophysiological mapping is an integral part of any functional neurosurgical procedure for treatment of movement disorders. Mapping strategies vary greatly among different surgical centers, but can be broadly categorized into those relying solely on macrostimulation to determine the threshold for clinical effects, and those employing additional recordings of neuronal activity through micro- or semimicroelectrodes. Microelectrode recordings provide physiological information about nuclear boundaries based on characteristic neuronal discharge patterns and stimulus responsiveness. This information has the advantage of being independent from patient cooperation and can also be obtained under general anaesthesia. Microelectrode recordings also allow parallel or sequential explorations by several passes through the target structure to delineate the optimal site for implantation, because they cause minimal microlesioning effects in contrast to larger macrostimulation probes. This chapter introduces the different techniques of electrophysiological mapping and discusses their risks and benefits for the three current targets of movement disorder surgery: the globus pallidus, ventrolateral thalamus, and subthalamic nucleus.

**Keywords:** deep brain stimulation, microelectrode recording, intra-operative stimulation, subthalamic nucleus, globus pallidus, VIM

## Introduction

The history of microelectrode recordings in functional stereotactic neurosurgery began in October 1961, when Mme. Denise Albe-Fessard, a renowned neurophysiologist at the Marey Institute in Paris, adapted her animal recording equipment to the stereotactic frame of Prof. Gerard Guiot and began a series of experiments with him to explore the thalamus and basal ganglia of patients treated for Parkinson's disease (PD; refs. [1] and [2]). They were the first to demonstrate that typical neuronal discharge patterns and characteristic evoked responses allow the precise identification of subcortical target structures for subsequent lesioning. This was a revolutionary discovery at a time when stereotactic surgery had to rely on indirect anatomical landmarks derived from pneumoencephalography and when stereotactic atlases were just beginning to emerge. Despite rapid progress in neuroimaging techniques, today intra-operative microrecording is still an integral part of functional neurosurgical procedures in many centers. By monitoring online the physiological signal of the tissue surrounding the microelectrode tip, which can be advanced on a sub-millimeter scale, one can identify nuclear boundaries with high precision. This spatial resolution is not achieved by radiological techniques. Microrecordings are usually combined with electrical stimulation as part of the intra-operative electrophysiological mapping procedure during lesional stereotaxy or the implantation of deep brain stimulation (DBS) electrodes.

The principle technique of extracellular recording has changed little over the past four decades. The renaissance of functional stereotaxy in the 1990s with the reintroduction of pallidotomy for treating advanced PD, and later DBS, has triggered commercial interest in this diagnostic procedure and several companies now offer reliable and comfortable solutions for intra-operative neurophysiological monitoring in functional stereotaxy. Microrecordings are therefore no longer a complicated technique for neurophysiologists who previously had to transfer their equipment and knowledge from the animal laboratory to the operating room, but have evolved into a routine neurophysiological procedure, that can be learned and applied by clinicians.

## Physiology

The recording of electrical brain activity began in 1875, when Richard Caton discovered that fluctuating currents could be recorded from within the brain *(3)*. Since then, we've learned that neurons are capable of generating electrical signals that propagate along their length and influence other neurons by direct electrical contact through gap junctions or chemically via synaptic neurotransmitter release. Neurons are organized into networks, in which their coordinated activity mediates a large diversity of behaviors. Extracellular recordings made by placing an electrode into the brain to measure voltage fluctuations to an indifferent reference electrode allow monitoring of electrical activity at various levels of the neuronal network which depend on the location and properties of the recording electrode. Lower-impedance macroelectrodes record the activity of large populations of neurons, which results in EEG-like signals that most likely reflect the temporal summation of slow dendritic currents. The oscillations of the local field potential therefore represent the synchronized synaptic activity of the population of neurons in the local area surrounding the recording electrode. Fast sodium action potentials do not significantly contribute to this field recording because of the low-pass (capacitative) filtering properties of the extracellular environment separating the recording electrode and the cell. Functional exploration of subcortical structures by means of macroelectrode techniques began to complement conventional electrical stimulation in the late 1940s and was soon routinely performed by many stereotactic neurosurgeons worldwide. Nevertheless, the results of macroelectrode recordings were heterogeneous and somewhat disappointing, since the relatively crude interpretation of the oscillatory signals allowed at best a rough differentiation between gray and white matter but not a precise delineation of the target structures. Recently, increased beta-oscillations have been described as a typical signature of local field potential recordings from the human basal ganglia in the parkinsonian state. Evidence suggests, that an increase in the power of beta-band activity may closely correlate with the macroelectrode entering the subthalamic nucleus (STN) in PD *(4)*. In the near future, this may help to develop field potential recordings as a useful tool for the electrophysiological guidance of electrode implantations.

By placing the tip of a high-impedance microelectrode less than a few hundred microns from a neuronal cell body one may register action potentials from a single cell. This is possible during an action potential in which a neuron transiently opens sodium channels allowing positively charged sodium ions to rush down the voltage gradient into the cell. A complex extracellular field potential builds up around the site of the largest membrane conductance and inactive parts of the cell membrane. The movement of ions into the cell creates a monophasic action potential in intracellular recordings. The corresponding extracellular current leads to a transient change in voltage between the extracellular recording electrode and the distant reference electrode, which is apparent as a typical "spike" in a voltage-time diagram. In contrast to intracellular recordings, extracellular spikes appear biphasic because the extracellular current flow is approximately proportional to the first derivative of the transmembrane potential over time.

The amplitude and shape of the extracellular spike further depends on a number of other factors, such as the geometry and size of the neuron, the distance and orientation of the recording electrode, and the summation of currents from simultaneously active neurons in the surrounding environment. Large cells with a soma diameter of 30 to 50 µm generate large extracellular spikes that can be traced over several hundred microns and "held" for relatively long recording periods. However, smaller cells that constitute the majority of neurons in the central nervous system, generate amplitudes of less than 200 µV, which can only be detected in the presence of background noise, when the microelectrode tip is immediately adjacent to the cell without injuring it. Thus, microrecordings within the constraints of a clinical setting will be dominated by activity of larger and more stable neurons. This sampling bias needs to be considered in the scientific interpretation of these recordings. However, for the clinical purpose of microrecording, this is not a serious limitation, because characteristic features such as the level of background noise, the temporal pattern of action potential firing or the density of these neuronal subsets, all help to identify the various structures reliably.

Despite their much smaller size one may occasionally record action potentials from axonal fibers rather than cell bodies. These axonal spikes are predominantly found within fiber bundles such as the pyramidal tract but may also be present within gray matter. Axonal spikes are typically triphasic (positive-negative-positive), but the negativity may be small depending on the position of the electrode tip, which often leads to the recording of a monophasic positive spike of short duration (< 1 millisecond). In contrast, spikes originating from the cell soma or axon hill are biphasic (either negative-positive or positive-negative depending on the cell type) and, with few exceptions, last more than 1 millisecond.

## Methods

In its simplest form, extracellular recording can be performed through a wire in the brain covered by insulation except for its very tip. Fluctuations in voltage between this wire and a reference electrode can then be measured. Because the fluctuations in the local field potential that occur in the brain are commonly less than a millivolt, the potential difference between the two electrodes must be amplified. The amplified signal is usually passed through a bandpass filter to remove biological and technical noise. Thereafter it can be displayed on an oscilloscope, played back as an audiosignal, or registered on tape recorders or PC-based recording systems. This setup is schematically summarized in Figure 6.1.

### Microelectrodes

Microelectrodes are commercially available from several companies, which have been approved for medical use according to the requirements of the FDA or CE-mark (Conformité Européenne). Commonly used electrodes consist of a thin tungsten or platin-iridium wire, which is coated by Parylene-C. Several lengths and diameters of electrode tips are available resulting in typical impedances between 0.5 and 2 MOhm. To extend the electrode for deep brain recordings it is inserted into stainless steel tubing. The tip of the electrode is very fragile and must never be touched or struck by other instruments in the operating room. To avoid mechanical damage during sterilization and intra-operative handling many electrodes are delivered with a protective tubing of the micro tip, which needs to be removed before recording.

An interesting alternative to conventional single core microelectrodes is the tetrode offered by Thomas Recording GmbH, Gießen, Germany. The tetrode

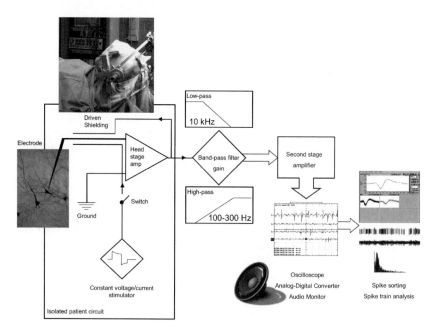

**Figure 6.1** Scheme of the equipment used for microelectrode recording and stimulation

consists of four platinum-tungsten fibers, which are combined by glass coating into a single electrode with a diameter of only 100 μm. At the tip of the microelectrode three recording sites are concentrically arranged around a central contact at distances of approximately 30 μm. This geometrical arrangement allows better isolation of individual neurons. Depending on the distance of a neuron to each of the four tetrode recording sites a typical signature of amplitude distributions can be found across the four channel recordings. With the use of appropriate postprocessing techniques such as multidimensional cluster analysis one may reliably identify the activity of up to 20 neurons in dense populations. This is especially attractive when microrecordings are performed for scientific purposes.

**Electronic Equipment**

In order to detect small neuronal signals in the presence of biological and technical noise, the principle of differential amplification is applied for microrecording. This method substracts remote electrical signals, most of which come from other electrical appliances in the operating room, which are equally picked up by the microelectrode and the reference electrode ("common mode rejection"). A number of additional technical solutions are available in commercial microrecording systems to improve the signal-to-noise ratio of neural recordings. Nevertheless, technical noise, especially AC main line hum (50 Hz in Europe or 60 Hz in the United States) may pose a challenge to microrecordings in the standard operating room, which is not specially shielded. To reduce electrical noise both the patient and equipment need to be properly grounded. The best grounding scheme is a "star" ground system, where all the local grounds are connected together, typically to the ground of the differential amplifier. All electrical appliances in the operating room, which are not strictly necessary, should be switched off or placed as far as possible from the microelectrode. The extension of the microelectrode, the cable connections to the prestage amplifier and all other extension cables must be shielded. The most common reason for an impaired recording, however, is the microelectrode itself. If the tip is damaged, weak, or noisy no signals at all may be recorded and the microelectrode must be exchanged. Additional sources of noise in the clinical setting are mechanical vibrations of the stereotactic frame induced by voluntary or involuntary (e.g., tremor) movements or speech of the patient.

After amplification the microrecording signal is bandpass filtered to improve the quality of the raw biological signal for postprocessing and graphical display. A stable baseline is obtained after high-pass filtering at 10 to 300 Hz. Low-pass filtering may distort the spike shape and should be carefully applied, if postprocessing of the data is intended, such as single unit detection by template matching. The most common setting for single or multiunit recordings is a bandpass between 100–300 Hz and 10 kHz. To record changes in neural background noise (e.g., light evoked responses in the optic tract), the filter must be "opened" to include the lower frequency components.

In commercial microrecording systems the signal is digitally converted and displayed on the computer screen. Simultaneously, the analog signal is fed into an audio amplifier and played via loudspeakers or headphones to allow the detection of typical discharge patterns by ear. The optical and acoustical recognition of characteristic neuronal signatures may be supplemented by online data analysis tools. A spike discriminator is used to distinguish the firing of an individual neuron from a group of simultaneously active cells and background noise. The output of the spike discriminator is a logic pulse each time the criteria for recognition of an individual spike are fulfilled. This signal can then be further processed to extract temporal features of neuronal firing, such as the mean firing rate, interspike interval histograms, burst statistics, and so forth. In its most simple form, the spike discriminator is based on a threshold trigger, where only spikes of a certain amplitude pass. The identification of single neuron activity using this approach is not very reliable as two or more neurons may be at a similar distance from the electrode and therefore generate approximately equal spike amplitudes. In this case the spike rate would be overestimated. Other more advanced methods of spike sorting include template matching or statistical approaches such as principle component analysis, which take into account additional features of a spike. Although the processing power of current PC systems allows these techniques to be applied online, this is rarely useful in the operating room where time is limited and because statistical analysis cannot replace neurophysiological experience in recognizing the pattern of typical neuronal signatures by visual inspection of the raw signal traces and the audiosignal. The clinical interpretation of microrecordings in this respect is very similar to electromyography, where quantitative approaches at best supplement the global impression derived by audiomonitoring by an experienced clinical neurophysiologist.

**Intra-operative Procedure**

*General Setup and Procedure (Figure 6.1)*
Microrecordings require an adaptation to the stereotactic frame to hold and guide the microelectrode along the intended trajectory. A headstage allows one to adjust a single trajectory in the $x$ and $y$ direction for multiple sequential microelectrode passes. Alternatively, the "Ben-Gun" system (developed by Alim Benabid) may be used, which consists of four concentrically arranged openings around a central opening placed in a cylinder that can hold up to five microelectrodes simultaneously at a defined distance of 2 to 3 mm. The electrodes are usually stabilized by guide tubes, which do not extend into the target area, and are advanced by a microdrive system. This may either be manually driven (micrometer screw, hydraulic microdrive) or operated by a remote controlled precision engine. The mechanical guiding system, the microelectrodes, cabling, and headstage amplifier are assembled under sterile conditions. After insertion into the brain the shielded recording lead of the microelectrode is connected to one input of the differential amplifier, the reference electrode (often the inner guide tube) is attached to the second input, and the indifferent or patient common ground lead is clipped to the stereotactic frame or guide tube adaptor. Multiple grounding of the patients should be avoided to reduce noise induced by ground loops. To avoid cerebrospinal leakage and subsequent brain shift during prolonged monitoring sessions, the burr hole is often sealed by fibrin glue.

The main unit of the recording system is placed outside the sterile field and is operated by another member of the surgical team (neurosurgeon, neurologist, or neurophysiologist) with training in microrecording. The microelectrodes are manually advanced to a defined distance from the anatomical target and then advanced by the microdrive to record from various levels along the trajectory. Recordings normally start several millimeters above the target to register typical changes in the discharge pattern as the electrode transverses different anatomical structures.

While the neuronal resting pattern is used to identify the boundaries of the target structure, the patient should remain relaxed and silent during the recordings. Depending on the target, the recording of resting activity may be supplemented by testing the sensory or motor responsiveness of the recorded cells. Microrecordings are usually followed by electrical stimulation along the same trajectories to evaluate the amplitude threshold for stimulation- induced adverse effects and the degree of symptomatic improvement with high-frequency stimulation in the awake patient.

### *Single- vs Multitrajectory Recording*

A "neurophysiological map" of the target area requires multiple electrode passes. A single trajectory may help to determine the length by which the microelectrode transverses a given anatomical target. It does not, however, allow one to determine where within the medio-lateral and anterior-posterior extent of the nucleus the electrode has passed. Many North American centers prefer sequential microelectrode passes, in which the next location is planned according to the results of the previous trajectory. The recording is terminated when a sufficient number of trajectories have been explored to delineate the target area. An alternative to the single electrode approach is the Ben-Gun method (used predominantly in Europe), which allows one to advance and monitor up to five microelectrodes simultaneously. This arrangement has the advantage of preventing brain shift between subsequent electrode passes, which may disturb the mapping procedure and may, in some hands, be more time efficient than the single microelectrode approach.

### *Stimulation*

Stimulation is mandatory before settling on a final location for the implantation of the DBS electrode. In the awake patient, stimulation and clinical examination help to verify the intended clinical response. Even in the anesthetized patient, it is possible to evaluate the amplitude threshold for certain adverse effects of stimulation (e.g., muscular contraction due to current diffusion into the pyramidal tract). To elicit a clinical response one has to use macrostimulation with currents in the milliampere range. Macrostimulation can be delivered in a number of different ways: through a dedicated electrode (often a radiofrequency lesioning probe), through the DBS electrode itself, through the low-impedance guide tube of the microelectrode or through the microelectrode itself. The latter approach is problematic, because passing a milliampere current through the high-impedance microelectrode leads to degradation of the microelectrode tip and can theoretically exceed the safe charge density range for neural tissue. The use of larger diameter macroelectrodes, on the other hand, may produce a microlesioning effect, which may interfere with clinical testing.

Macrostimulation is normally performed with the same pulse width and frequency as chronic DBS. It is practical to first establish the therapeutic window of stimulation by carefully raising current or voltage until adverse effects of stimulation are noted. Then the beneficial clinical effects of stimulation (reduction of rigidity, tremor, or bradykinesia) are evaluated. We use the same amplitude (1.5 mA) to compare efficacy at different sites and rate the degree of clinical improvement from baseline for each symptom on a semiquantitative scale. This allows us to determine the optimal site for the final electrode implantation from the ratio between beneficial and side effects. Typically, the site is chosen where the best clinical improvement can be observed at the lowest voltage/current and which offers the largest therapeutic width (i.e., voltage or current differences between the beneficial effects of stimulation and the development of side effects).

## Anesthesia

The implantation of DBS leads is normally performed in the awake patient, because anesthesia precludes testing of the full clinical response to stimulation. An exception is DBS in dystonic patients, who may not be able to lie in a supine position on the operating table during prolonged surgery and in whom severe dystonic spasms may interfere with the ability to discern dystonic movements from those caused by stimulation and invasion of the internal capsule. Such dystonic movements may sometimes also cause frame dislocation or fracture of the frame fixation. Moreover, the clinical response to stimulation is often delayed in dystonia and may require days or weeks of stimulation before one observes clear clinical benefit, and this renders the intra-operative evaluation of clinical efficacy unreliable as a predictor of the eventual postoperative response.

Neural spike activity has been recorded under general anesthesia with propofol from the pallidum of patients with dystonia *(5, 6)* and from the STN of patients with PD *(7)*. The level of anesthesia, however, may affect the neural recordings *(7)*. Deep anesthesia can entirely suppress spontaneous neural discharges. In addition, there is currently an ongoing debate as to whether propofol alters the firing frequency and discharge pattern of neurons *(5, 6)*. Visual evoked potentials may be obtained under general anesthesia to map the optic tract *(8)*. Although macrostimulation under anesthesia does not allow one to assess subjective side effects such as paresthesias or visual phosphenes, it is still useful to determine the threshold for capsular effects, although one must take into consideration that this threshold may be raised when the patient is under anesthesia.

So far only one small study has compared outcomes in patients with PD operated with and without general anesthesia. Maltete and colleagues *(9)* reported a slightly better clinical outcome in the group of patients operated when awake (73 vs 64% improvement in the off-period UPDRS motor score after surgery). Even without such comparative trials, the advantages of intra-operative testing during awake surgery are sufficiently obvious that one should use this option unless the condition of the patient (dystonia, spine deformities, age, anxiety, or claustrophobia) requires general anesthesia *(7)*.

# Target Specific Strategies of Electrophysiological Mapping

## Subthalamic Nucleus (STN)

### Microelectrode Recording (Figure 6.2)

The STN is an ideal target for identification by microelectrode recording, because it is largely surrounded by white matter. The abrupt increase in background noise and the appearance of large amplitude irregular or bursting spike activity cannot be missed, when the electrode tip is advanced into the STN from the surrounding white matter.

Recordings start typically 6 to 20 mm above the intended target, depending on local practices at each center. The recording pattern along the way to the STN depends on the obliquity of the planned trajectory. With a lateral approach, the electrode may miss the thalamus and advance through the corona radiata and internal capsule before entering the STN. We prefer a precoronal entry point approximately 3 to 4 cm lateral from the midline, which guides the trajectory at a safe distance along the wall of the lateral ventricle through the head of the caudate (20–40 mm above the target). Starting at 10 mm above the intended STN target one may still find spontaneous burst discharges of neurons within the anterior thalamus (Voa nucleus) or thalamic reticular formation. These neurons may show irregular low frequency

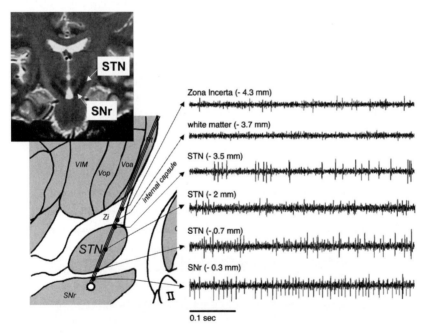

**Figure 6.2** Subthalamic nucleus (STN) and substantia nigra pars reticulata (SNr) present as a hypointense ovoid lateral to the red nucleus on a coronal T2-weighted MRI. The border between both structures is difficult to delineate despite high-resolution images. Examples of microrecordings at different depth along a single trajectory towards the anatomically predefined target (white circle) show the characteristic discharge pattern of zona incerta, white matter, STN, and SNr. STN activity could be recorded between 3.5 and 0.7 mm above the intended target. At the predefined target typical SNr units were found suggesting that it had been chosen too deep

discharges between 1 and 20 Hz but more characteristically short rhythmic bursts of few (typically two to five) spikes *(10, 11)*. Thalamic activity can extend for up to 6 to 7 mm above the STN target. After another 2 to 3 mm, during which low background activity with sparse low frequency and irregular spikes corresponding to neurons of the zona incerta are exhibited, the dorsal border of the STN is reached.

The STN has a high cellular density, which sometimes causes difficulties in isolating single unit activity. The entry into the STN is best identified by the steep (at least two- to threefold) increase in the amplitude of background noise. Single units typically exhibit an irregular or burst-like firing pattern with a mean frequency around 30 to 60 Hz *(11–19)*. Tremor-locked bursting activity at 4 to 6 Hz can be encountered within the dorsolateral region of the STN, where many cells are movement-responsive. The optimal target for the implantation of a DBS electrode corresponds to this "sensorimotor" region of the STN *(20–26)*. Some groups routinely assess responsiveness to active or passive movements to identify the sensorimotor part of the STN. Approximately 20 to 40% of units in the dorsolateral region of the STN are driven by passive joint movements. The representation of movements within STN follows a gross somatotopic organization with leg-related cells localized more medial and ventral compared to arm-related cells *(14, 27)*.

When the electrode is advanced further and reaches the ventral border of the STN, neuronal activity decreases again and the amplitude of background noise drops to the level of white matter (Figure 6.3). The electrode then traverses into the substantia nigra pars reticulata (SNr) at a variable distance of between 0 and 3 mm. Typically, neurons in the SNr have a more tonic firing pattern, a smaller spike amplitude and a higher mean firing rate of around 50 to 70 Hz, compared to STN neurons *(12, 14, 15, 17, 18)*. These characteristics and differences in background noise level reliably identify the SNr, compared to neuroimaging where the border between STN and SNr can be difficult to delineate due to the similar contrast of both structures on T2-weighted MRI.

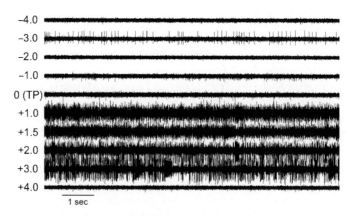

**Figure 6.3** Computer screen shot of microelectrode recordings at different levels along a trajectory towards the subthalamic nucleus. Note the marked increase in background noise, when the microelectrode enters the STN 1 mm below the intended target point (TP). Typical STN signals are recorded over a distance of 2 mm until the electrode leaves the nucleus at 4 mm below the target point

## Stimulation

High-frequency stimulation within the dorsolateral STN should produce a marked reduction of contralateral parkinsonian symptoms within the therapeutic range of 1 to 3 mA. Rigidity responds earliest to test stimulation and unlike bradykinesia does not depend on patient cooperation. Rest tremor is a very reliable indicator of stimulation effect but can fluctuate spontaneously. When present and continuous, it is considered a clinical sign well suited for monitoring the clinical response to test stimulation. A marked decrease in muscle tone is felt approximately 20 to 30 seconds after initiating stimulation with currents as low as 0-5-1 mA at optimal sites. Contralateral activating maneuvers such as finger tapping can be helpful to establish a stable baseline for clinical testing, especially if the patient had little rigidity before surgery or a microlesioning effect has already decreased contralateral signs.

Stimulation-induced dyskinesias are the only adverse effects that are acceptable at low threshold. They often resemble levodopa-induced peak-dose dyskinesias that the patient has already experienced and indicate optimal placement of the electrode. Other adverse effects result from current spread to neighboring structures *(28)* and may indicate a misplaced electrode if they are encountered at low threshold. Stimulation of the pyramidal tract lateral to the STN evokes tetanic contractions, typically of hand or face muscles, and are located closest to the anterolateral STN border. Speech should be monitored carefully, because dysarthria can often be heard before stimulation of corticobulbar fibers produces muscle contractions. Current spread posteriorly into the medial lemniscus produces paraesthesias, which usually habituate rapidly. Current diffusion medially causes oculomotor side effects due to stimulation of supranuclear oculomotor fibers. Eye signs can vary and may consist of dysconjugate contraversive gaze deviation, ipsilateral eye deviation, eyelid retraction, or mydriasis. Occasionally, contralateral eye deviations may be observed because part of the third nerve fibers, which run medial and ventral to the STN, cross at brainstem level. Conjugate gaze deviation provides less localizing information because it may result from medial current spread, lateral current spread into the internal capsule, or stimulation within the STN itself, which also contains an oculomotor region with saccade related neuronal activity *(29, 30)*. Other non-localizing adverse effects are nausea, dizziness, or anxiety. Autonomic symptoms such as flushing, ipsilateral sweating, or mydriasis are often encountered anterior or medial to the STN. Stimulation dorsal to the STN within the subthalamic white matter or zona incerta can reduce rigidity and tremor, but improves bradykinesia less and requires more current intensity to achieve similar clinical benefits *(26)*. Stimulation within the substantia nigra pars reticulata can worsen akinesia and inhibit the levodopa response, but this adverse effect is difficult to monitor intra-operatively.

## Target Selection (Figure 6.4)

We typically encounter STN activity along two to three of the five parallel microelectrode trajectories. The track with the longest pass through the STN (4 mm or more) is the first to be probed by test stimulation at the target level. We first assess the threshold for adverse effects by carefully raising the current until typical symptoms of current diffusion outside of the STN are noted. The type of stimulation induced adverse effects helps localize the position of the electrode relative to the STN (e.g., the observation of a dysconjugate

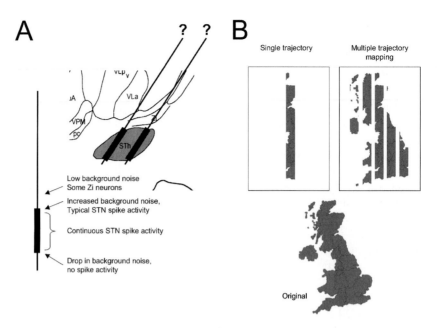

**Figure 6.4** It is not sufficient to determine the length of a single microrecording pass through the STN to obtain spatial information about the location within the nucleus, because two passes of equal length may localize to quite different regions of the STN (A). A useful map may only be reconstructed from multiple trajectories. This is schematically illustrated by a single and multiple trajectory "map" of the United Kingdom (B)

gaze deviation as the first symptom of current diffusion would indicate medial placement of the electrode). The amplitude threshold corresponds to the distance from the STN border. We consider adverse effects at a threshold of 3 mA or more (60 µs pulse width and 130 Hz frequency) acceptable and do not test beyond 5 mA, because they usually lie outside the therapeutic range of a well-placed electrode. Next, we assess the clinical benefit by stimulating with a fixed amplitude (1.5 mA) and rating the improvement for comparison of different sites. Ideally, one should observe at least a 70 to 90% reduction of contralateral rigidity with this stimulation setting. Depending on the results of the first test, one or several subsequent trajectories are also by stimulation explored. The target for implantation of the permanent DBS electrode is selected based on the best clinical improvement achieved and the threshold for inducing adverse effects above 3 mA. The quality and length of microrecordings is only exceptionally taken into account, if clinical testing is unreliable (e.g., in a confused patient or with a pronounced microlesioning effect). In experienced hands the entire electrophysiological mapping procedure requires approximately 30 minutes.

This or a similar approach is used by most DBS centers. Details may vary depending on the equipment and previous clinical experience. Some centers put more emphasis on identifying movement-related cells, others choose the longest pass with typical STN recordings for implantation of the DBS electrode and just stimulate to determine an acceptable threshold for adverse effects. Because clinical outcome depends on many factors other than just the electrophysiological mapping technique, it is impossible to objectively compare different approaches across groups. The criteria for implantation, however, can be analyzed within a single cohort of patients. Houeto and colleagues found no predictive value of the length of the STN microrecording path based on postoperative outcome *(31)*. They also described a better correlation between stimulation induced dyskinesias and outcome than with intra-operative decreases in bradykinesia or rigidity. Not all patients, however, experience dyskinesias with stimulation and some may not be cooperative enough to assess bradykinesia. This emphasizes the importance of an individualized approach, in which the available electrophysiological information is weighed depending on the clinical context.

**Nucleus Ventrointermedius Thalami (VIM)**

*Microelectrode Recording*

Thalamotomy for tremor targets the VIM nucleus of the ventrolateral thalamus where deep kinesthetic afferents, muscle spindle afferents, and cerebellar afferents converge. The VIM cannot be reliably distinguished from surrounding nuclei based on spontaneous discharge patterns but responses to active and passive movements may be helpful. With a typical double oblique (anterolateral) approach, the microelectrode traverses the dorsal parts of the ventralis anterior and posterior nucleus (Voa/Vop), where mostly tonically active units are encountered with a mean discharge rate around 18 Hz in PD *(32)*. These units can be driven by active movements *(33, 34)*. The transition into VIM is characterized by increasingly frequent proprioceptive units, which respond to passive joint movements, tendon pressure, or muscle palpation *(35)*. The posterior border of VIM is formed by the ventrocaudal nucleus (VC), which receives sensory afferents through the medial lemniscus. VC units respond to light touch in well defined cutaneous receptive fields. Voa/Vop, VIM, and VC contain individual somatotopic maps with the same mediolateral sequence of face, arm, and leg areas *(36, 37)*. Evaluating the receptive field of individual neurons can therefore provide information on the laterality of the trajectory.

Previous reports have emphasized the presence of tremor cells within the target region for thalamotomy *(38–41)*. However, rhythmic, tremor-locked neural activity can be encountered throughout the entire ventrolateral thalamic complex and does not provide reliable topographic information by itself *(11)*. Moreover, during audiomonitoring tremor cells may be confused with periodic low-threshold calcium spike bursts, which have a similar frequency but represent a physiological property of thalamic neurons *(11, 42)*.

*Stimulation*

Complete or near complete tremor suppression can be observed with currents as low as 0.5 mA. It may be necessary to evaluate rest tremor during provoking maneuvers such as mental calculation or counting backward, to increase tremor amplitude and to overcome spontaneous fluctuations in severity. Postural and intention tremor are best assessed with the arms held in the "wing-beating" position and during "finger-to-finger" pointing. Functional tests such as spiral drawing may be used to evaluate the impact of stimulation on fine motor skills. With lateral placements in VIM current spread to the pyramidal tract causes tetanic muscle contractions or dysarthria. Paraesthesias result from current diffusion into the posterior located ventrocaudal nucleus. When the electrode is within VIM at a safe distance to the VC, mild dysaesthesias may still be elicited by switching on stimulation, but should habituate rapidly within seconds. Stimulation below the thalamus close to or within the medial lemniscus produces widespread dysaesthesias of the contralateral hemibody at low threshold. Within the subthalamic area, the tremor suppressing effect of stimulation has to be carefully balanced against stimulation-induced dysmetria, which is best observed during "finger-to-finger" pointing *(43)*.

*Target Selection*
The usefulness of microrecordings in selecting the optimal target for thalamotomy or thalamic DBS implantation is strongly debated. Many centers plan the trajectory anatomically and just apply macrostimulation to verify tremor suppression and the absence of intolerable side effects *(44)*. In the literature, one cannot discern a difference in the outcomes reported by groups using or not using microelectrode recording. Electrophysiological mapping of the VIM may also be obsolete, because several recent reports document a better efficacy of DBS within the subthalamic area for severe postural and intention tremors *(43, 45–48)*.

We use the five track-microelectrode holder for thalamic electrode implantations, but only perform microrecordings to determine the ventral border of the ventrolateral thalamus. Our intended target lies 1 to 2 mm deeper within the subthalamic white matter *(43)*. Stimulation is then performed to compare the amplitude threshold for (near) complete tremor suppression across the different electrodes. We carefully assess for stimulation-induced dysmetria and other stimulation-induced adverse effects. Often tremor suppression is found at equally low thresholds for two or more of the microelectrodes. The profile of side effects, however, may vary even between neighboring trajectories and determine the final site of implantation.

**Internal Globus Pallidus (GPi)**

*Microelectrode Recording (Figure 6.5)*
The motor region of the GPi is the target for DBS in dystonia and selected cases of PD. This region corresponds to the ventral and posterior portion of the GPi. The borders of this area are formed laterally by the lamina medullaris

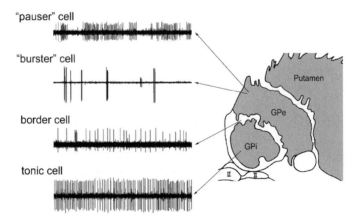

**Figure 6.5** Examples of spontaneous neuronal discharges recorded from external globus pallidus (GPe), border regions, and internal globus pallidus (GPi) in a patient suffering from Parkinson's disease. Bursting activity (either "burster" or "pauser" neurons) are characteristic for GPe, while GPi neurons show high-frequency, tonic activity

interna and the external globus pallidus (GPe), posteriorly and medially by the internal capsule, and ventrally by the ansa lenticularis and the optic tract. Anteriorly, the sensorimotor region merges with other nonmotor regions of the GPi and has no distinct border. For this reason, electrophysiological mapping normally aims at defining the lateral, medial, posterior, dorsal and ventral border of the GPi and identification of the internal capsule and the optic tract.

Depending on which distance from the target recordings are initiated, one can subsequently record from the caudate or putamen and GPe and GPi along a typical trajectory. Each region has its "signature" cell type *(49, 50)*. Neurons of the caudate and putamen have a low-frequency (1–5 Hz) irregular firing pattern. The characteristic sounds from the audiomonitor accounts for calling these units "popcorn cells." Frequently, striatal neurons may become active as the electrode is advanced, with neuronal activity gradually subsiding over a few seconds. Passing through the lamina medullaris externa one can find tonically active (~30 Hz) cells termed "border" cells. These types of units mark all borders around GPe and GPi and the laminae within the lentiform nucleus.

The firing pattern and frequency of neurons within the pallidal complex depends on the underlying disease and has to be discussed separately for PD and dystonia *(51, 52)*. In the parkinsonian state, distinct unit activity can be found within GPe and GPi. The GPe contains two types of units: low-frequency discharge bursting units ("burster cells") and higher-frequency units that are tonically active with intermittent pauses of variable duration ("pauser cells"). The transition from GPe to GPi is marked by a drop of background activity and identification of border cells, when passing the lamina medullaris interna. In PD, neurons in the GPi have a characteristic tonic, high-frequency discharge pattern with a mean frequency around 70 to 80 Hz *(53–56)*. In dystonia, the activity of GPi neurons is more "GPe-like," with lower frequency burst-like and irregular activity *(52, 57–59)*. In our own analysis of 269 units recorded from the GPe and GPi during dystonia surgery, we have found a mean discharge rate of $19 \pm 18$ Hz in GPe and $17 \pm 14$ Hz in GPi (Figure 6.6). A bursting-type discharge pattern was found in 69% of GPe neurons and 54% of GPi neurons, while the remaining units had an irregular or tonic pattern *(60)*. The higher proportion of bursting-type activity in GPe was statically significant, but the large overlap does not allow one to reliably distinguish the GPi from GPe in dystonia patients.

By further advancing the microelectrode beyond the ventral GPi border, the optic tract can be reached within 2 to 4 mm. Flashing light into the patient's eyes evokes fiber discharges that can be heard during audiomonitoring by a change in the amplitude and frequency of the background noise *(57)*. For this purpose, the tip of the microelectrode has to be inside or within a range of several hundred micrometers of the optic tract. We do not recommend this procedure and stopped using it early in our series because the region below the GPi is highly vascularized and the sharp-tipped microelectrodes carry a risk of bleeding. We normally discontinue recordings when the drop in background activity and the presence of border cells indicate leaving the GPi. On the other hand, it continues to be common practice in many other centers to identify the optic tract.

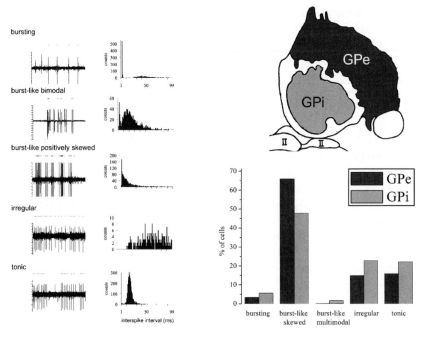

**Figure 6.6** The spontaneous activity of 269 single units was recorded from the external (GPe) and internal (GPi) globus pallidus in 11 patients with generalized dystonia. The discharge pattern was classified based on the interspike interval histograms into bursting, burst-like bimodal, burst-like positively skewed, irregular, and tonic activity. Examples for each type of activity are shown on the left. We found more frequently bursting or burst-like activity in GPe and irregular or tonic activity in GPi, but the overlap was large and did not allow unequivocal identification of each pallidal segment

*Stimulation*

In PD, stimulation is performed to determine the threshold for clinical benefits and adverse effects. Similar to the STN target, marked reductions in muscle tone, improvements in bradykinesia and sometimes stimulation-induced dyskinesias are observed within the sensorimotor GPi although such changes do not appear to be as common with intra-operative GPi stimulation as STN stimulation and the absence of such changes may therefore not necessarily indicate poor electrode localization. Stimulation-induced muscle contractions and phosphenes help to delineate the distance to the internal capsule and optic tract. At higher amplitudes, stimulation may elicit nausea and dizziness, but these effects are non-localizing.

The clinical benefit of DBS cannot be assessed during dystonia surgery, because prolonged stimulation (days to weeks) is often required to induce visible improvements in dystonic movements or postures. Moreover, many dystonia patients with prominent involuntary movements are operated under general anesthesia, which also precludes testing the perception of phosphenes. The threshold for pyramidal tract responses, however, can be determined and helps to establish a safe distance to the internal capsule.

*Target Selection*

The goal of electrophysiological mapping in PD is to identify a long path through the sensorimotor GPi. Microrecordings help to define this path by the presence of typical high-frequency tonic units and their driving by active or passive movements. The lateral border of GPi is marked by a smaller excursion through GPi and the presence of border cells. Even more laterally one would encounter only GPe unit activity. A safe distance to the internal capsule and optic tract is established by macrostimulation.

Mapping in dystonia is more difficult due to the overlapping neuronal signatures of GPe and GPi. We use five parallel microrecording trajectories and search for border cells and the drop in background activity marking the transition between both pallidal segments. Microrecordings are also helpful to define the ventral border of the GPi. We then carefully assess the stimulation threshold for capsular responses by raising the current until contractions are first visible, typically in face or hand muscles. We consider a threshold of 2.5 mA or more (120 μs pulse width, 130 Hz frequency) safe for implantation of the permanent DBS lead. To determine the final site of implantation we combine the *a priori* anatomical information from fast spin-echo inversion recovery MRI, which provides direct visualization of the GPi target and the optic tract, with the results of electrophysiological mapping. Our goal is to place the electrode immediately above or slightly medial to the optic tract within the most posterior aspect of the ventral GPi. The central trajectory of the Ben-Gun microelectrode holder is directed toward this anatomical target. If typical pallidal signals are recorded over a sufficiently long path with the medial or posterior electrode and the threshold of stimulation indicates a safe distance to the internal capsule, we may adjust the final implant site in either direction. If a low threshold for pyramidal tract responses is observed for the central trajectory, we normally move to the anterior electrode, which should increase the distance to the internal capsule. In our experience with 42 consecutive dystonia surgeries, the central trajectory was chosen for 64% of the DBS electrodes. The most common deviation from the central track occurred in the medial direction (20%), followed by the anterior direction (9%).

## Benefits and Risks of Microrecording

Movement disorder surgery is not a life-saving procedure but rather aims at restoring quality of life in a disabled person. The requirements of safety and quality of outcome are special in such elective procedure. When a patient is selected for movement disorder surgery, he or she is willing to accept a certain inherent risk of the neurosurgical procedure. In return, the patient expects the neurosurgeon to take all necessary measures to guarantee the best possible treatment result in his or her individual case. The controversy about the use of microelectrode recordings during movement disorder surgery resides within this risk–benefit dilemma. The proponents of microelectrode recording believe that this technique is essential to secure an optimal placement of lesions or DBS electrodes, improves efficacy of the treatment, and reduces adverse effects related to misplacement *(15, 56, 61–63)*. The most common arguments against microelectrode recording are safety aspects such as a potentially increased risk of bleeding or the lengthening of the surgical procedure. Unfortunately, there is little objective evidence to support either view. Unlike drugs, surgical techniques are difficult to evaluate in clinical trials. Microelectrode recordings can be performed in numerous ways. The interpretation of the data and the safety of the method may greatly depend on the quality of the instruments, the experience of the surgical team and a multitude of other surgical aspects such as the method of stereotactic planning. Surgical techniques are not strictly standardized, they are shaped to the individual needs of a center and subjected to an individual learning curve.

In many discussions about the pros and cons of microelectrode recordings, we have been presented with literature-based comparisons of the clinical outcome of those groups performing microelectrode recordings to those not using them. They seem to indicate superior results for the STN or GPi target in centres using microelectrodes, when presented by proponents of this technique *(15, 56, 61–63)*. Interestingly, in an older study, Hariz and Fodstad *(64)* came to the opposite conclusion based on their critical review of the literature and found groups performing movement disorder surgery without microelectrode recordings to have an equivalent outcome but a lower rate of adverse effects. These contradictory results and conclusions simply indicate that a review of the literature is not a valid approach to the problem. The way of performing surgery in centers that are being compared may differ in many aspects other than the simple fact of using a microelectrode or not. Moreover, there is no common benchmark for evaluating clinical outcome. In PD, it may be necessary to relate the clinical improvement with stimulation alone to the best medication "on" state to evaluate the quality of the surgical procedure in each individual case and reduce the variability induced by differences in levodopa responsiveness *(26)*. This information, however, is not always provided in the literature.

Theoretically, multiple brain penetrations should increase bleeding risk during microelectrode-guided interventions as compared to single trajectory, macrostimulation-guided implantations. Gorgulho and colleagues *(65)* found in their own series of 248 functional stereotactic procedures at the University of California at Los Angeles a trend between the occurrence of hemorrhages and multiple microelectrode passes, but no overall difference in the incidence of intracranial hemorrhages with (2.9%) or without microelectrode recordings (1.4%, $p = 0.65$). Voges et al. *(66)* retrospectively analyzed serious surgical adverse events of DBS implantation in 1183 patients from five German stereotactic centers. Intra-operative microelectrode-recording was applied in all centers but at different frequencies (two centers: <50% of cases; two centers >90% of cases; one center: all cases). No difference was found in the frequency of adverse events between the centers. The overall rate of asymptomatic intracranial hemorrhage was 1.6% and the incidence of symptomatic bleeding was 1.3%. This data is within the incidence range (0.6–5.7%, average: 2.7%) taken from previously published larger single-center studies, which have reported on microelectrode-guided surgery in series of more than 50 patients *(62, 67–71)* and the rate of 1.2% in a group using macrostimulation only *(72)*. In practical terms, microelectrode recordings are therefore unlikely to increase bleeding risk during movement disorder surgery beyond the generally accepted range of a 1 to 3% incidence of symptomatic hemorrhages for any functional stereotactic procedure.

Although no evidence from appropriately designed clinical trials exists, several practical arguments favor the use of microelectrode mapping during movement disorder surgery:

1. Modern neuroimaging techniques have substantially improved anatomical targeting in stereotactic neurosurgery. Nevertheless, the majority of neurosurgeons acknowledge the need for additional physiological verification of the radiologically defined target. Besides the inherent uncertainty of landmark-based, stereotactic targeting, brain shift during the procedure or small deviations of the introduced probe with respect to the precalculated trajectory are factors that are difficult to otherwise account for. Such small deviations from the intended target, however, may be decisive for the postoperative outcome. Therefore, movement disorders surgery is normally performed in awake patients and macrostimulation is considered the minimal requirement to test for clinical benefit and possible side effects at the anatomically predefined target.
2. Unfortunately, intra-operative clinical assessment during macrostimulation is not an easy task, even for experienced neurologists. A number of problems may confound the evaluation of stimulation effects. A substantial number of patients become confused or drowsy during the procedure and cannot cooperate sufficiently during clinical testing. Symptoms and signs may fluctuate or may be masked by prolonged medication effects and one may not be able to provoke them at the time of testing. Most importantly, the microlesioning effect after inserting a stimulating probe often reduces or abolishes signs necessary for clinical testing. Unfortunately, the microlesioning effect is not necessarily predictive for an optimal probe placement. If one is fortunate enough not to encounter any of these problems one may later experience difficulty when the response to stimulation does not correspond to the expected benefit. In such a case, the surgical team will have to decide whether to be satisfied with a moderate intra-operative improvement and stay with the anatomically predefined target or to extend surgery and explore an alternative trajectory for a better response. Multiple perforations with a macrostimulation probe, however, increase the risk of tissue damage and lead to a progressive microlesioning effect, which again impairs clinical comparison of the different targets.
3. Microelectrode recordings provide physiological information about nuclear boundaries that are independent from the cooperation of the patient. They can be performed under general anaesthesia, which is often necessary in patients with severe dystonia, who cannot easily be fixed in a stereotactic frame. The microlesioning effect is minimal when using microelectrodes. Therefore, several trajectories can be explored without compromising subsequent clinical testing during stimulation. Most centers using microelectrode recording in fact believe that several simultaneous or subsequent trajectories are essential to establish a physiological "map" of the target area that can be used to adjust the atlas based anatomy to the individual brain. Microrecordings are usually combined with stimulation either through the microelectrode itself or a microprobe, which is advanced to the target. Using the Ben-Gun method with five simultaneous parallel microelectrode trajectories, we often find very distinct clinical responses at stimulation sites that are only 2 mm apart. In our own experience, the central trajectory, which corresponds to the anatomically predefined target, is used for final implantation of the DBS electrode in only 60 to 70% of cases. The other implantation sites are equally distributed among the surrounding trajectories. Our decision to implant at a particular trajectory is

based on the presence of typical cell discharges in neural recordings and the ratio of benefit to adverse events during stimulation. If one assumes intra-operative stimulation to be predictive for postoperative clinical outcome, one must expect suboptimal electrode placement in approximately 30 to 40% of cases when relying on anatomical targeting and electrophysiological exploration of only a single trajectory. In a retrospective analysis of 50 pallidotomies, Guridi et al. *(56)* found an average deviation of 3 mm between the anatomically and physiologically defined target. In only 45% of the cases would an anatomically defined lesion have overlapped with the final lesion site. Tsao et al. *(73)* concluded from their series that in only 13 of 25 pallidotomies the lesion would have been confined to the GPi based on anatomical targeting. Finally, Alterman et al. *(61)* described a change from the initial anatomical target in 98% of their pallidotomies based on microelectrode recordings with a deviation by more than 4 mm in 12% of the cases. Even for the smaller STN, the mean deviation between anatomically defined target and physiologically defined target may differ between 1.5 and 2.6 mm *(63)*. Amirnov and colleagues *(62)* modified the predicted target in 58% of their STN implantation based on microelectrode recordings. Although these studies do not answer the ultimate question whether microelectrode recording improves clinical outcome, they demonstrate at the very least the uncertainty of anatomical targeting and of a "single trajectory approach."

In summary, we believe that physiological mapping of the target area using multiple microelectrode trajectories helps to improve the accuracy of electrode or lesion placement in movement disorder surgery without significantly increasing risk. The additional time required for microelectrode recording during surgery is well invested, given the amount of time one has to spend for postoperative adjustments of DBS parameters in patients with suboptimal electrode placement *(74)*.

## References

1. Albe-Fessard D, Hardy J, Vourch G, Hertzog E, Aleonard P, Derome P (1962) Dérivation d'activités spontanées et évoquuées dans les structures cérebrale profondes de l'homme. Revue Neurologique 106:89–105.
2. Guiot G, Hardy J, Albe-Fessard D (1962) [Precise delimitation of the subcortical structures and identification of thalamic nuclei in man by stereotactic electrophysiology.]. Neurochirurgia 5:1–18.
3. Caton R (1875) The electrical currents of the brain. BMJ 2:278.
4. Chen CC, Pogosyan A, Zrinzo LU, et al (2006) Intra-operative recordings of local field potentials can help localize the subthalamic nucleus in Parkinson's disease surgery. Exp Neurol 198(1):214–221.
5. Hutchison WD, Lang AE, Dostrovsky JO, Lozano AM (2003) Pallidal neuronal activity: implications for models of dystonia. Ann Neurol 53(4):480–488.
6. Steigerwald F, Hinz L, Pinsker MO, et al (2005) Effect of propofol anesthesia on pallidal neuronal discharges in generalized dystonia. Neurosci Lett 386(3):156–159.
7. Hertel F, Zuchner M, Weimar I, et al (2006) Implantation of electrodes for deep brain stimulation of the subthalamic nucleus in advanced Parkinson's disease with the aid of intraoperative microrecording under general anesthesia. Neurosurgery 59(5):E1138.
8. Krause M, Fogel W, Kloss M, Rasche D, Volkmann J, Tronnier V (2004) Pallidal stimulation for dystonia. Neurosurgery 55(6):1361–1370.

9. Maltete D, Navarro S, Welter ML, et al (2004) Subthalamic stimulation in Parkinson disease: with or without anesthesia? Arch Neurol 61(3):390–392.
10. Raeva S, Lukashev A, Lashin A (1991) Unit activity in human thalamic reticularis nucleus. I. Spontaneous activity. Electroencephalogr Clin Neurophysiol 79(2):133–140.
11. Magnin M, Morel A, Jeanmonod D (2000) Single-unit analysis of the pallidum, thalamus and subthalamic nucleus in parkinsonian patients. Neuroscience 96(3):549–564.
12. Hutchison WD, Allan RJ, Opitz H, et al (1998) Neurophysiological identification of the subthalamic nucleus in surgery for Parkinson's disease. Ann Neurol 44(4):622–628.
13. Magarinos-Ascone CM, Figueiras-Mendez R, Riva-Meana C, Cordoba-Fernandez A (2000) Subthalamic neuron activity related to tremor and movement in Parkinson's disease. Eur J Neurosci 12(7):2597–2607.
14. Rodriguez-Oroz MC, Rodriguez M, Guridi J, et al (2001) The subthalamic nucleus in Parkinson's disease: somatotopic organization and physiological characteristics. Brain 124(Pt 9):1777–1790.
15. Benazzouz A, Breit S, Koudsie A, Pollak P, Krack P, Benabid AL (2002) Intraoperative microrecordings of the subthalamic nucleus in Parkinson's disease. Mov Disord 17(Suppl 3):S145–S149.
16. Lopez-Flores G, Miguel-Morales J, Teijeiro-Amador J, et al (2003) Anatomic and neurophysiological methods for the targeting and lesioning of the subthalamic nucleus: Cuban experience and review. Neurosurgery 52(4):817–830.
17. Bejjani BP, Dormont D, Pidoux B, et al (2000) Bilateral subthalamic stimulation for Parkinson's disease by using three-dimensional stereotactic magnetic resonance imaging and electrophysiological guidance. J Neurosurg 92(4):615–625.
18. Sterio D, Zonenshayn M, Mogilner AY, et al (2002) Neurophysiological refinement of subthalamic nucleus targeting. Neurosurgery 50(1):58–67.
19. Pralong E, Ghika J, Temperli P, Pollo C, Vingerhoets F, Villemure JG (2002) Electrophysiological localization of the subthalamic nucleus in parkinsonian patients. Neurosci Lett 325(2):144–146.
20. Saint-Cyr JA, Hoque T, Pereira LC, et al (2002) Localization of clinically effective stimulating electrodes in the human subthalamic nucleus on magnetic resonance imaging. J Neurosurg 97(5):1152–1166.
21. Pollo C, Vingerhoets F, Pralong E, et al (2007) Localization of electrodes in the subthalamic nucleus on magnetic resonance imaging. J Neurosurg 106(1):36–44.
22. Lanotte MM, Rizzone M, Bergamasco B, Faccani G, Melcarne A, Lopiano L (2002) Deep brain stimulation of the subthalamic nucleus: anatomical, neurophysiological, and outcome correlations with the effects of stimulation. J Neurol Neurosurg Psychiatry 72(1):53–58.
23. Voges J, Volkmann J, Allert N, et al (2002) Bilateral high-frequency stimulation in the subthalamic nucleus for the treatment of Parkinson disease: correlation of therapeutic effect with anatomical electrode position. J Neurosurg 96(2):269–279.
24. Zonenshayn M, Sterio D, Kelly PJ, Rezai AR, Beric A (2004) Location of the active contact within the subthalamic nucleus (STN) in the treatment of idiopathic Parkinson's disease. Surg Neurol 62(3):216–225.
25. Godinho F, Thobois S, Magnin M, et al (2006) Subthalamic nucleus stimulation in Parkinson's disease: anatomical and electrophysiological localization of active contacts. J Neurol 253(10):1347–1355.
26. Herzog J, Fietzek U, Hamel W, et al (2004) Most effective stimulation site in subthalamic deep brain stimulation for Parkinson's disease. Mov Disord 19(9):1050–1054.

27. Romanelli P, Heit G, Hill BC, Kraus A, Hastie T, Bronte-Stewart HM (2004) Microelectrode recording revealing a somatotopic body map in the subthalamic nucleus in humans with Parkinson disease. J Neurosurg 100(4):611–618.
28. Volkmann J, Fogel W, Krack P (2000) Postoperatives neurologisches Management bei Stimulation des Nucleus subthalamicus. Aktuelle Neurol 27(Suppl 1):23–39.
29. Fawcett AP, Cunic D, Hamani C, et al (2007) Saccade-related potentials recorded from human subthalamic nucleus. Clin Neurophysiol 118(1):155–163.
30. Fawcett AP, Dostrovsky JO, Lozano AM, Hutchison WD (2005) Eye movement-related responses of neurons in human subthalamic nucleus. Exp Brain Res 162(3):357–365.
31. Houeto JL, Welter ML, Bejjani PB, et al (2003) Subthalamic stimulation in Parkinson disease: intraoperative predictive factors. Arch Neurol 60(5):690–694.
32. Molnar GF, Pilliar A, Lozano AM, Dostrovsky JO (2005) Differences in neuronal firing rates in pallidal and cerebellar receiving areas of thalamus in patients with Parkinson's disease, essential tremor, and pain. J Neurophysiol 93(6):3094–3101.
33. Lenz FA, Kwan HC, Dostrovsky JO, Tasker RR, Murphy JT, Lenz YE (1990) Single unit analysis of the human ventral thalamic nuclear group. Activity correlated with movement. Brain 113 (Pt 6):1795–1821.
34. Raeva SN (1990) Unit activity of the human thalamus during voluntary movements. Stereotactic and functional neurosurgery 54–55:154–158.
35. Kiss ZH, Davis KD, Tasker RR, Lozano AM, Hu B, Dostrovsky JO (2003) Kinaesthetic neurons in thalamus of humans with and without tremor. Exp Brain Res 150(1):85–94.
36. Lenz FA, Dostrovsky JO, Tasker RR, Yamashiro K, Kwan HC, Murphy JT (1988) Single-unit analysis of the human ventral thalamic nuclear group: somatosensory responses. J Neurophysiol 59(2):299–316.
37. Hua SE, Garonzik IM, Lee JI, Lenz FA (2000) Microelectrode studies of normal organization and plasticity of human somatosensory thalamus. J Clin Neurophysiol 17(6):559–574.
38. Jones MW, Tasker RR (1990) The relationship of documented destruction of specific cell types to complications and effectiveness in thalamotomy for tremor in Parkinson's disease. Stereotact Funct Neurosurg 54–55:207–211.
39. Lenz FA, Tasker RR, Kwan HC, et al (1988) Single unit analysis of the human ventral thalamic nuclear group: correlation of thalamic "tremor cells" with the 3-6 Hz component of parkinsonian tremor. J Neurosci 8(3):754–764.
40. Lenz FA, Kwan HC, Martin RL, Tasker RR, Dostrovsky JO, Lenz YE (1994) Single unit analysis of the human ventral thalamic nuclear group. Tremor-related activity in functionally identified cells. Brain 117(Pt 3):531–543.
41. Lenz FA, Normand SL, Kwan HC, et al (1995) Statistical prediction of the optimal site for thalamotomy in parkinsonian tremor. Mov Disord 10(3):318–328.
42. Ohara S, Taghva A, Kim JH, Lenz FA (2007) Spontaneous low threshold spike bursting in awake humans is different in different lateral thalamic nuclei. Exp Brain Res 180(2):281–8.
43. Herzog J, Hamel W, Wenzelburger R, et al (2007) Kinematic analysis of thalamic versus subthalamic neurostimulation in postural and intention tremor. Brain. 130(6):1608–25.
44. Gross RE, Krack P, Rodriguez-Oroz MC, Rezai AR, Benabid AL (2006) Electrophysiological mapping for the implantation of deep brain stimulators for Parkinson's disease and tremor. Mov Disord 21(Suppl 14):S259–S283.
45. Velasco F, Jimenez F, Perez ML, et al (2001) Electrical stimulation of the prelemniscal radiation in the treatment of Parkinson's disease: an old target revised with new techniques. Neurosurgery 49(2):293–306.
46. Plaha P, Patel NK, Gill SS (2004) Stimulation of the subthalamic region for essential tremor. J Neurosurg 101(1):48–54.

47. Kitagawa M, Murata J, Uesugi H, et al (2005) Two-year follow-up of chronic stimulation of the posterior subthalamic white matter for tremor-dominant Parkinson's disease. Neurosurgery 56(2):281–289.
48. Murata J, Kitagawa M, Uesugi H, et al (2003) Electrical stimulation of the posterior subthalamic area for the treatment of intractable proximal tremor. J Neurosurg 99(4):708–715.
49. Sterio D, Beric A, Dogali M, Fazzini E, Alfaro G, Devinsky O (1994) Neurophysiological properties of pallidal neurons in Parkinson's disease. Ann Neurol 35(5):586–591.
50. Lozano AM, Hutchison WD (2002) Microelectrode recordings in the pallidum. Mov Disord 17(Suppl 3):S150–S154.
51. Vitek JL (2002) Pathophysiology of dystonia: a neuronal model. Mov Disord 17(Suppl 3):S49–S62.
52. Vitek JL, Chockkan V, Zhang JY, et al (1999) Neuronal activity in the basal ganglia in patients with generalized dystonia and hemiballismus. Ann Neurol 46(1):22–35.
53. Vitek JL, Bakay RA, Hashimoto T, et al (1998) Microelectrode-guided pallidotomy: technical approach and its application in medically intractable Parkinson's disease. J Neurosurg 88(6):1027–1043.
54. Lozano A, Hutchison W, Kiss Z, Tasker R, Davis K, Dostrovsky J (1996) Methods for microelectrode-guided posteroventral pallidotomy. J Neurosurg 84(2):194–202.
55. Hutchison WD, Lozano AM, Davis KD, Saint-Cyr JA, Lang AE, Dostrovsky JO (1994) Differential neuronal activity in segments of globus pallidus in Parkinson's disease patients. Neuroreport 5(12):1533–1537.
56. Guridi J, Gorospe A, Ramos E, Linazasoro G, Rodriguez MC, Obeso JA (1999) Stereotactic targeting of the globus pallidus internus in Parkinson's disease: imaging versus electrophysiological mapping. Neurosurgery 45(2):278–287.
57. Merello M, Cerquetti D, Cammarota A, et al (2004) Neuronal globus pallidus activity in patients with generalised dystonia. Mov Disord 19(5):548–554.
58. Sanghera MK, Grossman RG, Kalhorn CG, Hamilton WJ, Ondo WG, Jankovic J (2003) Basal ganglia neuronal discharge in primary and secondary dystonia in patients undergoing pallidotomy. Neurosurgery 52(6):1358–1370.
59. Lenz FA, Suarez JI, Metman LV, et al (1998) Pallidal activity during dystonia: somatosensory reorganisation and changes with severity. J Neurol Neurosurg Psychiatry 65(5):767–770.
60. Hinz L, Steigerwald F, Fietzek U, Mehdorn H, Deuschl G, Volkmann J (2004) Pallidal neuronal activity in generalized dystonia. Mov Disord 19:S293.
61. Alterman RL, Sterio D, Beric A, Kelly PJ (1999) Microelectrode recording during posteroventral pallidotomy: impact on target selection and complications. Neurosurgery 44(2):315–321.
62. Amirnovin R, Williams ZM, Cosgrove GR, Eskandar EN (2006) Experience with microelectrode guided subthalamic nucleus deep brain stimulation. Neurosurgery 58(1 Suppl):102.
63. Zonenshayn M, Rezai AR, Mogilner AY, Beric A, Sterio D, Kelly PJ (2000) Comparison of anatomic and neurophysiological methods for subthalamic nucleus targeting. Neurosurgery 47(2):282–292.
64. Hariz MI, Fodstad H (1999) Do microelectrode techniques increase accuracy or decrease risks in pallidotomy and deep brain stimulation? A critical review of the literature. Stereotact Funct Neurosurg 72(2–4):157–169.
65. Gorgulho A, De Salles AA, Frighetto L, Behnke E (2005) Incidence of hemorrhage associated with electrophysiological studies performed using macroelectrodes and microelectrodes in functional neurosurgery. J Neurosurg 102(5):888–896.
66. Voges J, Hilker R, Bötzel K, et al (2007) 30-days complication rate following surgery performed for Deep-Brain-Stimulation. Mov Disord 22(10):1486–9.

67. Binder DK, Rau GM, Starr PA (2005) Risk factors for hemorrhage during microelectrode-guided deep brain stimulator implantation for movement disorders. Neurosurgery 56(4):722–732.
68. Goodman RR, Kim B, McClelland S 3rd, et al (2006) Operative techniques and morbidity with subthalamic nucleus deep brain stimulation in 100 consecutive patients with advanced Parkinson's disease. J Neurol Neurosurg Psychiatry 77(1):12–17.
69. Terao T, Takahashi H, Yokochi F, Taniguchi M, Okiyama R, Hamada I (2003) Hemorrhagic complication of stereotactic surgery in patients with movement disorders. J Neurosurg 98(6):1241–1246.
70. Umemura A, Jaggi JL, Hurtig HI, et al (2003) Deep brain stimulation for movement disorders: morbidity and mortality in 109 patients. J Neurosurg 98(4):779–784.
71. Lyons KE, Wilkinson SB, Overman J, Pahwa R (2004) Surgical and hardware complications of subthalamic stimulation: a series of 160 procedures. Neurology 63(4):612–616.
72. Blomstedt P, Hariz MI (2006) Are complications less common in deep brain stimulation than in ablative procedures for movement disorders? Stereotact Funct Neurosurg 84(2–3):72–81.
73. Tsao K, Wilkinson S, Overman J, et al (1998) Comparison of actual pallidotomy lesion location with expected stereotactic location. Stereotact Funct Neurosurg 71(1):1–19.
74. Okun MS, Tagliati M, Pourfar M, et al (2005) Management of referred deep brain stimulation failures: a retrospective analysis from 2 movement disorders centers. Arch Neurol 62(8):1250–1255.

# 7
# Complication Avoidance and Management in Deep Brain Stimulation Surgery

Philip A. Starr and Karl Sillay

## Abstract

A number of recent publications have reviewed complications of deep brain stimulation (DBS) implantation *(1–11)*. A summary of the author's peri-operative and device-related complications using Medtronic DBS hardware is provided in Table 7.1. This is based on a series of 637 new DBS leads in 358 patients implanted by a single surgeon (PAS). Procedures were performed with frame-based stereotaxy using MRI and microelectrode recording (MER). The total incidence of unexpected returns to the operating room for management of a complication was 59 surgical cases in 50 of the 358 operated patients, or 14%. Most of these re-operations were on the subcutaneous rather than intracranial parts of the hardware. The risk of requiring further intracranial surgery to replace a broken, misplaced, or infected lead was 5.9% per patient. This chapter provides a description of our current methods for complication avoidance and management.

**Keywords:** deep brain stimulation (DBS), surgical complications, hardware complications, stereotaxy, brain hemorrhage, infection

## Stroke

Stroke is the most serious potential complication of movement disorders surgery. Stroke is defined as a new neurologic deficit of vascular origin, lasting longer than 24 hours. Using this definition, the incidence of stroke in our series was nine cases, or 1.5% per lead and 2.5% per patient. Eight of the nine strokes were hemorrhagic strokes, and of these, three were likely venous infarctions based on the CT appearance (Figure 7.1). Four patients (1.1%) had a permanent neurologic deficit. Table 7.2 provides details of presumed etiologic factors and outcomes. The rate of stroke with permanent

**Table 7.1** Complications in 637 DBS implants in 358 patients implanted 1998–2006. The mean follow-up time was 54 months.

| Complication | No. of occurrences | No. of patients[‡] | Implanted leads (%) | Patients (%) |
|---|---|---|---|---|
| Hemorrhagic stroke (arterial or venous) | 8 | 8 | 1.3 | 2.2 |
| Ischemic stroke (capsular infarction) | 1 | 1 | 0.2 | 0.3 |
| Asymptomatic hemorrhage* | 15 | 15 | 2.4 | 4.2 |
| Stroke with permanent neurologic deficit | 4 | 4 | 0.6 | 1.1 |
| Chronic subdural hematoma | 1 | 1 | 0.2 | 0.3 |
| DBS lead fracture | 5 | 4 | 1.4 | 1.1 |
| Lead extender fracture | 3 | 3 | 0.5 | 0.8 |
| Poor initial lead position resulting in re-operation | 11 | 10 | 1.7 | 2.8 |
| Lead migration resulting in re-operation | 2 | 2 | 0.3 | 0.6 |
| Infection requiring removal of IPG and lead extender, and IV antibiotics | 8 | 8 | 1.6[†] | 2.2 |
| Infection requiring removal of all hardware including brain leads | 7 | 7 | 1.6[†] | 2.0 |
| Return to operating room for other exploration/repair of subcutaneous hardware[⊥] | 22 | 19 | 3.5 | 5.3 |
| Infection requiring IV antibiotics without hardware removal (both at frontal incision) | 2 | 2 | 0.3 | 0.6 |
| Major air embolus (prolonging the procedure or requiring its abandonment) | 3 | 3 | 0.5 | 0.8 |
| Intra-operative seizure (focal) | 1 | 1 | 0.2 | 0.3 |
| Postoperative seizures | 4 | 4 | 0.6 | 1.4 |
| Tense cerebrospinal fluid collection around IPG, not surgically treated | 2 | 2 | 0.3 | 0.6 |
| Postoperative aspiration pneumonia | 3 | 3 | 0.5 | 0.8 |
| Suicide attempt or psychiatric hospitalization within 6 months of surgery | 4 | 4 | 0.6 | 1.1 |
| TOTAL UNPLANNED INTRACRANIAL RE-OPERATIONS | 26 | 21 | 4.1 | 5.9 |
| TOTAL UNPLANNED RE-OPERATIONS | 59 | 50 | 9.3 | 14.0 |

[‡]The number of occurrences is greater than the number of patients affected for certain types of complications becuase there were multiple occurrences in on patient.

[†]To calculate a "per lead implant" infection rate, an infection involving a dual-channel IPG (Kinetra) was counted as affecting two leads, while an infection of a single-channel IPG was counted as affecting one lead.

*Threshold of detection was volume $>0.2$ cc.

[⊥]Problems included: sterile seroma around IPG, $N = 2$; hematoma around IPG, $N = 1$; hardware disconnection, $N = 3$; failure of wound to heal, $N = 1$; IPG malfunction, $N = 1$; elective repositioning of connector from cervical to cranial position, $N = 8$; lead extender replacement to address patient discomfort, $N = 2$; connector or IPG repositioning for threatened erosion, $N = 3$; repair DBS anchoring system, $N = 1$.

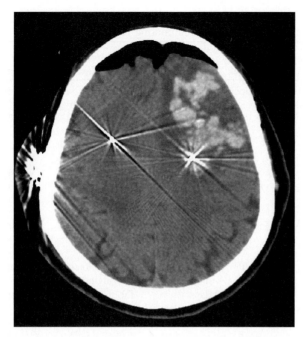

**Figure 7.1** Axial CT scan of a 75-year-old patient 10 hours after placement of bilateral subthalamic nucleus deep brain stimulators, showing an apparent venous infarction. The patient initially had no postoperative deficits, then evolved an aphasia, prompting urgent CT. No cortical veins were transgressed during the procedure, but significant intracranial air entry and a state of dehydration may have triggered a vein thrombosis

deficit in other large published series (>100 patients) has ranged from 0 *(7)* to 2.8% *(12)*.

Ischemic infarction is very infrequent following DBS surgery, occurring only once in our series. In contrast, delayed ischemic capsular infarction has been well described following pallidotomy *(13, 14)*, and is probably a more frequent complication of stereotactic lesioning surgery than of DBS.

Asymptomatic hemorrhage is more common than symptomatic hemorrhage, but is only detected if postoperative imaging is performed systematically. Our rate of asymptomatic hemorrhage, detected on routine postoperative MRI was 2.4% per lead. Most of the asymptomatic hematomas occurred subcortically, 25 to 35 mm superior to the target, corresponding to the location where the guide tube for the microelectrode terminated.

## Avoidance of Stroke

We recommend the following measures to reduce the incidence of stroke, both arterial and venous:

1. Maintain systolic pressure under 140 and mean arterial pressure (MAP) under 90. In any patient with pre-existing hypertension, place an arterial line and control blood pressure with a continuous intravenous drip.
2. Utilize a stereotactic surgical planning software package to plan the trajectory to the desired target that avoids MR- or CT-visible blood vessels, sulci, and ventricles. Use contrast-enhanced images to visualize venous structures.

**Table 7.2** Hemorrhagic stroke in 358 patients undergoing frame-based DBS electrode implants: presumed precipitating factors.

| Description of stroke | Surgical target | Time of occurrence | Presumed etiologic factors | Outcome |
|---|---|---|---|---|
| Rapidly evolving large basal ganglia hematoma | Gpi | Intra-operative | Crossing choroidal fissure during microelectrode recording, lateral to optic tract | Permanent hemiparesis |
| Frontal venous infarction | GPi | Intra-operative | Coagulation of a bridging vein | Permanent hemiparesis, aspiration pneumonia, death at 3 months post-surgery |
| Frontal venous infarction | GPi | 2 days post-surgery | Coagulation of a bridging vein | Full recovery |
| Thalamic hematoma | STN | 3 days post-surgery | Fit of severe coughing associated with a URI | Permanent worsening of gait and balance |
| Capsular hematoma | STN | Intra-operative | Rapid withdrawal of a microelectrode | Full recovery |
| Capsular hematoma | STN | Intra-operative | Unknown | Full recovery |
| Frontal venous infarction | STN | 10 hours post-surgery | Dehydration, large amount of intracranial air entry | Permanent speech impairment |
| Putaminal/capsular hematoma | GPi | Intra-operative | Microelectrode mapping | Full recovery |

GPi, globus pallidus internus; STN, subthalamic nucleus; URI, upper respiratory infection.

3. Avoid damage to or coagulation of venous structures.
4. Because dehydration is a risk factor for venous infarction, patients should be adequately hydrated. We hydrate with 1 L of intravenous crystalloid at the beginning of the case, subsequent to Foley catheter insertion.
5. Avoid entry of large amounts of intracranial air, because this may precipitate subdural hematoma or venous infarction. Subdural spaces should be filled with saline irrigation and sealed with gelfoam when instruments are not being passed.
6. During pallidal surgery, avoid passing instruments deep to the optic tract (OT), into the choroidal fissure. Currently, if we do not locate OT within 2 mm of the base of pallidum during MER, we do not continue more inferiorly.
7. Any Valsalva maneuver during or immediately after surgery carries a risk of hemorrhage. If a patient has an upper respiratory infection or any other reversible source of coughing, surgery should be postponed. If the patients has uncontrolled coughing or sneezing during awake surgery, consider sedating the patient or aborting the case.

8. Avoid rapid insertion or withdrawal (>0.5 mm/second) of instruments into or out of the brain.
9. During and at the end of the procedure, cover the cortical entry with gelfoam and fibrin glue to avoid subdural blood accumulation.

## Management of Stroke

If a new neurologic deficit occur during the procedure, surgery should be stopped immediately. The anesthesiologists are asked to redouble efforts at blood pressure control and ensure appropriate oxygenation. All instruments should be removed from the brain and the cortex inspected. If no surface bleeding is seen and no bleeding is seen from the cortical entry, the scalp should be rapidly closed, the headframe removed, and the patient is taken for a head CT scan.

During surgery, there may be more subtle signs of an intraparenchymal hemorrhage that is initially asymptomatic and may remain so depending on its final size and location. When we have observed blood coming from the subcortical guide tube after withdrawal of a stylet or microelectrode, a small hematoma is almost always observed on postoperative imaging at a depth corresponding to the termination of the guide tube. During MER, if a significant region of electrical silence is observed at a depth where neuronal tissue is predicted based on prior adjacent MER tracks, the cause may be a small hematoma. If either of these signs of potential hematoma formation is observed, we halt the procedure, closely observe the patient for subtle new neurologic deficit, while reconfirming strict blood pressure control. If no deficit occurs in 5 to 10 minutes, we proceed with surgery.

## Air Embolus

Transvenous air embolism is relatively frequent in DBS surgery, due mainly to patient positioning (head elevated above heart level). In addition, DBS is often performed on awake patients who are more likely to generate negative venous pressures during spontaneous respiration, compared with anesthetized patients under positive pressure ventilation. A significant air embolus may prolong a case, necessitate aborting the case or, if not promptly recognized by the surgeon and anesthesiologist, could prove fatal. Air embolism occurs most frequently during drilling of the bone or opening the dura. In the awake patient, its initial manifestation is usually coughing, followed by a decrease in end tidal C02. Hypoxia and a cardiac murmur may ensue if the problem is not promptly corrected.

### Steps to Prevent Air Embolism

1. Adequately hydrate the patient pre-operatively and intra-operatively.
2. Wax all bone edges (even if they are not bleeding).
3. Avoid entry into dural venous sinuses.

### Management of Air Embolism

1. Lower the head of the bed.
2. Flood the surgical field with saline.

3. Auscultate the heart.
4. If symptoms are ongoing or a cardiac murmur appears, compress the jugular veins and close the incision.

## Infection

A serious infection is defined as one that requires a return to the operating room for removal of all or part of the DBS hardware. The incidence of serious infection in our series was 15 cases, or 3.2% per lead and 4.2% per patient (Table 7.1). All of these infections have occurred subcutaneously, starting at the lead extender or the implanted pulse generator (IPG). The offending organism was *Staphylococcus aureus* in the majority of cases. Using traditional stereotaxy in a regular operating room, we have had no infections in the brain, and in fact cerebral abscess or cerebritis complicating DBS is only rarely reported *(15, 16)*. In our experience, infections at the frontal incision did not occur. It has been reported that linear incisions that directly cross the hardware anchoring site are associated with an increased risk of infection at the burr hole site *(11)*. When electrodes are implanted in an interventional MRI setting outside of a standard operating room, the incidence of intracranial infection may be higher *(17)*. Externalizing the electrodes for a period of postoperative testing, prior to permanent internalization, probably increases the risk of infection *(11)*.

Most of our infections presented with some combination of swelling, redness, pain, or drainage over the connector of the lead extender, or over the IPG. Of 15 infections, 13 presented within 1 to 8 weeks of surgery, although two presented as stitch abscess over an anchoring suture on the connector, 4 months and 2 years after implantation.

### Infection Avoidance

Our approach to avoidance of infection, in addition to meticulous attention to sterile technique follows:

1. Patients are instructed to shower the night pre-operatively using chlorhexidine scrub on the surgical sites.
2. Pre-operative prophylaxis with an anti-staphylococcal cephalosporin in the hour prior to skin incision, followed by a second dose given 3 hours later.
3. Shaving is done immediately prior to surgery with clippers rather than a razor.
4. Surgeons double glove for all procedures.
5. Cranial incisions are curvilinear rather than straight so as to avoid crossing the lead anchoring device.
6. Utilization of the lowest-profile hardware available, with recessing of larger components into a drilled bone trough in patients with thin skin.
7. Implants are removed from the sterile inner container by the implanting surgeon and placed directly from the box into the patient, with no other individuals handling the implants.
8. Where permanent anchoring sutures are used on the lead extenders or IPG, these are placed into deep fascial layers rather than more superficially in the dermis.
9. The IPG is placed directly onto the well-vascularized pectoralis fascia rather than into subcutaneous fat more superficially.

10. Surgery is performed efficiently to reduce operative time.
11. Copious irrigation of all incisions with bacitracin solution prior to closure.
12. Temporary externalization of the lead for postoperative testing is avoided.

**Infection Management**

The management of hardware infections has not been standardized. Several groups have reported that infections of any part of the device were ultimately treated with removal of all hardware in most cases, despite initial attempts at more localized treatment (5, 11, 18). Successful management of an unambiguous, culture-documented infection with intravenous antibiotics alone has been reported by Temel et al. (19) in two of four DBS device infections, but successful nonoperative treatment of infections in direct contact with hardware has not been widely replicated on other series, and cannot be recommended (20). We and others have had success with a lead-sparing partial hardware removal approach in selected cases where infection presents early and is localized to one hardware component (10, 16, 19). Our infection management algorithm follows:

1. For superficial infections at incision sites where hardware does not appear to be in direct contact with pus or necrotic tissue, the patient is treated with oral antibiotics and local wound care without hardware removal, and followed weekly with clinical examination until wounds are completely healed.
2. For infections where the lead extender or IPG are in direct contact with pus or necrotic tissue, the affected components are removed immediately on presentation, and the patient is treated with the appropriate IV antibiotics. If a localized infection around the pulse generator or lead extender is discovered early in its course, prompt removal of the IPG and lead extender alone, with sparing of the brain electrodes, has been successful in 70% of cases where this was attempted in our series.
3. When there is infection in direct contact with the brain lead or an infection along the extender or IPG showing extensive surrounding cellulites, we remove all DBS hardware on presentation.
4. Following partial or complete hardware removal, we wait at least 2 months following the completion of antibiotic therapy to re-implant devices.

## Sterile Fluid Collections

Four of our patients have presented within 1 month post-surgery with tense swellings around the IPG, which were fluctuant but painless and without redness or warmth. Surgical exploration of one of these revealed a sterile clear fluid collection consistent with cerebrospinal fluid (CSF). This appears to occur more frequently with burr hole-based anchoring methods that are not watertight (such as the Medtronic Stim-lock system), as CSF can "wick" along the hardware to accumulate in the pectoral cavity. Sealing the burr hole with gelfoam and fibrin glue prior to closure has reduced the incidence of these sterile collections. If a swelling around an IPG is not red, tender, or warm, and the incision is healing well, our practice is to observe it. Sterile fluid collections typically resolve spontaneously, or with application of a pressure dressing to the chest.

## Misplaced Electrodes

Utilizing current surgical techniques, even experienced stereotactic surgeons occasionally find that an electrode is misplaced. An example of a misplaced subthalamic nucleus (STN) electrode, and its subsequent proper positioning, is shown in Figure 7.2. At this time, there are no clear guidelines for what constitutes acceptable lead locations for movement disorders, other than that the electrode should be in a position to affect the motor territories of the relevant nuclei: the dorsolateral STN, posterolateral internal pallidum, or ventrolateral thalamus. Radiographically, we consider an electrode malpositioned if it is more than 2 mm from the intended location in the relevant axial plane on postoperative MRI. Clinically, an electrode may be considered malpositioned if it is radiographically well positioned, but fails to provide the expected clinical benefit despite multiple programming attempts, and/or produces simulation-induced side effects at thresholds low enough to interfere with clinical use. If an electrode is malpositioned on clinical grounds, we perform stereotactic insertion of a new lead under fluoroscopy, using the initial, malpositioned lead as an internal reference marker. MER is not used in this setting. MER is very difficult to interpret if a nearby lead has just been removed, because the resulting tissue edema alters neuronal discharge characteristics. In our series, 1.7% of implanted electrodes were ultimately replaced due to poor initial position (Table 7.1).

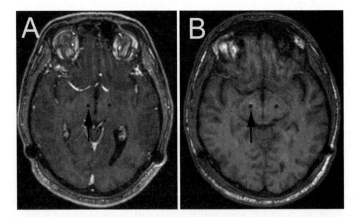

**Figure 7.2** Axial T1-weighted MRI scan of bilateral STN DBS leads showing (A) a poorly positioned right STN DBS electrode and (B) the same patient following stereotactic repositioning of the right electrode. The center of the round signal void is considered to represent the location of the lead (black arrows). The imaging plane is 4 mm inferior to the intercommissural line. (A) The initial right lead shown could be programmed to provide some motor benefit, but was associated with stimulation-induced mood depression. (B) The repositioned right lead provided improved motor benefits and was not associated with mood depression

## Long-term Hardware-Related Complications

In a long-term longitudinal analysis by Oh et al. *(5)*, the risk of having a hardware-related complication was 8.4% per lead implant per year. The major hardware complications are those associated with lead fracture, lead migration, and device erosion. Our experience with these complications is detailed in Table 7.1.

### Lead Fractures

Our series includes five lead fractures, two in the neck associated with a low lying lead extenders (occurring 10 months post-surgery), one under a titanium miniplate used to anchor the DBS electrode (occurring 2 years post-surgery), and two near the lead extender junction in the parietal area in a patient with very severe cervical dystonia, within a few months of surgery (Figure 7.3). The Medtronic models 3387 and 3389 may be relatively sensitive to motion-induced fracture because of the helical coiling of the wires. Other types of DBS electrodes now undergoing clinical testing may be less susceptible to this problem.

### Measures to Avoid Lead Fractures With Medtronic DBS Electrodes

Place the proximal part of the lead extender (the connector) under the scalp, not in the cervical area where mobility at the junction between the lead and the connector predisposes to fracture. In most patients, we place the connector posterior and slightly superior to the pinna of the ear. In patients with severe cervical dystonia with a strong phasic component, we now place the connection to the lead extender even more superiorly, at the vertex of the scalp. This reduces transmission of severe cervical spasms to the lead, which can occur with low parieto-occipital placement of the proximal lead extender (Figure 7.3).

1. Anchor the lead extender connector under the scalp, either using a silk suture to the underlying fascia, or by drilling a small trough in the skull to recess the connector.

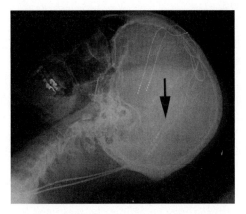

**Figure 7.3** Lateral skull X-ray showing a lead fracture near the junction of the lead with the lead extender (black arrow). The patient is 18 years old with severe juvenile-onset idiopathic generalized dystonia, involving violent neck spasms that generated motion at the distal lead, in spite of positioning the lead extender over skull. At lead replacement, the connection with the lead extender was placed over the skull vertex

2. If a patient is noted on follow-up to have a connector in the cervical area, either from migration or improper initial placement, we offer elective repositioning to a more rostral level to reduce the risk of delayed fracture. This usually requires re-tunneling of the connector from a parietal incision.
3. Although we initially used titanium miniplates to anchor DBS leads, we have abandoned this method due to the observation by ourselves and others of delayed fractures under the edge of the plate.

**Management of Lead Fractures**

To replace a fractured lead, we perform a new stereotactic procedure, and use fluoroscopy to visualize the initial lead and confirm placement of a new one at the same site. MER is not used. It may be possible to slide a new lead "freehand" down the prior gliotic lead track, after visualizing the initial lead on fluoroscopy and removing it, but we do not have experience with this.

**Lead Migration**

We have observed delayed lead migration in two early cases where the lead was anchored only with methylmethacrylate. Migration has not been observed following use of a titanium miniplate (approximately 100 leads) or use of the Medtronic Stim-lock burr hole cap (~500 leads). The most important steps to avoid delayed lead migration are:

1. Do not depend on methylmethacrylate alone to anchor the lead.
2. Leave redundant coils of lead under the frontoparietal scalp so that tension on the lead extender is not transmitted directly to the lead at its anchor point. Some redundant coils are normally necessary if the connector is placed under the parietal scalp and a 28 or 40 cm DBS leads are used.

Normally, a lead migration will require a new stereotactic procedure to re-insert the lead.

**Hardware Erosion**

Erosion of the skin over part of the device can occur insidiously and will never be completely eliminated with current DBS device designs. The following can help minimize the long-term erosion risk.

1. Use the lowest-profile hardware available. With regard to the Medtronic DBS system, avoid the original Medtronic burr hole cap as this has a profile that is both high and sharp, and avoid the use of the older Medtronic high-profile connectors in favor of the low profile connector.
2. In patients with thin scalps, drill a trough in the skull to recess the lead anchoring devices and the connector.
3. At the level of the pulse generator, any excess lead extender wire should be coiled underneath the IPG rather than above it.
4. An impending erosion may sometimes be prevented by prophylactic surgery. If, on a follow-up visit, the skin over the lead extender connector is noted to be very thin and avascular, we electively reposition the connector to a new location where a trough is drilled in the parietal bone.

## Management of Hardware Erosion

If erosion has just occurred, transposition without device removal may be attempted, but the most definitive treatment is to remove the part of the device that has eroded and replace it later after the skin has completely healed. If an erosion of a pulse generator occurs in a very thin individual, we replace the IPG in the abdomen rather than the chest.

## Rare but Spectacular Complications of DBS

### Inadvertant Thermal Lesioning

Inadvertent thermal lesioning around a DBS electrode has been reported following cardioversion *(21)*, diathermy *(22)*, and MRI using a body transmit coil *(23)*. Diathermy is a treatment of undocumented utility that involves the application of rapidly alternating electromagnetic current to produce "deep tissue heating." When applied near a DBS device, large radiofrequency lesions around the DBS contacts in the brain may occur which produce permanent brain damage. Exposure to diathermy is absolutely contraindicated in patients with deep brain electrodes.

MRI must be used with caution, following the manufacturer's guidelines, in the setting of implanted DBS devices. One permanent thermal brain injury due to MRI in a patient with deep brain stimulators has been reported. This occurred during a lumbar spine MRI in a 1.0 Tesla unit, using a body transmit coil, in a patient with a pulse generator in the abdomen and a long lead extender (23). Brain MRI is thought to be safe if performed at 1.5T using a transmit-receive head coil and protocols with low specific absorption rate. However, with currently available DBS devices, body MRI is contraindicated, as is brain MRI if not performed within the manufacturer's specifications.

### Electrolysis and Gas Production

Normally the current transmitted through a DBS contact is alternating current so that there is no net charge build-up on a contact. Malfunction of a pulse generator so as to produce a net direct current may result in electrolysis and the production of an intraparenchymal gas bubble presenting as an expanding mass lesion. This has been reported in the context of a malfunction of an external pulse generator that was used for several days of testing through an externalized lead *(24)*. The authors recommended that the duration of external test stimulation, if done at all, should be kept to a minimum.

### Damage to Lead or Lead Extender due to Patient Manipulation of the IPG

If the IPG is not sutured to the underlying pectoralis fascia, it may be possible for the patient to manually rotate the device within its subcutaneous pocket. One of our patients presented with a short circuit between three contacts of the DBS lead, and a new protuberance under the parietal scalp immediately superior to the connector of the lead extender. An X-ray showed a highly unusual coiling of the distal lead near its insertion into the connector. At surgical exploration, extensive twisting of both the lead extender and the lead were found, apparently due to the patient's repeated rotation of the IPG under the skin. This so-called "Twiddler's syndrome" has been well documented in the literature on cardiac pacemakers *(25)*.

## Postoperative Cognitive Decline in Patients With Parkinson's Disease (PD)

Even in the absence of stroke or other neurological complications, patients with advanced PD may be at risk for permanent cognitive decline following bilateral STN DBS *(26–28)*. The presence of significant cognitive impairment pre-operatively or advanced age increase the risk of this complication *(26)*. It is not yet clear if unilateral STN DBS or bilateral globus pallidus internus (GPi) DBS carry the same risk. Our current measures to avoid this complication are:

1. PD patients with significant cognitive dysfunction (Mini Mental Status score <24) are not offered surgery.
2. PD patients over 80 are very rarely accepted for surgery, unless their physical health and cognitive function are unusually good.
3. PD patients over 70, or patients under 70 who have mild cognitive dysfunction, are offered staged implants rather than simultaneous bilateral implants. Formal neuropsychological testing is done before and after the first implant. The second implant is not performed until full neuropsychological recovery from the first implant is documented.

## Troubleshooting the Lead That Doesn't Work

In a movement disorders surgery clinic, a frequent request for consultation concerns a patient who has an implanted DBS system and is not getting the expected or desired benefit. A detailed analysis of reasons for device failure has been published by Okun et al. *(29)*. In their series of 41 patients referred for "failed" DBS, the most common reasons for failure were misplaced electrodes. In general, there are five broad reasons for device "failure":

1. There is an electrical malfunction.
2. The electrode is poorly located in the brain.
3. The patient has a diagnosis that will not respond to DBS.
4. The patient has become tolerant to the therapeutic effect of DBS.
5. The patient is poorly programmed.

Initially, electrical malfunction should be ruled out by interrogating the battery, determining if the battery is generating adequate voltage, verifying that the system is turned on, and checking the current and impedance at each contact to rule out an open circuit. If all four contacts have developed an open circuit in a system that had previously been working, it is likely that the lead or lead extender is fractured. AP and lateral X-ray of the skull and neck can confirm this in most cases. In some cases, however, there is a lead fracture without X-ray visible separation between the strands.

If the electrical system is found to have appropriate impedances, location-specific stimulation-induced adverse effects are sought. The most common of these are dysarthria and paresthesia for thalamic or STN DBS, and dysarthria or visual phenomena for GPi DBS. If these are not produced at high voltage or are produced at voltages lower than typical therapeutic parameters for each target, the brain should be imaged to check for a misplaced DBS electrode (Figure 7.2).

If stimulation induced adverse effects and/or imaging indicate appropriate electrode location, then the patient's diagnosis should be revisited. Movement disorders for which DBS has been utilized but may only be marginally effective are atypical forms of parkinsonism, and some secondary dystonias. Some types of tremor that have been treated by DBS, such as post-traumatic tremor or MS-associated tremor, are less likely to be responsive to DBS than parkinsonian tremor and essential tremor (ET).

Even for patients with an "on-label" indication for DBS therapy, a possibility for long-term failure is physiologic tolerance to the therapeutic effect of stimulation. This problem arises primarily in thalamic DBS for ET, for which the incidence of tolerance has been reported at 10 to 30% *(30–34)*. At least some of these cases are probably due to true physiologic tolerance to a well-located electrode, rather than suboptimal electrode positioning. These cases are potentially treatable by lesioning through the DBS electrode *(35, 36)*. Some have argued that GPi DBS in PD also may manifest tolerance after several years *(37)*, but this may relate to suboptimal electrode placement rather than true tolerance to GPi DBS. Tolerance to the therapeutic effect of STN DBS in PD with respect to Sinemet-responsive symptoms has not been reported with follow-up of 4 *(38, 39)* and 5 *(40, 41)* years. However, as PD progresses, more Sinemet unresponsive symptoms such as postural instability, severe on-period freezing of gait, hypophonia, or cognitive impairment may manifest. These Sinemet unresponsive symptoms also tend to be resistant to DBS, resulting in a partial loss of benefit to the patient over time *(40)*. With regard to pallidal stimulation for idiopathic dystonia, long term tolerance has been reported anecdotally *(42)*. Currently no large series documents outcomes for DBS in dystonia at greater than 2 years following implantation, so the incidence of long-term tolerance to the therapeutic effect is unknown.

Finally, improper programming may be a source of long-term failure, particularly in PD *(29)*. This can be avoided if programming is performed by a movement disorders neurologist with expertise in DBS programming. Published guidelines for DBS programming in PD are available *(43, 44)*.

In conclusion, the most important peri-operative complications related to deep brain stimulator implant surgery are hemorrhagic stroke, intra-operative air embolus, device infection, and suboptimal placement of the brain electrode. The most common long-term complications are fracture of the brain electrode, and device erosion. Strategies for the avoidance and management of these complications are discussed.

## References

1. Hariz MI (2002) Complications of deep brain stimulation surgery. Mov Disord 17(Suppl 3):S162–S166.
2. Kondziolka D, Whiting D, Germanwala A, Oh M (2002) Hardware-related complications after placement of thalamic deep brain stimulator systems. Stereotact Funct Neurosurg 79:228–233.

3. Beric A, Kelly PJ, Rezai A, Stereo D, Mogilner A, Zonenshayn M, et al (2001) Complications of deep brain stimulation surgery. Stereotact Funct Neurosurg 77:73–78.
4. Umemura A, Jaggi JL, Hurtig HI, Siderowf AD, Colcher A, Stern MB, et al (2003) Deep brain stimulation for movement disorders: morbidity and mortality in 109 patients. J Neurosurg 98:779–784.
5. Oh MY, Abosch A, Kim SH, Lang AE, Lozano AM (2002) Long-term hardware-related complications of deep brain stimulation. Neurosurgery 50:1274–1276.
6. Joint J, Nandi D, Parkin S, Gregory R, Aziz T (2002) Hardware-related problems of deep brain stimulation. Mov Disord 17(Suppl 3):175–180.
7. Blomstedt P, Hariz MI (2006) Are complications less common in deep brain stimulation than in ablative procedures for movement disorders? Stereotact Funct Neurosurg 84(2–3):72–81.
8. Binder D, Rau G, Starr PA (2005) Risk factors for hemorrhage during microelectrode-guided deep brain stimulator implantation for movement disorders. Neurosurgery 56:722–732.
9. Voges J, Waerzeggers Y, Maarouf M, Lehrke R, Koulousakis A, Lenartz D, et al (2006) Deep-brain stimulation: long-term analysis of complications caused by hardware and surgery—experiences from a single centre. J Neurol Neurosurg Psychiatry 77(7):868–872.
10. Lyons KE, Wilkinson SB, Overman J, Pahwa R (2004) Surgical and hardware complications of subthalamic stimulation: a series of 160 procedures. Neurology 63(4):612–616.
11. Constantoyannis C, Berk C, Honey CR, Mendez I, Brownstone RM (2005) Reducing hardware-related complications of deep brain stimulation. Can J Neurol Sci 32(2):194–200.
12. Deep Brain Stimulation for Parkinson's Disease Study Group (2001) Deep-brain stimulation of the subthalamic nucleus or the pars interna of the globus pallidus in Parkinson's diseasee. New Engl J Med 345:956–963.
13. Lim JY, DeSalles AAF, Bronstein J, Masterman DL, Saver JL (1997) Delayed internal capsule infarctions following radiofrequency pallidotomy. J Neurosurg 87:955–960.
14. Baron MS, Vitek JL, Bakay RAE, Green J, Kaneoke Y, Hashimoto T, et al (1996) Treatment of advanced Parkinson's disease by posterior GPi pallidotomy: 1-year results of a pilot study. Ann Neurol 40:355–366.
15. Merello M, Cammarota A, Leiguarda R, Pikielny R (2001) Delayed intracerebral electrode infection after bilateral STN implantation for Parkinson's disease. Case report. Mov Disord 16(1):168–170.
16. Levy RM, Lamb S, Adams JE (1987) Treatment of chronic pain by deep brain stimulation: long term follow-up and review of the literature. Neurosurgery 21(6):885–893.
17. Martin A, Larson P, Ostrem J, Sootsman K, Weber O, Lindsey N, et al (2005) Placement of deep brain stimulator electrodes using real-time high field interventional MRI. Mag Res Med 54:1107–1114.
18. Umemura A, Jaggi JL, Dolinskas CA, Stern MB, Baltuch GH (2004) Pallidal deep brain stimulation for longstanding severe generalized dystonia in Hallervorden-Spatz syndrome. Case report. J Neurosurg 100:706–709.
19. Temel Y, Ackermans L, Celik H, Spincemaille GH, van der Linden C, Walenkamp GH, et al (2004) Management of hardware infections following deep brain stimulation. Acta Neurochir (Wien) 146(4):355–361.
20. Rezai AR, Kopell BH, Gross RE, Vitek JL, Sharan AD, Limousin P, et al (2006) Deep brain stimulation for Parkinson's disease: Surgical issues. Mov Disord 21(Suppl 14):S197–S218.

21. Yamamoto T, Katayama Y, Fukaya C, Kurihara J, Oshima H, Kasai M (2000) Thalamotomy caused by cardioversion in a patient treated with brain stimulation. Stereotact Funct Neurosurg 74:73–82.
22. Nutt JG, Anderson VC, Peacock JH, Hammerstad JP, Burchiel KJ (2001) DBS and diathermy interaction induces severe CNS damage. Neurology 56:1384–1386.
23. Henderson JM, Tkach J, Phillips M, Baker K, Shellock FG, Rezai AR (2005) Permanent neurological deficit related to magnetic resonance imaging in a patient with implanted deep brain stimulation electrodes for Parkinson's disease: case report. Neurosurgery 57(5):E1063; discussion E1063.
24. Radbauer C, Volc D, Standhardt H, Alesch F (2000) Pneumocephalus in a patient with deep brain stimulation (DBS)—a case report. Mov Disord 15(Suppl 3):58.
25. Castillo R, Cavusoglu E (2006) Twiddler's syndrome: an interesting cause of pacemaker failure. Cardiology 105(2):119–121.
26. Saint-Cyr JA, Trepanier LL, Kumar R, Lozano AM, Lang AE (2000) Neuropsychological consequences of chronic bilateral stimulation of the subthalamic nucleus in Parkinson's disease. Brain 123:2091–2108.
27. Smeding HM, Speelman JD, Koning-Haanstra M, Schuurman PR, Nijssen P, van Laar T, et al (2006) Neuropsychological effects of bilateral STN stimulation in Parkinson disease: a controlled study. Neurology 66(12):1830–1836.
28. Voon V, Kubu C, Krack P, Houeto J, Troster AI (2006) Deep brain stimulation: Neuropsychological and neuropsychiatric issues. Mov Disord 21(Suppl 14): S305–S327.
29. Okun MS, Tagliati M, Pourfar M, Fernandez HH, Rodriguez RL, Alterman RL, et al (2005) Management of referred deep brain stimulation failures: a retrospective analysis from 2 movement disorders centers. Arch Neurol 62(8):1250–1255.
30. Hariz MI, Shamsgovara P, Johansson F, Hariz G, Fodstad H (1999) Tolerance and tremor rebound following long-term chronic thalamic stimulation for Parkinsonian and essential tremor. Stereotact Funct Neurosurg 72:208–218.
31. Benabid AL, Benazzouz A, Hoffman D, Limousin P, Krack P, Pollak P (1998) Long-term electrical inhibition of deep brain targets in movement disorders. Mov Disord 119(Suppl 3):119–125.
32. Koller WC, Lyons KE, Wilkinson SB, Troster AI, Pahwa R (2001) Long-term safety and efficacy of unilateral deep brain stimulation of the thalamus in essential tremor. Mov Disord 16:464–468.
33. Papavassiliou E, Rau G, Heath S, Abosch A, Barbaro NM, Larson PS, et al (2004) Thalamic deep brain stimulation for essential tremor: relation of lead location to outcome. Neurosurgery 54:1120–1129.
34. Pahwa R, Lyons KE, Wilkinson SB, Simpson RK, Jr., Ondo WG, Tarsy D, et al (2006) Long-term evaluation of deep brain stimulation of the thalamus. J Neurosurg 104(4):506–512.
35. Oh MY, Hodaie M, Kim SH, Alkhani A, Lang AE, Lozano AM (2001) Deep brain stimulator electrodes used for lesioning: proof of principle. Neurosurgery 49:363–367.
36. Raoul S, Faighel M, Rivier I, Verin M, Lajat Y, Damier P (2003) Staged lesions through implanted deep brain stimulating electrodes: A new surgical procedure for treating tremor or dyskinesias. Mov Disord 18:933–938.
37. Houeto JL, Bejjani PB, Damier P, Staedler C, Bonnett AM, Pidoux B, et al (2000) Failure of long-term pallidal stimulation corrected by subthalamic stimulation in PD. Neurology 55:728–730.
38. Rodriguez-Oroz MC, Obeso JA, Lang AE, Houeto JL, Pollak P, Rehncrona S, et al (2005) Bilateral deep brain stimulation in Parkinson's disease: a multicentre study with 4 years follow-up. Brain 128(Pt 10):2240–2249.

39. Visser-Vandewalle V, van der Linden C, Temel Y, Celik H, Ackermans L, Spincemaille G, et al (2005) Long-term effects of bilateral subthalamic nucleus stimulation in advanced Parkinson disease: a four year follow-up study. Parkinsonism Relat Disord 11(3):157–165.
40. Krack P, Batir A, Blercom NV, Chabardes S, Fraix V, Ardouin C, et al (2003) Five year follow-up of bilateral stimulation of the subthalamic nucleus in advanced Parkinson's disease. New Engl J Med 349:1925–1934.
41. Schupbach WM, Chastan N, Welter ML, Houeto JL, Mesnage V, Bonnet AM, et al (2005) Stimulation of the subthalamic nucleus in Parkinson's disease: a 5 year follow up. J Neurol Neurosurg Psychiatry 76(12):1640–1644.
42. Krause M, Fogel W, Kloss M, Rasche D, Volkmann J, Tronnier V (2004) Pallidal stimulation for dystonia. Neurosurgery 55:1361–1370.
43. Krack P, Fraix V, Mendes A, Benabid AL, Pollak P (2002) Postoperative management of subthalamic nucleus stimulation for Parkinson's disease. Mov Disord 17(Suppl 3):S188–S197.
44. Volkmann J, Moro E, Pahwa R (2006) Basic algorithms for the programming of deep brain stimulation in Parkinson' disease. Mov Disord 21(Suppl 14):S284–S289.

# 8
# Mechanisms of Deep Brain Stimulation

Svjetlana Miocinovic, Cameron C. McIntyre,
Marc Savasta, and Jerrold L. Vitek

## Abstract

Chronic electrical stimulation of the brain, known as the deep brain stimulation (DBS), has become the preferred surgical treatment for advanced Parkinson's disease (PD). Despite its remarkable clinical success, the therapeutic mechanisms of DBS are still not completely understood, limiting opportunities to improve treatment efficacy and simplify selection of stimulation parameters. This chapter discusses three questions essential to understanding the mechanisms of DBS: (1) How does DBS affect individual neurons in the region around the electrode? (2) What are the neural elements that mediate the therapeutic effect of DBS? (3) How does DBS affect the cortico-thalamo-basal ganglia network? Results from electrophysiological experiments, biochemical analyses, computer modeling and imaging studies are integrated to provide an up to date understanding of DBS mechanisms. Early hypotheses proposed that stimulation inhibited neuronal activity at the site of stimulation, mimicking the effect of lesioning. Recent studies have challenged that view and suggested that while somatic activity near the DBS electrode is decreased by synaptic inhibition, DBS increases output from the stimulated nucleus by directly activating the axons of the local projection neurons. As a result, their intrinsic activity is replaced by high-frequency activity that is time-locked to the stimulus and more regular in pattern. The stimulation induced change in neuronal pattern prevents transmission of pathologic bursting and oscillatory activity within the basal ganglia network resulting in improved processing of sensorimotor information and reduction of disease symptoms. In addition to the targeted nucleus, surrounding structures are also stimulated by subthalamic DBS, which may contribute to its therapeutic effect.

**Keywords:** deep brain stimulation, Parkinson's disease, basal ganglia, subthalamic nucleus, globus pallidus, motor circuit, electrophysiology, neurochemistry, computer modeling

## Introduction

DBS is currently the main surgical therapy for treatment of advanced PD. Several features of DBS have made it the preferred surgical therapy for PD and other movement disorders and have permitted the exploration of its application for a wide variety of other neurological disorders. These include the reversibility of stimulation induced side effects, the ability to adjust stimulation parameters to achieve optimal therapeutic benefit and the fact that it can be performed bilaterally without the high incidence of side effects associated with bilateral ablative surgery. Despite its remarkable clinical success, the therapeutic mechanisms of DBS have eluded our understanding and continue to be debated. Understanding the mechanism underlying the beneficial effects of DBS would greatly improve current applications, provide the rationale for the development of new applications and new technology, and simplify the process of optimizing stimulation parameters for patients currently receiving this therapy.

This chapter discusses three questions essential to understanding the mechanisms of DBS: (1) How does DBS affect individual neurons in the region around the electrode? (2) What are the neural elements that mediate the therapeutic effect of DBS? (3) How does DBS affect the cortico-thalamo-basal ganglia network? We have focused our discussion on subthalamic nucleus (STN) DBS because this is the site most commonly targeted and because most work examining the mechanism of DBS has focused on this structure. The STN is currently the most widely used anatomical target for DBS electrode implantation in PD *(1)*, although other structures such as the thalamus *(2, 3)*, globus pallidus internus (GPi; refs. *4* and *5*), globus pallidus externus (GPe; ref. *6*), pedunculopontine nucleus *(7, 8)*, and motor cortex *(9, 10)* have also been shown to reduce PD symptoms, albeit to different degrees.

Since the inception of DBS as a clinical therapy, its mechanisms have been the focus of intense scientific study. The similarity between the clinical effects of DBS *(11, 12)* and those resulting from a lesion in the same nucleus *(13–15)* prompted the theory that DBS works by inhibiting neural output *(16, 17)*. These conclusions were based mostly on neural microrecordings where high-frequency stimulation (HFS) resulted in reduction of neural activity in the stimulated nucleus *(17, 18)*. However, some studies suggest a more complex mechanism of action that includes stimulation-induced activation of neural elements. Observations from a variety of experimental studies have now demonstrated changes in neuronal activity consistent with activation of output from the stimulated structure *(19–24)*. Although these studies seem in direct contradiction to earlier reports of inhibition at the stimulated site, modeling studies suggested that neurons can be inhibited at the stimulated site, while axons projecting from the inhibited neurons and those passing nearby are activated *(25, 26)*. This work prompted many to ask which neural elements would be stimulated by STN DBS and would they vary dependent on stimulation parameters and their location and orientation within the current field? It now appears that in addition to the direct stimulation of STN projection neurons, stimulation of fiber tracts and other nuclei surrounding the STN may also contribute to the beneficial effect of STN DBS on PD motor signs. It is also now apparent that the effects of stimulation permeate throughout the basal ganglia thalamocortical network. These findings have led to the hypothesis that stimulation may improve PD motor signs by regularizing or interrupting pathologic neuronal activity from the basal ganglia allowing cortical motor areas to function in a more normal fashion without interference from subcortical structures.

## Current Methodologies for Studying DBS Mechanisms

A variety of research modalities, each with their own strengths and weaknesses, have been employed to study the mechanism of DBS. Electrophysiological recordings of neuronal activity, biochemical analyses, computer modeling and imaging studies have all provided crucial pieces to the mechanism puzzle. The goal of this chapter is to integrate the complementing and contrasting results from these studies to provide an up to date understanding of DBS mechanisms.

### Neuronal Recordings

Neural recordings examining DBS mechanisms have been conducted on brain slices, anesthetized and awake animals, and PD patients undergoing DBS surgery. *In vitro* brain slice preparations have made it possible to record neural activity intracellularly and characterize the effect of stimulation on cell membrane properties and neuronal elements in the slice *(16, 27–31)*. Various pharmaceutical agents can easily be added to the slices to further characterize neural responses to these agents. Stimulation amplitude and current spread in a thin slice, however, may not accurately reflect *in vivo* conditions. Unlike *in vitro* experiments, *in vivo* studies have the advantage of preserving brain structure and anatomical connections and provide the ability to correlate neuronal activity to behavior. *In vivo* experiments record extracellular activity and their primary disadvantage is the presence of stimulus artifact due to saturation of the recording amplifier during stimulation. If the artifact is not removed, it can obscure activity during the first few milliseconds after a stimulus pulse. In some studies due to interference from large artifact neural activity was only recorded after stimulation had been discontinued. Post-stimulation activity, however, may not accurately reflect the neural response that occurs during stimulation. Methods to remove or reduce this artifact have been developed and have significantly improved these studies allowing one to assess the changes in neuronal activity during the time of stimulation *(32)*. A number of *in vivo* microelectrode recordings have been performed in human PD patients *(17, 18, 33–38)*, monkeys *(19, 39–43)*, and rats *(44–49)*. In addition to microelectrode recordings, studies have been conducted that have used the DBS electrode to record local field potentials in the targeted nucleus *(50–53)*. Although PD patients are naturally ideal subjects, they can only participate in microelectrode recordings during medically warranted procedures due to the invasiveness of deep brain recordings. As a result, most human microrecordings are done during DBS implantation surgery in the same nucleus where the DBS electrode is implanted. As an alternative, non human primates offer the advantage of similar brain anatomy and physiology, while also allowing one to carry out microrecordings in nuclei other than the implanted nucleus and to verify the location of these recordings as well as the location of the DBS lead. This work has provided invaluable information on the downstream effects of DBS. Rats have been used in a similar fashion and in several studies recordings have been made at multiple sites within the basal ganglia in this model. Rat and monkey models of PD are now commonly utilized in DBS studies and offer the advantage of detailed analyses at multiple sites during stimulation.

**Biochemical Studies**

Neurotransmitter analysis has also been used to help establish the mechanism underlying neuronal responses during stimulation (e.g., it can provide support for activation of certain pathways by finding increased levels of the neurotransmitter used by that pathway). Biochemical studies of DBS mechanisms include experiments that measure levels of neurotransmitters, second messengers and mRNA in specific nuclei throughout the basal ganglia. These studies are typically performed in rats, although there have been several reports of neurotransmitter measurements from human PD patients *(34, 54, 55)*. A microdialysis technique is utilized to measure these levels by extracting small fluid samples from the targeted region in either anesthetized or awake subjects *(23, 24, 56–63)*. The advantage of this method over neural recordings is that there is no interference from stimulation artifact during DBS; the downside is that temporal resolution is much poorer (samples are generally collected every 15 minutes). To achieve real-time monitoring, constant current amperometry can be employed to monitor changes in the level of neurotransmitter such as dopamine *(29)*. In this case, however, the presence of dopamine is only indirectly demonstrated using its electrochemical properties. Although the source of neurotransmitter cannot be determined with certainty, synaptic origin is commonly assumed.

*In situ* hybridization is another approach that has been used to study DBS mechanisms. This technique can investigate molecular changes in the basal ganglia, but requires that the animal is euthanized. Using this technique, changes in neuronal metabolic activity can be inferred by measuring levels of cytochrome oxidase subunit I (CoI) mRNA *(64, 65)*. Expression of neurotransmitter-related genes (e.g., GAD67, substance P and enkephalin) and immediate early gene encoded proteins (e.g., c-fos) can be used to monitor the cellular response to various experimental conditions *(65, 66)*. Short- or long-term adaptive mechanisms occurring in the brain in response to DBS can be studied with this approach.

**Computer Modeling**

Computer modeling studies simulate experiments in a highly controlled environment. Model neurons and neural circuits can be perturbed at will and their responses observed at the level of ionic channels, single neurons or the neural network. The goal of modeling studies is to explain experimental findings by reducing the complexity of the system and identifying those variables responsible for the observed phenomena. In addition, computer models can generate viable hypotheses that can be tested experimentally. Anatomically and biophysically realistic models of basal ganglia neurons and their interaction with detailed representations of DBS electric fields are currently available *(25, 26, 67)*. These field-neuron models can be used to predict the response of the various neuronal elements (soma, axon, dendrites) to stimulation. These data provide the necessary framework for the development of subject-specific DBS models that can be created by building a 3D representation of the subject's basal ganglia and reconstructing the DBS electrode position within the target site. The nuclei are then populated with model neurons and the calculated electric field is applied to individual cells. The response of model neurons to DBS can be correlated to the observed clinical effect in that particular patient or experimental animal.

**Imaging**

Imaging studies are a powerful way to examine the effect of DBS at the network level by simultaneously observing activity at multiple sites in the brain. The most popular studies use PET and functional MRI (fMRI) to observe changes in brain activity on the basis of changes in regional blood flow and blood oxygenation, respectively *(68)*. It is assumed that these increases or decreases in neuronal activity stem from changes in afferent synaptic or local interneuron activity, rather than from changes in output from the imaged region *(21)*. Imaging studies related to DBS are discussed in another chapter. In addition to imaging, cortical function during DBS can be studied with electroencephalographic and transcranial magnetic stimulation techniques *(53, 69–71)*.

There are many approaches to studying DBS mechanisms. Because methodological differences can affect observed responses, it is important to consider the state of the preparation (*in vitro* or *in vivo*; anesthetized or awake; normal or parkinsonian), stimulation parameters (current amplitude is the most difficult to compare across studies), stimulation duration (milliseconds vs hours), the type of stimulation electrode used, its relative size and exact location, all of which can significantly affect the volume of tissue affected by stimulation. Also, one cannot overemphasize the importance of a behavioral correlate in DBS experiments. Observed stimulation effects are relevant to therapeutic mechanisms of DBS only if they accompany improvement in disease symptoms. Valuable information can be obtained from experiments using brain slices, anesthetized, or non-parkinsonian subjects, but conclusions from those studies regarding DBS mechanisms underlying its therapeutic effect must be interpreted with caution. We have observed significantly different effects on neuronal activity with stimulation parameters that produced a therapeutic effect compared to those that did not *(19)*.

## Effect of DBS on Neuronal Activity

The nuclei of the basal ganglia are linked into a complex network through both inhibitory and excitatory connections. The input into this network comes mainly from the cerebral cortex and the thalamus, whereas the output is directed toward the cortex via the thalamus and the brainstem areas, primarily the PPN and midbrain extrapyramidal area. A stimulating electrode positioned in the brain exerts both local and distal effects. Local effects can be investigated by observing the neuronal response in the stimulated nucleus. Distal effects can be studied by examining the effect of DBS on sites downstream and upstream from the stimulated nucleus as the stimulation response spreads orthodromically and antidromically throughout the basal ganglia-thalamo-cortical circuit. Elucidation of the mechanisms of DBS requires understanding both the local and distal effects of stimulation.

## Neuronal Recordings in the Stimulated Nucleus

The STN is positioned at a central location within the basal ganglia and has direct influence over the major output structures of the basal ganglia, GPi and substantia nigra pars reticulata (SNr). STN neurons are spontaneously active due in part to the pacemaker activity of persistent sodium channels *(72)*. This activity is further modulated by excitatory synaptic connections from the cerebral cortex and to a lesser extent the thalamus, and inhibitory afferents from the GPe *(73)*. As a result, STN neurons discharge spontaneously at a frequency of about 20 Hz *(74)*. In PD they become hyperactive and spikes occur in a bursty and irregular manner, with an average firing rate of about 40 Hz *(75–78)*. This hyperactivity is thought to increase the inhibitory drive of the basal ganglia on the thalamus and suppress thalamic excitatory output, resulting in reduced cortical activity and the appearance of hypokinetic motor symptoms *(79)*. Based on this "rate" model of PD, lesions in the STN or GPi would reduce the excessive inhibition of the GPi and improve the motor signs associated with PD. In support of this hypothesis, lesions in either the STN or GPi are associated with improvement in PD motor signs.

The earliest hypotheses on DBS mechanisms attempted to reconcile the similarity in clinical outcome after a lesion and during DBS by proposing that HFS inhibited neurons and decreased output from the stimulated site. Consistent with this hypothesis, studies have shown that HFS in the STN suppresses the activity of STN neurons. Meissner et al. *(43)* recorded STN neuronal activity for several minutes before, during, and after HFS (100 µA amplitude, 130 Hz frequency, and 60 µs pulse width) that improved contralateral rigidity in parkinsonian monkeys. Removal of the stimulus artifact by a template subtraction method allowed neural activity to be recorded during stimulation with minimal loss of the recorded signal. They showed that therapeutic stimulation decreased the mean firing rate in the majority of STN neurons, from 19 to 8 Hz. Activity returned to baseline within 100 milliseconds following the end of the stimulus train. Meissner et al. *(43)* proposed that the decrease in the mean firing rate resulted from resetting the firing probability of STN neurons to virtually zero by each stimulus pulse. Neurons resumed activity after about 3 milliseconds following a stimulus pulse and returned to baseline after approximately 7 ms. Stimulation at 130 Hz corresponds to a 7.7-millisecond interpulse interval, meaning that the neurons were able to fire at their baseline rate for only a very short period of time, resulting in an overall reduction in the mean firing rate.

Further evidence in support of somatic inhibition in the stimulated nucleus during DBS comes from recordings in the STN and GPi in humans. The studies of STN DBS in humans showed that neuronal activity in almost all STN cells examined was reduced or completely inhibited during stimulation *(33, 37)*. About 50% of the cells were completely inhibited for approximately 150 milliseconds following a stimulus train while the remaining cells showed no consistent effect *(33)*. STN neuron firing rate was also decreased during stimulation by 77% on average *(37)*. Studies in rats have also shown that STN activity is inhibited during therapeutic STN DBS in both awake *(48)* and anesthetized animals *(44, 49)*. Similar results were also observed in pallidal neurons during GPi HFS in both human patients *(17, 18)* and parkinsonian monkeys *(40, 41)*.

The previously mentioned studies demonstrate that HFS reduces somatic activity of local neurons, so the question arises as to what causes this apparent inhibition and more importantly how relevant is this local observation in explaining the therapeutic effects of DBS. Because electrical stimulation is generally thought to excite neurons, mechanisms proposed to explain the observed inhibition were depolarization block—cessation of activity due to increase in membrane potential and inactivation of sodium channels *(16, 45)*, and synaptic inhibition—stimulation-induced activation of inhibitory presynaptic terminals *(80)*. Support for the depolarization block hypothesis comes mainly from *in vitro* experiments. STN cells have been shown to increase firing during the initial stimulation period after which they fail to respond, suggesting inactivation of sodium channels *(29, 31)*. Contrary to these observations however, another *in vitro* study found that STN HFS can generate spike bursts time-locked to stimulus pulses *(27)*. In vivo studies favor the synaptic inhibition hypothesis, and the fact that *in vitro* slices are disconnected from their inhibitory inputs could explain the different results observed in the two types of studies. In an *in vivo* situation, depolarization block is unlikely because STN HFS reduces but does not completely block neuronal activity *(37, 43, 49)*, inhibition can occur even after a single stimulus pulse *(33)*, and both inhibition and recovery from inhibition occur at latencies consistent with GABAergic postsynaptic current kinetics *(43)*. Furthermore, *in vitro* STN HFS can either excite or inhibit STN neurons through a synaptically mediated mechanism *(30, 46)*. Indeed, a small number of STN neurons have also been excited *in vivo*, which could result from activation of excitatory afferents that are also present in the STN *(49)*. Stimulation induced synaptic inhibition could also explain inhibitory effects seen during GPi HFS because the GPi also receives strong inhibitory connections from GPe. Interestingly, one study on thalamic DBS has shown that thalamic neurons that receive predominantly excitatory afferents can be excited by stimulation *(80)*.

**Neural Recordings in Downstream Nuclei**

In the previous section, evidence was presented that DBS inhibits somatic activity in the stimulated nucleus. However, inhibition of somatic activity does not necessarily reflect reduced output from the nucleus. Indeed, several experimental studies have suggested that output is increased from the stimulated nucleus *(19, 39, 47)* leaving us to explain this apparent paradox and bringing into question the mechanism underlying this dissociation. One explanation is that axons are excited, while the cell soma is suppressed. Axons are the neural elements most easily excited by extracellular stimulation, and they are likely to be activated by DBS. It is difficult to directly record axonal activity; however, axonal firing can be indirectly monitored by recording from cells receiving afferent activity from the stimulated nucleus. STN neurons send excitatory glutamatergic projections to the GPe and the two output structures of the basal ganglia, GPi and SNr. Recordings in these target nuclei reflect downstream effects of DBS, which are of crucial importance to our understanding the mechanisms of DBS.

Taking this approach, Hashimoto et al. *(19)* demonstrated that neuronal activity in GPe and GPi increased in response to STN DBS suggesting increased output from the STN (Figure 8.1). The experimental setup in awake, parkinsonian monkeys closely resembled the human DBS system. Monkeys

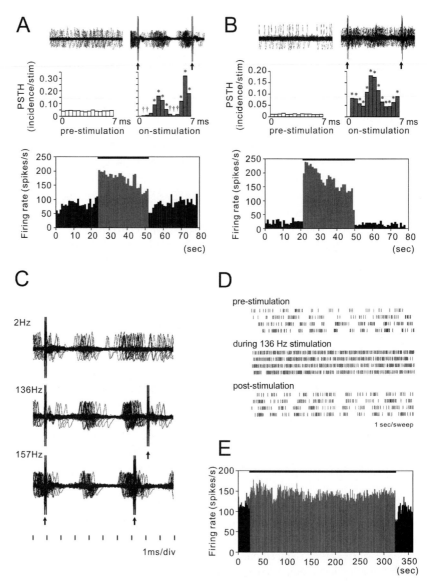

**Figure 8.1** (A, B) Examples of neuronal responses occurring during STN stimulation in a GPi and GPe cell of a parkinsonian monkey. Top traces show analog signal overlays of 100 sweeps made by triggering at 10-millisecond intervals in the pre-stimulation period (before start of stimulation) and by triggering on the stimulation pulse in the on-stimulation period. Arrows indicate residual stimulation artifacts after artifact template subtraction. Middle traces display PSTHs reconstructed from successive 7.0-millisecond time periods in the pre-stimulation period and from the interstimulus periods, in the on-stimulation period. The first PSTH bin is omitted in the on-stimulation period because of signal saturation and residual stimulation artifacts. *Significant increase at $p < 0.01$; †significant decrease at $p < 0.01$; Wilcoxon signed rank test. Bottom plots represent the mean firing rate calculated every 1 second on the basis of the PSTH, illustrating the time course of the firing rate. Thick bars indicate the stimulation period. (C) Overlay of 50 sweeps of neuronal activity of a GPi cell during 2 Hz (top), 136 Hz (middle), and 157 Hz (bottom) stimulation at 3.0 V (R370). Depolarization (negative potential) is shown as an upward deflection. Each stimulation frequency is associated with excitation peaks at 2.5 to 4.0 milliseconds and 5.5 to 7.0 millisecond after the onset of stimulation. Short-latency excitation was greater and more tightly coupled to each

were implanted with a scaled down version of a clinical DBS electrode (four contacts with 0.75 mm diameter, 0.5 mm height, and 0.5 mm separation between the contacts) and an implantable pulse generator. Therapeutic stimulation parameters resulted in reduction of contralateral rigidity and bradykinesia and increased spontaneous movement. Microelectrode recordings were performed in GPe and GPi during both therapeutic and nontherapeutic stimulation, and peri-stimulus time histograms were constructed. During therapeutically effective stimulation, a majority of neurons showed a significant increase in the average firing rate. In addition there was a consistent pattern of response of these neurons to STN stimulation with two consistent peaks of increased activity in the post-stimulus time histogram occurring at 3 and 6.5 milliseconds. Surrounding the excitatory peaks were periods of inhibition, especially pronounced in GPi neurons, which is not surprising because they receive GABAergic connections from the GPe. The precise pattern and latency of the responses resulted in regularization of GPe and GPi activity. During therapeutically ineffective stimulation, the overall firing rate and pattern of GPi activity did not change significantly. These results suggest that therapeutic STN DBS activates subthalamo-pallidal projections and changes the discharge pattern of GP neurons from an irregular to a stimulus-synchronized, more regular pattern of activity, which the authors hypothesized was responsible for the reduction in parkinsonian symptoms. Similar excitatory latencies in GPe and GPi neurons during STN stimulation in monkeys were observed by Kita et al. *(42)*. This study also showed that the excitatory response in GPe neurons was glutamatergic while GPi inhibition was GABAergic and originating from GPe. The inhibitory GPi response seen in this study was more pronounced than those observed in the Hashimoto et al. *(19)* study. The relative importance of inhibitory GPe–GPi connections compared to excitatory STN–GPi connections in non-parkinsonian animals stimulated with small electrodes and long pulses could contribute to the observed differences. In PD increased inhibitory striatal output to GPe reduces GPe firing and therefore weakens GPe–GPi connection, but strengthens STN–GPi pathway. In further support of the "output activation" hypothesis in non-human primates, Anderson et al. *(39)* showed that GPi stimulation suppressed thalamic activity and we have observed a suppression of STN neuronal activity during stimulation in GPe (Vitek et al., unpublished observations). These observations are consistent with activation of inhibitory GABAergic GPi projections to thalamic neurons.

Recordings in nuclei receiving STN projections in rats generally support the notion that STN output is activated by DBS, although results vary across studies. Shi et al. *(48)* simultaneously recorded at multiple locations within the basal ganglia and found nearly equal numbers of excitatory and inhibitory responses in GP (rat analog of primate GPe) and SNr during STN

**Figure 8.1** (continued) stimulation pulse during higher-frequency stimulation. Arrows indicate residual stimulation artifacts after artifact template subtraction. (D) Rasters of GPi neuronal activity (R370). The firing changed from an irregular pattern with varying ISIs into a high-frequency regular pattern with most ISIs occurring at 4 or 8 milliseconds during 136 Hz, 3.0 V stimulation. (E) An example of the time course of the change in firing rate of a GPi neuron during prolonged 136 Hz STN stimulation. Increased mean discharge rates in this neuron were sustained during the 5 minutes stimulation period

DBS, which improved treadmill locomotion in parkinsonian rats (50–175 μA, 130 Hz, 60 μs, intermittent 3 seconds on, 2 seconds off cycle). Similarly, in normal, anesthetized rats, Maurice et al. *(47)* showed that STN DBS causes inhibition of SNr neurons at low amplitudes (20–80 μA), but excitation at higher amplitudes (100–240 μA). The authors suggested that inhibitory effects were likely due to activation of inhibitory pallidonigral fibers or GABAergic intranigral neurons, whereas excitatory effects resulted from direct activation of subthalamo-nigral projections. However, several studies, also in normal, anesthetized rats, showed the opposite effect, a decrease in SNr firing during high-amplitude STN DBS (400 μA; ref. *49*) and long-lasting inhibition in SNr and entopeduncular nucleus (EP; rat analog of primate GPi) immediately following high-amplitude STN DBS (300–500 μA; refs. *44* and *45*). Benazzouz et al. *(44)*, however, also found a long-lasting excitation in GPe, which would be consistent with activation of excitatory STN output. Differences in stimulation amplitudes, exact stimulation sites, and anesthesia methods likely contribute to the variable results seen in these studies. These differences however, also attest to the complex pattern of excitation and inhibition that is likely to emerge in response to stimulation and the importance of considering the effects of stimulation on polysynaptic pathways (e.g., STN-GPe-SNr) and fiber tracts surrounding the stimulation site (e.g., nigrostriatal, pallidothalamic, pallidonigral, and cerebellothalamic in the case of STN DBS).

Several studies in human PD patients, where recordings could be made in downstream nuclei, also support the output activation hypothesis *(34–36)*. Galati et al. *(34)* recorded an increase in firing frequency and more regularity in the firing pattern of SNr neurons during therapeutic STN DBS. However, Maltete et al. *(38)* reported a decrease in the overall SNr firing during STN stimulation, although they also recorded inhibition-excitation-inhibition pattern of neural activity in the 7-millisecond interpulse interval. Similar to what was observed in the rat studies, smaller electrodes and lower stimulus amplitudes used by Maltete et al., *(38)* may have preferentially activated pallido-subthalamic synaptic afferents, which inhibited STN spontaneous firing. Therapeutic efficacy of these stimulation parameters was not evaluated so they could have been subthreshold for direct activation of a sufficient number of STN-SNr axons necessary to see an overall increase in the activity of SNr neurons *(25)*. Montgomery *(35)* reported a reduction in thalamic neuronal activity 3.5 to 5 milliseconds following a stimulus pulse during GPi DBS, consistent with orthodromic activation of GPi output leading to inhibition of thalamic neurons. In addition, human PET studies showed an increase in blood flow in the region of GPi during STN DBS *(81)* and an increase in cortical blood flow during thalamic DBS both consistent with activation of output from the stimulated site *(21)*. Similarly, an fMRI study found an increase in blood oxygen level-dependent signal in the GPi of patients undergoing STN DBS *(20)*. These results and others from fMRI studies regarding the mechanisms of DBS are discussed in another chapter in this volume.

Reviewing the experimental data it would appear that although cell bodies in the stimulated nucleus are inhibited and/or bridled, the axons of these projection neurons are activated. This causes downstream excitation when glutamatergic STN neuron axons are activated; inhibition, when GABAergic GPi neuron axons are activated; or a combination of excitation and inhibition, when polysynaptic pathways are involved. For example, the GPi response to

STN DBS is influenced by direct excitatory STN-GPi projections and indirect inhibitory STN-GPe-GPi pathway. The role of antidromic axonal activation should also be considered, such as the activation of afferent cortical projections during STN DBS, which may affect cortical and subsequently striatal activity *(42, 70)* as well as activation of GPe-STN projections with axon collaterals to GPi. In summary, neural recording studies suggest that DBS inhibits local cell bodies likely by activating inhibitory presynaptic terminals. At the same time it also activates projection axons of the local neurons, fibers of passage, and surrounding fiber pathways resulting in a complex pattern of excitatory and inhibitory effects, which modulate not only local basal ganglia activity but the basal ganglia thalamocortical network as a whole. The particular changes that take place in this network with therapeutic stimulation and their role in the alleviation of parkinsonian motor signs remain to be determined.

**Neurochemical and Gene Expression Studies**

Neurochemical and gene expression studies of STN DBS in large part support conclusions from single cell recording studies and provide further evidence for network wide changes during stimulation. Microdialysis studies in normal anesthetized rats detected elevated levels of glutamate in both SNr and GP (rat analog of primate GPe) and GABA in SNr during STN HFS consistent with increased output from STN *(23, 24)*. This increase was also frequency dependent closely mimicking the frequency-response curve seen in clinical applications of DBS *(23)*. In parkinsonian rats, basal levels of glutamate and GABA in GP *(63)* and SNr *(56, 63)* were higher than in normal rats consistent with STN hyperactivity (excessive striatal indirect pathway activity could be responsible for increase in GABA seen in GP). During STN DBS in anesthetized parkinsonian animals, there was an increase in GABA in the SNr, but contrary to the response in normal rats, no increase in glutamate was detected (500 µA; ref. *63*). Lesioning GP eliminated the increase in GABA, suggesting that pallidal neurons constitute a major source of GABA in the SNr, although additional pathways, such as inhibitory striatonigral projections and/or SNr neuron collaterals, may also be involved *(44, 63)*. Because no increase in glutamate was detected in the GP the authors suggested that pallidonigral fibers were stimulated directly by STN DBS (rather than via subthalamo-pallidal afferents).

In a subsequent study in awake, parkinsonian and intact rats, the effects of STN DBS on biochemical changes in SNr were also investigated (Figure 8.2; ref. *56*). At high stimulation amplitudes, which induced forelimb dyskinesias (75–200 µA) glutamate and GABA increased in the SNr of intact rats, but only glutamate increased in parkinsonian rats. At lower stimulation amplitudes (<60 µA), GABA but not glutamate increased in parkinsonian animals (no change was seen in intact rats). This is consistent with findings from neural recording experiments, which showed an increase in SNr activity with high-amplitude stimulation and a decrease in activity with low amplitude stimulation *(47)*. Activation of the STN–SNr pathway by high-amplitude stimulation appears to be responsible for limb dyskinesia observed in both normal and hemiparkinsonian rats. These experiments were not designed to investigate therapeutic effects, but human studies suggest that the same mechanisms are responsible for amelioration of PD symptoms *(34)*.

## A. STN HFS I > 60μA

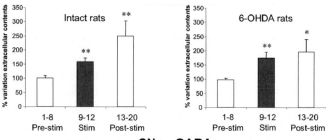

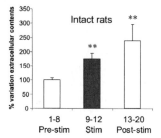
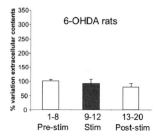

## B. STN HFS I < 60μA

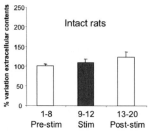
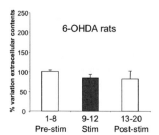

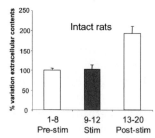
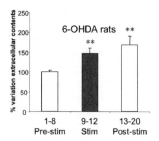

**Figure 8.2** Extracellular glutamate and GABA collected in the SNr ipsilateral to stimulation in intact and 6-OHDA-lesioned rats under basal conditions and during 1 hour of STN-HFS with (A) an intensity which induces forelimb dyskinesia (I >60μA) or (B) with an intensity below threshold for forelimb dyskinesia (I >60μA). The pre-stimulation period (pre-stim) corresponds to the mean ± SEM of the eight "pre-stim" dialysates collected at 15-minute intervals, the stimulation period (stim) indicated by the black horizontal bar, corresponds to the mean ± SEM of the four fractions

Comparison of microdialysis results from rats and humans shows some parallels, but also indicates that more than one mechanism may be responsible for therapeutic effects in the two species. Results from normal rats show an increase of pallidal glutamate during STN DBS, consistent with an increase in STN output. Contrary to expectations, a similar increase in pallidal glutamate was not seen in parkinsonian animals, or in human PD patients during STN DBS *(54)*. An increase in cGMP, considered to be a secondary messenger in the glutamatergic signaling pathway, was detected in the human study and was accompanied by improvement in clinical symptoms *(54, 55)*. One potential explanation for the lack of increase in glutamate in the parkinsonian state is that glutamate levels are already high and further increases are difficult to detect *(63)*. In support of this argument STN DBS in human PD patients produced an increase in cGMP and an increase in firing rate in the SNr *(34)*.

Changes in glutamate, GABA and dopamine levels have also been measured in the striatum during STN DBS. The small number of subthalamic projections to the striatum probably cannot account for these changes *(73)*. One hypothesis is that one would need a multitude of stimulation induced changes throughout the network to account for all these changes. Studies to address the underlying etiology of these changes have found higher levels of glutamate and GABA in the striatum of parkinsonian rats compared to normal rats. These levels are further increased in both hemispheres during unilateral STN DBS; furthermore, these changes appear to be modulated by dopamine antagonists *(58)*. Microdialysis and amperometry studies have shown that dopamine and dopamine metabolites are also increased in the striatum during STN DBS of normal *(29, 57)* and parkinsonian rats *(57, 61)*. Several hypotheses have been offered to explain this observation. The first is that STN DBS inhibits SNr neurons, which in turn disinhibit SNc neurons increasing SNc activity and subsequent release of dopamine in the striatum *(61)*. A second explanation is that STN DBS results in activation of nigrostriatal dopaminergic fibers that pass just dorsal to the STN *(29)*. STN also sends some axons directly to SNc so that direct activation of dopaminergic SNc neurons is another possible explanation for these findings. Consistent with these hypotheses, stimulation in the entopeduncular nucleus, which has no direct connections with the striatum or SN and no nearby dopaminergic fiber tracts, does not result in an increase in striatal dopamine *(60)*.

Recently, it has been shown that STN-HFS modifies the response to acute L-DOPA administration in partially dopaminergically denervated (DA PL) rats on striatal extracellular concentrations of dopamine and its metabolites. Indeed, L-DOPA treatment significantly increases striatal dopamine levels in

**Figure 8.2** (continued) nine to 12 and the post-stimulation period (Post-stim) to eight fractions (13–20). The mean ± SEM of the eight pre-stim dialysates, collected before STN-HFS, was used to determine baseline levels. Results are expressed as a percentage of variation of this baseline value. Each percentage for each period corresponds to the mean variations ± SEM calculated for five to eight animals. In A, note that Glu levels increased in both intact and 6-OHDA-lesioned rats, whereas GABA levels increased only in intact animals. In B, note that Glu levels in the SNr were not significantly affected by STN-HFS in the SNr in either intact or 6-OHDA-lesioned rats, whereas GABA levels increased only in 6-OHDA-lesioned animals. *$p < 0.05$; **$p < 0.01$, versus baseline values. Error bars indicate the SEM

intact and DA PL animals, with the maximal effect observed 1 hour after L-DOPA injection. This increase is more pronounced in DA PL rats (ipsilateral to the lesion) than in intact animals. It remains fairly stable 1 hour after the maximal effect of L-DOPA and then decreases towards the basal values. STN-HFS in intact rats has no effect on the maximal L-DOPA-induced increase in striatal extracellular dopamine concentration or the return to basal values, the profiles observed being similar to those for non-stimulated intact animals. Conversely, STN-HFS amplifies the L-DOPA-induced increase in striatal dopamine levels during the stimulation period (1 hour) in DA PL rats, and this increase is sustained throughout the post-stimulation period (2.5 hours), without the return to basal levels observed in stimulated intact and non-stimulated rats. These recent neurochemical data suggest that that STN-HFS interferes with DA turnover, in DA PL rats probably by modulating DA uptake and synthesis, suggesting a prolonged smooth DA action and adaptive mechanisms for alleviating L-DOPA-related motor fluctuations such as the wearing-off phenomenon, thereby shedding light on possible mechanisms of STN-HFS in PD *(59)*.

While animal studies offer an attractive explanation for improvement of PD symptoms with STN DBS by showing a significant increase in striatal dopamine, there has been no evidence that a similar process occurs in humans. Several PET studies using [11C]raclopride to measure dopamine binding have failed to show changes during STN DBS, suggesting that the therapeutic effects of STN stimulation are not mediated by striatal dopamine release *(82–85)*. However, the discrepancy in the results between human and animal studies may stem from methodological differences used to measure neurotransmitter levels. For example, the detection threshold is higher for PET than for microdialysis and constant potential amperometry studies, because such dopamine release may be detected by one method but not another *(29)*. Another possibility is that advanced-stage PD patients may have fewer SNc neurons available to release dopamine and when such patients are imaged using PET techniques one may be less likely to observe a change in dopamine levels sufficient to be detected by this technique.

Molecular studies measuring levels of protein and gene expression suggest that stimulation-induced changes occur throughout the basal ganglia nuclei and cortical receiving areas. Decreased levels of CoI mRNA are found in the STN during stimulation in both normal and parkinsonian rats and are consistent with the hypothesis that stimulation suppresses STN neuronal activity *(64, 65, 86)*. In parkinsonian rats STN stimulation returned levels of CoI *(64)* and neurotransmitter-related genes *(65)* towards those seen in normal rats. Short-term STN stimulation decreased levels of glutamate decarboxylase 67 kDa isoform (GAD67), a marker of GABA neuron activity, in SNr and EP, but not in GP *(65)*; however, chronic stimulation (4 days) reduced GAD67 in GP as well, showing that STN DBS involves long-term adaptive processes *(86)*. A decrease in GAD67 indicates reduced activity in the nuclei downstream from the STN, which is contrary to studies demonstrating increased STN output. However, as seen previously in rat experiments STN stimulation at low current amplitudes such as used in this study may result in inhibition of basal ganglia output structures that may not represent what occurs during STN stimulation at therapeutic stimulation parameters. The expression of immediate early genes serves as an indicator of change in neuronal activity. STN DBS induces rapid changes in expression of immediate early gene encoded proteins such as c-Fos, c-Jun, and Krox-24 in multiple STN projection sites *(66)*. Consistent with neural recording experiments, these studies suggest that STN activity is reduced during stimulation, but at the same time projection sites experience transsynaptic modulation of neuronal activity consistent with activation of STN output.

**Computer Models of DBS**

Although it might seem improbable that a neuron can be inhibited and activated at the same time during extracellular electrical stimulation, both experimental *(87, 88)* and computer modeling *(25, 89)* studies support this concept. The key physiological feature that explains this apparent paradox is that when a cell is exposed to extracellular stimulation, the stimulation-induced action potential initiates in the axon rather than the cell body. In that case, inhibition of the cell body can occur coincident with axonal activation. A modeling study of thalamocortical neurons stimulated by DBS found that the position of the neuron with respect to the electrode determines the neuron's output firing characteristics *(25)*. A neuron close to the stimulating electrode will have its spontaneous activity suppressed by activation of inhibitory presynaptic terminals, but its axon will be directly activated. As a result, the neuron will generate spikes that are time-locked to the stimulus frequency. A neuron positioned further away from the electrode will still be influenced by inhibitory synapses because axonal terminals are the most excitable neural elements *(90, 91)*. However, the stimulus will be subthreshold for direct axonal activation and the neural output will resemble that of the cell body, which can be total or partial inhibition.

If a neuron's position with respect to the electrode determines its response to stimulation, how are neurons in and around the STN affected by STN DBS? Miocinovic et al. *(26)* created a comprehensive computer model simulating the monkey STN DBS experiments described by Hashimoto et al. (Figure 8.3; ref. *19*). The goal was to quantify the number of STN projection neurons and adjacent pallidothalamic fibers that were activated during therapeutically effective vs ineffective stimulation in two parkinsonian macaques. To correlate simulation results to the behavioral outcomes of each animal, a detailed and anatomically accurate model of the each monkeys' basal ganglia was constructed. The 3D anatomical nuclei were reconstructed from histological sections through the nuclei from these animals. A virtual DBS electrode was positioned within the STN in the same location as that placed experimentally, whose position was verified histologically. Populations of STN projection neurons and pallidothalamic fibers were placed in their anatomically correct positions and orientations within the 3D nuclei. The model neuron geometries were based on actual reconstructions of STN and GPi neurons and fibers and their biophysical properties reflected the firing characteristics of neurons in a parkinsonian monkey. Voltage generated in the tissue by the active DBS electrode was calculated with a finite element model and applied to the model of STN neurons and pallidothalamic fibers to determine the effect of stimulation on these neuronal elements.

The voltage field generated by the DBS electrode is a 3D phenomenon and its effect on individual neurons and fibers depends on the cell's position

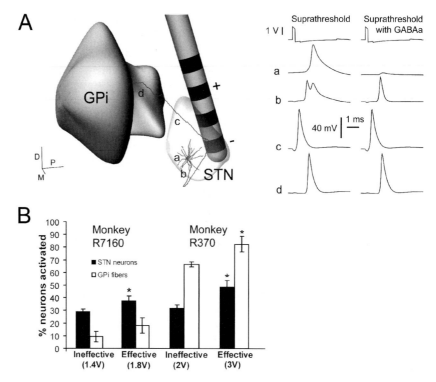

**Figure 8.3** (A) 3D model of an STN projection neuron responding to extracellular stimulation. Lowercase letters indicate location in the STN neuron where the transmembrane voltage was recorded. a, soma; b, 1st node of Ranvier; c, 30th node of Ranvier; d, 50th node of Ranvier. The action potential is initiated in the axon and propagated toward the cell body and axonal terminals in the GPi. Traces in the top row represent stimulus voltage waveforms applied to the neuron. The four traces below show response to a suprathreshold DBS pulse (1.8 V) in a model with (right) and without (left) inhibitory somatic synapses. (B) Computer simulation of neural activation in two parkinsonian monkeys during clinically effective and ineffective STN DBS. Percent of activated STN neuron output axons and GPi (LF) fibers was averaged over three randomized populations. Asterisks indicate significant difference between clinically ineffective and effective stimulation ($p < 0.05$; $t$-test)

and orientation within the field. The stimulation of model neurons and axons results in a complex polarization profile along each neuronal element related to the second order derivative of extracellular voltage. As expected, based on this model, the stimulation-induced action potential was initiated in the axon. The decoupling of somatic and axonal activity was clearly present in the STN projection neurons. Inhibitory afferents suppressed spontaneous somatic activity in proportion to synaptic strength. However, the axonal firing and hence the neuronal output was largely unaffected by these inhibitory inputs. The neuron was considered activated if its axonal terminal fired in response to at least 80% of stimulus pulses. In both monkeys, about 50% of model STN neuron axons were activated during therapeutic stimulation and this increase was significant compared to clinically ineffective stimulation. In one monkey, a large number of GPi fibers running dorsal to the STN were activated by effective stimulation while in the other animal only a few GPi axons were activated while using effective stimulation parameters. These predictions were compared to and confirmed by the experimental recordings. The position of the DBS electrode was determined to be a critical feature and submillimeter movements produced a significant change in simulation results. The implications of pallidothalamic fiber activation and electrode location on STN DBS mechanisms are reviewed later.

## Therapeutic Target of STN DBS

When considering therapeutic mechanisms of DBS, the primary focus has been on the response of the neurons in the stimulated site (i.e., target nucleus neurons). However, stimulation effects can and do spread outside the borders of the anatomical nuclei. This finding is especially true for the STN, which is a small nucleus surrounded by several major fibers tracts *(73)*. Neural recordings and biochemical studies in rats have suggested that pallidonigral and nigrostriatal fiber tracts are likely activated during STN DBS and may contribute to its therapeutic effects. In a computer simulation of STN DBS in a monkey, a significant activation of pallidothalamic fibers was observed at therapeutic stimulation intensity. This fiber tract, also known as the lenticular fasciculus (LF), or H2 field of Forel, runs dorsal to the STN carrying inhibitory fibers from the GPi to the motor thalamus. The LF and the zona incerta (ZI), which is a small nucleus dorsal to the LF, have been implicated as possible therapeutic targets because of their proximity to active DBS electrode contacts. Similarly, the activation of passing cerebellothalamic fibers has been suggested as a possible mechanism in treatment of essential tremor by STN DBS *(92)*. Interestingly, the GPi nucleus itself is also an effective target for DBS electrode implantation in PD. The potential role of activation of fiber bundles running near or within the GPi remains to be determined, but are likely to play a role in its therapeutic effect similar to the hypothesis that activation of adjacent fiber pathways during STN DBS provide a component to its therapeutic benefit.

The role of electrode location in mediating therapeutic benefit of STN DBS has been debated with some arguing that optimal stimulation requires the effective contact to be within the STN while others argue that optimal stimulation requires a volume of activation that includes the white matter region dorsal to the STN *(93–95)*. The DBS electrode has four contacts and in each patient it is determined empirically which contact provides maximum relief of symptoms with minimum side effects. Intra-operative neurophysiological data, brain atlases and postoperative imaging can be used to determine the location of the active contact with respect to the target site and the surrounding structures. The accuracy of these methods remains to be determined, but they can give an approximate idea of the location of the active contact. If bipolar stimulation is used, the location of the cathode is most relevant because cathodic stimuli are more effective in activating axons.

Numerous studies have supported the hypothesis that the optimal contact for therapeutic stimulation is located near the dorsal border of the STN, where stimulation effects are likely to extend into the LF and ZI *(93, 95–104)*. The dorsolateral portion of the STN projects to cortical motor areas and is considered the "motor" area of the nucleus. As such, one would argue that stimulation in this region would produce the greatest therapeutic benefit for motor symptoms. However, during stimulation current likely spreads outside the motor area and affects passing fiber tracts. It is not clear if stimulation of the structures dorsal to STN is more therapeutic than stimulation of the STN itself, or if the combined stimulation of multiple structures nearby makes the STN such a successful target for PD. Although several studies have found that stimulation dorsal to the STN was less effective than stimulation at the dorsal border of the nucleus *(93, 95)*, another study comparing stimulation in the STN to the dorsal border of the STN versus the caudal ZI found that stimulation in the ZI was the most effective site *(94)*. Support for the argument that stimulation in ZI may be equally or more effective than in the STN is derived from reports of the involvement of ZI in locomotor activity and the observation that stimulation in the ZI in rats normalized dopamine-depletion induced molecular changes in a manner similar to that reported with STN stimulation *(64, 105)*. Despite these intriguing results, the major deficiency of these studies is the inaccuracy in contact location estimation and inability to quantify the effective current spread.

Previous studies have implied based on the presumed location of the active contact that structures adjacent to the site of stimulation are also activated; however, it is not known precisely how far stimulation spreads and how this varies with different stimulation parameters (amplitude, pulse width, frequency). A computer modeling study quantified the spread of stimulation during STN DBS in a human PD patient and correlated it to clinical outcomes *(67)*. The location of electrode contacts was reconstructed from postoperative MRI, and a 3D brain atlas was warped to the patient's MRI to identify anatomical structures and their location with respect to the electrode. The patient-specific volume of tissue activated (VTA) was constructed using theoretical models of the DBS voltage field and neural (axonal) response to extracellular stimulation. The patient was clinically evaluated for rigidity, bradykinesia, and corticospinal tract activation at various stimulation parameter settings. The VTAs accurately predicted the spread of stimulation into the internal capsule for stimulus parameters that activated corticospinal fibers as measured by electromyography. Two separate contacts provided relief of rigidity and bradykinesia, and both of their VTAs included the LF and ZI. Improvement of rigidity was also correlated with spread of stimulation into the thalamus, the ZI, and the LF, but not the STN (contact closest to the STN induced side effects so it was clinically ineffective). While this study analyzed a single patient, its conclusions agree with previous clinical studies and suggest that the ZI and LF are activated during STN DBS and may provide a significant contribution to the beneficial effects observed with STN stimulation. The exact contribution of each, however, remains unclear. Results from monkey experiments indicate that large-scale stimulation of LF may not be necessary for the therapeutic effect *(26, 83)*. Similarly, lesions of the STN in both humans *(106)* and monkeys *(14, 107)* also suggest that altering STN output clearly has a therapeutic effect on PD motor signs. All these studies provide some critical clues to the optimal site of stimulation, yet therapeutic stimulation needs to be investigated in a larger cohort of patients and animal subjects if we are to determine the optimal site for DBS in PD and whether or not this may vary based on individual patient symptomatology.

## Effect of DBS on the Network

The classical model of the basal ganglia *(108)* predicts that destruction of nigrostriatal dopaminergic neurons as occurs in PD leads to hyperactivity of the STN. This causes excessive activity in the GPi and subsequent inhibition of thalamocortical projections thought to result in the motor signs associated with PD. Both STN and GPi lesioning reduce hyperactivity in the STN-GPi circuit thereby removing excessive pallido-thalamic inhibition and suppression of thalamo-cortical output which results in alleviation of parkinsonian symptoms. Although this model can explain the improvement in parkinsonian motor signs seen with lesions in the STN and GPi, it does not explain the improvement in dyskinesia seen with GPi lesions or the improvement in some parkinsonian motor signs following thalamotomy. This has led to the hypothesis that patterns of neuronal activity may be more important than changes in rate for the development of parkinsonian motor signs. Consistent with this hypothesis, STN DBS increases STN output and the mean discharge rate of GPi neurons, yet similarly to GPi lesions, leads to improvement in motor function.

The key to this apparent paradox is the stimulation frequency necessary to achieve therapeutic effect. A proposed mechanism of DBS consistent with an increase in neural output from the STN is that stimulation overrides pathological neuronal discharge by imposing a more regular higher frequency neuronal activity from the STN to the GPi *(19, 22, 109)*. Both experimental *(19, 28)* and modeling *(110)* studies have shown that HFS replaces intrinsic irregular activity with one that is time-locked to the stimulus. Only frequencies above 100 Hz provide symptom relief while frequencies below 20 Hz often worsen symptoms probably because this just adds spikes to an already irregular pattern of spontaneous firing. Neurochemical studies have also shown that low-frequency stimulation does not lead to the neurochemical and molecular changes seen with HFS *(23, 66)*. It has been suggested that regularization of GPi firing by STN DBS reduces the disorder (entropy) in neuronal signals (A. Dorval, personal communication) and restores the responsiveness of thalamocortical cells to synaptic inputs (e.g., sensorimotor information) despite increased inhibitory drive *(111)*.

Because an action potential that responds to extracellular stimulation begins in the axon, stimulation at frequencies greater that the neuron's own spontaneous rate can override the neuron's intrinsic output. There are two possible mechanisms by which this may occur. First, antidromic stimulus-initiated action potentials can collide with othrodromic soma-initiated spikes blocking this irregular pattern of activity from being conducted down the axon. Second, antidromic invasion of the soma prevents the cell from discharging spontaneously due to the refractory period associated with such activity. In both cases irregular orthodromic activity is replaced by a more regular pattern of discharge. Even though this tonic, high-frequency firing pattern is not considered normal, it is seemingly devoid of informational content and results in an 'informational lesion', preventing the pathological activity from being transmitted within the basal ganglia *(110)*. Interestingly, in dystonia, where intrinsic pathologic GPi firing rates are lower than in PD, therapeutic DBS frequencies may also be lower *(112, 113)*.

Our analysis of the current DBS experimental data supports the concept that the neural pattern, rather than firing rate, is an important determinant of the pathologic state of PD and the therapeutic effects seen with DBS *(19, 22, 109)*. In addition to an increase in the mean rate and irregularity of neuronal discharge in the basal ganglia, PD is also characterized by the development of rhythmic, oscillatory activity *(76, 78)*. Most notably, synchronized bursting is present between STN and GPe *(50, 114, 115)*, and STN oscillatory frequencies in the 15 to 30 Hz (beta) range tend to predominate *(116)*. Similar to the effect of L-dopa, STN DBS appears to suppress abnormal beta rhythms in the GPi *(117)*, but it is unclear if reduction of beta activity is necessary for symptom improvement *(51)*. STN DBS has been shown to decrease oscillatory and burst activity in the STN and its target nuclei *(19, 43, 48)*. As a result, reduction of pathologic activity and its transmission, and the subsequent improvement in information processing could be responsible for amelioration of motor symptoms during DBS.

Stimulation may induce both short- and long-term changes in the network. This is exemplified by the period of time necessary to achieve full reduction of symptoms once stimulation is initiated and the prolonged therapeutic effect once stimulation is stopped *(118)*. Recording experiments show that neural activity at the site of stimulation or in the site receiving projections from the stimulated site returns to baseline within milliseconds or seconds after stimulation stops. Yet, it may take minutes, hours, or even days for symptoms to worsen. Similarly, when stimulation is initiated, improvement in gait may take hours to occur whereas tremor may disappear almost instantly. To account for this observation one would seemingly need to propose that there are changes occurring within the network over different timelines. Molecular studies also indicate that there are both short- and long-term adaptive changes occurring in response to stimulation *(86)*. To understand this process it will be necessary to perform experiments over long time periods while simultaneously recording from multiple neurons at multiple sites.

## Conclusions

Early hypotheses on DBS mechanisms proposed that stimulation inhibited neuronal activity at the site of stimulation, thereby mimicking the effect of lesioning. Recent studies have challenged this view and suggested that while somatic activity near the DBS electrode is decreased by synaptic inhibition, DBS increases output from the stimulated nucleus by directly activating the axons of the local projection neurons. As a result, their intrinsic activity is replaced by high-frequency activity that is time-locked to the stimulus and more regular in pattern. The stimulation-induced change in neuronal patterns prevents transmission of pathologic bursting and oscillatory activity within the basal ganglia network resulting in improved processing of sensorimotor information and reduction of motor symptoms. In addition to the targeted nucleus, stimulation of surrounding structures by STN DBS may also contribute to its therapeutic effect.

The mechanism of DBS is likely not simply a matter of inhibition or excitation, rather it involves complex changes throughout the entire basal ganglia-thalamo-cortical network. Understanding this process will be critically important if we are to reach the full potential of this powerful tool and will in turn lead us to technological advancements and improvements in our understanding of the physiologic signature of PD and other movement disorders.

# References

1. Kleiner-Fisman G, Herzog J, Fisman DN, et al (2006) Subthalamic nucleus deep brain stimulation: summary and meta-analysis of outcomes. Mov Disord 21(Suppl 14): S290–S304.
2. Benabid AL, Pollak P, Gervason C, et al (1991) Long-term suppression of tremor by chronic stimulation of the ventral intermediate thalamic nucleus. Lancet 337(8738):403–406.
3. Benabid AL, Pollak P, Louveau A, Henry S, de Rougemont J (1987) Combined (thalamotomy and stimulation) stereotactic surgery of the VIM thalamic nucleus for bilateral Parkinson disease. Appl Neurophysiol 50(1–6):344–346.
4. Bejjani B, Damier P, Arnulf I, et al (1997) Pallidal stimulation for Parkinson's disease. Two targets? Neurology 49(6):1564–1569.
5. Kumar R, Lozano AM, Montgomery E, Lang AE (1998) Pallidotomy and deep brain stimulation of the pallidum and subthalamic nucleus in advanced Parkinson's disease. Mov Disord 13(Suppl 1):73–82.
6. Vitek JL, Hashimoto T, Peoples J, DeLong MR, Bakay RA (2004) Acute stimulation in the external segment of the globus pallidus improves parkinsonian motor signs. Mov Disord 19(8):907–915.
7. Mazzone P, Lozano A, Stanzione P, et al (2005) Implantation of human pedunculopontine nucleus: a safe and clinically relevant target in Parkinson's disease. Neuroreport 16(17):1877–1881.
8. Plaha P, Gill SS (2005) Bilateral deep brain stimulation of the pedunculopontine nucleus for Parkinson's disease. Neuroreport 16(17):1883–1887.
9. Canavero S, Paolotti R, Bonicalzi V, et al (2002) Extradural motor cortex stimulation for advanced Parkinson disease. Report of two cases. J Neurosurg 97(5):1208–1211.
10. Pagni CA, Altibrandi MG, Bentivoglio A, et al (2005) Extradural motor cortex stimulation (EMCS) for Parkinson's disease. History and first results by the study group of the Italian neurosurgical society. Acta neurochirurgica 93:113–119.
11. Benazzouz A, Gross C, Feger J, Boraud T, Bioulac B (1993) Reversal of rigidity and improvement in motor performance by subthalamic high-frequency stimulation in MPTP-treated monkeys. Eur J Neurosci 5(4):382–389.
12. Limousin P, Pollak P, Benazzouz A, et al (1995) Effect of parkinsonian signs and symptoms of bilateral subthalamic nucleus stimulation. Lancet 345(8942):91–95.
13. Aziz TZ, Peggs D, Sambrook MA, Crossman AR (1991) Lesion of the subthalamic nucleus for the alleviation of 1-methyl-4-phenyl-1,2,3,6-tetrahydropyridine (MPTP)-induced parkinsonism in the primate. Mov Disord 6(4):288–292.
14. Bergman H, Wichmann T, DeLong MR (1990) Reversal of experimental parkinsonism by lesions of the subthalamic nucleus. Science 249(4975):1436–1438.
15. Patel NK, Heywood P, O'Sullivan K, McCarter R, Love S, Gill SS (2003) Unilateral subthalamotomy in the treatment of Parkinson's disease. Brain 126(Pt 5): 1136–1145.
16. Beurrier C, Bioulac B, Audin J, Hammond C (2001) High-frequency stimulation produces a transient blockade of voltage-gated currents in subthalamic neurons. J Neurophysiol 85(4):1351–1356.
17. Dostrovsky JO, Levy R, Wu JP, Hutchison WD, Tasker RR, Lozano AM (2000) Microstimulation-induced inhibition of neuronal firing in human globus pallidus. J Neurophysiol 84(1):570–574.
18. Wu YR, Levy R, Ashby P, Tasker RR, Dostrovsky JO (2001) Does stimulation of the GPi control dyskinesia by activating inhibitory axons? Mov Disord 16(2):208–216.
19. Hashimoto T, Elder CM, Okun MS, Patrick SK, Vitek JL (2003) Stimulation of the subthalamic nucleus changes the firing pattern of pallidal neurons. J Neurosci 23(5):1916–1923.

20. Jech R, Urgosik D, Tintera J, et al (2001) Functional magnetic resonance imaging during deep brain stimulation: a pilot study in four patients with Parkinson's disease. Mov Disord 16(6):1126–1132.
21. Perlmutter JS, Mink JW, Bastian AJ, et al (2002) Blood flow responses to deep brain stimulation of thalamus. Neurology 58(9):1388–1394.
22. Vitek JL (2002) Mechanisms of deep brain stimulation: excitation or inhibition. Mov Disord 17(Suppl 3):S69–S72.
23. Windels F, Bruet N, Poupard A, Feuerstein C, Bertrand A, Savasta M (2003) Influence of the frequency parameter on extracellular glutamate and gamma-aminobutyric acid in substantia nigra and globus pallidus during electrical stimulation of subthalamic nucleus in rats. J Neurosci Res 72(2):259–267.
24. Windels F, Bruet N, Poupard A, et al (2000) Effects of high frequency stimulation of subthalamic nucleus on extracellular glutamate and GABA in substantia nigra and globus pallidus in the normal rat. Eur J Neurosci 12(11):4141–4146.
25. McIntyre CC, Grill WM, Sherman DL, Thakor NV (2004) Cellular effects of deep brain stimulation: model-based analysis of activation and inhibition. J Neurophysiol 91(4):1457–1469.
26. Miocinovic S, Parent M, Butson CR, et al (2006) Computational analysis of subthalamic nucleus and lenticular fasciculus activation during therapeutic deep brain stimulation. J Neurophysiol 96(3):1569–1580.
27. Garcia L, Audin J, D'Alessandro G, Bioulac B, Hammond C (2003) Dual effect of high-frequency stimulation on subthalamic neuron activity. J Neurosci 23(25):8743–8751.
28. Garcia L, D'Alessandro G, Fernagut PO, Bioulac B, Hammond C (2005) Impact of high-frequency stimulation parameters on the pattern of discharge of subthalamic neurons. J Neurophysiol 94(6):3662–3669.
29. Lee KH, Blaha CD, Harris BT, et al (2006) Dopamine efflux in the rat striatum evoked by electrical stimulation of the subthalamic nucleus: potential mechanism of action in Parkinson's disease. Eur J Neurosci 23(4):1005–1014.
30. Lee KH, Roberts DW, Kim U (2003) Effect of high-frequency stimulation of the subthalamic nucleus on subthalamic neurons: an intracellular study. Stereotact Funct Neurosurg 80(1–4):32–36.
31. Magarinos-Ascone C, Pazo JH, Macadar O, Buno W (2002) High-frequency stimulation of the subthalamic nucleus silences subthalamic neurons: a possible cellular mechanism in Parkinson's disease. Neuroscience 115(4):1109–1117.
32. Hashimoto T, Elder CM, Vitek JL (2002) A template subtraction method for stimulus artifact removal in high-frequency deep brain stimulation. J Neurosci Meth 113(2):181–186.
33. Filali M, Hutchison WD, Palter VN, Lozano AM, Dostrovsky JO (2004) Stimulation-induced inhibition of neuronal firing in human subthalamic nucleus. Exp Brain Res Experimentelle Hirnforschung 156(3):274–281.
34. Galati S, Mazzone P, Fedele E, et al (2006) Biochemical and electrophysiological changes of substantia nigra pars reticulata driven by subthalamic stimulation in patients with Parkinson's disease. Eur J Neurosci 23(11):2923–2928.
35. Montgomery EB Jr (2006) Effects of GPi stimulation on human thalamic neuronal activity. Clin Neurophysiol 117(12):2691–2702.
36. Pralong E, Debatisse D, Maeder M, Vingerhoets F, Ghika J, Villemure JG (2003) Effect of deep brain stimulation of GPI on neuronal activity of the thalamic nucleus ventralis oralis in a dystonic patient. Neurophysiologie clinique 33(4):169–173.
37. Welter ML, Houeto JL, Bonnet AM, et al (2004) Effects of high-frequency stimulation on subthalamic neuronal activity in parkinsonian patients. Arch Neurol 61(1):89–96.
38. Maltete D, Jodoin N, Karachi C, et al (2007) Subthalamic stimulation and neuronal activity in the substantia nigra in Parkinson's disease. J Neurophysiol 97(6):4017–4022.

39. Anderson ME, Postupna N, Ruffo M (2003) Effects of high-frequency stimulation in the internal globus pallidus on the activity of thalamic neurons in the awake monkey. J Neurophysiol 89(2):1150–1160.
40. Bar-Gad I, Elias S, Vaadia E, Bergman H (2004) Complex locking rather than complete cessation of neuronal activity in the globus pallidus of a 1-methyl-4-phenyl-1, 2,3,6-tetrahydropyridine-treated primate in response to pallidal microstimulation. J Neurosci 24(33):7410–7419.
41. Boraud T, Bezard E, Bioulac B, Gross C (1996) High frequency stimulation of the internal Globus Pallidus (GPi) simultaneously improves parkinsonian symptoms and reduces the firing frequency of GPi neurons in the MPTP-treated monkey. Neurosci Lett 215(1):17–20.
42. Kita H, Tachibana Y, Nambu A, Chiken S (2005) Balance of monosynaptic excitatory and disynaptic inhibitory responses of the globus pallidus induced after stimulation of the subthalamic nucleus in the monkey. J Neurosci 25(38):8611–8619.
43. Meissner W, Leblois A, Hansel D, et al (2005) Subthalamic high frequency stimulation resets subthalamic firing and reduces abnormal oscillations. Brain 128 (Pt 10):2372–2382.
44. Benazzouz A, Gao DM, Ni ZG, Piallat B, Bouali-Benazzouz R, Benabid AL (2000) Effect of high-frequency stimulation of the subthalamic nucleus on the neuronal activities of the substantia nigra pars reticulata and ventrolateral nucleus of the thalamus in the rat. Neuroscience 99(2):289–295.
45. Benazzouz A, Piallat B, Pollak P, Benabid AL (1995) Responses of substantia nigra pars reticulata and globus pallidus complex to high frequency stimulation of the subthalamic nucleus in rats: electrophysiological data. Neurosci Lett 189(2):77–80.
46. Lee KH, Chang SY, Roberts DW, Kim U (2004) Neurotransmitter release from high-frequency stimulation of the subthalamic nucleus. J Neurosurg 101(3):511–517.
47. Maurice N, Thierry AM, Glowinski J, Deniau JM (2003) Spontaneous and evoked activity of substantia nigra pars reticulata neurons during high-frequency stimulation of the subthalamic nucleus. J Neurosci 23(30):9929–9936.
48. Shi LH, Luo F, Woodward DJ, Chang JY (2006) Basal ganglia neural responses during behaviorally effective deep brain stimulation of the subthalamic nucleus in rats performing a treadmill locomotion test. Synapse 59(7):445–457.
49. Tai CH, Boraud T, Bezard E, Bioulac B, Gross C, Benazzouz A (2003) Electrophysiological and metabolic evidence that high-frequency stimulation of the subthalamic nucleus bridles neuronal activity in the subthalamic nucleus and the substantia nigra reticulata. Faseb J 17(13):1820–1830.
50. Brown P, Oliviero A, Mazzone P, Insola A, Tonali P, Di Lazzaro V (2001) Dopamine dependency of oscillations between subthalamic nucleus and pallidum in Parkinson's disease. J Neurosci 21(3):1033–1038.
51. Foffani G, Ardolino G, Egidi M, Caputo E, Bossi B, Priori A (2006) Subthalamic oscillatory activities at beta or higher frequency do not change after high-frequency DBS in Parkinson's disease. Brain Res Bull 69(2):123–130.
52. Foffani G, Priori A, Egidi M, et al (2003) 300-Hz subthalamic oscillations in Parkinson's disease. Brain 126(Pt 10):2153–2163.
53. Marsden JF, Limousin-Dowsey P, Ashby P, Pollak P, Brown P (2001) Subthalamic nucleus, sensorimotor cortex and muscle interrelationships in Parkinson's disease. Brain 124(Pt 2):378–388.
54. Stefani A, Fedele E, Galati S, et al (2005) Subthalamic stimulation activates internal pallidus: evidence from cGMP microdialysis in PD patients. Ann Neurol 57(3):448–452.
55. Stefani A, Fedele E, Galati S, et al (2006) Deep brain stimulation in Parkinson's disease patients: biochemical evidence. J Neural Trans 70:401–408.
56. Boulet S, Lacombe E, Carcenac C, et al (2006) Subthalamic stimulation-induced forelimb dyskinesias are linked to an increase in glutamate levels in the substantia nigra pars reticulata. J Neurosci 26(42):10,768–10,776.

57. Bruet N, Windels F, Bertrand A, Feuerstein C, Poupard A, Savasta M (2001) High frequency stimulation of the subthalamic nucleus increases the extracellular contents of striatal dopamine in normal and partially dopaminergic denervated rats. J Neuropathol Exp Neurol 60(1):15–24.
58. Bruet N, Windels F, Carcenac C, et al (2003) Neurochemical mechanisms induced by high frequency stimulation of the subthalamic nucleus: increase of extracellular striatal glutamate and GABA in normal and hemiparkinsonian rats. J Neuropathol Exp Neurol 62(12):1228–1240.
59. Lacombe E, Carcenac C, Boulet S, et al (2007) High-frequency stimulation of the subthalamic nucleus prolongs the increase in striatal dopamine induced by acute L-DOPA in dopaminergic denervated rats. Eur J Neurosci In press.
60. Meissner W, Harnack D, Hoessle N, et al (2004) High frequency stimulation of the entopeduncular nucleus has no effect on striatal dopaminergic transmission. Neurochem Int 44(4):281–286.
61. Meissner W, Harnack D, Paul G, et al (2002) Deep brain stimulation of subthalamic neurons increases striatal dopamine metabolism and induces contralateral circling in freely moving 6-hydroxydopamine-lesioned rats. Neurosci Lett 328(2):105–108.
62. Meissner W, Harnack D, Reese R, et al (2003) High-frequency stimulation of the subthalamic nucleus enhances striatal dopamine release and metabolism in rats. J Neurochem 85(3):601–609.
63. Windels F, Carcenac C, Poupard A, Savasta M (2005) Pallidal origin of GABA release within the substantia nigra pars reticulata during high-frequency stimulation of the subthalamic nucleus. J Neurosci 25(20):5079–5086.
64. Benazzouz A, Tai CH, Meissner W, Bioulac B, Bezard E, Gross C (2004) High-frequency stimulation of both zona incerta and subthalamic nucleus induces a similar normalization of basal ganglia metabolic activity in experimental parkinsonism. Faseb J 18(3):528–530.
65. Salin P, Manrique C, Forni C, Kerkerian-Le Goff L (2002) High-frequency stimulation of the subthalamic nucleus selectively reverses dopamine denervation-induced cellular defects in the output structures of the basal ganglia in the rat. J Neurosci 22(12):5137–5148.
66. Schulte T, Brecht S, Herdegen T, Illert M, Mehdorn HM, Hamel W (2006) Induction of immediate early gene expression by high-frequency stimulation of the subthalamic nucleus in rats. Neurosci 138(4):1377–1385.
67. Butson CR, Cooper SE, Henderson JM, McIntyre CC (2007) Patient-specific analysis of the volume of tissue activated during deep brain stimulation. NeuroImage 34(2):661–670.
68. Ceballos-Baumann AO (2003) Functional imaging in Parkinson's disease: activation studies with PET, fMRI and SPECT. J Neurol 250(Suppl 1):I15–I23.
69. Ashby P, Kim YJ, Kumar R, Lang AE, Lozano AM (1999) Neurophysiological effects of stimulation through electrodes in the human subthalamic nucleus. Brain 122(Pt 10):1919–1931.
70. Ashby P, Paradiso G, Saint-Cyr JA, Chen R, Lang AE, Lozano AM (2001) Potentials recorded at the scalp by stimulation near the human subthalamic nucleus. Clin Neurophysiol 112(3):431–437.
71. Baker KB, Montgomery EB Jr, Rezai AR, Burgess R, Luders HO (2002) Subthalamic nucleus deep brain stimulus evoked potentials: physiological and therapeutic implications. Mov Disord 17(5):969–983.
72. Bevan MD, Wilson CJ (1999) Mechanisms underlying spontaneous oscillation and rhythmic firing in rat subthalamic neurons. J Neurosci 19(17):7617–7628.
73. Hamani C, Saint-Cyr JA, Fraser J, Kaplitt M, Lozano AM (2004) The subthalamic nucleus in the context of movement disorders. Brain 127(Pt 1):4–20.
74. Wichmann T, Bergman H, DeLong MR (1994) The primate subthalamic nucleus. I. Functional properties in intact animals. J Neurophysiol 72(2):494–506.

75. Benazzouz A, Breit S, Koudsie A, Pollak P, Krack P, Benabid AL (2002) Intraoperative microrecordings of the subthalamic nucleus in Parkinson's disease. Mov Disord 17(Suppl 3):S145–S149.
76. Bergman H, Wichmann T, Karmon B, DeLong MR (1994) The primate subthalamic nucleus. II. Neuronal activity in the MPTP model of parkinsonism. J Neurophysiol 72(2):507–520.
77. Hutchison WD, Allan RJ, Opitz H, et al (1998) Neurophysiological identification of the subthalamic nucleus in surgery for Parkinson's disease. Ann Neurol 44(4):622–628.
78. Magnin M, Morel A, Jeanmonod D (2000) Single-unit analysis of the pallidum, thalamus and subthalamic nucleus in parkinsonian patients. Neuroscience 96(3):549–564.
79. DeLong MR (1990) Primate models of movement disorders of basal ganglia origin. Trends Neurosci 13(7):281–285.
80. Dostrovsky JO, Lozano AM (2002) Mechanisms of deep brain stimulation. Mov Disord 17(Suppl 3):S63–S68.
81. Hershey T, Revilla FJ, Wernle AR, et al (2003) Cortical and subcortical blood flow effects of subthalamic nucleus stimulation in PD. Neurology 61(6):816–821.
82. Abosch A, Kapur S, Lang AE, et al (2003) Stimulation of the subthalamic nucleus in Parkinson's disease does not produce striatal dopamine release. Neurosurgery 53(5):1095–1102; discussion 102–105.
83. Hilker R, Voges J, Ghaemi M, et al (2003) Deep brain stimulation of the subthalamic nucleus does not increase the striatal dopamine concentration in parkinsonian humans. Mov Disord 18(1):41–48.
84. Strafella AP, Sadikot AF, Dagher A (2003) Subthalamic deep brain stimulation does not induce striatal dopamine release in Parkinson's disease. Neuroreport 14(9):1287–1289.
85. Thobois S, Fraix V, Savasta M, et al (2003) Chronic subthalamic nucleus stimulation and striatal D2 dopamine receptors in Parkinson's disease—A [(11)C]-raclopride PET study. J Neurol 250(10):1219–1223.
86. Bacci JJ, Absi el H, Manrique C, Baunez C, Salin P, Kerkerian-Le Goff L (2004) Differential effects of prolonged high frequency stimulation and of excitotoxic lesion of the subthalamic nucleus on dopamine denervation-induced cellular defects in the rat striatum and globus pallidus. Eur J Neurosci 20(12):3331–3341.
87. Nowak LG, Bullier J (1998) Axons, but not cell bodies, are activated by electrical stimulation in cortical gray matter. I. Evidence from chronaxie measurements. Experimentelle Hirnforschung 118(4):477–488.
88. Nowak LG, Bullier J (1998) Axons, but not cell bodies, are activated by electrical stimulation in cortical gray matter. II. Evidence from selective inactivation of cell bodies and axon initial segments. Experimentelle Hirnforschung 118(4):489–500.
89. McIntyre CC, Grill WM (1999) Excitation of central nervous system neurons by nonuniform electric fields. Biophysic J 76(2):878–888.
90. Baldissera F, Lundberg A, Udo M (1972) Stimulation of pre- and postsynaptic elements in the red nucleus. Experimentelle Hirnforschung 15(2):151–167.
91. Gustafsson B, Jankowska E (1976) Direct and indirect activation of nerve cells by electrical pulses applied extracellularly. J Physiol 258(1):33–61.
92. Stover NP, Okun MS, Evatt ML, Raju DV, Bakay RA, Vitek JL (2005) Stimulation of the subthalamic nucleus in a patient with Parkinson disease and essential tremor. Arch Neurol 62(1):141–143.
93. Herzog J, Fietzek U, Hamel W, et al (2004) Most effective stimulation site in subthalamic deep brain stimulation for Parkinson's disease. Mov Disord 19(9):1050–1054.
94. Plaha P, Ben-Shlomo Y, Patel NK, Gill SS (2006) Stimulation of the caudal zona incerta is superior to stimulation of the subthalamic nucleus in improving contralateral parkinsonism. Brain 129(Pt 7):1732–1747.

95. Yokoyama T, Ando N, Sugiyama K, Akamine S, Namba H (2006) Relationship of stimulation site location within the subthalamic nucleus region to clinical effects on parkinsonian symptoms. Stereotact Funct Neurosurg 84(4):170–175.
96. Godinho F, Thobois S, Magnin M, et al (2006) Subthalamic nucleus stimulation in Parkinson's disease: anatomical and electrophysiological localization of active contacts. J Neurol 253(10):1347–1355.
97. Hamel W, Fietzek U, Morsnowski A, et al (2003) Deep brain stimulation of the subthalamic nucleus in Parkinson's disease: evaluation of active electrode contacts. J Neurol Neurosurg Psychiatry 74(8):1036–1046.
98. Lanotte MM, Rizzone M, Bergamasco B, Faccani G, Melcarne A, Lopiano L (2002) Deep brain stimulation of the subthalamic nucleus: anatomical, neurophysiological, and outcome correlations with the effects of stimulation. J Neurol Neurosurg Psychiatry 72(1):53–58.
99. Nowinski WL, Belov D, Pollak P, Benabid AL (2005) Statistical analysis of 168 bilateral subthalamic nucleus implantations by means of the probabilistic functional atlas. Neurosurgery 57(4 Suppl):319–330; discussion 30.
100. Saint-Cyr JA, Hoque T, Pereira LC, et al (2002) Localization of clinically effective stimulating electrodes in the human subthalamic nucleus on magnetic resonance imaging. J Neurosurg 97(5):1152–1166.
101. Starr PA, Christine CW, Theodosopoulos PV, et al (2002) Implantation of deep brain stimulators into the subthalamic nucleus: technical approach and magnetic resonance imaging-verified lead locations. J Neurosurg 97(2):370–387.
102. Voges J, Volkmann J, Allert N, et al (2002) Bilateral high-frequency stimulation in the subthalamic nucleus for the treatment of Parkinson disease: correlation of therapeutic effect with anatomical electrode position. J Neurosurg 96(2):269–279.
103. Yelnik J, Damier P, Demeret S, et al (2003) Localization of stimulating electrodes in patients with Parkinson disease by using a three-dimensional atlas-magnetic resonance imaging coregistration method. J Neurosurg 99(1):89–99.
104. Zonenshayn M, Sterio D, Kelly PJ, Rezai AR, Beric A (2004) Location of the active contact within the subthalamic nucleus (STN) in the treatment of idiopathic Parkinson's disease. Surg Neurol 62(3):216–225; discussion 25–26.
105. Perier C, Vila M, Feger J, Agid Y, Hirsch EC (2000) Functional activity of zona incerta neurons is altered after nigrostriatal denervation in hemiparkinsonian rats. Exp Neurol 162(1):215–224.
106. Alvarez L, Macias R, Lopez G, et al (2005) Bilateral subthalamotomy in Parkinson's disease: initial and long-term response. Brain 128(Pt 3):570–583.
107. Guridi J, Herrero MT, Luquin R, Guillen J, Obeso JA (1994) Subthalamotomy improves MPTP-induced parkinsonism in monkeys. Stereotact Funct Neurosurg 62(1–4):98–102.
108. Alexander GE, Crutcher MD (1990) Functional architecture of basal ganglia circuits: neural substrates of parallel processing. Trends Neurosci 13(7):266–271.
109. Montgomery EB Jr, Baker KB (2000) Mechanisms of deep brain stimulation and future technical developments. Neurologic Res 22(3):259–266.
110. Grill WM, Snyder AN, Miocinovic S (2004) Deep brain stimulation creates an informational lesion of the stimulated nucleus. Neuroreport 15(7):1137–1140.
111. Rubin JE, Terman D (2004) High frequency stimulation of the subthalamic nucleus eliminates pathological thalamic rhythmicity in a computational model. J Comp Neurosci 16(3):211–235.
112. Tagliati M, Shils J, Sun C, Alterman R (2004) Deep brain stimulation for dystonia. Expert Rev Med Devices 1(1):33–41.
113. Alterman R, Shils J, Miravite J, Tagliati M (2007) Lower stimulation frequency can enhance tolerability and efficacy of pallidal deep brain stimulation for dystonia. Mov Disord 22(3):366–368.

114. Magill PJ, Bolam JP, Bevan MD (2001) Dopamine regulates the impact of the cerebral cortex on the subthalamic nucleus-globus pallidus network. Neuroscience 106(2):313–330.
115. Plenz D, Kital ST (1999) A basal ganglia pacemaker formed by the subthalamic nucleus and external globus pallidus. Nature 400(6745):677–682.
116. Levy R, Ashby P, Hutchison WD, Lang AE, Lozano AM, Dostrovsky JO (2002) Dependence of subthalamic nucleus oscillations on movement and dopamine in Parkinson's disease. Brain 125(Pt 6):1196–1209.
117. Brown P, Mazzone P, Oliviero A, et al (2004) Effects of stimulation of the subthalamic area on oscillatory pallidal activity in Parkinson's disease. Exp Neurol 188(2):480–490.
118. Temperli P, Ghika J, Villemure JG, Burkhard PR, Bogousslavsky J, Vingerhoets FJ (2003) How do parkinsonian signs return after discontinuation of subthalamic DBS? Neurology 60(1):78–81.

# 9
# Functional Imaging of Deep Brain Stimulation: fMRI, SPECT, and PET

Robert Jech

## Abstract

This chapter gives an overview of the relevant literature concerning functional imaging and deep brain stimulation (DBS). Although there is no doubt about the clinical effects of DBS, knowledge concerning its mechanism of function is limited. Methods of functional imaging such as functional MRI (fMRI), single photon emission computed tomography (SPECT), and positron emission tomography (PET) to measure cerebral blood flow or fluorodeoxyclucose metabolism may help us understand the mechanisms of neurostimulation at the site of stimulation and also provide a global view of what is happening in the rest of the brain. Under review are typical patterns of activation/deactivation in the ipsi- and contralateral hemispheres at subcortical and cortical levels while stimulating the subthalamic nucleus (STN), ventral intermediate nucleus of thalamus (VIM) and globus pallidus interna (GPi), while working on different types of tasks. The site of stimulation usually becomes overactivated, which indirectly supports a mechanism of locally increased neuronal activity which than spreads by orthodromic and/or antidromic fashion into areas not being directly stimulated by the DBS electrode. As follows from comparisons with neurostimulation in on and off modes, DBS usually leads to a normalization of pathological patterns of brain activations. Despite similar clinical effects, the mechanisms of DBS are different from those of stereotactic lesions. However, the majority of available studies have produced many contradictory results due to significant methodological differences between studies.

**Keywords:** functional imaging, fMRI, regional cerebral blood flow, SPECT, PET, Parkinson's disease, essential tremor, dystonia, deep brain stimulation, DBS, STN, ventral intermediate nucleus, globus pallidus, thalamus, sensorimotor cortex.

From: *Current Clinical Neurology: Deep Brain Stimulation in Neurological and Psychiatric Disorders*
Edited by: D. Tarsy, J.L. Vitek, P.A. Starr, and M.S. Okun © Humana Press, Totowa, NJ

The primary motivation for the use of the fMRI technique during DBS is to better understand the pathophysiological mechanisms of this kind of therapy. Like PET and SPECT, its purpose is to offer a macroscopic view of the functional state of the basal ganglia and cortex in the course of neurostimulation. fMRI is also a promising tool for searching specific patterns that make predicting the future development of the disease, including any adverse complications, possible. However, our knowledge does not yet extend that far. Despite the ready availability of fMRI, the threat of the potential biological risks involved *(1–3)* is the main reason for the continuing low numbers of fMRI-examined patients.

While the microrecording of single-cell activity or the local detection of neuromediators provide a direct reflection of neuronal activity, functional imaging of activation or deactivation only gives an indirect idea of neuronal activity based on local metabolic turnover or regional cerebral blood flow (rCBF; ref. *4*). As for blood oxygenation level-dependent (BOLD)-fMRI, activation is caused by rCBF increases, and higher local blood volume containing a higher concentration of oxygen *(5)*. Hence, as a matter of principle, neither fMRI nor other rCBF imaging methods can define what neuronal processes occur at the site of neurostimulation because whatever activation or deactivation is observed in functional imaging is not necessarily equivalent to neuronal excitation or inhibition.

The techniques of functional imaging of DBS with fMRI, as distinct from rCBF SPECT, [$^{15}$O]H$_2$O PET, or [$^{18}$F] fluorodeoxyglucose (FDG)-PET techniques differ in many technical details, in particular in the paradigm of the investigation. As for perfusion and metabolic studies, what we see most often is a rating for the DBS effect on the resting rCBF or resting-state metabolism *(6–11)*. Some authors, however, have studied rCBF changes with the use of motor *(12–17)* or cognitive tasks *(18, 19)*. The effects of DBS are usually assessed by using various contrasts in multifactorial linear models. fMRI studies frequently use unilateral alternating on/off switching of DBS, lasting a few tens of seconds while the patient performs no active movement *(20–22)*. The results are often not comparable due to the different types of neurostimulation that are employed.

While PET and SPECT are prone to the risk of exposure to ionizing radiation, MRI is generally regarded as a safe diagnostic method. The presence of an implanted intracerebral electrode, however, makes MRI a potentially dangerous technique namely because of risks of thermal damage or electrode displacement *(1, 21, 23–25)*. Apparently for reasons of MRI-related biological hazards, PET is far more frequently used to study DBS effects than fMRI. Paradoxically, in patients with an implanted electrode, routine MRI brain scanning is frequently used, mainly to control its correct placement *(26, 27)*. Despite the presence of the metallic electrode, MRI can be regarded as safe even in patients treated by DBS, provided a number of technical precautions are taken *(2, 3)*. Technical issues and safety risks of MRI in patients treated by DBS are discussed in detail in the Chapter 22.

Apart from thermal risks, the biological effects of induced currents are another aspect of safety which must be kept in mind *(28)*. The currents are present not only while the MR gradient coils are in operation but also mainly as a result of radiofrequency pulses. According to Georgi et al. *(ref. 3)*, neuronal function is unlikely to be affected due to the very high frequency of induced currents. However, interaction with neuronal activity cannot be completely ruled out.

Worse still for fMRI, susceptibility artifacts develop at the site of the implanted electrode contacts that are often larger than the stimulated nucleus *(22, 29, 30)*. In addition, artifacts caused by the metallic material of the connector and conductors of the external cable may largely deform the image. Unfortunately, susceptibility artifacts that cause undesirable image distortion are typical, particularly in the echo-planar sequence commonly used for fMRI. This is the main reason why fMRI cannot be evaluated in some parts of the brain.

Another limitation of fMRI studies is that they are usually confined to a few hours or days while the implanted electrodes are still externalized. DBS needs an external neurostimulator to be placed outside the strong magnetic field to function correctly. The only mode of stimulation that can be used in these conditions is a bipolar mode of stimulation. In contrast, PET and SPECT can use the monopolar mode of stimulation, the most common contact setting which is used for chronic DBS. Moreover, the pre-fMRI period is usually too short to find the optimal contacts and stimulation parameters that will be used for chronic DBS. fMRI performed days after the implantation of electrodes is also hampered by the potential for a microlesion effect and focal edema around the electrodes, conditions that often take days to subside. Acute microlesions and edema in themselves affect the function of motor circuits and modify clinical symptoms. Furthermore, edema has adverse effects on the detection of the BOLD signal, which is essential for fMRI. The question then is whether we are studying the same DBS mechanism when using fMRI as with PET and SPECT performed months after the operation with the patient optimized and adapted to chronic DBS.

## STN DBS

### Acute STN DBS in a Resting State Visualized by fMRI

The statistical comparison of fMRI examinations with DBS switched on and off allows us to study the immediate effects of DBS (Figure 9.1). As a rule, the patient is lying at rest with eyes closed. We first tested this technique on three patients with Parkinson's disease (PD) who were examined on day 3 after electrodes were implanted into the STN. Unilateral STN DBS was switched on and off every 48 seconds. DBS caused a local BOLD signal increase in the thalamus including the area of the STN in all three patients *(29)*. In two cases, activation was also present in the GP. No such activation was noted in the third patient, in whom STN DBS subsequently led to only temporary improvement. The entire group, later joined by five other PD patients who had responded favorably to DBS therapy, exhibited thalamic and GP activation in response to unilateral STN DBS *(31)*. The immediate effects of acute DBS were also studied by other researchers. Unilateral STN DBS switched on and off every 30 seconds was found to activate the ventrolateral part of the ipsilateral thalamus and putamen *(32)*. In another study, STN DBS unilaterally switched on each time for a period of 32 seconds caused hyperactivation in the posterior part of the ipsilateral GP externa and putamen of all five PD patients enrolled in the study *(22)*. On the contrary, in a recent study of four PD patients who had unilateral STN DBS (after previous contralateral pallidotomy), no significant difference was noted in the fMRI results when STN DBS was repeatedly switched on and off *(30)*.

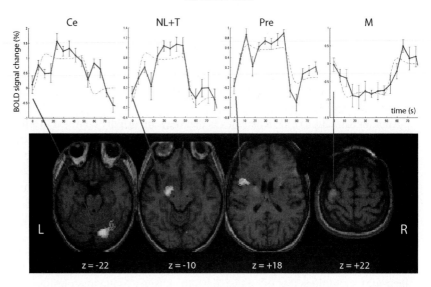

**Figure 9.1** Manifestations of acute STN DBS in a 1.5 T fMRI scan of a PD patient (woman, 63 years, PD duration 12 years, UPDRS III: OFF = 53, ON = 30). Bipolar left-sided DBS was switched on and off every 48 seconds (130 Hz, 60 μs, 3.2 V) with right-sided DBS switched off throughout the procedure. The patient lay at rest with eyes closed. With DBS on, there was activation in the ipsilateral thalamus (T), nucleus lentiformis (NL), ipsilateral premotor cortex (Pre), and contralateral cerebellum (Ce), and simultaneous hypoactivation mainly affecting the ipsilateral primary motor cortex (M). $P < 0.05$, False Discovery Rate corrected. (To view this figure in color, see insert)

## *fMRI Artifacts or Biological Signal?*

BOLD signal changes caused by periodically switching the neurostimulator on and off need not be consistent with changes in neuronal activity. They may simply be an artifact, conceivably arising from direct stimulation of a blood vessel responsible for a local increase in perfusion. Findings from PET studies performed during transcranial magnetic stimulation are at variance with this mechanism. Both hyperactivation *(33)* and hypoactivation *(34)* can be detected in the stimulated region. If transcranial magnetic stimulation leads to neuronal membrane excitation or inhibition by induced electric current *(35)*, i.e., by the same mechanism as in electric stimulation, it is hard to imagine why the same type of stimulus used in different areas of the cerebral cortex should affect blood vessels in opposite ways. In the event simple vasodilatation occurred as a reaction to the electromagnetic stimulus, a uniform response pattern would be expected instead.

It is also unlikely that a local BOLD signal increase should be due to a current flow artifact, although electric currents may cause susceptibility artifacts which can be visualized using MRI *(36)*. If that were the case, we should also have noticed significant signal changes in the phantom experiment. Neither the site of the electrode nor its vicinity showed any signs of signal fluctuation that correlated with the stimulator being switched on and off *(31)*. It would seem equally improbable that local temperature changes would account for the area of activation. Even if there had been a significant local radio-frequency temperature increase during fMRI, it would have been continuous from the beginning to the end of the examination. Consequently, a BOLD signal change induced in this way could not have correlated with the course of the stimulation task to become visualized as an activated area. While correction for motor artifacts may not have eliminated all problems arising from head movements, it is unlikely that the motor artifacts would increase the signal solely in the predicted areas such as the thalamus or basal ganglia.

## fMRI Local and Distant Effects of STN DBS

As already mentioned, an artifact arising at the electrode contacts precludes observation of what is happening in the stimulated nucleus. In fact, magnetic field distortion around the implanted electrode is the reason for partial displacement of the image of the nucleus activity from its actual position. In some patients, the cluster of activation was found close to some of the contacts *(29)*, which might reflect the STN BOLD signal activity. Assuming the hypothesis that areas of fMRI activation develop indirectly as a result of increased neuronal activity, it is not clear why hyperactivation should be present during DBS. From the therapeutic point of view, there is no difference between a thermolesion and DBS. Certain authors postulated early that high-frequency DBS should cause long-term depolarization and thereby local inhibition *(37–39)*. However, according to others, what appears to occur in the nucleus is excitation or simultaneous excitation and inhibition *(40–44)*. If there is a predominant blockade during DBS, the site of stimulation should show hypoactivation similar to that of therapeutic thermolesions *(45–47)* rather than the type of hyperactivation we and some other authors observed *(6, 12, 29)*. The BOLD signal increase during stimulation provides indirect evidence of increased metabolic turnover. This may then reflect an effect of stimulation spreading via orthodromic and/or antidromic activation into areas that are not being stimulated directly with the DBS electrode. Hyperactivation of the thalamus, upper part of the midbrain, and GP as seen during STN DBS *(22, 29)* may well point to stimulation propagating along anatomical connections. With respect to the glutamatergic projection from the STN, these structures ought to be hypoactivated when the STN is inactivated. However, according to some researchers, there occurs an increase in the neuronal activities of the GP and substantia nigra pars reticulata *(41)* as well as an increase in the local concentration of glutamate *(42, 48)*, which would suggest excitation spreading from the STN during stimulation in this structure.

During STN DBS, some patients have shown activation in remote subcortical and cortical areas known to be anatomically connected with the stimulated nucleus. With STN DBS, hyperactivity was noted not only in the basal ganglia, but also in the ipsilateral premotor cortex, dorsolateral prefrontal cortex (DLPFC), brainstem and contralateral cerebellum *(22, 29, 31, 32)*. Some patients showed signs of deactivation of the primary sensorimotor cortex and supplementary motor area (SMA; refs. *31* and *32*). In one patient, right-side DBS led to depressive dysphoria accompanied by increased BOLD signal in the upper prefrontal cortex, anterior cingulate and anterior thalamus. The implanted electrode contact lay dorsolateral to the STN *(32)*.

### Chronic STN DBS in a Resting State Visualized by PET and SPECT

The effects of STN DBS have been repeatedly studied using rCBF PET and SPECT or FDG PET. Patients were examined in a resting state after a sufficiently long (hours or days) adaptation to DBS. Some clinical manifestations such as rigidity disappear within seconds after switching STN DBS on, but it often takes hours/days to achieve the full therapeutic effect. Also, after STN DBS has been switched off, the different symptoms reappear with varying progression *(49)*. Moreover, a study of the chronic effects of DBS is free from the risk of interference by transient phenomena such as transitory paraesthesia, which is likely to appear in many patients immediately after switching STN DBS on and then disappear spontaneously within seconds.

During discontinued medication, the brain resting-state of glucose metabolism in PD is characterized by a specific pattern: bilateral hyperactivation of the GP, thalamus, and pons and simultaneous hypoactivation of the prefrontal, premotor, and parietal regions *(50–53)*. This pattern of glucose metabolism, described as a PD-related covariance pattern, correlates with a similar pattern of resting-state rCBF, and exhibits stable reproducibility *(54)*.

Chronic STN DBS leads to increased metabolic activity *(6, 9)* and rCBF *(8, 12)* of the thalamus or subthalamus. As the frequency of stimulation increases, there is a linear increase in subthalamic perfusion *(55)*. Findings such as these make us question the theory of neuronal inhibition or depolarization block as a DBS mechanism. When studying DBS effects close to the electrode, other authors have conversely found only non-significant increases of rCBF *(15)*, no change *(56)*, or even a drop in glucose metabolism *(11, 57)* similar to that observed after STN lesions *(45)*.

With STN DBS, glucose activity decreased in the GP and putamen *(6, 11)*. However, most of the other FDG PET and rCBF studies found no changes in this area. There are exceptions: three studies describe an increase in the regional resting-state rCBF in the GP while STN DBS was on *(12)* with simultaneous increase *(7)* or decrease *(8)* of rCBF in some areas of the frontal lobe.

According to a longitudinal study, a STN DBS-related increase in rCBF was present at 5 and even 42 months after implantation. rCBF in the rostral SMA, DLPFC, and premotor cortex later showed an even greater increase. Moreover, rCBF also increased in the GP, thalamus, midbrain, pons, and cerebellum *(7)*, which may be consistent with the functional reorganization of the cortico-subcortical circuits attributable to progression of PD. Chronic STN DBS is unlikely to slow down PD progression since the dopaminergic activity of the caudate nucleus and putamen continues to abate at a rate of 9.5 to 12.9% annually *(58)*.

A STN DBS-related increase in cortical activity has also been observed by other authors. They have found increased rCBF of the DLPFC *(10)*, and enhanced glucose metabolism in the mesial frontal cortex and in some regions of the parietal and temporal lobes *(9, 11, 57)*. Therefore, rCBF changes appear to reflect the clinical effect of DBS. For example, it was only in responders that STN DBS led to an increase and, thereby, to the normalization of abnormally reduced rCBF in the frontal, parietal and occipital lobes *(59)*. Also, many remote DBS effects may have been related to cognitive, behavioral, or affective disorders that are likely to appear in some STN DBS-treated patients *(60)*.

Opinions differ as to the resting activity of the cingulate. While some have noted an increase of rCBF in the anterior cingulate *(56)*, others found no change *(10)* or even a decrease in this area *(12, 13)*, including a local drop in glucose metabolism *(11)*. The differences appear to result from different methodological approaches, some of which studied PD patients with different spectra of clinical symptoms while others studied STN DBS effects with or without dopaminergic medication.

However, many authors concur in their views concerning resting activity in the primary motor and/or sensorimotor regions. With STN DBS on, both rCBF *(12, 13, 15)* and glucose metabolism show a decline *(6, 11, 57)*. Besides, the rCBF decline correlates with a decrease of stimulation frequency, thus indirectly proving STN modulatory effects on motor cortex function *(55)*. STN DBS-induced decrease in rCBF and glucose metabolic activity has also been described in the cerebellum, mainly in the vermis area *(6, 11)* as well as in the cerebellar hemispheres *(9, 13, 57)*. Lower resting-state activity in the motor circuits may possibly be due to decreased proprioceptive feedback as a result of decreased rigidity or resting tremor, or conceivably due to a reduction of abnormal synchronized oscillations in the motor circuits *(61)*.

**Motor Tasks in fMRI**

During sequential motor tasks with the thumb successively touching the fingers of the same hand, or during repetitive opening and closing of the hand, PD patients in a hypodopaminergic state reveal a number of substantial changes in activation patterns when compared with healthy controls. Patients with advanced PD show a stronger BOLD signal in the primary sensorimotor cortex, lateral premotor cortex, inferior parietal cortex, anterior cingulate, and caudal portion of the SMA. Hyperactivation in these areas is probably a compensatory counteraction of the deactivated areas such as the rostral portion of the SMA and right DLPFC *(62)*. A similar situation was observed during discontinued antiparkinsonian medication in early-phase PD while patients performed a self-paced single joystick movement task analyzed by means of event-related fMRI *(63)*. Even asymptomatic carriers of the mutated Parkin gene exhibit greater BOLD activity in the anterior cingulate and premotor cortex, as seen in movements relying on internal cues *(64)*. In this way, hyperactivity of the frontal premotor and frontomesial cortex, essential in the planning and execution of complex voluntary movements *(62, 65)*, may arise from either dysfunction or compensatory activation of those areas.

*STN DBS Effects on Motion-Related fMRI Activity*

When studying DBS effects on brain motion-related activity, the sequential motor task is executed twice, with STN DBS unilaterally switched on and off *(31, 66)*. While moving a hand contralateral to the stimulated nucleus, one patient treated with STN DBS showed a decrease in motion-related activity in the primary sensorimotor cortex of the stimulated hemisphere accompanied by cerebellar hypoactivation in the hemisphere contralateral to DBS. Three variants of bipolar stimulation were used successively for this study; however, only one stimulation triggered activation in the anterior insula, putamen, and caudate nucleus of the stimulated hemisphere *(66)*. In our group of eight PD patients, we also noted a decrease in motion-related activity during STN DBS (Figure 9.2). The decrease was significant in the primary sensorimotor cortex

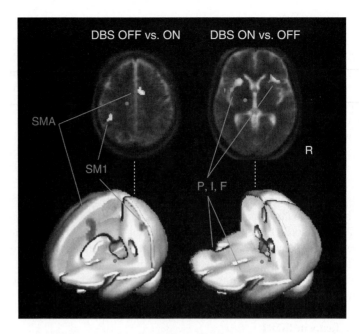

**Figure 9.2** Effects of left-sided STN DBS on motion-related activity in eight patients with PD scanned with 1.5 T fMRI after overnight discontinuation of L-DOPA. During fMRI, patients executed sequential movements with the fingers of the right-hand (the motor and resting phases changed periodically every 48 seconds). With DBS on, motion-related activity decreased in the primary sensorimotor cortex (SM1) and supplementary motor area (SMA), and increased in the putamen, insula and inferolateral frontal cortex (P, I, F). $P < 0.001$, uncorrected. (To view this figure in color, see insert)

of the stimulated hemisphere (i.e., contralateral to the moving hand) while activity in the SMA of the contralateral hemisphere (ipsilateral to the moving hand) abated simultaneously. This appears to reflect normalization of the function of those areas. We also observed a bilateral activation in the insula, in the inferolateral prefrontal cortex, and in the putamen, while cerebellar activity remained unchanged *(31)*. Because STN DBS also has some beneficial effect on ipsilateral extremities *(67, 68)*, we studied STN DBS effects on motion-related activity of the ipsilateral hand. With DBS on, we found hypoactivation in the SMA of both hemispheres without a change in activity of the primary sensorimotor cortex or cerebellum. Hence, this finding suggests that unilateral STN DBS does influence the function of both hemispheres *(31)*.

**Motor Tasks in PET and SPECT**

The findings from rCBF studies of PD patients during the execution of sequential motor tasks are similar to results of fMRI. rCBF PET and SPECT studies which showed, in particular, increased motion-related activity of the lateral premotor cortex and inferolateral parietal cortex in comparison with healthy controls, in what might be compensation for the hypoactivation of the DLPFC and mesial frontal cortex *(69)*. The execution of self-initiated movements led to a substantially lower activation of the DLPFC, mesial frontal and parietal cortices *(70)*. On the contrary, the ipsilateral hemisphere of the cerebellum is an area which has shown increased motion-related activity *(71)*.

Most PET and SPECT studies of PD concurrently describe a decrease in motion-related activity of the SMA *(69, 70, 72–75)*, an area participating in movement planning and initiation, i.e., functions that obviously are affected in PD. SMA hypoactivation appears to be caused by excessive inhibition from the thalamo-cortical projections, which may perhaps relate to manifestations of akinesia *(76)*. Only one study found increased SMA activity in PD *(65)*, namely during the execution of long sequences of overtrained finger movements.

## STN DBS Effects on Motion-Related rCBF

A large number of studies deal with the effects of unilateral or bilateral STN DBS on rCBF during motion execution in patients with PD. What they describe is normalization of the abnormal pattern of cortical activation, which are found while DBS is switched off and dopaminergic medication is discontinued. To put this in simple terms, STN DBS leads to hyperactivation of the fronto-striato-thalamic circuits along with simultaneous modulation of the activity of the primary and secondary motor areas.

Effective left-sided STN DBS with the right hand in motion was found to increase rCBF in the anterior cingulate, the left primary sensorimotor cortex, and the right cerebellum. As subsequent more detailed analysis revealed, the cause of the difference lay not in cortical hyperactivation during the motion but in its decrease during the resting phase of the task *(13)*. However, decreasing motion-related rCBF of the primary motor cortex, ipsilaterally *(12)* or contralaterally *(14)* to STN DBS has been observed previously.

Increased rCBF caused by unilateral STN DBS was observed bilaterally in prefrontal cortex including DLPFC, in the left thalamus and putamen. Such changes were observed not only in the execution of a sequential joystick movement but also while the motion was merely imaginary *(14)*. Also, in another study authors using unilateral high-frequency STN DBS found increased motion-related rCBF in the DLPFC *(15)*, while bilateral STN DBS caused increased rCBF in the GP *(17)*.

The changes in SMA activity are somewhat contradictory. Ceballos-Baumann et al. *(12)* found, in the course of a motor task with STN DBS on as distinct from DBS off, increased rCBF of premotor cortex and rostral SMA together with simultaneous hypoactivation in the caudal SMA. In another study a motion-related rCBF decrease was found in the rostral SMA *(14)*. Other authors then found rCBF in the SMA increased *(15, 16)*, which correlated positively with motor improvement as seen in the speed of joystick movement *(17)*. In addition, STN DBS led to suppression of rCBF fluctuations in the SMA, which co-varied previously with the extent of joystick movements. The authors interpreted this that different levels of brain activation reflect mechanisms to achieve similar levels of behavioral performance *(16)*. With unilateral STN DBS, they also noted an increase in motion-related rCBF in those brain areas which were previously hypoactive, while other hypoactivated areas became active to a point that resembled normal functioning.

A closer look at the above studies reveals some methodological differences. While most authors compare the effects of STN DBS unilaterally (or bilaterally) switched on or off, others compare the pattern of brain activation under different conditions; that is, in a state of effective and ineffective stimulation *(15–17)*. Another weakness of most imaging studies (including fMRI) is that the changes in motion-related activation need not be related to DBS; they may simply be manifestations of differences in motor performance. Other discrepancies may arise from differences between patients in the study group exhibiting a different spectrum or intensity of clinical symptoms. Moreover, many findings are difficult to interpret because it is not always possible to differentiate between what is pathologically abnormal and what is a sign of functional adaptation. Consequently, comparisons between stimulator conditions, regardless of the presence of resting tremor, may lead to false conclusions. Hypoactivation of the primary sensorimotor cortex may thus be a consequence of suppressed tremor rather than a straightforward effect of DBS *(77)*.

### *STN DBS Effects on rCBF in Cognitive Tasks*

Apart from studying the effects of STN DBS on motion-related brain activity, several studies have focused on speech and cognitive function. Most PD patients have problems with speech *(78)*, which tends to be monotonous, quiet, and irregularly accelerated. STN DBS can make dysarthria worse or, to some extent, better *(79–81)*. The results of a rCBF PET study aimed at speech production and silent articulation suggested that parkinsonian dysarthria is associated with insufficient activation of the orofacial primary motor cortex and the cerebellum in the presence of excessive activation of the premotor cortex, SMA, and DLPFC. With STN DBS on, there was partial improvement of speech while functional imaging showed a pattern almost resembling that of healthy persons *(82)*.

As for cognitive executive tasks, two were used during STN DBS: the Stroop task and the verbal fluency task *(18, 19)*. Worsened performance was repeatedly seen while the PD patients were coping with both tasks. Further deterioration is often noted using STN DBS *(83–86)*. The Stroop task is a response conflict task that requires patients to name the font color of color words printed in an incongruent ink. A worse performance in this test induced by switching DBS on led to a bilateral rCBF decrease in the anterior cingulate and right ventral striatum. This finding documents that STN stimulation may have an impact on non-motor striato-thalamo-cortical circuits *(18)*. In a verbal fluency test, stimulated patients produced significantly fewer words than with DBS off. Affected at the same time, regional rCBF while STN DBS was switched on decreased in the right orbitofrontal cortex and the frontotemporal circuits of the left hemisphere, i.e., areas activated during word production *(19)*.

## STN DBS Compared With L-dopa Effects

Although STN DBS and treatment with L-dopa both produce similar improvement in PD symptoms, DBS fails to restore dopamine synthesis *(87, 88)*. Nevertheless, the consequences of both interventions on motor circuits are similar in several ways *(6, 89)*. In a study comparing the effects of DBS and L-dopa using FDG PET, both led to decreased metabolism in the putamen, GP, primary sensorimotor cortex, and cerebellar vermis *(6)*. This is in agreement with a previous study describing an L-dopa-related decrease of rCBF in putamen and thalamus *(90)*. Conversely, with STN DBS, the resting activation of the thalamus and GP became higher as proven in both rCBF *(7, 8, 12)* and fMRI studies *(22, 29)*.

Effects of STN DBS and L-dopa treatment do differ in some aspects. As distinct from effects of L-dopa, STN DBS resulted in increased metabolic activity in the thalamus together with the adjacent subthalamus and in decreased metabolism of the ventromedial prefrontal cortex *(6)*. These differences therefore reflect their different mechanisms of action on the thalamus and cognitive functions. Using rCBF PET, other authors comparing L-dopa and DBS reached somewhat different conclusions. After L-dopa, the thalamus and caudate nucleus were more active and the inferolateral prefrontal cortex, midbrain and cerebellum were less active than with DBS *(89)*. However, there was a methodological difference between the two studies. In Goerendt et al.'s study in 2006, the patients were tested when solving a spatial search task designed to guarantee a stable cognitive-behavioral state.

To some extent, it is difficult to compare DBS and L-dopa effects on primary sensorimotor cortical function. This is due to the different influence of L-dopa on cortical activity. While early PD patients who execute hand motions showed lower primary sensorimotor cortex activity *(63)*, other authors *(91, 92)* found an increase in cortical activity afer L-dopa intake. The discrepant results may have been due to differences in the motor tasks or to the duration of previous long-term antiparkinsonian medication. Whereas in Haslinger et al.'s study in 2001 patients had been taking L-dopa chronically, only L-dopa-naive patients were enrolled in the study by Buhmann et al. (2003). This is also congruent with the findings of a SPECT study *(93)* in which the resting-state rCBF of the primary sensorimotor cortex changed differently in response to L-dopa in groups of naive and chronically treated patients. Since DBS electrodes are usually implanted in PD patients with motor fluctuations after several years of exposure to L-dopa, the reported DBS effects on the primary sensorimotor cortex are similar. Switching DBS on led to a decrease in its resting *(6, 11–13, 15, 57)* but also motion-related activities *(14, 31, 66)*.

## Ventral Intermediate Nucleus (VIM) DBS

Tremor has been explored with fMRI in a number of studies. Patients with essential tremor, manifested typically while maintaining a sustained posture, showed abnormally increased activation in the primary contralateral sensorimotor cortex, GP, and thalamus simultaneously with bilateral activation of the cerebellar hemispheres, dentate and red nuclei. Activation in the cerebellar hemisphere and red nucleus was significantly higher in patients with essential tremor than in controls whose tremor was mimicked by passive wrist oscillations *(94)*. A similar conclusion had previously also been reached in a rCBF PET study *(95)*.

PD patients with resting tremor, as distinct from those without tremor, exhibited increased glucose metabolism in the pons, in the thalamus bilaterally, and in the premotor and sensorimotor cortical areas of the left hemisphere *(96)*. Patients with exclusively unilateral parkinsonian tremor were found to have increased metabolic activity in the anterior ventrolateral nuclei of the contralateral thalamus, with metabolic fluctuations correlating positively with tremor amplitude *(97)*. This particular study, also noted hyperactivation of the cerebellum and contralateral sensorimotor cortex in connection with parkinsonian tremor.

Consequently, despite obvious clinical differences between parkinsonian and essential tremor, both types were found to exhibit increased activity in subcortical cerebello-thalamic and cortical sensorimotor areas.

**Functional Imaging in Ventrointermediate (VIM) DBS for Essential Tremor**

Two patients with essential tremor exposed in a resting state to alternating unilateral on and off DBS of the VIM nucleus every 30 seconds showed an ipsilateral BOLD signal increase in the thalamus close to the stimulation electrode. At the same time, there was activation of the primary sensory cortex, possibly in connection with transient paraesthesia while VIM DBS was activated (20). Similarly, another three patients with essential tremor exhibited fMRI signs of increased activity in the thalamus and primary sensorimotor cortex ipsilateral to VIM DBS. In addition, there was hyperactivation in the contralateral cerebellar hemisphere (Figure 9.3; ref. 31). A similar fMRI pattern was observed in one tremor-affected patient with IgM paraproteinaemic demyelinating neuropathy, which may have been a separate type or just a variant of essential tremor (98).

rCBF PET study of essential tremor patients yielded similar results. With VIM DBS switched on, rCBF increased in the thalamus, close to the stimulating electrode. This was accompanied by a significant rCBF increase in the ipsilateral SMA and by a non-significant elevation in the ipsilateral motor cortex and contralateral cerebellum (99). In another PET study exploring the effects of unilateral effective, ineffective and no DBS, hyperactivity in the primary motor cortex was observed during effective VIM DBS (100). A growing amplitude of stimulation paralleled a linear increase of rCBF in the thalamus along with a non-linear rCBF change in the ipsilateral primary sensorimotor cortex. As the stimulation frequency increased, rCBF of this cortical region was reported to increase linearly (101). All these studies thus appear to provide evidence of DBS excitatory effects at the site of stimulation, and of functional connectivity between the VIM nucleus and ipsilateral primary sensorimotor cortex and contralateral cerebellum. Hypoperfusion of the parieto-insular vestibular cortex, which was found in one study, may be a functional correlate of postural instability (100), such as occasionally occurs in some patients treated with VIM DBS.

It is worth mentioning a comparison of the impact of VIM and STN DBS on the primary sensorimotor cortex. While its resting-state activity increases during VIM DBS, stimulation of the STN has an entirely opposite effect (6, 11–13, 15, 31). This is perhaps related to different anatomical connections as the STN has an indirect influence on the motor cortex via the GP and thalamus (102). A possible explanation for these disparate findings is that during VIM DBS, while excitatory thalamocortical projections cause an activation of primary sensorimotor cortex, a different situation occurs during STN DBS which, in functional imaging, increases GP activation (7, 8, 12, 22, 29, 32). GPi via pallidothalamic pathways may cause increased synaptic activity of thalamus leading to suppression of thalamocortical activity because of the inhibitory effect of GPi on the thalamus (103). This reduced input from thalamus would cause decreased activity in the cortex in areas to which this portion of the thalamus projects. This may be why in a resting state the activity of the primary sensorimotor cortex decreases during STN DBS and increases during VIM DBS.

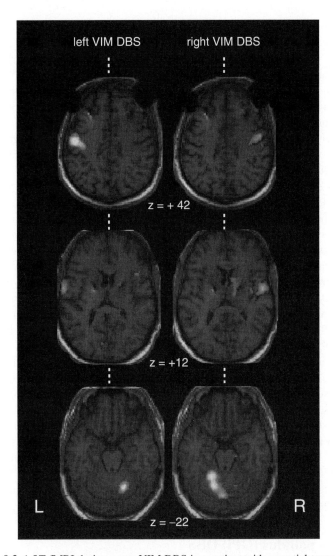

**Figure 9.3** 1.5 T fMRI during acute VIM DBS in a patient with essential tremor (man, 58 years, tremor duration 20 years). Unilateral bipolar DBS was switched on and off every 48 seconds (130 Hz, 60 µs, 3 V) while the patient lay at rest with eyes closed. Unilateral stimulation of the left and right VIM nucleus activated mirror subcortical and cortical areas. $P < 0.05$, False Discovery Rate corrected. (To view this figure in color, see insert)

**Functional Imaging in VIM DBS for Parkinsonian Tremor**

The results of VIM DBS in patients treated for parkinsonian tremor are difficult to interpret. For functional imaging the patients are usually examined at rest, i.e., in a situation likely to induce resting tremor. VIM DBS in such patients leads to its inhibition. Hence, comparisons between rCBF while DBS is on or off will hardly decide which is due to the suppression of the rhythmic oscillations or kinesthetic feedback and which is connected with the direct effects of DBS. There is no such problem in rating VIM DBS effects in essential tremor because patients are usually examined with their extremities at rest when no tremor appears *(76)*. The differences observed between these two types of tremor in VIM DBS functional imaging are probably associated with this phenomenon. This is because VIM DBS effects on the ipsilateral primary sensorimotor cortex and contralateral cerebellum in parkinsonian tremor are the opposite of those which occur in essential tremor. With VIM DBS on and with parkinsonian tremor suppressed, only reduced rCBF was observed in those regions. Changes in tremor acceleration correlated with activations of the ipsilateral primary sensorimotor cortex and SMA cortex positively, while fluctuations in tremor frequency showed a negative correlation with the contralateral dentate nucleus and pontine activations *(104)*. Therapeutic thalamotomy also resulted in decreased rCBF of the ipsilateral primary sensorimotor and premotor cortex, probably because of the inhibition of the thalamo-cortical oscillations *(105)*.

Another two studies mentioned reduced activity in the cerebello-thalamo-cortical circuits in response to VIM DBS *(106, 107)*. The inhibition of resting tremor was associated with a bilateral decline in rCBF in the cerebellum, ipsilateral somatosensory cortex, SMA and caudate nucleus *(106)*. Yet another study showed a decrease in cerebellar rCBF during effective high-frequency VIM DBS. Ineffective low-frequency, similar to effective high-frequency, stimulation only led to hypoactivation of the ipsilateral somatosensory cortex *(107)*. VIM DBS-related deactivation of cortical regions was also observed in another study of patients with parkinsonian tremor. Ipsilateral motor cortex and SMA were deactivated, as were the prefrontal cortex and anterior cingulate bilaterally *(108)*. In contrast, the authors found no decline in cerebellar rCBF. These variations probably arise from methodological differences and from the enrollment of PD patients with slightly different clinical symptoms.

Two studies found activity changes at the site of the stimulation electrode while VIM DBS was on. In both cases, there was an increase in thalamic activity. fMRI of one PD patient showed a local increase in the BOLD signal *(29)*. A PET study of eight PD patients revealed an increase of rCBF *(104)*. These results also tend to support the theory that local excitation occurs at the site of the DBS.

## Globus pallidus (GPi) DBS

The effects of GPi DBS using fMRI have not yet been studied. In contrast, a number of authors have explored the effects of GPi DBS or pallidotomy on glucose metabolism and regional brain perfusion. The findings show some differences relative to whether patients with PD or generalized dystonia were under study.

### Functional Imaging in GPi DBS for PD

GPi DBS in PD patients in a resting state caused an increase in regional glucose metabolism in ipsilateral premotor cortex and both hemispheres of the cerebellum *(109)* along with simultaneous reduction of abnormal PD-related covariance pattern *(52)*. This appears to have been due to normalization of abnormal resting metabolic activity of the cortico-striato-pallido-thalamo-cortical circuitry. According to another study, DBS increased resting rCBF of the ipsilateral putamen and rostral SMA, accompanied by improvements in rigidity and akinesia *(110)*.

GPi DBS also influenced rCBF during a motor task in which the patient was instructed to move the cursor with a digital tablet. With DBS, there was hyperactivation of the anterior cingulate, primary sensorimotor cortex (contralateral to moving hand), and bilateral SMA. Improved motor performance correlated with increased rCBF in the sensorimotor cortex, ventrolateral thalamus, and cerebellum *(111)*. GPi DBS effects on SMA function were similar to those of a lesion since an increase in rCBF in the SMA during hand motion was also observed in connection with unilateral pallidotomy *(112–114)*. However, other remote effects were different. Thermolesion of the GPi was not followed by increased rCBF of the primary sensorimotor cortex nor was there any DLPFC activation during DBS.

By contrast, in another study the authors found no GPi DBS-related brain rCBF changes either at rest or during hand movements *(15)*. Their methods were substantially different from those used in other studies. This particular study was designed merely to explore the short-term effects of effective (130 Hz) and ineffective (2 Hz) stimulation while other studies monitored effects for at least 12 hours from the start of stimulation while comparing the state with DBS on and off *(109, 111)*.

**Functional Imaging in GPi DBS for Generalized Dystonia**

Patients with genetically confirmed (DYT1) generalized dystonia, subjected to FDG PET in a resting state, were found to have increased regional metabolism of the basal ganglia, cerebellum and SMA *(115, 116)*. During a motor task involving joystick movement, they exhibited increased rCBF in the rostral SMA, premotor cortex, DLPFC, anterior cingulate, putamen and cerebellum, and simultaneous decreased rCBF in the primary sensorimotor cortex *(117, 118)*, in the caudal SMA, and in posterior cingulate *(117)*. Both were studies of patients with idiopathic generalized dystonia. This is partially congruent with the outcome of a study measuring rCBF in a group of six patients with primary generalized dystonia five of whom were DYT1 positive. Unlike normal controls, they found increased motion-related rCBF in the DLPFC and other prefrontal areas *(119)*.

During left-sided GPi DBS, the same group of patients showed increased resting regional rCBF in the left GPi (i.e., at the site of stimulation), in the left thalamus and in the right caudate. Activation was also noted in the right cerebellar hemisphere as well as in different parts of the frontal, parietal and temporal lobes of both hemispheres. At the same time, rCBF was decreased in the primary motor cortex *(119)*. This means that abnormal resting-state rCBF became even more accentuated in response to GPi DBS. However, it may also mean that DBS leads to excitation, which then propagated along anatomic pathways toward different areas of cerebral cortex. In contrast, the execution of a movement was accompanied by a decrease and consequently a normalization of the abnormal hyperactivity of the prefrontal areas. This is also in agreement with the published case of a patient with idiopathic generalized dystonia and bilateral GPi DBS, who showed signs of suppressed motion-related rCBF of prefrontal areas while neurostimulators were switched on. Suppressed activation of the primary motor cortex was also observed in this case *(120)*.

Another SPECT study designed to detect resting-state rCBF in five dystonic patients with GPi DBS bilaterally switched on, revealed individually variable hyper- or hypoactivation in different brain regions *(121)*. The variable results were probably due to the enrollment of patients with various types of dystonia.

## Conclusions

DBS has been repeatedly studied by means of functional imaging. Beside rCBF studies using SPECT and PET, it has also proved feasible, despite technical difficulties, to study DBS effects with fMRI. While there is not any doubt about the clinical effects of DBS, relatively very little is known about its mechanisms. Thus, methods of functional imaging help us understand the processes associated with neurostimulation, not only at the site of stimulation, but also in providing a global view of what is happening in the rest of the brain. Studies on the most frequent targets for DBS, STN, VIM, and GPi have found that, besides local metabolic changes in the stimulated nucleus, there are also functional changes in remote subcortical regions, cerebral cortex, or cerebellum. The site of stimulation usually becomes activated which indirectly supports a mechanism of locally increased neuronal activity related to increased synaptic or axonal activity. Consequently, despite similar clinical effects, the mechanisms of DBS markedly differ from those of stereotactic lesions.

Subcortical regions co-activated during neurostimulation while the patient is in a resting state are the thalamus (in the case of VIM DBS) and the thalamus and globus pallidus (in the case of STN DBS). The cerebral cortex may be influenced directly by way of thalamocortical connections (as in case of VIM DBS) or indirectly after being relayed by way of the thalamus as in case of STN or GPi DBS. In cerebral cortex there are motor and sensory areas whose activity is frequently affected by DBS. It follows from comparisons with neurostimulation switched on and off, that DBS usually leads to improvement of pathological pattern of brain activations or, more precisely, to a state of activation more closely resembling images obtained in healthy subjects, regardless of which nucleus is stimulated or of the actual movement disorder. In addition, neurostimulation of the STN, VIM or GPi may influence functions in the non-stimulated hemisphere reaching even beyond the motor system. Observed changes in activation have appeared unilaterally or bilaterally in the mesial, dorsolateral or inferolateral parts of the frontal lobes, in areas involved mainly in affective and cognitive processing.

However, it must be recognized that the majority of studies have also produced contradictory results. Examined closely, there are often great methodological differences. While many authors have compared effects of neurostimulation unilaterally or bilaterally, DBS switched on or off, others have compared patterns of cerebral activation under different conditions such as during states of effective and ineffective stimulation. Moreover, rCBF SPECT and PET studies are usually carried out weeks or even months after stabilization of the clinical state when optimal parameters of neurostimulation have been achieved. By contrast, fMRI studies can only be carried out soon after implantation of the intracerebral electrode which confines them to studying the acute effects of DBS. Discrepancies may also be due to differences among patients who exhibit different types or severity of clinical symptoms. Finally, the motor task is another variable which needs to be considered. Besides functional imaging in a resting state, while no movements are being performed, DBS is often studied in relation to control of voluntary movements. The difficulty with most imaging studies is that changes in motion-related activation need not be related to DBS; they may simply be manifestations of differences in motor performance. In spite of these caveats, functional imaging has contributed greatly to our knowledge of DBS and in the future fMRI, perfusion SPECT and PET will retain an important role in the research of the mechanisms of neurostimulation.

*Acknowledgments*: Supported by grant from the Czech Ministry of Health (IGA MZ CR 1A/8629-5) and from the Czech Ministry of Education (research program MSM 0021620849)

## References

1. Rezai AR, Finelli D, Nyenhuis JA, et al (2002) Neurostimulation systems for deep brain stimulation: in vitro evaluation of magnetic resonance imaging-related heating at 1.5 tesla. J Magn Reson Imaging 15(3):241–250.
2. Rezai AR, Phillips M, Baker KB, et al (2004) Neurostimulation system used for deep brain stimulation (DBS): MR safety issues and implications of failing to follow safety recommendations. Invest Radiol 39(5):300–303.
3. Georgi JC, Stippich C, Tronnier VM, Heiland S (2004) Active deep brain stimulation during MRI: a feasibility study. Magn Reson Med 51(2):380–388.
4. Jueptner M, Weiller C (1995) Review: does measurement of regional cerebral blood flow reflect synaptic activity? Implications for PET and fMRI. Neuroimage 2(2):148–156.
5. Chen W, Ogawa S (2000) Principles of BOLD Functional MRI. In: Moonen CTW, Bandettini PA, eds. Functional MRI. Berlin: Springer-Verlag, pp. 103–114.
6. Asanuma K, Tang C, Ma Y, et al (2006) Network modulation in the treatment of Parkinson's disease. Brain.
7. Sestini S, Ramat S, Formiconi AR, Ammannati F, Sorbi S, Pupi A (2005) Brain networks underlying the clinical effects of long-term subthalamic stimulation for Parkinson's disease: a 4-year follow-up study with rCBF SPECT. J Nucl Med 46(9):1444–1454.
8. Hershey T, Revilla FJ, Wernle AR, et al (2003) Cortical and subcortical blood flow effects of subthalamic nucleus stimulation in PD. Neurology 61(6):816–821.
9. Hilker R, Voges J, Weisenbach S, et al (2004) Subthalamic nucleus stimulation restores glucose metabolism in associative and limbic cortices and in cerebellum: evidence from a FDG-PET study in advanced Parkinson's disease. J Cereb Blood Flow Metab 24(1):7–16.
10. Haegelen C, Verin M, Broche BA, et al (2005) Does subthalamic nucleus stimulation affect the frontal limbic areas? A single-photon emission computed tomography study using a manual anatomical segmentation method. Surg Radiol Anat 27(5):389–394.
11. Trost M, Su S, Su P, et al (2006) Network modulation by the subthalamic nucleus in the treatment of Parkinson's disease. Neuroimage 31(1):301–307.
12. Ceballos-Baumann AO, Boecker H, Bartenstein P, et al (1999) A positron emission tomographic study of subthalamic nucleus stimulation in Parkinson disease: enhanced movement-related activity of motor-association cortex and decreased motor cortex resting activity. Arch Neurol 56(8):997–1003.
13. Payoux P, Remy P, Damier P, et al (2004) Subthalamic nucleus stimulation reduces abnormal motor cortical overactivity in Parkinson disease. Arch Neurol 61(8):1307–1313.

14. Thobois S, Dominey P, Fraix V, et al (2002) Effects of subthalamic nucleus stimulation on actual and imagined movement in Parkinson's disease: a PET study. J Neurol 249(12):1689–1698.
15. Limousin P, Greene J, Pollak P, Rothwell J, Benabid AL, Frackowiak R (1997) Changes in cerebral activity pattern due to subthalamic nucleus or internal pallidum stimulation in Parkinson's disease. Ann Neurol 42(3):283–291.
16. Grafton ST, Turner RS, Desmurget M, et al (2006) Normalizing motor-related brain activity: subthalamic nucleus stimulation in Parkinson disease. Neurology 66(8):1192–1199.
17. Strafella AP, Dagher A, Sadikot AF (2003) Cerebral blood flow changes induced by subthalamic stimulation in Parkinson's disease. Neurology 60(6):1039–1042.
18. Schroeder U, Kuehler A, Haslinger B, et al (2002) Subthalamic nucleus stimulation affects striato-anterior cingulate cortex circuit in a response conflict task: a PET study. Brain 125(Pt 9):1995–2004.
19. Schroeder U, Kuehler A, Lange KW, et al (2003) Subthalamic nucleus stimulation affects a frontotemporal network: a PET study. Ann Neurol 54(4):445–450.
20. Rezai AR, Lozano AM, Crawley AP, et al (1999) Thalamic stimulation and functional magnetic resonance imaging: localization of cortical and subcortical activation with implanted electrodes. Technical note. J Neurosurg 90(3):583–590.
21. Jech R, Ruzicka E, Tintera J, Urgosik D (2003) Reply: fMRI during deep brain stimulation. Mov Disord 18(4):461–462.
22. Phillips MD, Baker KB, Lowe MJ, et al (2006) Parkinson disease: pattern of functional MR imaging activation during deep brain stimulation of subthalamic nucleus—initial experience. Radiology 239(1):209–216.
23. Baker KB, Nyenhuis JA, Hrdlicka G, Rezai AR, Tkach JA, Shellock FG (2005) Neurostimulation systems: assessment of magnetic field interactions associated with 1.5- and 3-Tesla MR systems. J Magn Reson Imaging 21(1):72–77.
24. Finelli DA, Rezai AR, Ruggieri PM, et al (2002) MR imaging-related heating of deep brain stimulation electrodes: in vitro study. AJNR Am J Neuroradiol 23(10):1795–1802.
25. Baker KB, Tkach J, Phillips MD (2006) In vitro studies of MRI-related heating of neurostimulation systems. Magn Reson Imaging 24(5):677–679; author reply 9–80.
26. Dormont D, Cornu P, Pidoux B, et al (1997) Chronic thalamic stimulation with three-dimensional MR stereotactic guidance. AJNR Am J Neuroradiol 18(6):1093–1107.
27. Yelnik J, Damier P, Demeret S, et al (2003) Localization of stimulating electrodes in patients with Parkinson disease by using a three-dimensional atlas-magnetic resonance imaging coregistration method. J Neurosurg 99(1):89–99.
28. Tronnier VM, Staubert A, Hahnel S, Sarem-Aslani A (1999) Magnetic resonance imaging with implanted neurostimulators: an in vitro and in vivo study. Neurosurgery 44(1):118–125; discussion 25–26.
29. Jech R, Urgosik D, Tintera J, et al (2001) Functional magnetic resonance imaging during deep brain stimulation: a pilot study in four patients with Parkinson's disease. Mov Disord 16(6):1126–1132.
30. Arantes PR, Cardoso EF, Barreiros MA, et al (2006) Performing functional magnetic resonance imaging in patients with Parkinson's disease treated with deep brain stimulation. Mov Disord 21(8):1154–1162.
31. Jech R, Urgosik D, Tintera J, Sieger T, Roth J, Ruzicka E (2002) Effects of deep brain stimulation of the STN and Vim nuclei under resting state and during simple movement tasks: A functional MRI study at 1.5 Tesla. Mov Disord 17:S173–S.
32. Stefurak T, Mikulis D, Mayberg H, et al (2003) Deep brain stimulation for Parkinson's disease dissociates mood and motor circuits: a functional MRI case study. Mov Disord 18(12):1508–1516.

33. Paus T, Jech R, Thompson CJ, Comeau R, Peters T, Evans AC (1997) Transcranial magnetic stimulation during positron emission tomography: a new method for studying connectivity of the human cerebral cortex. J Neurosci 17(9):3178–3184.
34. Paus T, Jech R, Thompson CJ, Comeau R, Peters T, Evans AC (1998) Dose-dependent reduction of cerebral blood flow during rapid-rate transcranial magnetic stimulation of the human sensorimotor cortex. J Neurophysiol 79(2):1102–1107.
35. Rothwell JC (1997) Techniques and mechanisms of action of transcranial stimulation of the human motor cortex. J Neurosci Methods 74(2):113–122.
36. Bodurka J, Bandettini PA (2002) Toward direct mapping of neuronal activity: MRI detection of ultraweak, transient magnetic field changes. Magn Reson Med 47(6):1052–1058.
37. Tai CH, Boraud T, Bezard E, Bioulac B, Gross C, Benazzouz A (2003) Electrophysiological and metabolic evidence that high-frequency stimulation of the subthalamic nucleus bridles neuronal activity in the subthalamic nucleus and the substantia nigra reticulata. Faseb J 17(13):1820–1830.
38. Filali M, Hutchison WD, Palter VN, Lozano AM, Dostrovsky JO (2004) Stimulation-induced inhibition of neuronal firing in human subthalamic nucleus. Exp Brain Res 156(3):274–281.
39. Benabid AL, Benazzouz A, Hoffmann D, Limousin P, Krack P, Pollak P (1998) Long-term electrical inhibition of deep brain targets in movement disorders. Mov Disord 13(Suppl 3):119–25.
40. Shen KZ, Zhu ZT, Munhall A, Johnson SW (2003) Synaptic plasticity in rat subthalamic nucleus induced by high-frequency stimulation. Synapse 50(4):314–319.
41. Hashimoto T, Elder CM, Okun MS, Patrick SK, Vitek JL (2003) Stimulation of the subthalamic nucleus changes the firing pattern of pallidal neurons. J Neurosci 23(5):1916–1923.
42. Bruet N, Windels F, Carcenac C, et al (2003) Neurochemical mechanisms induced by high frequency stimulation of the subthalamic nucleus: increase of extracellular striatal glutamate and GABA in normal and hemiparkinsonian rats. J Neuropathol Exp Neurol 62(12):1228–1240.
43. McIntyre CC, Savasta M, Kerkerian-Le Goff L, Vitek JL (2004) Uncovering the mechanism(s) of action of deep brain stimulation: activation, inhibition, or both. Clin Neurophysiol 115(6):1239–1248.
44. Vitek JL (2002) Mechanisms of deep brain stimulation: excitation or inhibition. Mov Disord 17(Suppl 3):S69–S72.
45. Trost M, Su PC, Barnes A, et al (2003) Evolving metabolic changes during the first postoperative year after subthalamotomy. J Neurosurg 99(5):872–878.
46. Hesselmann V, Maarouf M, Hunsche S, et al (2006) Functional MRI for immediate monitoring stereotactic thalamotomy in a patient with essential tremor. Eur Radiol 16(10):2229–2233.
47. Eidelberg D, Moeller JR, Ishikawa T, et al (1996) Regional metabolic correlates of surgical outcome following unilateral pallidotomy for Parkinson's disease. Ann Neurol 39(4):450–459.
48. Windels F, Bruet N, Poupard A, Feuerstein C, Bertrand A, Savasta M (2003) Influence of the frequency parameter on extracellular glutamate and gamma-aminobutyric acid in substantia nigra and globus pallidus during electrical stimulation of subthalamic nucleus in rats. J Neurosci Res 72(2):259–267.
49. Temperli P, Ghika J, Villemure JG, Burkhard PR, Bogousslavsky J, Vingerhoets FJ (2003) How do parkinsonian signs return after discontinuation of subthalamic DBS? Neurology 60(1):78–81.
50. Lozza C, Baron JC, Eidelberg D, Mentis MJ, Carbon M, Marie RM (2004) Executive processes in Parkinson's disease: FDG-PET and network analysis. Hum Brain Mapp 22(3):236–245.
51. Eidelberg D, Edwards C (2000) Functional brain imaging of movement disorders. Neurol Res 22(3):305–312.

52. Eidelberg D, Moeller JR, Dhawan V, et al (1994) The metabolic topography of parkinsonism. J Cereb Blood Flow Metab 14(5):783–801.
53. Moeller JR, Nakamura T, Mentis MJ, et al (1999) Reproducibility of regional metabolic covariance patterns: comparison of four populations. J Nucl Med 40(8):1264–1269.
54. Ma Y, Tang C, Spetsieris PG, Dhawan V, Eidelberg D (2006) Abnormal metabolic network activity in Parkinson's disease: test-retest reproducibility. J Cereb Blood Flow Metab.
55. Haslinger B, Kalteis K, Boecker H, Alesch F, Ceballos-Baumann AO (2005) Frequency-correlated decreases of motor cortex activity associated with subthalamic nucleus stimulation in Parkinson's disease. Neuroimage 28(3):598–606.
56. Sestini S, Scotto di Luzio A, Ammannati F, et al (2002) Changes in regional cerebral blood flow caused by deep-brain stimulation of the subthalamic nucleus in Parkinson's disease. J Nucl Med 43(6):725–732.
57. Hilker R, Voges J, Thiel A, et al (2002) Deep brain stimulation of the subthalamic nucleus versus levodopa challenge in Parkinson's disease: measuring the on- and off-conditions with FDG-PET. J Neural Transm 109(10):1257–1264.
58. Hilker R, Portman AT, Voges J, et al (2005) Disease progression continues in patients with advanced Parkinson's disease and effective subthalamic nucleus stimulation. J Neurol Neurosurg Psychiatry 76(9):1217–1221.
59. Antonini A, Marotta G, Benti R, et al (2003) Brain flow changes before and after deep brain stimulation of the subthalamic nucleus in Parkinson's disease. Neurol Sci 24(3):151–152.
60. Temel Y, Kessels A, Tan S, Topdag A, Boon P, Visser-Vandewalle V (2006) Behavioural changes after bilateral subthalamic stimulation in advanced Parkinson disease: a systematic review. Parkinsonism Relat Disord 12(5):265–272.
61. Goldberg JA, Boraud T, Maraton S, Haber SN, Vaadia E, Bergman H (2002) Enhanced synchrony among primary motor cortex neurons in the 1-methyl-4-phenyl-1,2,3,6-tetrahydropyridine primate model of Parkinson's disease. J Neurosci 22(11):4639–4653.
62. Sabatini U, Boulanouar K, Fabre N, et al (2000) Cortical motor reorganization in akinetic patients with Parkinson's disease: a functional MRI study. Brain 123 (Pt 2):394–403.
63. Haslinger B, Erhard P, Kampfe N, et al (2001) Event-related functional magnetic resonance imaging in Parkinson's disease before and after levodopa. Brain 124 (Pt 3):558–570.
64. Buhmann C, Binkofski F, Klein C, et al (2005) Motor reorganization in asymptomatic carriers of a single mutant Parkin allele: a human model for presymptomatic parkinsonism. Brain 128(Pt 10):2281–2290.
65. Catalan MJ, Ishii K, Honda M, Samii A, Hallett M (1999) A PET study of sequential finger movements of varying length in patients with Parkinson's disease. Brain 122(Pt 3):483–495.
66. Hesselmann V, Sorger B, Girnus R, et al (2004) Intraoperative functional MRI as a new approach to monitor deep brain stimulation in Parkinson's disease. Eur Radiol 14(4):686–690.
67. Germano IM, Gracies JM, Weisz DJ, Tse W, Koller WC, Olanow CW (2004) Unilateral stimulation of the subthalamic nucleus in Parkinson disease: a double-blind 12-month evaluation study. J Neurosurg 101(1):36–42.
68. Alberts JL, Elder CM, Okun MS, Vitek JL (2004) Comparison of pallidal and subthalamic stimulation on force control in patient's with Parkinson's disease. Motor Control 8(4):484–499.
69. Samuel M, Ceballos-Baumann AO, Blin J, et al (1997) Evidence for lateral premotor and parietal overactivity in Parkinson's disease during sequential and bimanual movements. A PET study. Brain 120(Pt 6):963–976.

70. Jahanshahi M, Jenkins IH, Brown RG, Marsden CD, Passingham RE, Brooks DJ (1995) Self-initiated versus externally triggered movements. I. An investigation using measurement of regional cerebral blood flow with PET and movement-related potentials in normal and Parkinson's disease subjects. Brain 118 (Pt 4):913–933.
71. Rascol O, Sabatini U, Fabre N, et al (1997) The ipsilateral cerebellar hemisphere is overactive during hand movements in akinetic parkinsonian patients. Brain 120 (Pt 1):103–110.
72. Jenkins IH, Fernandez W, Playford ED, et al (1992) Impaired activation of the supplementary motor area in Parkinson's disease is reversed when akinesia is treated with apomorphine. Ann Neurol 32(6):749–757.
73. Piccini P, Lindvall O, Bjorklund A, et al (2000) Delayed recovery of movement-related cortical function in Parkinson's disease after striatal dopaminergic grafts. Ann Neurol 48(5):689–695.
74. Playford ED, Jenkins IH, Passingham RE, Nutt J, Frackowiak RS, Brooks DJ (1992) Impaired mesial frontal and putamen activation in Parkinson's disease: a positron emission tomography study. Ann Neurol 32(2):151–161.
75. Rascol O, Sabatini U, Chollet F, et al (1992) Supplementary and primary sensory motor area activity in Parkinson's disease. Regional cerebral blood flow changes during finger movements and effects of apomorphine. Arch Neurol 49(2):144–148.
76. Ceballos-Baumann AO (2003) Functional imaging in Parkinson's disease: activation studies with PET, fMRI and SPECT. J Neurol 250(Suppl 1):I15–I23.
77. Hershey T, Mink JW (2006) Using functional neuroimaging to study the brain's response to deep brain stimulation. Neurology 66(8):1142–1143.
78. Ramig LO, Countryman S, Thompson LL, Horii Y (1995) Comparison of two forms of intensive speech treatment for Parkinson disease. J Speech Hearing Res 38(6):1232–1251.
79. Limousin P, Krack P, Pollak P, et al (1998) Electrical stimulation of the subthalamic nucleus in advanced Parkinson's disease. N Engl J Med 339(16):1105–1111.
80. Pinto S, Ozsancak C, Tripoliti E, Thobois S, Limousin-Dowsey P, Auzou P (2004) Treatments for dysarthria in Parkinson's disease. Lancet Neurol 3(9):547–556.
81. Rousseaux M, Krystkowiak P, Kozlowski O, Ozsancak C, Blond S, Destee A (2004) Effects of subthalamic nucleus stimulation on parkinsonian dysarthria and speech intelligibility. J Neurol 251(3):327–334.
82. Pinto S, Thobois S, Costes N, et al (2004) Subthalamic nucleus stimulation and dysarthria in Parkinson's disease: a PET study. Brain 127(Pt 3):602–615.
83. Jahanshahi M, Ardouin CM, Brown RG, et al (2000) The impact of deep brain stimulation on executive function in Parkinson's disease. Brain 123(Pt 6):1142–1154.
84. Dujardin K, Defebvre L, Krystkowiak P, Blond S, Destee A (2001) Influence of chronic bilateral stimulation of the subthalamic nucleus on cognitive function in Parkinson's disease. J Neurol 248(7):603–611.
85. Pillon B, Ardouin C, Damier P, et al (2000) Neuropsychological changes between "off" and "on" STN or GPi stimulation in Parkinson's disease. Neurology 55(3):411–418.
86. Saint-Cyr JA, Trepanier LL, Kumar R, Lozano AM, Lang AE (2000) Neuropsychological consequences of chronic bilateral stimulation of the subthalamic nucleus in Parkinson's disease. Brain 123(Pt 10):2091–2108.
87. Hilker R, Voges J, Ghaemi M, et al (2003) Deep brain stimulation of the subthalamic nucleus does not increase the striatal dopamine concentration in parkinsonian humans. Mov Disord 18(1):41–48.
88. Strafella AP, Sadikot AF, Dagher A (2003) Subthalamic deep brain stimulation does not induce striatal dopamine release in Parkinson's disease. Neuroreport 14(9):1287–1289.

89. Goerendt IK, Lawrence AD, Mehta MA, Stern JS, Odin P, Brooks DJ (2006) Distributed neural actions of anti-parkinsonian therapies as revealed by PET. J Neural Transm 113(1):75–86.
90. Feigin A, Fukuda M, Dhawan V, et al (2001) Metabolic correlates of levodopa response in Parkinson's disease. Neurology 57(11):2083–2088.
91. Buhmann C, Glauche V, Sturenburg HJ, Oechsner M, Weiller C, Buchel C (2003) Pharmacologically modulated fMRI—cortical responsiveness to levodopa in drug-naive hemiparkinsonian patients. Brain 126(Pt 2):451–461.
92. Mattay VS, Tessitore A, Callicott JH, et al (2002) Dopaminergic modulation of cortical function in patients with Parkinson's disease. Ann Neurol 51(2):156–164.
93. Hershey T, Black KJ, Carl JL, McGee-Minnich L, Snyder AZ, Perlmutter JS (2003) Long term treatment and disease severity change brain responses to levodopa in Parkinson's disease. J Neurol Neurosurg Psychiatry 74(7):844–851.
94. Bucher SF, Seelos KC, Dodel RC, Reiser M, Oertel WH (1997) Activation mapping in essential tremor with functional magnetic resonance imaging. Ann Neurol 41(1):32–40.
95. Wills AJ, Jenkins IH, Thompson PD, Findley LJ, Brooks DJ (1995) A positron emission tomography study of cerebral activation associated with essential and writing tremor. Arch Neurol 52(3):299–305.
96. Antonini A, Moeller JR, Nakamura T, Spetsieris P, Dhawan V, Eidelberg D (1998) The metabolic anatomy of tremor in Parkinson's disease. Neurology 51(3):803–810.
97. Kassubek J, Juengling FD, Hellwig B, Knauff M, Spreer J, Lucking CH (2001) Hypermetabolism in the ventrolateral thalamus in unilateral Parkinsonian resting tremor: a positron emission tomography study. Neurosci Lett 304(1–2):17–20.
98. Ruzicka E, Jech R, Zarubova K, Roth J, Urgosik D (2003) VIM thalamic stimulation for tremor in a patient with IgM paraproteinaemic demyelinating neuropathy. Mov Disord 18(10):1192–1195.
99. Perlmutter JS, Mink JW, Bastian AJ, et al (2002) Blood flow responses to deep brain stimulation of thalamus. Neurology 58(9):1388–1394.
100. Ceballos-Baumann AO, Boecker H, Fogel W, et al (2001) Thalamic stimulation for essential tremor activates motor and deactivates vestibular cortex. Neurology 56(10):1347–1354.
101. Haslinger B, Boecker H, Buchel C, et al (2003) Differential modulation of subcortical target and cortex during deep brain stimulation. Neuroimage 18(2):517–524.
102. Kopell BH, Rezai AR, Chang JW, Vitek JL (2006) Anatomy and physiology of the basal ganglia: implications for deep brain stimulation for Parkinson's disease. Mov Disord 21(Suppl 14):S238–S246.
103. Parent A, Hazrati LN (1995) Functional anatomy of the basal ganglia. I. The cortico-basal ganglia-thalamo-cortical loop. Brain Res 20(1):91–127.
104. Fukuda M, Barnes A, Simon ES, et al (2004) Thalamic stimulation for parkinsonian tremor: correlation between regional cerebral blood flow and physiological tremor characteristics. Neuroimage 21(2):608–615.
105. Boecker H, Wills AJ, Ceballos-Baumann A, et al (1997) Stereotactic thalamotomy in tremor-dominant Parkinson's disease: an H2(15)O PET motor activation study. Ann Neurol 41(1):108–111.
106. Parker F, Tzourio N, Blond S, Petit H, Mazoyer B (1992) Evidence for a common network of brain structures involved in parkinsonian tremor and voluntary repetitive movement. Brain Res 584(1–2):11–17.
107. Deiber MP, Pollak P, Passingham R, et al (1993) Thalamic stimulation and suppression of parkinsonian tremor. Evidence of a cerebellar deactivation using positron emission tomography. Brain 116(Pt 1):267–279.
108. Wielepp JP, Burgunder JM, Pohle T, Ritter EP, Kinser JA, Krauss JK (2001) Deactivation of thalamocortical activity is responsible for suppression of parkinsonian

tremor by thalamic stimulation: a 99mTc-ECD SPECT study. Clin Neurol Neurosurg 103(4):228–231.
109. Fukuda M, Mentis MJ, Ma Y, et al (2001) Networks mediating the clinical effects of pallidal brain stimulation for Parkinson's disease: a PET study of resting-state glucose metabolism. Brain 124(Pt 8):1601–1609.
110. Davis KD, Taub E, Houle S, et al (1997) Globus pallidus stimulation activates the cortical motor system during alleviation of parkinsonian symptoms. Nat Med 3(6):671–674.
111. Fukuda M, Mentis M, Ghilardi MF, et al (2001) Functional correlates of pallidal stimulation for Parkinson's disease. Ann Neurol 49(2):155–164.
112. Samuel M, Ceballos-Baumann AO, Turjanski N, et al (1997) Pallidotomy in Parkinson's disease increases supplementary motor area and prefrontal activation during performance of volitional movements an H2(15)O PET study. Brain 120(Pt 8):1301–1313.
113. Grafton ST, Waters C, Sutton J, Lew MF, Couldwell W (1995) Pallidotomy increases activity of motor association cortex in Parkinson's disease: a positron emission tomographic study. Ann Neurol 37(6):776–783.
114. Ceballos-Baumann AO, Obeso JA, Vitek JL, et al (1994) Restoration of thalamo-cortical activity after posteroventral pallidotomy in Parkinson's disease. Lancet 344(8925):814.
115. Eidelberg D, Moeller JR, Antonini A, et al (1998) Functional brain networks in DYT1 dystonia. Ann Neurol 44(3):303–312.
116. Trost M, Carbon M, Edwards C, et al (2002) Primary dystonia: is abnormal functional brain architecture linked to genotype? Ann Neurol 52(6):853–856.
117. Ceballos-Baumann AO, Passingham RE, Warner T, Playford ED, Marsden CD, Brooks DJ (1995) Overactive prefrontal and underactive motor cortical areas in idiopathic dystonia. Ann Neurol 37(3):363–372.
118. Playford ED, Passingham RE, Marsden CD, Brooks DJ (1998) Increased activation of frontal areas during arm movement in idiopathic torsion dystonia. Mov Disord 13(2):309–318.
119. Detante O, Vercueil L, Thobois S, et al (2004) Globus pallidus internus stimulation in primary generalized dystonia: a H215O PET study. Brain 127(Pt 8):1899–1908.
120. Kumar R, Dagher A, Hutchison WD, Lang AE, Lozano AM (1999) Globus pallidus deep brain stimulation for generalized dystonia: clinical and PET investigation. Neurology 53(4):871–874.
121. Yianni J, Bradley K, Soper N, et al (2005) Effect of GPi DBS on functional imaging of the brain in dystonia. J Clin Neurosci 12(2):137–141.

# Part II

# Deep Brain Stimulation in Movement Disorders

# 10
# Thalamic Deep Brain Stimulation and Essential Tremor

Kelly E. Lyons and Rajesh Pahwa

## Abstract

Essential tremor (ET) is one of the most common movement disorders and is characterized by an action or postural tremor of the hands, which can also affect the head, voice, trunk, and lower limbs. ET can cause significant functional disability that makes activities of daily living such as eating, drinking and writing difficult and in some cases nearly impossible. Although ET can occur at any age, it is more common with advancing age. It is estimated that up to five of every 100 persons over 60 years of age are affected *(1)*. Current first-line pharmacological treatment includes primidone and beta adrenergic blockers such as propranolol. Second-line pharmacological therapies include benzodiazepines, gabapentin, and topiramate. In some patients, botulinum toxin injections provide some benefit but outcomes have been inconsistent. In general, pharmacological therapies are effective in only about 50% of ET patients *(2)*. For ET patients with medication-resistant tremor that causes significant disability but who do not have significant cognitive, behavioral/psychiatric, or other medical conditions that preclude surgery, deep brain stimulation (DBS) of the ventral intermediate nucleus (VIM) of the thalamus is a worthwhile treatment option.

**Keywords:** deep brain stimulation, DBS, essential tremor, thalamic stimulation

## DBS of the Thalamus

During the performance of thalamotomy in the 1960s, it became apparent that intra-operative high-frequency stimulation (>100 Hz) of the VIM nucleus of the thalamus dramatically reduced tremor *(3, 4)*. Stimulation was therefore often used intra-operatively to help identify the appropriate target for thalamotomy. In an attempt to reduce the adverse effects and complications occurring with thalamotomy, particularly after bilateral procedures, Benabid and his colleagues implanted DBS electrodes into the thalamus as a treatment for tremor *(5)*. Many investigators have since reported the safety and efficacy of chronic thalamic stimulation for ET (Table 10.1; refs. *6–16*) and VIM DBS has since

**Table 10.1** Selected studies of thalamic deep brain stimulation for the treatment of essential tremor (% improvement compared to baseline).

| Author, year | n (uni/bi) | Age (years) | Follow-up (months) | Overall tremor | Hand tremor | Functional ability* | Activities of daily living |
|---|---|---|---|---|---|---|---|
| Koller et al., 1997 *(9)* | 29/0 | 67 | 3, 6, 12 | — | ~60% | 48–63% | — |
| Pahwa et al., 2006 *(17)* | 15/7 | 71 | 60 | 46–78% | 65–86% | 35–57% | 36–51% |
| Limousin et al., 1999 *(11)* | 28/9 | 63 | 3, 12 | 55% | >75% | 44% | 80% |
| Sydow et al., 2003 *(16)* | 12/7 | 62 | 80 | 41% | 50–70% | 37% | 39% |
| Koller et al., 2001 *(10)* | 25/0 | 72 | 40.2 | 50% | 78% | — | — |
| Putzke et al., 2004 *(18)* | 29/23 | 72 | 3, 12, 24, 36 | — | >83% | — | >63% |

Uni, unilateral; bi, bilateral; *, writing, drawing, pouring.

become the surgery of choice for the treatment of medication-resistant ET. These studies are reviewed in the remainder of this chapter.

Benabid and his colleagues reported multiple studies regarding the efficacy of VIM DBS for the treatment of tremor in the early 1990s *(6–8)*. In 1993, they described 13 ET patients of which 68% had good or excellent tremor relief after VIM DBS *(7)*. They subsequently reported an additional 20 ET patients, including 13 with bilateral VIM DBS and two with contralateral thalamotomy, who underwent VIM DBS *(8)*. The majority of patients, at 3 months and also at their last follow-up visit of at least 6 months, had marked improvement in tremor, although benefit deteriorated in 18.5% of cases over time. This deterioration occurred most often in patients with action tremor. Adverse effects related to stimulation were relatively mild and included paresthesia, dysarthria, disequilibrium, contralateral dystonia, and hypersalivation.

Koller et al. *(9)* reported the first North American multi-center study examining the effects of unilateral thalamic DBS in 29 ET patients 3 and 12 months after surgery. At 3 months, 23 of the 29 ET patients reported marked improvement, three reported moderate improvement, one reported mild improvement, and two patients were unchanged. There was a significant improvement of approximately 60% in contralateral hand tremor and 43 to 68% improvement in activities of daily living such as writing, drawing spirals, drawing straight lines, pouring liquids, and bringing liquids to the mouth at 3 and 12 months. Complications were reported for the combined cohorts of ET patients ($n = 29$) and patients with parkinsonian tremor ($n = 24$). Surgical complications included a lead dislodgement during surgery requiring repeat surgery and generalized seizures in one patient. Adverse effects due to stimulation were mild and controlled by adjusting stimulation parameters. These included paresthesia (79%), headache (11%), disequilibrium (9%), paresis (8%), gait disorder (6%), dystonia (6%), dysarthria (4%), and localized pain (3%). Other complications related to the device that occurred during the first year included skin infections in two patients, pulse generator malfunction in one patient, and skin erosion from the extension wire in one patient.

Pahwa and colleagues *(17)* recently reported the long-term safety and efficacy of thalamic DBS in 26 of the 29 ET patients reported in the prior study by Koller et al. *(9)*. Sixteen patients with unilateral procedures completed patient global assessments at 5 years that indicated that 15 patients were improved compared to baseline and one patient was unchanged. Five-year follow-up data from the tremor rating scale were available for 15 patients with unilateral procedures. In these patients there was 75% improvement in targeted hand tremor, 46% improvement in overall tremor, 51% improvement in activities of daily living, 57% improvement in drawing, and 44% improvement in pouring. Seven ET patients who received bilateral implantation completed the 5-year follow-up. Global ratings indicated that all patients were improved compared to baseline. Tremor rating scale scores revealed 65% improvement in left-handed tremor, 86% improvement in right-handed tremor, 78% improvement in overall tremor, and a 36% improvement in activities of daily living. Of 45 patients with either ET or parkinsonian tremor, 27% required surgical revisions other than implantable pulse generator replacements while adverse events related to stimulation occurred in 10%. The most common adverse events in unilaterally operated ET patients included paresthesia (56%), pain (33%), asthenia (22%), dysarthria, incoordination, abnormal thinking and headache each in 17%, depression and hallucinations each in 11%, and dysphagia, hypertonia, increased salivation, insomnia, hypophonia and somnolence each in 6%. In ET patients operated bilaterally, the most common adverse events were dysarthria (63%), incoordination (38%), pain, paresthesia, asthenia, insomnia, abnormal gait, hypophonia and somnolence each in 25%, and dysphagia and abnormal thinking each in 13%.

Limousin and colleagues *(11)* reported a multi-center European study of 37 ET patients evaluated 3 and 12 months after thalamic DBS. At 12 months, postural and action tremor of the upper and lower extremities were significantly improved compared to baseline. Activities of daily living also remained significantly improved by 80% at 12 months compared to baseline. Adverse events were reported for the entire cohort of 111 patients with parkinsonian tremor and ET. One patient was not operated due to breathing problems in the operating room. Three patients died due to unrelated causes and one had a stroke 3 months after surgery. Three patients had hematomas that resolved without intervention and two patients had subcutaneous hematomas. Infection occurred in two patients which required temporary removal of the system. Stimulation related adverse events were mild and reversible with stimulation parameter adjustments. They included dysarthria in five unilaterally and two bilaterally implanted patients, disequilibrium in three bilaterally operated patients, and dystonia in one patient.

Sydow and colleagues *(16)* reported long-term follow-up assessment of 19 ET patients (12 unilateral, seven bilateral) of the 37 patients enrolled in the study by Limousin et al. *(11)*. A significant overall tremor improvement of 41% was maintained 6.5 years following thalamic DBS. Importantly, although overall tremor was significantly improved compared to baseline at 6.5 years, the improvement was 14% less than that reported at 1 year compared to baseline. Upper limb action tremor was significantly improved by 71% at 12 months and 50% at 6.5 years compared to baseline and upper limb postural tremor was improved by 83% at 12 months and 70% at 6.5 years compared to baseline. Activities of daily living were significantly improved by 39% at 6.5 years; representing a reduction of 41% compared to the improvement seen at 12 months. The most common adverse events were paresthesia ($n = 6$), dysarthria ($n = 4$; most with bilateral DBS), gait disorders ($n = 3$), headache ($n = 2$), and other pain ($n = 5$). Infection, erosion and skin irritation each occurred in two patients, repositioning was necessary due to unsatisfactory effects in one patient, loss of effect occurred in two patients, intermittent stimulation occurred in one patient, and five needed battery replacements after a mean of 70 months. One patient experienced severe dystonia, which led to discontinuation of stimulation.

Rehncrona et al. *(15)* examined two cohorts of ET patients from the Limousin et al. *(11)* study, which included 18 patients 2 years after thalamic DBS and 13 patients 6 to 7 years after thalamic DBS. They used a randomized, double-blind, cross-over design to evaluate patients in the stimulation on and stimulation off conditions at each follow-up visit. At 2 years, there was 67% improvement in upper limb postural and action tremor in the stimulation on compared to the stimulation off condition. The stimulation off condition did not differ from baseline. At 6 to 7 years after implant, there was a 67% improvement in both the stimulation on and off conditions compared to baseline for upper limb postural tremor and a 50% improvement in upper limb action tremor with stimulation on compared to stimulation off, which was slightly worsened compared to baseline. Total tremor scores were improved by 49% at 2 years and 47% 6 to 7 years postoperatively in the stimulation on compared to the stimulation off condition. Similarly, writing, drawing, and pouring was improved by 75% at 2 years and 55% at 6 to 7 years with stimulation on compared to the stimulation off condition. The authors concluded that thalamic DBS can successfully suppress action and postural tremor for at least 6 years after implant.

Putzke and colleagues *(18)* reported their experience with unilateral and bilateral thalamic DBS for ET in 35 patients 3 months after surgery, 27 patients after 1 year, 23 patients after 2 years, and seven patients after 3 years. At all follow-up visits there was at least an 83% improvement in upper extremity tremor and at least a 63% improvement in activities of daily living. They observed no worsening of tremor over time. Adverse events included dysarthria in 40%, disequilibrium in 31%, motor disturbance (eye deviation, pulling, or tightness) in 24%, and paresthesia in 16%. Eight leads were repositioned due to loss of effect, two leads were replaced due to breakage, and one patient experienced infection requiring device removal. Similarly, in a long-term study of 25 ET patients followed for an average of 40 months (range 22–69 months) after unilateral thalamic DBS, Koller et al. *(10)* reported that a significant improvement in total tremor of 50% was maintained at the longest follow-up, as was an improvement of 78% in targeted hand tremor. Surgical adverse events included seizures in one patient. Device complications included lead replacement due to loss of effect in six patients, lead fracture in one patient, lead migration in one patient, extension wire erosion in three patients, a pulse generator shocking sensation in one patient, and system removal due to loss of effect in one patient. Stimulation-related adverse events were mild and resolved with programming adjustments. These included paresthesia (84%), headache (60%), paresis (24%), dysarthria (16%), disequilibrium (16%), facial weakness (12%), and gait disorder, dystonia, dizziness, and cognitive deficits each in 8% of patients.

The American Academy of Neurology (AAN) Practice Parameter concerning therapies for ET *(19)* concluded that DBS of the VIM thalamic nucleus effectively reduces contralateral limb tremor in medically refractory ET. Furthermore, they recommended that DBS of the VIM thalamic nucleus may be used to treat medically refractory limb tremor in ET (Level C).

## Unilateral vs. Bilateral Stimulation

Pahwa et al. *(14)* reported results of staged bilateral thalamic DBS in nine ET patients. The patients had a 35% improvement in total tremor scores after the first surgery and an additional 34% improvement 1 year after the second surgery. Combined postural and kinetic hand tremor scores for the target limb were improved by 68% after the first surgery and by 75% on the opposite side after the second surgery. Five patients had head tremor at baseline; only two had head tremor after the initial surgery and only one after bilateral DBS. The most common side effects were paresthesia, dysarthria, and disequilibrium. Dysarthria was assessed by a speech pathologist in six patients before and after surgery with the left stimulator on, the right stimulator on, and both stimulators on. Three patients had increased dysarthria compared to baseline with one stimulator turned on. This effect was similar with either the right or left side on. With both stimulators on, the dysarthria score was further increased. One patient had increased dysarthria only with bilateral stimulation and two patients had no changes in dysarthria with unilateral or bilateral stimulation.

Ondo et al. *(13)* compared unilateral and bilateral thalamic DBS in 11 ET patients. Upper extremity tremor contralateral to the initial surgery improved by 68%, while the opposite side improved by 77% after the second surgery. Activities of daily living were improved by 45% after the initial surgery, which increased to 59% after the second surgery. Unilateral DBS improved head tremor by 30%, whereas a 65% improvement resulted after the second implant. The most common side effects were balance difficulty in five patients and speech difficulty, which occurred in only one patient after the initial procedure but in five additional patients after the second procedure.

The AAN Practice Parameter concerning therapies for ET *(19)* concluded that thalamic DBS suppresses only contralateral limb tremor and that bilateral DBS is necessary to suppress tremor in both upper limbs. However, they found no evidence for a synergistic therapeutic effect on limb tremor with bilateral DBS and insufficient data regarding the risk–benefit ratios of unilateral versus bilateral DBS. They further stated that side effects are more frequent with bilateral DBS and that bilateral thalamotomy is not recommended.

## Head Tremor

Berk and Honey *(20)* reported two ET patients who underwent bilateral thalamic DBS for isolated head tremor. They reported complete resolution of head tremor 9 months after surgery. Aside from this case report, no studies have reported thalamic DBS that was performed specifically for head tremor. However, several studies have examined effects of DBS on head tremor in patients who received unilateral and/or bilateral thalamic DBS for treatment of disabling hand tremor (Table 10.2).

Koller et al. *(21)* reported the effects of unilateral thalamic DBS in 38 ET patients at 3 months, 22 at 6 months, and 20 at 1 year. There were significant improvements in head tremor of 52% at 3 months, 35% at 6 months, and 50% 12 months after surgery. At the 12-month evaluation, head tremor remained improved in 75% of patients, was unchanged in 20% of patients, and was worsened in 5% of patients compared to baseline. There was also significant improvement in total tremor scores at all follow-up visits. Similarly, Ondo et al. *(12)* reported a 55% improvement in head tremor in 14 ET patients 3

**Table 10.2** Selected studies of thalamic deep brain stimulation for the treatment of essential head tremor (% improvement compared to baseline).

| Author, year | N (uni/bi) | Follow-up (months) | Head tremor |
|---|---|---|---|
| Koller et al., 1999 *(21)* | | | |
| Unilateral | 20/0 | 12 | 50%* |
| Limousin et al., 1999 *(11)* | | | |
| Unilateral | 28 | 12 | 15% |
| Bilateral | 9 | 12 | 85%* |
| Sydow et al., 2003 *(16)* | 19 | 80 | 58%* |
| Unilateral | 12 | 80 | 45% |
| Bilateral | 7 | 80 | 85% |
| Obwegeser et al., 2000 *(22)* | | | |
| Unilateral | 11 | 11 | 38%* |
| Bilateral | 11 | 12 | 95%* |
| Ondo et al., 2001 *(13)* | | | |
| Unilateral | 11 | 3 | 30% |
| Bilateral | 11 | 3 | 65%* |
| Putzke et al., 2005 *(23)* | | | |
| Bilateral | 13 | 24 | 90%* |

*, reported as significantly improved.

months after unilateral thalamic DBS for hand tremor but this improvement did not reach statistical significance.

Limousin and colleagues *(11)* reported a nonsignificant improvement in head tremor of 15% in 28 ET patients with unilateral thalamic DBS and a significant 85% improvement 12 months after surgery in four ET patients operated bilaterally. From the same cohort, Sydow et al. *(16)* reported a significant improvement in head tremor of 58% when the entire cohort of 19 patients was examined 6.5 years after thalamic DBS. When examining unilaterally and bilaterally operated patients separately, there was a 45% improvement in head tremor 6.5 years after unilateral thalamic DBS in 12 ET patients and an 85% improvement in seven ET patients with bilateral thalamic DBS.

Ondo et al. *(13)* reported 11 patients with staged bilateral thalamic DBS of which nine had head tremor. In these patients, head tremor was nonsignificantly improved by 30% after unilateral thalamic DBS and significantly improved by 65% after bilateral thalamic DBS. Obwegeser et al. *(22)* reported very similar results in 11 ET patients both after unilateral and bilateral stimulation. There was 38% improvement in head tremor 11 months after unilateral thalamic DBS and 95% improvement in head tremor 12 months after bilateral thalamic DBS. Finally, Putzke et al. *(23)* reported a significant improvement of at least 90% in head tremor at one, 3, 12, and 24 months after staged bilateral thalamic DBS.

Considering these data, the AAN Practice Parameter concerning therapies for ET *(19)* concluded that there is inconsistent and insufficient evidence to make recommendations about the use of unilateral or bilateral thalamic DBS for essential head tremor.

**Voice Tremor**

Only a few studies have examined the effects of thalamic DBS on voice tremor (Table 10.3). Carpenter et al. *(24)* studied the effects of thalamic stimulation on voice tremor in seven ET patients (five unilateral, two bilateral) who had

**Table 10.3** Selected studies of thalamic deep brain stimulation for the treatment of essential voice tremor (% improvement compared to baseline).

| Author, year | N(uni/bi) | Follow-up (months) | Voice tremor |
|---|---|---|---|
| Limousin et al., 1999 *(11)* | | | |
|     Unilateral | 28 | 12 | 33% |
|     Bilateral | 9 | 12 | 40% |
| Sydow et al., 2003 *(16)* | | | |
|     Unilateral | 12 | 80 | 25% |
|     Bilateral | 7 | 80 | 60% |
| Obwegeser et al., 2000 *(22)* | | | |
|     Unilateral | 11 | 11 | 28% |
|     Bilateral | 11 | 12 | 83%* |
| Putzke et al., 2005 *(23)* | | | |
|     Bilateral | 13 | 24 | 65%* |

*, reported as significantly improved.

undergone thalamic DBS for hand tremor and had voice tremor before surgery. Voice assessments were conducted an average of 18 months (1–32 months) after surgery. They included patient and speech clinician global ratings as well as acoustic assessments. Voice tremor was improved significantly only in patients who had severe symptoms and did not parallel improvement in hand tremor. There were no notable differences between unilateral and bilateral patients. Overall, four of seven patients had documented improvement in voice tremor.

Limousin and colleagues *(11)* reported a 33% decrease in voice tremor in 28 ET patients 12 months after unilateral thalamic DBS and a 40% decrease in nine ET patients 12 months after bilateral thalamic DBS; however, improvements in voice tremor were not significant after either unilateral or bilateral implants. Sydow and colleagues *(16)* reported no significant change in voice tremor in 12 unilateral and seven bilateral thalamic DBS patients after 1 or 6 years of follow-up. In a study of staged bilateral thalamic DBS, Obwegeser et al. *(22)* reported no significant change in voice tremor in 12 ET patients 11 months after unilateral thalamic DBS. However, 12 months after the second implant, these 12 patients demonstrated a significant improvement of 83% in voice tremor. Dysarthria was a common adverse effect and was more prevalent after the second implant. Finally, Putzke et al. *(23)* reported a significant improvement in voice tremor at 1, 3, 12, and 24 months after staged bilateral thalamic DBS.

The AAN Practice Parameter concerning therapies for ET *(19)* concluded that there is inconsistent and insufficient evidence to make a recommendation about the use of unilateral or bilateral thalamic DBS for essential voice tremor.

## Thalamotomy vs. Thalamic DBS

Thalamic DBS has largely replaced thalamotomy as the surgery of choice for disabling, medication-resistant ET. The advantages of thalamic DBS compared to thalamotomy include the reversibility of the procedure, lack of destruction of brain tissue, ability to adjust stimulation parameters to increase efficacy or reduce side effects, and the reduced morbidity associated with bilateral procedures. The disadvantages of thalamic DBS include increased costs, implantation of a foreign material (which increases the potential for infection), additional surgical procedures to replace the battery, possible need for replacement of other system hardware due to breakage or malfunction, and the additional time, effort, and follow-up visits required to optimize stimulation parameters.

Several studies have compared the safety and efficacy of thalamic DBS and thalamotomy. Tasker and colleagues *(25)* retrospectively compared 19 tremor patients who underwent thalamic DBS (16 parkinsonian, three ET) to 26 tremor patients who had thalamotomy (23 parkinsonian, three ET) all of whom were followed for at least 3 months. Efficacy was similar between the two groups with 42% of both groups having complete tremor resolution and 79% of those with DBS vs 69% of those with thalamotomy having marked reduction in tremor. Of the patients with thalamotomies, 15% required repeat surgery while no patients with DBS required repeat surgery. The most common adverse events were ataxia, dysarthria, and gait disturbance, which occurred in 42% of the patients with thalamotomy and in 26% of patients with DBS.

Pahwa and coworkers *(26)* also retrospectively compared 17 ET patients who underwent thalamotomy to 17 ET patients who underwent thalamic DBS. The average follow-up for the thalamotomy group was 2.2 months and the average follow-up in the thalamic DBS group was 3.1 months. The two groups were matched according to age, sex, side of surgery, and severity of tremor. Efficacy was similar in the two groups with total tremor ratings improving 49% with thalamotomy and 50% with thalamic DBS. Surgical complications were more prevalent in the thalamotomy group with five patients having asymptomatic hemorrhages, and one patient having a symptomatic hemorrhage, while there were no hemorrhages in the thalamic DBS group. Cognitive problems occurred in 29% of the thalamotomy patients and in none of those with DBS. Patients with DBS had higher rates of paresthesia, dizziness, disequilibrium, and dysarthria but with reprogramming of the stimulation parameters, these side effects were eliminated. In the thalamotomy group, two patients had repeat surgery due to lack of benefit; in the thalamic DBS group there were six additional surgeries including four lead replacements, one pulse generator malfunction, and one battery replacement. In addition, in one patient the DBS system was explanted and a thalamotomy was performed due to lack of benefit.

Finally, Schuurman and colleagues *(27)* conducted a randomized prospective study that compared thalamic DBS and thalamotomy for treatment of tremor. In this study, six ET patients underwent thalamotomy and seven ET patients underwent thalamic DBS. Tremor reduction was similar for the two groups. Adverse events were more common in the thalamotomy group (50%), consisting of dysarthria, gait and balance difficulty, and cognitive deterioration compared to the thalamic DBS group in which only one patient (14.3%) had gait and balance disturbance. In each of the studies cited previously, it was concluded that thalamic DBS and thalamotomy were equivalent in terms of efficacy but that thalamic DBS was uniformly considered to be the treatment of choice due to the ability to adjust stimulation parameters in order to improve efficacy and reduce adverse effects.

The AAN Practice Parameter concerning therapies for ET *(19)* concluded that both DBS and thalamotomy effectively suppress tremor in ET. Further, they state that DBS is associated with fewer adverse events than thalamotomy. However, the decision to use either procedure depends on each patient's circumstances and the risk for intra-operative complications compared to feasibility of stimulator monitoring and adjustments.

## Summary

VIM DBS is a safe, effective treatment for disabling, medication-resistant ET. Multiple studies have demonstrated significant efficacy of both unilateral and bilateral thalamic DBS in controlling upper extremity tremor. Head and voice tremor have also been significantly reduced with thalamic DBS but bilateral procedures have produced more dramatic effects than unilateral procedures. Several reports have demonstrated that the effects of thalamic DBS are maintained long term. However, in several studies there was some loss of benefit over time. It is unclear if this loss of benefit is due to disease progression and consequent worsening of tremor, tolerance to stimulation, or some other factor. Adverse stimulation-related events are typically mild and can generally be eliminated with adjustments of the stimulation parameter settings. Adverse events such as dysarthria and gait and balance disturbance have been shown to be more common with bilateral procedures. Device complications such as lead misplacement, migration, or fracture; extension wire erosion; and pulse generator malfunction may occur and often require additional surgical procedures. Battery replacement is typically necessary every 3 to 6 years depending on usage patterns and stimulation parameter settings. Thalamic DBS and thalamotomy have been shown to have comparable efficacy; however, adverse events have been shown to be more common with thalamotomy. In general, DBS of the thalamus is considered the surgical treatment of choice for ET patients with disabling, medication-resistant tremor.

## References

1. Pahwa R, Lyons KE (2003) Essential tremor: differential diagnosis and current therapy. Am J Med 115(2):134–142.
2. Lyons KE, Pahwa R, Comella CL, et al (2003) Benefits and risks of pharmacological treatments for essential tremor. Drug Saf 26(7):461–481.
3. Hassler R, Riechert T, Mundinger F, Umbach W, Ganglberger JA (1960) Physiological observations in stereotaxic operations in extrapyramidal motor disturbances. Brain 83:337–350.
4. Ohye C, Kubota K, Hongo T, Nagao T, Narabayashi H (1964) Ventrolateral and subventrolateral thalamic stimulation. Motor effects. Arch Neurol 11:427–434.
5. Benabid AL, Pollak P, Louveau A, Henry S, de Rougemont J (1987) Combined (thalamotomy and stimulation) stereotactic surgery of the VIM thalamic nucleus for bilateral Parkinson disease. Appl Neurophysiol 50(1–6):344–346.
6. Benabid AL, Pollak P, Gervason C, et al (1991) Long-term suppression of tremor by chronic stimulation of the ventral intermediate thalamic nucleus. Lancet 337(8738):403–406.
7. Benabid AL, Pollak P, Seigneuret E, Hoffmann D, Gay E, Perret J (1993) Chronic VIM thalamic stimulation in Parkinson's disease, essential tremor and extra-pyramidal dyskinesias. Acta Neurochirurgica Supplementum 58:39–44.
8. Benabid AL, Pollak P, Gao D, et al (1996) Chronic electrical stimulation of the ventralis intermedius nucleus of the thalamus as a treatment of movement disorders. J Neurosurg 84(2):203–214.

9. Koller W, Pahwa R, Busenbark K, et al (1997) High-frequency unilateral thalamic stimulation in the treatment of essential and parkinsonian tremor. Ann Neurol 42(3):292–299.
10. Koller WC, Lyons KE, Wilkinson SB, Troster AI, Pahwa R (2001) Long-term safety and efficacy of unilateral deep brain stimulation of the thalamus in essential tremor. Mov Disord 16(3):464–468.
11. Limousin P, Speelman JD, Gielen F, Janssens M (1999) Multicentre European study of thalamic stimulation in parkinsonian and essential tremor. J Neurol Neurosurg Psychiatry 66(3):289–296.
12. Ondo W, Jankovic J, Schwartz K, Almaguer M, Simpson RK (1998) Unilateral thalamic deep brain stimulation for refractory essential tremor and Parkinson's disease tremor. Neurology 51(4):1063–1069.
13. Ondo W, Almaguer M, Jankovic J, Simpson RK (2001) Thalamic deep brain stimulation: comparison between unilateral and bilateral placement. Arch Neurol 58(2):218–222.
14. Pahwa R, Lyons KL, Wilkinson SB, et al (1999) Bilateral thalamic stimulation for the treatment of essential tremor. Neurology 53(7):1447–1450.
15. Rehncrona S, Johnels B, Widner H, Tornqvist AL, Hariz M, Sydow O (2003) Long-term efficacy of thalamic deep brain stimulation for tremor: double-blind assessments. Mov Disord 18(2):163–170.
16. Sydow O, Thobois S, Alesch F, Speelman JD (2003) Multicentre European study of thalamic stimulation in essential tremor: a six year follow up. J Neurol Neurosurg Psychiatry 74(10):1387–1391.
17. Pahwa R, Lyons KE, Wilkinson SB, et al (2006) Long-term evaluation of deep brain stimulation of the thalamus. J Neurosurg 104(4):506–512.
18. Putzke JD, Wharen RE Jr, Obwegeser AA, et al (2004) Thalamic deep brain stimulation for essential tremor: recommendations for long-term outcome analysis. Can J Neurol Sci 31(3):333–342.
19. Zesiewicz TA, Elble R, Louis ED, et al (2005) Practice parameter: therapies for essential tremor: report of the Quality Standards Subcommittee of the American Academy of Neurology. Neurology 64(12):2008–2020.
20. Berk C, Honey CR (2002) Bilateral thalamic deep brain stimulation for the treatment of head tremor. Report of two cases. J Neurosurg 96(3):615–618.
21. Koller WC, Lyons KE, Wilkinson SB, Pahwa R (1999) Efficacy of unilateral deep brain stimulation of the VIM nucleus of the thalamus for essential head tremor. Mov Disord 14(5):847–850.
22. Obwegeser AA, Uitti RJ, Turk MF, Strongosky AJ, Wharen RE (2000) Thalamic stimulation for the treatment of midline tremors in essential tremor patients. Neurology 54(12):2342–2344.
23. Putzke JD, Uitti RJ, Obwegeser AA, Wszolek ZK, Wharen RE (2005) Bilateral thalamic deep brain stimulation: midline tremor control. J Neurol Neurosurg Psychiatry 76(5):684–690.
24. Carpenter MA, Pahwa R, Miyawaki KL, Wilkinson SB, Searl JP, Koller WC (1998) Reduction in voice tremor under thalamic stimulation. Neurology 50(3):796–798.
25. Tasker RR (1998) Deep brain stimulation is preferable to thalamotomy for tremor suppression. Surg Neurol 49(2):145–153; discussion 153–144.
26. Pahwa R, Lyons KE, Wilkinson SB, et al (2001) Comparison of thalamotomy to deep brain stimulation of the thalamus in essential tremor. Mov Disord 16(1):140–143.
27. Schuurman PR, Bosch DA, Bossuyt PM, et al (2000) A comparison of continuous thalamic stimulation and thalamotomy for suppression of severe tremor. N Engl J Med 342(7):461–468.

# 11

# Thalamic Deep Brain Stimulation for Other Tremors

Erwin B. Montgomery, Jr.

## Abstract

Deep brain stimulation (DBS) is approved by the U.S. Food and Drug Administration (FDA) for unilateral placement in the ventrolateral nucleus of the thalamus (VL) for the treatment of essential tremor (ET) and tremor due to Parkinson's disease (PD). There is also evidence that VL DBS is effective for tremor secondary to other causes such as multiple sclerosis (MS), post-anoxic and post-traumatic action tremor, and miscellaneous tremors from other causes. In this chapter, experience with VL DBS for tremor due to conditions other than ET or PD are reviewed. It also discusses surgical approaches that may be unique to non-ET and non-PD patients. VL DBS is discussed as a safe, effective treatment for the reduction of tremor due to a wide variety of disorders. The issue of cost-effectiveness is also addressed. Finally, some implications of VL DBS for non-ET, non-PD, and other "off-label" indications will be considered.

**Keywords:** tremor, multiple sclerosis, stroke, deep brain stimulation, DBS, thalamus

## Introduction

DBS is approved by the U.S. FDA for unilateral placement in the VL for the treatment of ET and tremor due to PD. However, there is evidence that VL DBS is also effective for tremor secondary to other causes such as MS, post-anoxic and post-traumatic action tremor, and tremor from other causes. The methodologies and devices used are essentially identical to those used for ET and PD. The precise mechanism by which DBS effects its therapeutic response is unknown *(1, 2)*. It is clear that the success of DBS has forced a reconsideration of current theories of pathophysiology of movement disorders, particularly with respect to PD *(3, 4)*. In the future similar studies may contribute to a better understanding of cerebellar physiology and pathophysiology thought to underlie other causes of tremor that will hopefully lead to more effective treatments.

In the interim, physicians caring for patients with tremor due to conditions other than ET and PD are confronted with the fact that there are few effective alternative treatments. Despite this, there are inconsistencies in referral patterns, which require explanation. For example, at the Cleveland Clinic Foundation from 1997 to 2003, many patients with cerebellar outflow tremor due to MS underwent VL DBS but from 2003 to 2007 not a single patient with MS was referred to the University of Wisconsin-Madison for VL DBS. What are possible explanations for this discrepancy? Do physicians at the University of Wisconsin-Madison know either more or less about DBS for tremor than physicians at the Cleveland Clinic Foundation? Was new knowledge acquired subsequent to 2003? Are MS patients different in Wisconsin compared to Ohio? Was the decision simply a matter of physician preference that differed between Wisconsin and Ohio? Was the decision a matter of insurance preferences that differ in Wisconsin and Ohio?

In this chapter, experience with VL DBS for tremor due to neurological disorders other than ET or PD are reviewed. There is a discussion of some aspects of the surgical approach that may be unique to non-ET and non-PD patients. Other implications of VL DBS for non-ET and non-PD for other "off-label" indications are also discussed.

## General Experience of VL DBS for MS

VL DBS has been performed in a number of patients with disorders other than ET or PD. The majority of these patients have undergone VL DBS for cerebellar outflow tremor due to MS. Tremor is a common and often very disabling complication of MS. According to some series, at least 50% of MS patients suffer from significant tremor *(5)*. However, it is rare for a patient with MS to have tremor as their sole disability. Consequently, it is important to keep the expectations of VL DBS in perspective. The primary objective of VL DBS in MS is to improve tremor. Its effectiveness for treatment of the cerebellar ataxia very commonly associated with tremor is uncertain but the presumption has been that it is not effective. The degree to which reduced tremor contributes to patient independence and improved quality of life is difficult to assess. Keeping expectations for VL DBS within the perspective of the total disability experienced by the patient has proven to be problematic when considering the value and appropriateness of VL DBS.

It is important to stipulate to patients in advance what the measure of successful DBS will be. Some published studies have used changes in the Extended Disability Status Scale (EDSS) scale as the best measure of success *(6)*. These scales are commonly used in clinical studies of MS and are considered by some to be the standard. Most studies have found no significant improvement in the EDSS scores in MS patients after VL DBS *(6)*. However, the EDSS and other similar outcome measures have typically been used when studying the natural history of MS and effects of therapeutic measures used to affect natural history. It is uncertain whether such measures are appropriate for assessment of the acute changes produced by VL DBS. Other measures such as independence, neuropsychological function, quality of life, or patient satisfaction have also not demonstrated significant improvements following VL DBS in MS patients *(6–9)*. Consequently, many investigators have been pessimistic about the value of DBS for MS tremor. However, when tremor scores alone are examined, nearly every study has concluded that VL DBS significantly reduces tremor *(5–15)*. Summarizing, the outgives appear to include: (1) relief of tremor, (2) increase in function, (3) improvement in quality of life, (4) cost effectiveness, and (5) the duration of improvement of these outgives. Table 11.1 summarizes many of the published reports on VL DBS for cerebellar outflow tremor secondary to MS.

Montgomery et al. had a modest expectation for reduction of tremor in the limb contralateral to VL DBS in the "cup task," which measures the amplitude

**Table 11.1** Summary of published literature on the efficacy of VL DBS for cerebellar outflow tremor secondary to MS.

| Article reference | Type of study | Number of subjects | Outcomes |
|---|---|---|---|
| Brice and McLellan *(36)* | Retrospective, unblinded, and uncontrolled | Two; follow-up 5 and 6 months | Tremor described as "strikingly" diminished |
| Nguyen and Degas *(37)* | Retrospective, unblinded, and uncontrolled | One; follow-up 17 months | Tremor described as changing from severe to slight |
| Seigfried and Lippitz *(38)* | Retrospective, unblinded, and uncontrolled | Nine (among other types of tremor); follow-up not reported | All described as improving, not specified for patients with MS |
| Benabid et al. *(39)* | Retrospective, unblinded, and uncontrolled | Four (among other types of tremor); follow-up from 3 to more than 6 months | Results not specified for patients with multiple sclerosis |
| Geny et al. (ref. *40*; may include patients from Nguyen and Degas *[37]*) | Retrospective, unblinded, and uncontrolled | 13; mean follow-up 13 months | Tremor improved by 69%; patients described as more functional but no change in Extended Disability Status Scale |
| Whittle et al. *(41)* | Retrospective, unblinded, and uncontrolled | Five; follow-up not reported | Eight subjects taken to surgery but only five implanted, these were the patients that demonstrated intra-operative reduction of tremor with stimulation |
| Hay *(42)* | Retrospective, unblinded, and uncontrolled | One; follow-up 2 months | Tremor described as improved |
| Montgomery et al. *(11)* | Retrospective, unblinded, and uncontrolled | 15; follow-up from 3 to 12 months | Mean tremor on the cup task preoperatively was 4 out of 4 which improved to 0.8 under optimal stimulation |
| Taha et al. *(43)* | Retrospective, unblinded, and uncontrolled | Two; follow-up approximately 10 months | Tremor improved in all patients to a tremor grade of 2 out of 4 but pre-operative scores not reported |
| Schuurman et al. *(13)* | Prospective, random assignment to VL DBS or thalamotomy and unblinded | Five (five other patients were assigned to thalamotomy), follow-up at 6 months | Frenchay Activities Index: statistically significant improvement; tremor severity; pre-operatively two patients with grade 3 out of 4 tremor, three patients with grade 4; post-operatively one patient with grade 0 tremor; one patient with grade 1; one patient with grade 2; two patients with grade 3 |

(continued)

**Table 11.1** (continued)

| Article reference | Type of study | Number of subjects | Outcomes |
|---|---|---|---|
| Matsumoto et al. (9) | Retrospective, unblinded, and uncontrolled | Three (three others had thalamotomy); follow-up to 12 months | All had significant improvement in tremor scores (results not specified by type of surgery), no improvement in the Extended Disability Status Scale |
| Hooper et al. (7) | Prospective, unblinded, and uncontrolled | 15; mean follow-up 12 months | Statistically significant improvement in the severity of tremor ($p = 0.02$) in the Modified Fahn Tremor Rating Scale and improvement in hand function ($p = 0.02$); no change in disability, handicap, neuropsychological function, and independence using the Kurtzke Functional Systems Scale, Extended Disability Status Scale, Functional Independence Measure, London Handicap Scale, Handicap Questionnaire, Fatigue Severity Scale |
| Berk et al. (8) | Prospective, blinded, and uncontrolled | 12; follow-up 12 months | 70% reduction in action tremor at 2 months and 67% at 1 year, no significant changes in the SF-36 |
| Schulder et al. (6) | Retrospective, unblinded, and uncontrolled | Nine; mean follow-up 32 months | Tremor scores averaged 5.4 before surgery, 1.7 at 6 months after surgery, and 2.1 at late follow-up; Extended Disability Status Scale scores averaged 7.2 before surgery, 6.8 at 6 months after surgery, and 7.8 at late follow-up |
| Wishart et al. (15) | Literature review and retrospective, unblinded, and uncontrolled report of authors' case series | Four; mean follow-up 22 months | All improved with tremor scores of 3 out of 4 to scores of 0 in two patients and 1 in two patients |
| Nandi and Aziz (44) | Retrospective, unblinded, and uncontrolled | 10; mean follow-up 15 months | Custom method for measuring tremor, group improvement by 64% in postural tremor and 36% in intention (action) tremor |
| Bittar et al. (ref. 12; may include patients from Nandi and Aziz [44]) | | 10 (10 patients underwent thalamotomy); mean follow-up 14.6 months | The mean improvement in postural tremor at 16.2 months following surgery was 78%, compared with a 64% improvement after thalamic stimulation (14.6 month follow-up; $p > 0.05$) |
| Foote et al. (26) | Retrospective, unblinded, and uncontrolled | One; at least 6 months | 50% reduction in tremor with ventrointermediate thalamic (VIM) DBS and 63% with combined VIM and ventroanterior/ventroposterior VL DBS |
| Herzog et al. (45) | Retrospective, unblinded, and uncontrolled. Objective to identify the optimal stimulation location was thought to be the subthalamic area rather than thalamus | 11; follow-up not specified | 62 to 76% improvement in tremor rating scale |

of limb tremor as a subject reaches for a cup and brings it to their lips *(7)*. This measure was chosen because it reflects an important activity of daily living *(11)*. Using the Clinical Tremor Rating Scale (CTRS), Montgomery et al. demonstrated impressive reduction in tremor using the cup task *(11)*. In addition to tremor others have reported improved upper extremity function during VL DBS *(7, 8)*. Schulder et al. *(6)* found no significant improvement in the EDSS (mean pre-surgery scores of 7.2, mean 6 months post-surgery scores of 6.8, and mean late post-surgery scores of 7.8), but did find significant improvement in tremor specific ratings (mean pre-surgery scores of 5.4, mean 6 months post-surgery scores of 1.7, and mean late post-surgery scores of 2.1).

The emphasis on tremor reduction in the dominant upper extremity is reflected in the selection criteria used by most centers. That is, the tremor must be functionally limiting without significant weakness or sensory loss in the targeted limb. This is because weakness or sensory loss may contribute to tremor but are unlikely to improve after VL DBS. Patients are advised that DBS does not cure the underlying neurological disorder and that MS may progress despite VL DBS surgery. The decision to proceed with VL DBS surgery should consider whether a major reduction in tremor is sufficient to justify the surgical risk of DBS, estimated as a 2 to 3% risk of a significant and/or persistent neurological complication. Most centers require the MS to be relatively stable at the time of surgery. At our institution, the patient may not have had a significant neurological exacerbation in the preceding 6 months. We also require that speech and swallowing not be significantly compromised because exacerbation of speech and swallowing deficit had been a significant complication of ablative thalamotomy.

**Long-Term Efficacy of VL DBS for MS**

There are relatively few long-term follow-up studies of longer than 1 year following surgery (Table 11.1). A common belief had been that efficacy would wane. To address this issue, we carried out a retrospective chart review of 25 consecutive patients with MS. The long-term efficacy of VL DBS was assessed by comparing the subject's worst and best scores during sessions of DBS adjustment during their last clinic visit. Notwithstanding the caveats appropriate to such limited and potentially biased retrospective studies, some interesting observations were made. In the absence of better data, these may serve to guide patient management. Figure 11.1 shows the best CTRS score achieved after DBS adjustment during the last visit and the time between the last visit and the date of DBS surgery. If benefits were temporary, then subjects furthest out from DBS surgery would be expected to have the greatest tremor. This was not the case including some subjects who had gone more than 1000 days since surgery (Figure 11.1). A correlation analysis demonstrated no significant relationship between the best scores and the time since surgery. Figure 11.2 shows the individual differences between the worst and best scores at the time of the last clinic visit. All but two subjects showed improvement with effective DBS and six subjects had absence of tremor during the cup task.

Previous retrospective studies concerning long-term efficacy of DBS in MS have relied on the patient and/or caregiver's global assessment often couched in the question of whether the patient would undergo the surgery again or

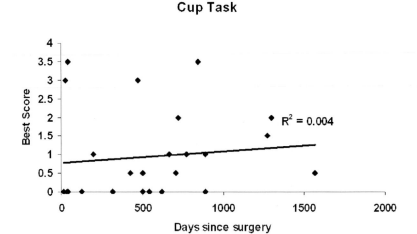

**Figure 11.1** The best CTRS scores during the cup task for individual patients at the time of their last clinic visit prior to the retrospective review measured as days since DBS implant surgery. The lowest score indicates the least tremor

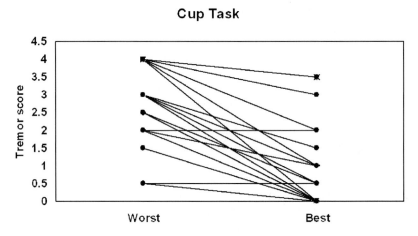

**Figure 11.2** Comparison between the best and worst CTRS scores during the cup task for individual patients at the time of their last clinic visit prior to the retrospective review

whether, in retrospect, the surgery was worthwhile *(16)*. We conducted a more detailed retrospective telephone survey to determine long-term efficacy in 21 consecutive patients who underwent VL DBS for MS tremor. A copy of the interview form is available from the author. Three patients were lost to follow-up. Of the 18 responses, 11 surveys were completed by the patient and seven by the caregiver. The mean (SD) time between DBS surgery and completing the survey was 45 (13.3) months. Because of the relatively small number of subjects and difficulty quantifying the clinical results, the results of the interview allow only a limited number of cautious conclusions. Twelve patients continued to use the stimulator while six patients stopped using DBS. In the six patients who stopped, the reason was not that "it did not help the tremor."

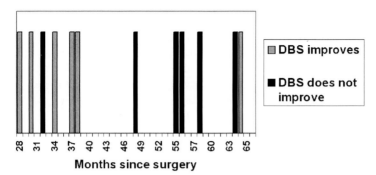

**Figure 11.3** The relationship between the time since surgery and the impression that VL DBS improved or did not improve the patient's quality of life based on the telephone interview. As can be seen, most patients that had surgery within the preceding 40 months claimed an improved quality of life in contrast to those patients whose surgery was longer than 40 months from the date of the survey

Of the 12 patients that continued to use DBS, six claimed an improved quality of life while six did not improve. Of the six that did not report an improved quality of life, four thought they would have an improved quality of life if they could get to the doctor for more frequent follow-up visits. Figure 11.3 shows the duration between the date of surgery and completion of the questionnaire. Most patients up to 40 months following DBS surgery generally describe an improvement in quality of life. More detailed results of the survey are available from the author.

**Conundrum**

Interpretation of the experiences described earlier leads to several reasonable conclusions. First, there is consistency in the observation that VL DBS significantly reduces tremor and that the benefit is sustained over time in a subset of patients who respond to this therapy. However, the question remains how to translate reduction in tremor to improvement in functional disabilities. Second, VL DBS does not consistently improve scores on global tests of functioning in MS patients such as the EDSS. It is an open question whether such global measures are appropriate to evaluate the effect of VL DBS for an isolated symptom such as tremor. Third, in a majority of patients, VL DBS does not improve patient or caregiver assessments of quality of life. Although, in our retrospective telephone survey, two-thirds of patients and/or caregivers reported that VL DBS did not improve long-term quality of life, most continued to use DBS. In addition, two-thirds of those still using VL DBS but reporting no improvement in quality of life said they thought that further stimulator adjustments would have helped. Although this is highly uncertain, it suggests that for many patients quality of life may be related more to access to follow-up programming than to the inherent efficacy of VL DBS.

The observations described earlier indicate the complexity of medical decision making, the results of which will be quite different depending on which of the elements described earlier are given the greatest weight. For example, if one considers only a significant and sustained reduction in tremor that impairs the ability of the patient to eat or drink, the data argues in favor of VL DBS. If one considers only the effects of VL DBS on the EDSS it is reasonable to conclude that VL DBS should not be recommended.

Medical decisions involve issues of cost in addition to issues of effectiveness. The data reviewed here only relate to issues of effectiveness. A physician's decision regarding whether to recommend VL DBS involves an assessment of cost and a perspective regarding how to factor in costs. Costs, and consequently medical decisions, include financial as well as medical, social, ethical, and moral considerations *(17)*. Medical costs must also include the risks of performing surgery as well as the cost of continued disability if surgery is not performed. Regardless of one's position on this issue, many physicians feel the right and/or obligation to consider costs in their recommendations to patients *(18–20)*.

As used to date, the EDSS and quality of life measures are too blunt as instruments to be used in the consideration of VL DBS for an individual patient. On the other hand, the evidence concerning reduction of tremor is more relevant and we believe the experience thus far is compelling. Consider a young man with severe cerebellar outflow tremor due to MS who underwent dominant-side VL DBS and experienced remarkable improvement of contralateral upper extremity function. He was advised to turn the stimulator off at bedtime and to turn it back on during the day in order to preserve battery life and avoid tolerance. However, the patient did the opposite. DBS controlled the tremor sufficiently so that he could use a telephone, feed himself finger-foods and bring a cup with a lid and straw to his mouth. Having this control available at night allowed the patient to care for himself independently, even at a time when functional demands were less. He no longer required 24 hour nursing support, his independence at night was a significant boost to his self-esteem, and costs were reduced.

This author believes that the limited and possibly flawed available data, which suggests improved quality of life for 40 months, to be sufficiently compelling to offer VL DBS to patients with cerebellar outflow tremor due to MS within the criteria discussed earlier. Additionally, we feel that insurer denial on the basis that VL DBS for non-ET or non-PD tremor is experimental or investigational is not persuasive. The author has previously described his opinion of the use of only level 1 evidence-based medicine criteria as a misrepresentation and disservice to evidence-based medicine and patient care *(17)*.

## Unique Pre-operative and Postoperative Issues Related to Non-ET and Non-PD Tremor

Clinical experience with VL DBS in patients with MS and post-traumatic action tremor illustrates a number of unique issues. First, patients with these tremors develop a number of habits that, while helpful in the presence of severe tremor, may become counterproductive once the tremor is under control. For example, patients often make very rapid limb movements to reach their target. They do so because they wish to reach the target successfully on their first attempt. They learn that if they must make several secondary, corrective movements the tremor will become worse. Some patients appear to "swat" at the target. Our experience suggests that following successful VL DBS such rapid movements to the target become less effective than slower purposeful movements. These patients may therefore require a period of retraining following DBS to modify strategies previously adopted prior to surgery.

Some patients attempt to minimize their tremor by reducing the degrees of freedom about limb joints. They typically do so by rigidly holding their arm in adduction against the chest in order to limit involuntary proximal movements of the elbow and shoulder. Continued use of this posture after surgery limits their use of the limb when the tremor is under control. In such cases, referral to an occupational therapist is helpful.

Another problem that frequently occurs in patients with action tremor, especially when secondary to MS, is the rapid development of tolerance to the DBS settings, which can occur within hours to days. Often, minimal changes, such as even a small reduction rather than increase in stimulation voltage, can regain tremor control. However, this often necessitates frequent visits for programming, which can be problematic for patients with the neurologic co-morbidities typically associated with MS. This may result in dissatisfaction with DBS and may play some role in the therapeutic nihilism present in some physicians with respect to use of VL DBS for these tremors.

The mechanisms for tolerance are uncertain. To avoid tolerance, most patients with MS tremor are advised to turn the stimulator off at times when dependence on tremor control is minimal such as during the night. Another option is to implant impulse generators that allow the patient and/or caregiver some control over the stimulation parameters. In this way, the patient and/or caregivers would be able to make small periodic adjustments in stimulation parameters in order to regain control if the patient develops tolerance.

Another issue unique for the MS patient is the risk for exacerbation of MS symptoms coincident with the DBS procedure. Because clinical experience is limited, a precise estimation of this risk is problematic. Montgomery et al. *(11)* suggested that the risk was approximately 10%. In their review of the literature, Wishart et al. *(15)* reported that six of 27 patients experienced an exacerbation of MS following DBS. For this reason, some centers have adopted as a surgical candidacy requirement the absence of any significant exacerbation of the MS within the previous 6 months, operationally defined as a significant and acute worsening of existing symptoms or the development of new symptoms and signs. A progressive worsening of cerebellar outflow tremor is not considered an exacerbation.

Patients with tremor secondary to other causes, particularly MS, are likely to have other concomitant neurological problems. The presence of dysphagia or dysarthria is particularly significant as there is considerable risk for exacerbation of these symptoms with VL DBS, particularly when carried out bilaterally. Consequently, the presence of significant dysphagia or dysarthria is considered a relative contraindication to VL DBS.

There has been considerable debate concerning the distinction between tremor and ataxia. The latter is generally considered poorly responsive to VL DBS. Unfortunately, there is little if any objective data that bears on this issue. The experience of this author is that ataxia is associated with greater proximal limb involvement compared to tremor. In general, proximal tremor is more difficult to control with VL DBS than distal tremor. It is therefore the practice of this author to discourage DBS in patients with marked and limiting proximal tremor. It is possible that proximal tremor has greater bilateral representation thereby making unilateral DBS less effective for its control. The output of the cerebellum is via the brachium conjunctivum, which bifurcates into two divisions near the level of the red nucleus that may play a role in posture *(21)*. The ascending division projects to the VL nucleus of the thalamus en route to cortex. The descending division projects to the brainstem and mediates stereotypic bilateral upper and lower proximal flexion responses to microstimulation of the deep cerebellar nuclei *(21)*. Perhaps this descending pathway, which is unaffected by DBS, has a greater effect on proximal muscle coordination.

## Surgical Issues Unique to Non-ET and Non-PD Tremor

The surgical methods for VL DBS have been reviewed elsewhere *(22)*. However, several comments are indicated. First, targeting within VL thalamus is different for some types of cerebellar outflow tremors than for tremor associated with ET or PD. Tremor in ET or PD tends to be more distal compared to the more proximal tremor associated with cerebellar outflow lesions. Consequently, DBS for these conditions should target the region representing the proximal musculature, which is more lateral in VL thalamus compared to representation of the distal musculature. For these reasons and others this author strongly recommends the use of intraoperative microelectrode recording to determine the optimal target.

## DBS for Tremors Other Than MS

VL DBS has been demonstrated to be effective in a number of other causes of tremor. These include: post-stroke tremor *(23)*, post-traumatic tremor *(24, 25)*, spinocerebellar degeneration *(27, 28)*, a variant of Behr's syndrome *(29)*, Holmes midbrain tremor secondary to brainstem hemorrhage or tumors *(30–33)*, and peripheral neuropathy secondary to monoclonal gammopathy *(34)*. In the author's limited experience, patients with post-traumatic or post-anoxic cerebellar outflow tremor do better than patients with MS tremor due to the non-progressive nature of the post-traumatic or post-anoxic disabilities.

## "Off-label" vs "Experimental" Use of DBS and Insurance Coverage

The DBS systems currently used for VL DBS for non-ET and non-PD tremor are the same systems that have received approval from the FDA for PD, tremor, and dystonia. Consequently, the use of these systems for non-ET and non-PD tremor meets the standard definition of "off-label" use. Such use is not necessarily experimental or investigational but often falls within the limits of standard and accepted medical therapy.

Evidence-based medicine is sometimes misused to deny "off-label" uses, which are based on case experience or experts utilizing logical inference. There may be many reasons for the lack of such data such as the unfeasibility of controlled trials or lack of sponsors to financially support such studies. This is particularly true for cerebellar outflow tremors due to rare causes such as anoxic brain injury. This author recently participated in VL DBS for cerebellar outflow tremor in a patient with galactosemia who did remarkably well. It may not be feasible to conduct randomized control studies in such circumstances. However, the insistence on level 1 evidence is against the original intent of evidence-based medicine *(17)*. The original concept of evidence-based medicine recognized the legitimacy of case reports and case series, as well as expert opinion *(17)*.

## DBS as "Symptomatic" Rather Than "Disease-Specific" Treatment

The issue of appropriate clinical indications can be viewed from a different perspective. One could reasonably consider VL DBS a symptomatic rather than a disease specific treatment. An analogy would be in considering the use of a new analgesic medication, which is clearly a symptomatic therapy. One would not require separate clinical trials for every possible cause of pain. Rather, physicians must use judgment to extrapolate useful indications based on the mechanism of action of the drug and a demonstration of efficacy across a broad spectrum of etiologies.

To take another example, globus pallidus DBS is effective across a broad range of etiologies including PD, dystonia, tardive dyskinesia, and Tourette's syndrome. The argument has therefore been made to consider globus pallidus DBS a symptomatic form of treatment rather than a disease-specific treatment *(35)*. The efficacy of VL DBS for a wide variety of cerebellar outflow tremors similarly supports the notion of a symptomatic therapy.

## References

1. McIntyre CC, Savasta M, Walter BL, Vitek JL (2004) How does deep brain stimulation work? Present understanding and future questions. J Clin Neurophysiol 21:40–50.
2. Montgomery EBJ, T GJ (2007) Mechanisms of action of deep brain stimulation (DBS). Neurosci Biobehav Rev in press.
3. Montgomery EB Jr (2006) Effects of GPi stimulation on human thalamic neuronal activity. Clin Neurophysiol 117:2691–2702.
4. Montgomery EBJ Subthalamic neuronal activity in Parkinson's Disease and epilepsy subjects. Parkinsonism Related Disord in press.
5. Cavallo M, Eleopra R, Biguzzi S, Sarubbo S (2006) Deep brain stimulation in the management of multiple sclerosis tremor. Neurolog Sci 27(Suppl 4):s331–s334.
6. Schulder M, Sernas T, Karimi R (2003) Thalamic stimulation in patients with multiple sclerosis: long-term follow-up. Stereotact Funct Neurosurg 80:48–55.
7. Hooper J, Taylor R, Pentland B, Whittle I (2002) A prospective study of thalamic deep brain stimulation for the treatment of movement disorders in multiple sclerosis. Brit J Neurosurg 16:102–109.
8. Berk C, Carr J, Sinden M, Martzke J, Honey C (2002) Thalamic deep brain stimulation for the treatment of tremor due to multiple sclerosis: a prospective study of tremor and quality of life. J Neurosurg 97:815–820.
9. Matsumoto J, Morrow D, Kaufman K, et al (2001) Surgical therapy for tremor in multiple sclerosis: an evaluation of outcome measures. Neurology 57:1876–1882.
10. Schulder M, Sernas T, Mahalick D, Adler R, Cook S (1999) Thalamic stimulation in patients with multiple sclerosis. Stereotact Funct Neurosurg 72:196–201.

11. Montgomery EBJ, Baker KB, Kinkel RP, Barnett G (1999) Chronic thalamic stimulation of the tremor of multiple sclerosis. Neurology 53:625–628.
12. Bittar R, Hyam J, Nandi D, et al (2005) Thalamotomy versus thalamic stimulation for multiple sclerosis tremor. J Clin Neurosci 12:638–642.
13. Schuurman P, Bosch D, Bossuyt P, et al (2000) A comparison of continuous thalamic stimulation and thalamotomy for suppression of severe tremor. N Engl J Med 342:461–468.
14. Patwardhan R, Minagar A, Kelley R, Nanda A (2006) Neurosurgical treatment of multiple sclerosis. Neurol Res 28:320–325.
15. Wishart H, Roberts D, Roth R, et al (2003) Chronic deep brain stimulation for the treatment of tremor in multiple sclerosis: review and case reports. J Neurol Neurosurg Psychiatry 74:1392–1397.
16. Tasker RR, Munz M, Junn F, et al (1997) Deep brain stimulation and thalamotomy for tremor compared. Acta Neurochir 68(Suppl):49–53.
17. Montgomery EBJ, Turkstra LS (2003) Evidenced based medicine: let's be reasonable. J Med Speech Lang Pathol 11:ix–xii.
18. Albin RL, Frey KA (2003) Initial agonist treatments in Parkinson disease: a critique. Neurology 62:390–394.
19. Montgomery EBJ (2003) Agonists versus levodopa in PD: the thrilla of whitha. Neurology 61:1462.
20. Albin RL, Frey KA (2003) Agonists versus levodopa in PD: the thrilla of whitha. Neurology 61:1462–1463.
21. Schultz W, Montgomery Jr EB, Marine R (1979) Proximal limb movements in response to microstimulation of primate dentate and interpositus nuclei mediated by brainstem structures. Brain 102:127–146.
22. Baker KB, Boulis NM, Rezai AR, Montgomery Jr EB (2004) Target selection using microelectrode recordings. In: Israel Z, Burchiel K, eds. Microelectrode Recordings in Movement Disorders Surgery. New York: Thieme Medical Press, pp. 138–151.
23. Katayama Y, Yamamoto T, Kobayashi K, Oshima H, Fukaya C (2003) Deep brain and motor cortex stimulation for post-stroke movement disorders and post-stroke pain. Acta Neurochir Suppl 87:121–123.
24. Martinez-Manas R, Rumia J, Valldeoriola F, Ferrer E, Tolosa E (2002) Thalamic neuro inhibition in the treatment of post traumatic tremor. Rev Neurol 34:258–261.
25. Umemura A, Samadani U, Jaggi JL, Hurtig HI, Baltuch GH (2004) Thalamic deep brain stimulation for posttraumatic action tremor. Clin Neurol Neurosurg 106:280–283.
26. Foote KD, Seignourel P, Fernandez HH, et al (2006) Dual electrode thalamic deep brain stimulation for the treatment of posttraumatic and multiple sclerosis tremor. Neurosurgery 58(4 Suppl 2):280–285.
27. Shimojima Y, Hashimoto T, Kaneko K, et al (2005) Thalamic stimulation for disabling tremor in a patient with spinocerebellar degeneration. Stereotact Funct Neurosurg 83:131–134.
28. Pirker W, Back C, Gerschlager W, Laccone F, Alesch F (2003) Chronic thalamic stimulation in a patient with spinocerebellar ataxia type 2. Mov Disord 18:222–225.
29. Schramm P, Scheihing M, Rasche D, Tronnier VM (2005) Behr syndrome variant with tremor treated by VIM stimulation. Acta Neurochirgica (Wien) 147:679–683.
30. Piette T, Mescola P, Henriet M, Cornil C, Jacquy J, Vanderkelen B (2004) A surgical approach to Holmes' tremor associated with high-frequency synchronous bursts. Rev Neurol (Paris) 160:707–711.
31. Nikkhah G, Prokop T, Hellwig B, Lucking CH, Ostertag CB (2004) Deep brain stimulation of the nucleus ventralis intermedius for Holmes (rubral) tremor and associated dystonia caused by upper brainstem lesions. Report of two cases. J Neurosurg 100:1079–1083.

32. Samadani U, Umemura A, Jaggi JL, Colcher A, Zager EL, Baltuch GH (2003) Thalamic deep brain stimulation for disabling tremor after excision of a midbrain cavernous angioma. Case report. J Neurosurg 98:888–890.
33. Pahwa R, Lyons KE, Kempf L, Wilkinson SB, Koller WC (2002) Thalamic stimulation for midbrain tremor after partial hemangioma resection. Mov Disord 17:404–407.
34. Ruzicka E, Jech R, Zarubova K, Roth J, Urgosik D (2003) VIM thalamic stimulation for tremor in a patient with IgM paraproteinaemic demyelinating neuropathy. Mov Disord 18:1192–1195.
35. Montgomery EBJ (2004) Deep brain stimulation for hyperkinetic disorders. Neurosurgical Focus 17:E1.
36. Brice J, McLellan L (1980) Suppression of intention tremor by contingent deep-brain stimulation. Lancet 1(8180):1221–1222.
37. Nguyen JP, Degos JD (1993) Thalamic stimulation and proximal tremor. A specific target in the nucleus ventrointermedius thalami. Arch Neurol 50:498–500.
38. Siegfried J, Lippitz B (1994) Chronic electrical stimulation of the VL-VPL complex and of the pallidum in the treatment of movement disorders: personal experience since 1982. Stereotact Funct Neurosurg 62:71–75.
39. Benabid AL, Pollak P, Gao D, et al (1996) Chronic electrical stimulation of the ventralis intermedius nucleus of the thalamus as a treatment of movement disorders. J Neurosurg 84:203–214.
40. Geny C, Nguyen JP, Pollin B, et al (1996) Improvement of severe postural cerebellar tremor in multiple sclerosis by chronic thalamic stimulation. Mov Disord 11:489–494.
41. Whittle IR, Hooper J, Pentland B (1998) Thalamic deep-brain stimulation for movement disorders due to multiple sclerosis. Lancet 10:109–110.
42. Hay SR (1999) Thalamic deep brain stimulation for treatment of visual symptoms in multiple sclerosis. Clin Eye Vision Care 11:121–131.
43. Taha JM, Janszen MA, Favre J (1999) Thalamic deep brain stimulation for the treatment of head, voice, and bilateral limb tremor. J Neurosurg 91:68–72.
44. Nandi D, Aziz TZ (2004) Deep brain stimulation in the management of neuropathic pain and multiple sclerosis tremor. J Clin Neurophysiol 21:31–39.
45. Herzog J, Hamel W, Wenzelburger R, et al (2007) Kinematic analysis of thalamic versus subthalamic neurostimulation in postural and intention tremor. Brain 130:1608–1625.

# 12
# Thalamic Deep Brain Stimulation for Parkinson's Disease Tremor

Daniel Tarsy, Efstathios Papavassiliou, Kelly E. Lyons, and Rajesh Pahwa

## Abstract

Thalamic deep brain stimulation (DBS) was introduced for the treatment of Parkinson's disease (PD) tremor and essential tremor (ET) in the late 1980s. Its remarkable success for these indications was followed by the introduction of DBS in other brain targets for the treatment of PD and dystonia. With the advent of subthalamic DBS for PD, the use of thalamic DBS for PD tremor has markedly declined. However, thalamic DBS is effective for PD tremor and remains a valid option in selected older patients with tremor predominant PD who do not have other disabling features of PD.

**Keywords:** tremor, Parkinson's disease, deep brain stimulation, DBS

## Introduction

Several nomenclatures have been used for nuclei of the motor thalamus (1–4). Hassler's terminology (1) is commonly used in the current clinical movement disorders literature. The motor thalamus lies ventrally and anterior to posterior, consists of the lateral polaris (Lpo), which receives input from the globus pallidus interna (GPi) and substantia nigra pars reticulata (SNr); the ventralis oralis anterior (Voa) and ventral oralis posterior (Vop), which receive input from the GPi; and the ventral intermediate nucleus (VIM), which receives input from the cerebellum and lemniscal system (5). The relative contribution of cerebellar and lemniscal inputs to the VIM is uncertain and depends in part on whether human or monkey data are used (5). The ventralis caudalis (Vc) lies posterior to motor thalamus and receives lemniscal and spinothalamic sensory input. In the Anglo-American nomenclature, the ventral anterior (VA) nucleus includes Lpo and Voa; the ventrolateral nucleus (VL) includes Vop and VIM; and the ventral posterior nucleus is equivalent to Vc.

Microelectrode recordings obtained during stereotactic surgery have identified thalamic neurons that burst at a frequency identical to the patient's tremor frequency (6). These are located in the ventral motor thalamus but also in other thalamic nuclei, medial GPi, putamen, caudate, and subthalamic nucleus (STN). In the thalamus, these have been particularly well studied in Vc, VIM, Voa, and Vop where they correlate with electromyographic recordings of tremor *(7)*. Subsequently, VIM has been accepted as the target of choice for the treatment of tremor *(8)*. Neuronal bursts in VIM also occur in response to active or passive movement of small joints *(9, 10)*. Intra-operative identification of these movement sensitive neurons has been helpful in locating thalamic sites for optimal placement of surgical lesions or stimulating electrodes for the treatment of tremor. Surgical ablation and high-frequency stimulation of areas in the VIM that contain "tremor cells" successfully abolish tremor. However, the pathophysiologic role of these "tremor cells" in causing tremor is uncertain because similar tremor bursts are identified in the GPi *(11)* and STN *(12)* and lesions in those areas also abolish tremor.

Before the introduction of levodopa, thalamotomy was the most common surgical procedure for the treatment of PD tremor. This was because of its lower morbidity compared with pallidotomy and striking benefit for tremor. However, evaluation of surgical results was typically qualitative rather than quantitative and controlled studies comparing procedures were not carried out in that era. The surgical target for thalamotomy was usually VIM but sometimes included Vop for control of rigidity. After pharmacologic treatment became available for PD and ET, medication-resistant tremors continued to provide a valid indication for thalamotomy *(13)*. Unilateral thalamotomy produced long-term effective treatment of contralateral tremor in up to 85% of patients but with a high incidence of transient complications lasting up to 3 months in as many as 60% of patients and a lower but substantial incidence of permanent complications, especially involving speech, in up to 23% of treated patients *(14)*.

## DBS

DBS has been a novel and rapidly expanding method for treatment of PD *(15, 16)*. Three targets have been used in PD: VIM, GPi, and STN. In the 1960s, intra-operative stimulation was used to identify VIM just before creating an ablative lesion. Low-frequency stimulation was known to activate or drive tremor while high-frequency stimulation in the same location suppressed tremor *(17–19)*. This technique was used during surgery to identify the proper site for thalamic lesioning *(19–21)*. The high frequency of adverse effects associated with bilateral thalamotomy motivated Benabid et al. to perform the first implantations of thalamic stimulators for the treatment of parkinsonian and ET *(21, 22)*. Benabid et al. carefully studied the effect of varying pulse frequency, current intensity, pulse width, polarity, and pulse duration on tremor control. Because of the dramatic efficacy and safety of thalamic DBS, the use of DBS in other brain targets such as GPi and STN was subsequently explored to control other parkinsonian symptoms.

## Thalamic Stimulation for Tremor in PD

### Background

Although tremor is often a major and very visible feature of PD, in most patients it is not necessarily a disabling symptom. Historically, the experience of thalamotomy was that even after successful alleviation of tremor, patients were often left with functional disability due to persistent bradykinesia, which was unrelieved by the procedure. However, in some cases, PD tremor is disabling, especially if there is a significant postural or kinetic component which interferes with manual activity. Some disabling postural tremors in PD, such as re-emergent tremor *(23)*, are easily overlooked because they do not appear until a new position of the hand has been assumed for several seconds.

Adverse effects on speech and cognitive function associated with thalamotomy motivated a search for alternative approaches for surgical treatment of tremor. Historically, chronic thalamic stimulation had already been used for the treatment of chronic pain. Andy *(20)* suggested that chronic thalamic stimulation might be preferable to ablation for treatment of tremor, especially in elderly, poor-risk patients. He implanted chronic electrodes and stimulated at 50 to 125 Hz in several thalamic nuclei in nine patients with a variety of motor disorders. He treated five patients with parkinsonian tremor, three of whom were targeted in VIM *(20)*. In most cases, stimulation was limited to 30 to 60 minutes three or four times daily but three patients underwent continuous stimulation. Results in PD tremor were "fair to excellent" but duration of follow-up was unstated. Siegfried and Lippitz *(24)* carried out VIM DBS in 40 patients with PD tremor, most of whom had undergone previous contralateral thalamotomy. Twenty-nine experienced complete tremor control. Tasker *(25)* also reported on chronic thalamic stimulation at 60 Hz in a small number of patients, one of whom had parkinsonian tremor, but with poor and short-lived results.

Benabid and his colleagues studied VIM stimulation further and concluded that it could be used as chronic therapy in patients with PD or ET who had previously undergone contralateral thalamotomy in order to avoid the potential adverse effects of bilateral thalamotomy. In their initial report, six patients with PD with previous thalamotomy were implanted in contralateral VIM *(22)* and stimulated at up to 130 Hz. Three patients were greatly improved and were connected to permanent stimulators thereby inaugurating the era of DBS for the long-term treatment of movement disorders. VIM DBS has also been extensively used for treatment of medication-resistant ET, which is primarily a postural or kinetic tremor and therefore more disabling than most parkinsonian tremors. Numerous studies have been carried out documenting the effect of VIM DBS in ET involving the extremities, head, and voice *(21, 26–36)*, which are not reviewed in this chapter but have been reviewed in detail elsewhere *(37, 38)*.

**Patient Selection**

Proper patient selection is crucial for the successful surgical treatment of movement disorders in general and PD tremor in particular. General requirements for stereotactic surgery in PD include good general health, ability to undergo and cooperate with the demands of stereotactic surgery while awake, no uncontrolled psychiatric or behavioral disorder, and no significant dementia. In the case of DBS, patients must be willing and able to return for reprogramming of the implantable pulse generator. VIM DBS should be considered for treatment of PD tremor if it is the major disabling feature of the disease, has a significant re-emergent or action component that interferes with activities of daily living, is refractory to pharmacologic treatment and is unilateral. Importantly, unlike medication-resistant bradykinesia or rigidity, medication refractory PD tremor does respond to VIM DBS. Bradykinesia, rigidity, and postural instability should be minor or absent. Similar to thalamotomy, VIM DBS improves rigidity only slightly and has no effect on bradykinesia or gait disorder. A particular advantage for VIM DBS in this setting is that advanced age is not an absolute contraindication because it is a simpler and shorter procedure than GPi or STN DBS as it does not require microelectrode recording, requires fewer postoperative programming visits, and is less likely to cause adverse cognitive effects.

### The Problem of Progressive Parkinsonism After Thalamic DBS for Tremor

Because GPi and STN DBS also effectively suppress PD tremor, the role of VIM DBS for this indication has declined, especially if other signs of PD are prominent *(38, 39)*. However, the question remains as to whether VIM DBS should still be considered an appropriate consideration for patients with stable tremor-dominant PD who lack significant bradykinesia, rigidity, or gait disturbance. The answer to this question relies on the natural progression of PD following VIM DBS. Lyons et al. *(40)* followed nine PD patients for a mean of 40 months after unilateral VIM DBS. Tremor remained significantly improved compared to the baseline on-medication condition but Unified Parkinson's Disease Rating Scale (UPDRS) motor scores at the longest follow-up with stimulation were not different from baseline on-medication scores. Several patients became significantly disabled because of their other parkinsonian symptoms and five patients required additional surgical procedures to maintain good tremor control. Tarsy et al. *(41)* followed nine patients with tremor-dominant PD for a mean of 5.5 years after VIM DBS (five unilateral; four bilateral), three of whom had tremor-dominant PD. Tremor suppression improved and remained stable without significantly increased akinesia, rigidity, or gait disturbance. However, there was a significant increase in levodopa and dopamine agonist dose requirement and a global assessment of PD progression showed moderate worsening *(41)*. In a 5-year follow-up study *(42)* of the North American multicenter trial of VIM DBS for essential and parkinsonian tremor *(26)*, 15 of 19 patients with PD were followed for 5 years. Significant bradykinesia and rigidity were present in addition to severe tremor. With stimulation, tremor was improved by at least 82% at 5 years compared to baseline. Rehncrona et al. *(43)* followed 16 patients with tremor-dominant PD for 2 years and 12 patients for 6 to 7 years after unilateral VIM DBS. Tremor was equally suppressed at 2 and 6 to 7 years after surgery, while UPDRS motor scores and mean levodopa intake were significantly increased at 6 to 7 years with stimulators off. Putzke et al. *(44)* followed 23 patients with tremor-dominant PD for a mean period of 18.7 months following unilateral or bilateral VIM DBS. Tremor control was stable. Although UPDRS was not recorded, mean levodopa equivalent daily dose did not increase. These follow-up studies are limited because only two *(43, 44)* were limited to patients with tremor-dominant PD and follow-up motor assessments were usually carried out while patients were on medication, potentially masking signs of progressive parkinsonism.

### The Importance of Tremor in PD

Tremor is one of the more obvious and visible features of PD; however, it is generally not as functionally disabling as other parkinsonian features. This is because PD tremor is usually present when the affected limb is at rest and suppresses during voluntary movements. In this situation, severe resting tremor may therefore be more of a cosmetic than functional concern. In some individuals, this may still constitute a valid indication for surgery, such as the actively employed individual who feels self-conscious socially or in his workplace because of tremor. In some patients there is a significant component of postural or re-emergent tremor in addition to the rest tremor that does, in fact, disturb motor function *(23)*. Bilateral VIM DBS for PD is generally not recommended due to adverse effects on speech and balance that may already be present in PD *(32)*. Therefore, PD patients with bilateral tremor being considered for DBS should undergo STN DBS.

Although it was initially reported that VIM DBS is more effective for distal than proximal tremor *(21, 45)*, uniform benefits for rest, kinetic, distal postural, and proximal postural tremor have also been demonstrated in PD *(27, 46)*. Lower limb, midline, and even ipsilateral resting tremor may also be relieved in some patients *(27)*. If lower extremity tremor is the principle indication for VIM DBS a more lateral site in VIM may need to be chosen for electrode implantation *(47)*.

Severity, distribution, and type of tremor should be documented by use of standard tremor rating scales such as the UPDRS motor scale *(48)* and Tremor Rating Scale *(49)*, supplemented by standard tasks such as writing, drawing a spiral, drawing a straight line between lines, and pouring water from one cup to another *(26)*. Tremor severity in operated patients has typically been 3 to 4 out of 4 in the UPDRS tremor subscale, moderate to marked and present most of the time.

## Results of VIM DBS for Treatment of Tremor in PD

In the early report by Benabid et al. *(21)* of VIM DBS for tremor, 26 patients with disabling PD tremor were implanted, 21 of whom had undergone no previous neurosurgery. Eight patients underwent bilateral VIM DBS implanted simultaneously. A Radionics 2.3-mm diameter electrode was used initially and later switched to a Medtronic 1.2-mm diameter electrode. The correct target was determined to be where stimulation at 100 Hz or higher suppressed tremor with the lowest possible voltage. Stimulation at lower frequencies either had no effect or aggravated the tremor. Electrodes were connected to an extension lead externalized over the scalp and test stimulation was carried out over at least 1 week. Once stimulation effects were deemed satisfactory, a programmable stimulator, the Medtronic Itrel I or Itrel II, was implanted in the subclavicular region and stimulation was maintained at 130 Hz. Contralateral upper limb tremor was totally suppressed in 23 and markedly improved in nine cases out of 34 thalami stimulated. Similar to the effects of thalamotomy, rigidity was slightly improved but there was no effect on akinesia. A microlesion effect lasting for 1 to 10 days occurred in some patients. Adverse effects were mild and stimulation-related including limb or face paresthesia, limb dystonia, and dysmetria. Dysarthria and gait disequilibrium occurred in six patients, five of whom had either bilateral DBS or a previous thalamotomy, and could be controlled by reducing the intensity of one or both stimulators.

Subsequent studies by Benabid and colleagues *(31, 33, 50)* involving up to 91 patients with PD documented improvement for up to at least 3 to 6 months postoperatively. There was good to excellent tremor suppression in 88% of PD patients. Resting tremor was better controlled than postural or action tremor, distal better than proximal or axial tremor, and upper better than lower extremity tremor *(45)*. Stimulation voltage had to be increased over the first several weeks following surgery, likely because of increases in tissue impedance. There was a subsequent need to increase stimulus voltage to control action tremor in some patients, more commonly in ET than PD. This was attributed to tolerance, possibly supported by the rebound increase in tremor which occurred in some patients when the stimulator was turned off. However, despite the observation of rebound tremor, tolerance evidenced by reduced clinical effect or need for increased stimulus voltage, has been reported in some *(51)* but not all studies *(22, 41)*.

Subsequent studies with more prolonged follow-up have confirmed the beneficial therapeutic effect of VIM DBS on PD tremor, which, similar to earlier studies, has been effective in approximately 90% of patients *(26, 29, 40, 41, 46, 52–54)*. In most studies, PD patients have had tremor predominant forms of PD. In the North American prospective multicenter trial, 24 PD patients were implanted with VIM thalamic stimulators and were evaluated using a double-blind assessment at 3 months and open follow-up assessments at 6, 9, and 12 months following surgery *(26)*. There was a statistically significant and clinically dramatic decrease in contralateral tremor compared to baseline with total resolution of tremor in 14 of 24 PD patients. However, by contrast with ET patients in the same study, functional activities of daily living (ADLs) such as handwriting, dressing, and cutting food were not improved, likely due to lack of improvement in parkinsonian bradykinesia. A single center study of 19 patients using similar methodology and examiner-blinded assessment at 3 months produced similar results with regard to both tremor and ADLs *(29)*. A European prospective multicenter trial (13 sites) assessed 73 PD patients in an unblinded fashion for 12 months following surgery *(30)*. There was a significant decrease in contralateral tremor, which was similar in magnitude to the North American trial. However, by contrast with the North American trial, ADLs were improved in the European study. Other studies have confirmed that subjective global disability ratings improve similarly in PD patients compared with ET patients *(46, 55)*. Although tremor is clearly improved and most studies have shown improved ADLs following VIM DBS, quality-of-life measures have not been extensively studied following VIM DBS *(56)* by contrast with effects on quality of life after other surgical treatments of PD *(57)*.

In one multicenter trial, VIM stimulation appeared to improve contralateral akinesia in addition to tremor *(30)*. However, akinesia was mild preoperatively, may have been difficult to assess in the presence of severe tremor, and very likely appeared to improve postoperatively due to improved tremor. In other studies, akinesia has shown little or no change following VIM DBS *(27, 28, 33)*. Gait and balance in PD patients have shown only minor and inconsistent improvement *(58–60)*. In one study, levodopa-induced dyskinesia was improved following thalamic DBS in five affected patients *(28, 61)*, but subsequent analysis of thalamic stimulation sites concluded that effects on dyskinesia were more likely due to more medial and deeper electrode placement closer to the centromedian and parafascicular nuclei *(62)*.

## Adverse Effects of VIM DBS

Adverse effects associated with VIM DBS in short-term studies have been related to regional effects of stimulation, hardware-related complications, and neurological consequences of intracerebral electrode implantation.

### *Regional Effects of Stimulation*

In Benabid et al.'s early reports *(21)*, adverse effects were mild and limited to stimulation effects such as paresthesia, limb dystonia, and dysmetria, which could be controlled by stimulation adjustment. Dysarthria and gait disequilibrium were uncommon and nearly always limited to patients receiving bilateral stimulation or those that had undergone previous contralateral thalamotomy. Paresthesia is a very common and expected adverse effect, occurring in 13 to 27% of PD patients *(42)*. It is nearly always limited to several seconds after the IPG is turned on and is due to the spread of current to Vc, the thalamic sensory receiving immediately posterior to VIM. Dysmetria and gait disequilibrium are attributable to DBS effects on Vop, the pallidal receiving nucleus immediately anterior to VIM. The incidence of serious paresthesia was only 2.5% in the Medtronic clinical investigation of DBS for tremor *(63)*. The higher frequency of dysarthria, dysmetria, and disequilibrium in patients undergoing bilateral VIM DBS has been documented *(32, 41)* and is more common in patients with PD than ET *(42)*. Although these adverse effects can usually be managed by adjustments in stimulator parameters, tremor suppression on at least one side of the body may become compromised as a result *(32)*.

### *Hardware-Related Complications*

Recently, longer-term studies following DBS have shown a higher incidence of hardware complications than occurred in previous shorter-term studies *(64, 65)*. Oh et al. *(64)* reported a 33-month retrospective study of 79 patients with 124 electrode implants, 38 of which were in thalamus. Overall, 25.3% of patients had hardware-related complications including lead fractures, lead migrations, open circuits, erosions and/or infections, foreign body reactions, and cerebrospinal fluid leaks. The hardware-related complication rate per electrode year was 8.4% and many occurred as late complications, possibly explaining the lower rates of hardware complications reported in shorter-term studies. Joint et al. *(65)* prospectively studied their experience over 3 years and reported a 20% occurrence rate of hardware-related problems in 49 operated patients with 79 implants, 14 of which were in thalamus. These included lead fractures, lead erosion, IPG malfunction, and lead misplacement. Useful references providing detailed methodology for troubleshooting hardware complications are available *(66, 67)* and are discussed elsewhere in this book. DBS technology is rapidly evolving and procedural and equipment modifications such as moving the electrode connector away from the cervical region to the scalp, use of low profile connectors, and use of microplate and screw fixation at the burr hole instead of a silicone burr ring and cap may reduce hardware complications *(27, 68)*, although a more recent survey showed a 13.9% incidence of hardware-related complications *(68)*. In an autopsy study of six PD patients with thalamic DBS, pathological examination up to 70 months following electrode implantation showed only a thin inner capsule of connective tissue and mild fibrillary gliosis around the lead track and active contact electrode *(69)*. Explantation of the intracerebral electrode is only occasionally necessary and is indicated in the presence of active infection or skin erosion unresponsive to medical management or skin grafting. If explantation should be required but reimplantation is not feasible, limited experience suggests it may be possible to generate a permanent thalamotomy using the DBS electrode to create a radiofrequency lesion prior to its removal (69, 70).

*Neurologic Adverse Effects*
Transient mild postoperative headache is common and attributable to the stereotaxic frame and skull fixation bolts. Intra-operative focal or generalized seizures are uncommon and not more frequent than during other stereotactic neurosurgical procedures. Permanent neurologic adverse effects of VIM DBS are uncommon. The most potentially serious neurologic adverse effect is intracranial hemorrhage. Benabid and coworkers (33) reported six intracerebral microhematomas in 177 operations, three of which were symptomatic. The incidence of documented intracranial hemorrhage was 2% in the North American and 5% in the European trials (26, 30). The incidence of intracranial hemorrhage among 266 patients in the Medtronic clinical investigation of DBS treatment of tremor was 2.6% (63). Hemorrhages include subdural and intracerebral hematomas. Many intracerebral hematomas are asymptomatic, may be limited to a region along the electrode tract, and are discovered only by postoperative brain imaging. There was only one immediate postoperative death among 266 patients enrolled in the Medtronic clinical trial of DBS for treatment of tremor (63). Detailed neuropsychological testing has shown no significant change in cognitive function following thalamic stimulation (56, 71, 72), although mild deficits in verbal fluency have been documented (33, 73).

## VIM DBS Compared With Thalamotomy

Speech and cognitive deficits and tremor recurrence rates of 4 to 22% following thalamotomy (74) motivated Benabid and colleagues to consider VIM DBS a potentially safer treatment for PD (33). Increasing thalamotomy size to prevent recurrence only served to increase the frequency of neurologic morbidity (75). It has been suggested that VIM DBS is less helpful for rigidity and levodopa-induced dyskinesia than VIM thalamotomy (76). This is likely because historically aggressive ablative lesions often included the Vop in addition to the VIM. There is universal agreement that neither procedure significantly improves akinesia.

There have been relatively few head to head studies comparing VIM DBS and thalamotomy. In a retrospective, non-randomized study, Tasker (47) compared 16 PD patients who underwent VIM DBS with 23 PD patients who underwent thalamotomy. Follow-up was more than 1 year in 60% of patients. Clinical outcome was assessed in an unblinded fashion using a semiquantitative scale. Outcomes were similar in the two groups with complete abolition of contralateral tremor in 42% of both groups and virtually complete abolition of tremor in 79% of VIM DBS patients and 69% of thalamotomy patients. Tremor recurred in 5% of VIM DBS cases and 15% of thalamotomy cases. No VIM DBS case required repeat surgery while 23% of thalamotomy cases had to be repeated in order to achieve a satisfactory response. Preoperative levodopa-induced dyskinesia improved in one-half of patients in each group. The major difference between the two groups was in complication rates.

Intracerebral hemorrhage occurred in 4% of the thalamotomy cases and in none of the VIM DBS cases. Permanent ataxia occurred in 15% and permanent paresthesia in 34% of thalamotomy cases. By contrast, stimulation induced ataxia and paresthesia occurred in 5% and 47% of VIM DBS cases respectively but could be alleviated by programming adjustments in all cases. Modern studies of unilateral thalamotomy have shown little postoperative cognitive change *(76)*.

There is only one published prospective, randomized study comparing VIM and thalamotomy in patients with PD *(77)*. In this study, which also included patients with ET and multiple sclerosis, 22 patients with PD were assigned to VIM DBS and 23 to thalamotomy. The follow-up period was 2 years but the main analyses were carried out at 6 months. Outcomes were assessed in an unblinded fashion using an ADL scale, a subjective patient assessment of functional status, and several tremor rating scales. In PD patients, improvement in ADL scores was significantly greater following VIM DBS than thalamotomy. Improvement in PD tremor was similar in the two treatment groups but adverse events were much more common in the thalamotomy group. Tremor was suppressed completely in 20 of 21 VIM DBS cases compared with 20 of 23 thalamotomy cases. Adverse effects were nearly all stimulator related in the VIM DBS cases except for one case each of hematoma, infection at the IPG site, and intracerebral hemorrhage. By contrast, permanent adverse effects occurred in 16 of 23 PD patients undergoing thalamotomy including cognitive deterioration, dysarthria, gait or balance disturbance, and arm ataxia. Neuropsychological outcomes were not reported in this study.

## Conclusions

VIM DBS is highly effective for the treatment of resting or postural tremor in PD. It is safer than thalamotomy and can be carried out bilaterally with less risk for speech or gait impairment than thalamotomy. According to the only available prospective randomized study, *(77)* it is also more effective for restoring upper extremity function than thalamotomy. Nearly all adverse effects such as paresthesia, dysmetria, gait disturbance, and dysarthria are transient stimulation effects and can be managed by altering stimulation parameters. Serious infectious complications such as meningitis and brain abcess have been exceedingly rare and no long-term tissue damage around the electrodes has been reported. Although hardware problems such as lead fractures, lead migration, skin erosions, scalp infection, infection at the IPG site, and IPG failure have been uncommon in short-term follow-up studies, they have occurred in up to 27% of patients *(68)* in recent longer-term studies. As discussed earlier, new procedural and technical advances have begin to reduce the frequency of these hardware complications.

In PD patients, the only indication for VIM DBS is control of unilateral, functionally disabling tremor that has failed medical management. Patients with disabling, tremor-dominant PD with stable or very slowly progressive akinesia may be potentially good candidates for thalamic DBS, particularly if they are frail or elderly patients who may not tolerate STN or GPi DBS. If PD appears to be progressive and disability is due to bradykinesia, gait disturbance, motor fluctuations, or levodopa-induced dyskinesia, STN or GPi DBS rather than VIM DBS are more appropriate.

*Acknowledgements*: We appreciate the support of the Olender Foundation, the Grand Circle Foundation, and the assistance of Patricia Ryan, Lisa Scollins, Linda Paul, Dawn Mechanic, Kristin Corapi, Siobhan O' Herron, and Shannon Donovan.

## References

1. Hassler R (1959) Introduction to Stereotaxis with an Atlas of the Human Brain. Stuttgart: Thieme.
2. Walker AE (1982) Normal and pathological physiology of the human thalamus. In: Schaltenbrand G, Walker AE, eds. Stereotaxy of the Human Brain: Anatomical, Physiological, and Clinical Applications. Stuttgart: Thieme, pp. 181–217.
3. Jones EG (1990) Correlation and revised nomenclature of ventral nuclei in the thalamus of human and monkey. Stereotact Funct Neurosurg 54/55:1–20.
4. Hirai T, Jones EG (1989) A new parcellation of the human thalamus on the basis of histochemical staining. Brain Res Rev 14:1–34.
5. Krack P, Dostrovsky J, Ilinsky I, Kultas-Ilinsky K, Lenz F, Lozano A, Vitek J (2002) Surgery of the motor thalamus: problems with the present nomenclatures. Mov Disord 17 (Suppl 3):S2–S8.
6. Albe-Fessard D, Arfel G, Guiot G (1962) Activities electriques characteristiques de quelques structures cerebrales chez l'homme. Ann Chir 17:1185–1214.
7. Lenz FA, Tasker RR, Kwan HC, et al (1988) Single unit analysis of the human ventral thalamic nuclear group: correlation of thalamic "tremor cells" with the 3–6 Hz component of parkinsonian tremor. J Neuroscience 8:754–764.
8. Hua SE, Garonzik IM, Lee JI, Lenz FA (2003) Thalamotomy for tremor. In: Tarsy D, Lozano AM, Vitek JL, eds. Surgical Treatment of Parkinson's Disease and Other Movement Disorders. Totowa, NJ: Humana Press, pp. 99–113.
9. Ohye C, Narabayashi H (1979) Physiological study of presumed ventralis intermedius neurons in the human thalamus. J Neurosurg 50:290–297.
10. Lenz FA, Kwan HC, Dostrovsky JO, Tasker RR, Murphy JT, Lenz YE (1990) Single unit analysis of the human ventral thalamic nuclear group. Brain 113:1795–1821.
11. Hutchison WD, Lozano AM, Tasker RR, Lang AE, Dostrovsky JO (1997) Identification and characterization of neurons with tremor-frequency activity in human globus pallidus. Exp Brain Res 113:557–563.
12. Bergman NH, Wichmann T, Karmon B, DeLong MR (1994) The primate subthalamic nucleus: II. Neuronal activity in the MPTP model of parkinsonism. J Neurophysiol 72:507–520.
13. Kelly PJ, Gillingham FJ (1980) The long-term results of stereotaxic surgery and L-dopa therapy in patients with Parkinson's disease. J Neurosurg 53:332–337.
14. Hallett M, Litvan I (1999) A task force on surgery for Parkinson's eisease. Evaluation of surgery for Parkinson's disease. Neurology 53:1910–1921.
15. Starr PA, Vitak JL, Bakay RAE (1998) Deep brain stimulation for movement disorders. Neurosurg Clin N Am 9:381–402.
16. Obeso JA, Benabid AL, Koller WC (2000) Deep brain stimulation for Parkinson's disease and tremor. Neurology 55(suppl 6):S1–S66.
17. Hassler R, Riechart T, Munginer F, et al (1960) Physiological observations in stereotaxic operations in extrapyramidal motor disturbances. Brain 83: 337–350.
18. Ohye C, Kubota K, Hooper HE, et al (1964) Ventrolateral and subventrolateral thalamic stimulation. Arch Neurol 11:427–434.
19. Cooper IS, Upton ARM, Amin I (1980) Reversibility of chronic neurologic deficits. Some effects of electrical stimulation of the thalamus and internal capsule in man. Appl Neurophysiol 43:244–258.

20. Andy OJ (1983) Thalamic stimulation for control of movement disorders. Appl Neurophysiol 46:107–111.
21. Benabid AL, Pollak P, Gervason C, et al (1991) Long-term suppression of tremor by chronic stimulation of the ventral intermediate thalamic nucleus. Lancet 337:403–406.
22. Benabid AL, Pollak P, Loveau A, Henry S, Rougemont J (1987) Combined (thalamotomy and stimulation) stereotactic surgery of the VIM thalamic nucleus for bilateral Parkinson disease. Appl Neurophysiol 50:344–346.
23. Jankovic J, Schwartz KS, Ondo W (1999) Re-emergent tremor of Parkinson's disease. J Neurol Neurosurg Psychiatry 67:646–650.
24. Siegfried J, Lippitz B (1994) Chronic electrical stimulation of the VL-VPL complex and of the pallidum in the treatment of movement disorders: personal experience since 1982. Stereotact Funct Neurosurg 62:71–75.
25. Tasker RR (1986) Effets sensitifs et moteurs de la stimulation thalamique chez l'homme. Applications Cliniques. Rev Neurol 142:316–326.
26. Koller W, Pahwa R, Busenbark K, Hubble J, Wilkinson S, Lang A, Tuite P, Sime E, Lozano A, Hauser R, Malapira T, Smith D, Tarsy D, Miyawaki E, Norregaard T, Kormos T, Olanow CW (1997) High-frequency unilateral thalamic stimulation in the treatment of essential and parkinsonian tremor. Ann Neurol 42:292–299.
27. Obwegeser AA, Uitti RJ, Witte RJ, Lucas JA, Turk MF, Wharen Jr RE (2001) Quantitative and qualitative outcome measures after thalamic deep brain stimulation to treat disabling tremors. Neurosurgery 48:274–284.
28. Blond S, Caparros-Lefebvre D, Parker F, et al (1992) Control of tremor and involuntary movement disorders by chronic stereotactic stimulation of the ventral intermediate thalamic nucleus. J Neurosurg 77:62–68.
29. Ondo W, Jankovic J, Schwartz K, et al (1998) Unilateral thalamic deep brain stimulation for refractory essential tremor and Parkinson's disease tremor. Neurology 51:1063–1069.
30. Limousin P, Speelman JD, Gielen F, et al (1999) Multicentre European study of thalamic stimulation in parkinsonian and essential tremor. J Neurol Neurosurg Psychiatry 66:289–296.
31. Benabid AL, Pollak P, Siegneuret E, Hoffmann D, Gay E, Perret J (1993) Chronic VIM thalamic stimulation in Parkinson's disease, essential tremor, and extrapyramidal dyskinesias. Acta Neurochir 58(suppl):39–44.
32. Ondo W, Almaguer M, Jankovic J, Simpson RK (2001) Thalamic deep brain stimulation. Comparison between unilateral and bilateral placement. Arch Neurol 58:218–232.
33. Benabid AL, Pollak P, Gao D, et al (1996) Chronic electrical stimulation of the ventralis intermedius nucleus of the thalamus as a treatment of movement disorders. J Neurosurg 84:203–214.
34. Hubble JP, Busenbark KL, Wilkinson S, Penn RD, Lyons K, Koller WC (1996) Deep brain stimulation for essential tremor. Neurology 46:1150–1153.
35. Taha JM, Janszen MA, Favre J (1999) Thalamic deep brain stimulation for the treatment of head, voice, and bilateral limb tremor. J Neurosurg 91:68–72.
36. Carpenter MA, Pahwa R, Miyawaki KL, Wilkinson SB, Seral JP, Koller WC (1998) Reduction in voice tremor under thalamic stimulation. Neurology 50:796–798.
37. Deuschl G, Bain P (2002) Deep brain stimulation for tremor: patient selection and evaluation. Mov Disord 17(Suppl 3):S102–S111.
38. Tarsy D, Norregaard T, Hubble J (2003) Thalamic deep brain stimulation for Parkinson's disease and essential tremor. In: Tarsy D, Lozano AM, Vitek JL, eds. Surgical Treatment of Parkinson's Disease and Other Movement Disorders. Totowa, NJ: Humana Press, pp. 153–161.
39. Krack P, Benazzouz A, Pollak P, Limousin P, Piallat B, Hoffmann D. Xie J, Benabid AL (1998) Treatment of tremor in Parkinson's disease by subthalamic nucleus stimulation. Mov Disord 13:907–914.

40. Lyons KE, Koller WC, Wilkinson SB, Pahwa R (2001) Long term safety and efficacy of unilateral deep brain stimulation of the thalamus for Parkinson tremor. J Neurol Neurosurg Psychiatry 71:682–684.
41. Tarsy D, Scollins L, Corapi K, O'Herron S, Apetauerova D, Norregaard T (2005) Progression of Parkinson's disease following thalamic deep brain stimulation for tremor. Stereotact Funct Neurosurg 83:222–227.
42. Pahwa R, Lyons K, Wilkinson SB, et al (2006) Long-term evaluation of deep brain stimulation of the thalamus. J Neurosurg 104:506–512.
43. Rehncrona S, Johnels B, Widner H et al (2001) Long-term safety and efficacy of thalamic deep brain stimulation of the thalamus for parkinsonian tremor. J Neurol Neurosurg Psychiatry 71:682–684.
44. Putzke JD, Wharen RE Jr, Wszolek ZK, et al (2003) Thalamic deep brain stimulation for tremor-predominant Parkinson's disease. Parkinsonism Relat Disord 10:81–88.
45. Benabid AL, Benazzouz A, Hoffmann D, Limousin P, Krack P, Pollak P (1998) Long-term electrical stimulation of deep brain targets in movement disorders. Mov Disord 13 (suppl 3):119–125.
46. Hubble JP, Busenbark KL, Wilkinson S, et al (1997) Effects of thalamic deep brain stimulation based on tremor type and diagnosis. Mov Disord 12:337–341.
47. Tasker RR (1998) Deep brain stimulation is preferable to thalamotomy for tremor suppression. Surg Neurol 49:145–154.
48. Fahn S, Elton RL (1987) Unified rating scale for Parkinson's disease. In: Fahn S, Marsden CD, eds. Recent Developments in Parkinson's Disease. Florham Park, NY: Macmillan, pp. 153–163, 293–304.
49. Fahn S, Tolosa E, Marin C (1993) Clinical rating scale for tremor. In: Jankovic J, Tolosa E, eds. Parkinson's Disease and Movement Disorders, second edition. Baltimore: Williams & Wilkins, pp. 225–234.
50. Benabid AL, Benazzouz A, Gao D, et al (1999) Chronic electrical stimulation of the ventralis intermedius nucleus of the thalamus and of other nuclei as a treatment for Parkinson's disease. Tech Neurosurg 5:5–30.
51. Hariz MI, Shamsgovara P, Johansson F, Hariz GM, Fodstad H (1999) Tolerance and tremor rebound following long-term chronic thalamic stimulation for parkinsonian and essential tremor. Stereotact Funct Neurosurg 72:208–218.
52. Blond S, Siegfried J (1991) Thalamic stimulation for the treatment of tremor and other movement disorders. Acta Neurochirurgica Suppl 52:109–111.
53. Albanese A, Nordera GP, Caraceni T, et al (1999) Longterm ventralis intermedius thalamic stimulation for parkinsonian tremor. Italian Registry for Neuromodulation in Movement disorders. Adv Neurol 80:631–634.
54. Pollak P, Benabid AL, Limousin P, Benazzouz A (1997) Chronic intracerebral stimulation in Parkinson's disease. Adv. Neurol 74:213–220.
55. Hariz GM, Bergenheim AT, Hariz MI, Lindberg M (1998) Assessment of ability/disability in patients treated with chronic thalamic stimulation for tremor. Mov Disord 13:78–83.
56. Troster AI, Fields JA (2003) The role of neuropsychological evaluation in the neurosurgical treatment of movement disorders. In: Tarsy D, Lozano AM, Vitek JL, eds. Surgical Treatment of Parkinson's Disease and Other Movement Disorders. Totowa: Humana Press, pp. 213–240.
57. Gray A, McNamara I, Aziz T, Gregory R, Bain P, Wilson J, Scott R (2002) Quality of life outcomes following surgical treatment of Parkinson's disease. Mov Disord 17:68–75.
58. Burleigh AL, Horak FB, Burchiel JK, Nutt JG (1993) Effects of thalamic stimulation on tremor, balance, and step initiation. A single subject study. Mov Disord 8:519–524.
59. Defebvre L, Blatt JL, Blond S, et al (1996) Effect of thalamic stimulation in Parkinson disease. Arch Neurol 53:898–903.

60. Pinter MM, Murg M, Alesch F, et al (1999) Does deep brain stimulation of the nucleus ventralis intermedius affect postural control and locomotion in Parkinson's disease? Mov Disord 14:958–963.
61. Caparros-Lefebvre D, Blond S, Vermersch P, et al (1993) Chronic thalamic stimulation improves tremor and levodopa-induced dyskinesias in Parkinson's disease. J Neurol Neurosurg Psychiatry 56:268–273.
62. Caparros-Lefebvre D, Blond S, Feltin MP, Pollak P, Benabid AL (1999) Improvement of levodopa induced dyskinesias by thalamic deep brain stimulation as related to slight variation in electrode placement: possible involvement of the centre median and parafascicularis complex. J Neurol Neurosurg Psychiatry 67:308–314.
63. Medtronic, Inc (2002) Deep brain stimulation for the treatment of tremor using the Medtronic Model 3387 DBS™ lead and the Itrel® II Model 7424 implantable pulse generator. Final Report.
64. Oh MY, Abosch A, Kim SH, Lang AE, Lozano AM (2002) Long-term hardware-related complications of deep brain stimulation. Neurosurgery 50:1268–1276.
65. Joint C, Nandi D, Parkin S, Gregory R, Aziz T (2002) Hardware-related problems of deep brain stimulation. Mov Disord 17(Suppl 3):S175–S180.
66. Kumar R (2003) Methods of programming and patient management with deep brain stimulation. In: Tarsy D, Lozano AM, Vitek JL, eds. Surgical Treatment of Parkinson's Disease and Other Movement Disorders. Totowa, NJ: Humana Press, pp. 189–212.
67. Volkmann J, Herzog J, Kopper F, Deuschl G (2002) Introduction to the programming of deep brain stimulators. Mov Disord 17(Suppl 3):S181–S187.
68. Voges J, Waerzeggers Y, Maarouf M, et al (2006) Deep-brain stimulation: long-term analysis of complications caused by hardware and surgery-experiences from a single centre. J Neurol Neurosurg Psychiatry 77:868–872.
69. Oh MY, Hodaie M, Kim SH, Alkhani A, Lang AE, Lozano AM (2001) Deep brain stimulator electrodes used for lesioning: proof of principle. Neurosurgery 49:363–369.
70. Kumar R, McVicker JM (2000) Radiofrequency lesioning through an implanted deep brain stimulating electrode: treatment of tolerance to thalamic stimulation in essential tremor. Mov Disord 15(Suppl 3):69.
71. Caparros-Lefebre D, Blond S, Pecheux N, Pasquier F, Petit H (1992) Evaluation neuropsychologique avant et après stimulation thalamique chez 9 parkinsoniens. Rev Neurol 148:117–122.
72. Troster AI, Fields JA, Pahwa R, et al (1999) Neuropsychological and quality of life outcome after thalamic stimulation for essential tremor. Neurology 53:1174–1780.
73. Hirai T, Miyazaki M, Nakajima H, et al (1983) The correlation between tremor characteristics and the predicted volume of effective lesions in stereotaxic nucleus ventralis intermedius thalamotomy. Brain 106:1001–1018.
74. Stellar S, Cooper IS (1968) Mortality and morbidity in cryothalamectomy for parkinsonism. A statistical study of 2,868 consecutive operations. J Neurosurg 28:459–467.
75. Pollak P, Fraix V, Krack P, Moro E, Mendes A, Chabardes S, Koudsie A, Benabid AL (2002) Treatment results: Parkinson's disease. Mov Disord 17(Suppl 3):S75–S83.
76. Lund-Johansen M, Hugdahl K, Wester K (1996) Cognitive function in patients with Parkinson's disease undergoing stereotaxic thalamotomy. J Neurol Neurosurg Psychiatry 60:564–571.
77. Schuurman PR, Bosch DA, Bossuyt PMN, et al (2000) A comparison of continuous thalamic stimulation and thalamotomy for suppression of severe tremor. N Engl J Med 342:461–468.

# 13

# Globus Pallidus Deep Brain Stimulation for Parkinson's Disease

Frances Weaver, Kenneth Follett, and Matthew Stern

## Abstract

Deep brain stimulation (DBS) has become the treatment of choice for patients with Parkinson's disease (PD) who are experiencing unmanageable complications of long-term medical therapy. The two established sites for DBS for PD are the subthalamic nucleus (STN) and the globus pallidus interna (GPi). Although most providers have already decided that STN is the preferred site for DBS, only one small, randomized trial has compared STN to GPi DBS, finding no difference between the two procedures in improving motor function following surgery. This chapter reviews the literature on the use of unilateral and bilateral GPi on patient outcomes including motor function, quality of life, medication use, and adverse events. The available data suggests that both GPi and STN DBS are effective interventions for PD. Target choice may be dependent on patient characteristics such as age or symptom profile. Large, randomized controlled trials continue to be needed to inform these decisions.

**Keywords:** deep brain stimulation, DBS, globus pallidus, subthalamic nucleus, Parkinson's disease, movement disorders

## Introduction

It has long been recognized that the basal ganglia are a useful target for surgery in the treatment of movement disorders. Studies by Meyers and others in the 1930s involved surgery in the pallidothalamic pathways, the caudate nucleus and the GPi *(1)*. However, high morbidity and mortality rates limited these strategies. Surgeons began performing pallidotomies in the late 1940s with better success, but then shifted to thalamotomy as an apparently safer procedure in the 1960s. Surgery was all but abandoned in the 1970s after levodopa was introduced. However, complications of levodopa therapy eventually fueled a search for better treatments and surgical approaches have enjoyed a renaissance. In the 1990s, unilateral pallidotomy became the most common surgery used for movement disorders worldwide *(2)*.

With the advent of DBS and the ability to modulate abnormal neuronal discharge using electrical stimulation, the use of pallidotomy decreased dramatically in the late 1990s. By 2000 it had already become a niche surgery. Neurosurgeons in Europe and North America quickly adopted DBS as the preferred surgical treatment for PD and other movement disorders. The advantages of DBS include the ability to safely perform surgery bilaterally for a bilateral disease and to target different structures for stimulation without the risks associated with ablative surgery.

Studies of DBS in the GPi suggest that stimulation may activate axons that produce GABAergic inhibition of the GPi neurons. Further, it may be that high-frequency nonphysiologic stimulation may override existing, highly abnormal GPi neuronal discharges with an uninterpretable but less noxious signal sent to afferent structures (3). GPi stimulation can improve all of the cardinal symptoms of PD including tremor, bradykinesia, rigidity, and levodopa-induced dyskinesias. It also has a direct anti-dyskinetic effect. Antiparkinson medications are usually not reduced following GPi DBS. In fact, stimulation of the GPi may allow for increased doses of levodopa to address ongoing PD symptoms by relief of dose-limiting dyskinesias.

A small study by Bejjani et al. (4) examined the effects of GPi stimulation in different portions of the GPi. Stimulation in the dorsal GP resulted in improved gait, akinesia, and ridgity but also was able to induce dyskinesias. Contacts that induced dyskinesias were within or very close to the external pallidum. Posteroventral GP stimulation resulted in worsened gait and akinesia, decreased rigidity, but dramatically reduced levodopa induced dyskinesias. Krack et al. (5) reported similar findings. To some extent location of GPi stimulation should be tailored to each patient's specific symptoms; but Krack et al. recommend a compromise between these opposite effects by stimulating through contacts located at an intermediate point between dorsal and ventral GPi.

## Review of Studies Utilizing Unilateral or Bilateral GPi DBS

There are only a few published studies of the outcomes of unilateral GPi DBS and results have been variable. Other papers have reported on both unilateral and bilateral GPi patients (6, 7) or unilateral GPi following a previous ablative procedure such as unilateral pallidotomy (8). A larger number of studies have reported on outcomes of bilateral GPi DBS. Reported outcomes typically utilize subscales of the Unified Parkinson's Disease Rating Scale (UPDRS), including the motor (part III) and activities of daily living (ADLs; part II) scores, timed measurements of motor function, changes in medication use, neuropsychological outcomes, and adverse events. Findings for each of these outcomes are described below.

### Impact on Motor Outcomes

Six studies specifically reported UPDRS motor scores off medications for patients undergoing unilateral GPi DBS (Table 13.1).Pahwa et al. (7) reported an average 46% improvement in motor function in two patients following unilateral stimulation. Similarly, Vingerhoets et al. (9) reported a 45% improvement in

**Table 13.1** Unilateral and Bilateral GPi DBS Studies^.

| First author | Year | Country | N | Mean age | % Male | Follow-up period (months) | Mean baseline UPDRS motor | Follow-up UPDRS motor& | % Change |
|---|---|---|---|---|---|---|---|---|---|
| UNILATERAL STUDIES | | | | | | | | | |
| Pahwa | 1997 | USA | 2 | 51.5 | 50 | 3 | 38 | 20.5 | 46 |
| Gross | 1997 | France | 7 | na | 100 | 12 | 53.4 | 37.0 | 31 |
| Vingerhoets | 1999 | Belgium | 20 | 54.9 | 70 | 3 | 23.0 ± 14.2 | 12.7 ± 9.3 | 45 |
| Kumar | 2000 | Canada, Europe | 5 | na | na | 6 | 38.9 ± 2.5 | 25.8 ± 6.8 | 37 |
| Loher | 2002 | Europe | 9 | 65.1 | 60 | 12 | 57.2 ± 13.7 | 35.3 ± 6.9 | 38.3 |
| Visser-Vandewalle | 2003 | Europe | 26 | 56.2 | 77 | 3, 32.7 | 26.5 ± 9.2 | 13.1 ± 6.1 | 50.7 |
| BILATERAL STUDIES | | | | | | | | | |
| Pahwa | 1997 | USA | 3[1] | 57 | 100 | 3 | 48 ± 12.77 | 15.3 ± 11.78 | 68.1 |
| Limousin | 1997 | France | 6 | 50 | 83 | na | 43* | 26 ± 11 | 40 |
| Krack | 1998 | France | 5 | 51 | 80 | 6 | 53.6 ± 10.4 | 32.5 ± 12.4 | 39.4 |
| Ghika | 1998 | Switzerland | 6 | 55 | na | 3,6,12,15,18,24 | 66.0 | 31.0 | 53.0 |
| Brown[2] | 1999 | Europe | 6 | 50.7 | 67 | 8.3 (ave) | 54.2 ± 9.2 | 27.2 ± 12.0 | 49.8 |
| Durif[3] | 1999 | France | 6 | 64 | 33 | 6 | 36 ± 2 | 23 ± 5 | 36.1 |
| Pillon (Greenoble) | 2000 | France | 8 | 52.5 | 75 | 3 | 55.4 ± 8.5 | 37.1 ± 13.3 | 33.0 |
| Pillon (Paris) | 2000 | France | 5 | 55.2 | 60 | 6 | 41.6 ± 14.1 | 27.0 ± 12.5 | 35.1 |
| Kumar | 2000 | Canada, Europe | 22[4] | 52.7 | 68 | 6 | 53.4 ± 3.3 | 37.1 ± 3.8 | 31 |
| Krause[5] | 2001 | Germany | 6 | 58.5 | na | 6 | 43.8 ± 8.2 | 39.2 ± 4.9 | 10.5 |
| Volkmann | 2001 | Germany | 11 | 56.6 | na | 6 | 52.5 ± 14.16 | 22.9 ± 15.48 | 56.4 |
| Parkinson's Disease Study Group | 2001 | Europe, Canada, USA | 38 | 55.7 | 71 | 6 | 50.8 ± 11.6 | 33.9 ± 12.3 | 33.3 |
| Loher | 2002 | Europe | 10[6] | 64.6 | 50 | 3, 12 | 63.4 ± 17.4 | 40.3 ± 10.3 | 36.4 |
| Minguez-Castellanos | 2005 | Spain | 10 | 59.0 | 70 | 12 | 63.4 ± 18.65 | 39.6 ± 15.69 | 35 |
| Rodriquez-Oroz | 2005 | Europe | 20 | 55.8 | 65 | 12, 3 to 4 years[7] | 51.7 ± 13.6 | 29.2 ± 14.9 | 43.5 |
| Anderson | 2005 | USA | 10 | 61 | na | 12 | 50 ± 23 | 30 ± 17 | 39 |

^All studies that reported p-values were significant at $P < 0.05$ or better except Durif, 1999 ($p = 0.27$). Six studies did not provide p-values.
*Calculated based on other information available; note that one patient did not complete 6-month assessment.
&The 6-month assessment was used or the closest assessment in time to 6 months.
1. Results for 3 patients with bilateral GPi only. Measured with meds on/stim on
2. Motor score ranged from 0 to 108 (scores were rescaled in calculation), otherwise assumed 0 to 104.
3. This study included one patient who underwent unilateral implantation.
4. The demographic information is based on 22 patients. Of these, 17 underwent bilateral surgery (and five had unilateral surgery). Outcome data are presented only for the 17 bilateral cases.
5. Information provided through e-mail correspondence with author; one patient was lost to follow-up.
6. There were 16 cases total, of which 10 were bilateral DBS cases.
7. Three to 4-year UPDRS score = 31.7 ± 12.8; 38.7% improvement over baseline.
na, information was not available.

UPDRS motor scores 3 months following unilateral GPi. Loher et al. *(10)* tested nine patients who received unilateral GPi at 3 and 12 months post-surgery. The improvement was the same at both 3 and 12 months (38%). Kumar et al. *(11)* reported a 37% improvement over baseline scores of 38.9 on the UPDRS motor scale for five subjects while Gross et al. *(12)* reported a 31% improvement for seven patients who underwent unilateral GPi. Visser-Vandewalle et al. *(13)* performed posteroventral pallidal stimulation in 26 patients with PD. At baseline, these patients had an average UPDRS motor off medication score of 26.5 ± 9.2. These scores improved by almost 51% (mean 13.1 ± 6.1) 3 months after surgery. However, when these patients were re-evaluated an average of 32.7 months later, UPDRS scores had actually worsened over baseline by 8.3% (mean 28.7 ± 7.6). The authors explained this worsening as a function of disease progression that outweighed the benefits of unilateral GPi over time. Of note, the baseline data suggest that the subjects in the Loher and Gross studies were more impaired before surgery than those in the Visser-Vandewalle study. On the other hand, patients were followed for only 12 months in the Loher study but for an average of more than 2.5 years in the Visser-Vandewalle study.

Several studies have reported on motor outcomes following bilateral GPi DBS *(7, 10, 11, 14–25)*. Table 13.1 provides information about the characteristics of subjects, and baseline and follow-up UPDRS motor scores. Most studies were conducted in Europe, had very small sample sizes (only three studies had 20 or more subjects), and follow-up was 1 year or less in all but two studies. Across these studies, the average improvement in UPDRS motor scores over baseline was 40%, although improvement ranged from a low of 10.5% *(20)* to a high of 68% *(7)*. Ghika et al. *(16)*, reporting on outcomes at 24 months, found that improvement in motor function declined only slightly from 53% at 6 months to 50% at 2 years. Rodriquez-Oroz et al. *(24)* followed subjects between 3 to 4 years following GPi DBS and also found a mild decline in motor function after the initial gains recorded at 1 year (43.5% at 12 months to 38.7% at 3–4 years). Although the data are very limited, these two studies suggest slight waning of motor improvement over time.

## Impact on PD Medication Use

Only two of the unilateral GPi DBS studies reported medication dose in levodopa equivalents following intervention (Table 13.2). The dose was essentially unchanged in one study *(10)* but increased significantly (53.8%) in the other *(13)*. In a meta-analysis of bilateral DBS trials, change in PD medications as a result of DBS was examined *(26)*. Effect sizes for nine bilateral GPi DBS studies ranged from −0.60 to 0.40 and the mean effect size was −0.02 (95% CI: −0.29–0.26) indicating that on average there was no change in medication dose. The effect size was negative in three studies (indicating that doses actually increased following DBS), positive in three other studies, and essentially unchanged in the remaining three. In two long-term follow-up studies of bilateral GPi DBS, one reported a slight decrease in medication dose while the other reported a 32% increase in levodopa equivalents from baseline *(24)*. Although due to the small number of studies, small sample sizes and conflicting results it is difficult to draw definite conclusions regarding medication dosing following GPi DBS, GPi DBS appears to have had no consistent effect on medication dose in these studies.

**Table 13.2** Levodopa equivalents and UPDRS ADL scores before and after GPi DBS.

| Author/year (bilateral, unless noted) | N | Medication (levodopa equivalents) Baseline | Follow-up | % Change | UPDRS–II (ADL scores; off medication/on stimulation) Baseline | Follow-up | % Change |
|---|---|---|---|---|---|---|---|
| Pahwa, 1997 (unilateral) | 2 | na | na | na | 30 | 23.5 | −21.6 |
| Pahwa, 1997 (bilateral) | 3 | na | na | na | 25.3 ± 4.5 | 21 ± 4.58 | −17 |
| Ghika, 1998 | 6 | 1080 | 960 | −11 | 31 | 8 | −74.2 |
| Krack, 1998 | 5 | 865 ± 366 | 1110 ± 444 | 28.3 | 27.8 ± 8.2 | 15.0 ± 6.4 | −46 |
| Durif, 1999 | 10 | 1200 ± 260 | 1275 | 0.06 | na | na | na |
| Vingerhoets, 1999 (unilateral) | 20 | 780 ± 278 | na | na | 8.8 ± 5.4 | 4.4 ± 3.8 | 50 |
| Kumar, 2000 (unilateral) | 5 | na | na | na | 26.9 ± 2 | 14.5 ± 5.2 | −44 |
| Kumar, 2000 (bilateral) | 17 | na | na | na | 30.0 ± 1.7 | 18.4 ± 1.8 | −39 |
| Pillon, 2000 (Greenoble) | 8 | 744 ± 264 | 873 ± 478 | 17.3 | na | na | na |
| Pillon, 2000 (Paris) | 5 | 850 ± 514 | 725 ± 308 | 14.7 | na | na | na |
| Krause, 2001 | 6 | na | na | na | 17.4 ± 1.5 | 18.0 ± 1.4 | +0.6 |
| Deep Brain Stimulation for Parkinson's Disease Study Group, 2001 | 38 | 1090.9±543 | 1120±537 | 0.15 | 27.9±7.4 | 17.9±8.4 | −34 |
| Volkmann, 2001 | 11 | 836 + 391 | 700 + 311 | −16.3 | 21.0 + 6.72 | 9.5 + 7.8 | −54.8 |
| Loher, 2002 (unilateral) | 9 | 1235.5* | 1233.5* | 0 | 30.8 + 7.1 | 20.4 + 4.2 | −33.6 |
| Loher, 2002 (bilateral) | 16 | 1235.5* | 1233.5* | 0 | 34.9 + 8.6 | 22.3 + 6.4 | −36 |
| Visser-Vandewalle, 2003 (unilateral) | 26 | 788 + 262 | 1212 + 409 | 53.8 | na | na | na |
| Rodriguez-Oroz, 2005 | 20 | 1074 + 462 | 1242 + 528 | 15.6 | 26.8 + 8.9 | 18.1 + 9.2 | −32.5 |
| Minguez-Castellanos, 2005 | 10 | 762 + 24.22 | 827 + 337 | +9.0 | 29.2 + 6.44 | 20.1 + 8.16 | −32 |

*Levodopa equivalents were combined for unilateral and bilateral cases.
na, information was not available.

Because GPi DBS does not exacerbate levodopa-induced dyskinesias, most providers have not tried to reduce medication dose. In fact, medication is sometimes increased as the patient becomes able to tolerate larger doses, and the medication may help other symptoms of PD not adequately managed with DBS. At this point, there is insufficient information to know whether antiparkinson medications can or should be reduced in patients who have undergone GPi DBS. There is also some evidence that stimulation of the pallidum sometimes induces dyskinesia but, as already discussed, this is probably an effect of dorsal GPi stimulation *(27)*.

### ADLs (UPDRS Part II)

Across unilateral and bilateral GPi DBS studies, all except one have reported improved ADL scores off medication/on stimulation compared with preoperative off medication scores (Table 13.2; ref. *20*). Younger patients (mean age 55 years or less) had greater improvement in ADL scores than older patients *(26)*. Although the number of studies is small, ADL scores for the on-medication/on-stimulation state were significantly improved in the GPi studies compared with preoperative on-medications scores, whereas improvement in the on-medication/on-stimulation state was not observed after STN DBS *(26)*. It is possible that anti-parkinson medication and GPi DBS may have an additive effect in PD patients *(28)*.

## Impact on Quality of Life

### Self-Reported Motor Function

A commonly used data collection tool in the area of movement disorders is the use of patient self-reported diaries. In 30-minute intervals over a 24-hour period, patients are asked to indicate which of four categories best reflects his/her physical functioning. These categories include: asleep, off (e.g., unable to move or very slow movements), on (good functioning), and on with troublesome dyskinesias. Although this information is frequently collected in clinical trials of medications in PD, it is rarely reported in DBS studies. We identified three studies that reported use of diaries in patients who underwent GPi DBS. The results of these three studies were very similar. Pahwa et al. *(7)* report an improvement in good on time from 21% at baseline to 65% three months after DBS for two unilateral and three bilateral cases. Similarly, both the Deep Brain Stimulation for Parkinson's Disease Study Group *(22)* and Rodriquez-Oroz et al. *(24)* report similar improvements in on time from 28 to 64% and from 26 to 69%, respectively. Unfortunately, none of these studies reported the actual number of hours of on time reported by each patient. However, if we assume that the average person has 16 hours of awake time a day, these subjects averaged 3.5 to 4.5 hours of on time per day prior to GPi DBS which improved to 10 to 11 hours a day; a gain of between 5.5 and 7.5 hours in a good functioning on state.

It is important to note that the magnitude of the improvement in on time following DBS is considerably greater than increases in on time noted with most drugs which have been tested as adjuncts to levodopa in PD. Most studies of medication use in PD report improvements in on time of only 1 to 3 hours *(29, 30)*. While this may be a consequence of the usual severity of PD in DBS treated patients, it represents a considerable improvement in function and may be more meaningful to patients than the other measures of PD, which are used in rating patients.

### Neuropsychological Outcomes of DBS

Quality of life has been increasingly recognized as an important outcome to assess in any intervention. Several disease specific quality of life measures have been developed for PD. The most frequently reported is the PD questionnaire (PDQ-39; ref. *31*). In our review of GPi studies, we did not find a single study that used the PDQ-39. A few studies reported on the Beck Depression

Inventory. Troster *(32)*, Volkmann *(21)*, and Vingerhoets *(9)* all reported trends in reduced symptoms of depression following DBS. Burchiel et al. *(28)* reported a 49% improvement in depression. Vingerhoets et al. *(9)* used the Sickness Impact Profile to assess patient quality of life. They found positive trends in the psychosocial dimension of the scale. Sleep and eating also improved and components of the physical dimension, ambulatory, body care, and movement also improved. Although it appears that quality of life is improved as a result of GPi DBS, there is little available data to support this. Future studies should include a quality of life assessment such as the PDQ-39 as part of the test battery.

## Adverse Events Associated with GPi DBS

Complications or adverse events in DBS are usually categorized into three groups: hardware-related complications, surgical complications, and stimulation- and target-related complications. Infections, skin erosions, lead breaks, lead migration, and hardware failure are all considered hardware complications *(33)*. In the largest published study of GPi DBS to date, 41 patients experienced two lead migrations, one infection, one lead break, and one seroma *(22)*. Volkmann *(21)* reported one lead migration and two skin erosions in 11 patients. The Deep Brain Stimulation for Parkinson's Disease study group *(22)* reported nine procedure-related complications including four intracranial hemorrhages, three instances of hemiparesis (secondary to hemorrhage), one patient with seizure, and one patient with dysarthria. Stimulation-induced complications reported in GPi DBS include confusion, depression, increased akinesia, and induction or aggravation of gait and speech problems *(33)*. Many of these complications are transient or can be eliminated by adjusting stimulation parameters. Krause et al. *(20)* reported on several severe events including one patient with severe depression requiring hospitalization, two patients who experienced strongly increased libido who were hospitalized psychiatrically, two cases of severe dysarthria, and one severe psychotic reaction attributed to initiating a new medication rather than stimulation. This study appears to be exceptional, as most other GPi DBS studies in PD have described less severe and more transient events or complications. Most recently, Blomstedt et al. *(34)* report on complications in both DBS and ablative movement disorder procedures. They found eight adverse events in five of 11 GPi DBS procedures, including two hardware complications, two cases of dysarthria, and single instances of hypophonia, vasovagal reaction, and confusion.

Although the data are limited, it is believed that postoperative psychiatric symptoms in GPi DBS are less common than after STN DBS *(35)*. Because there are far fewer studies of GPi DBS than STN DBS, comparison between these surgical targets is difficult. In addition, some convention is needed to standardize the reporting of adverse events or complications in order to make comparison across studies easier.

## Current Status of GPi DBS in PD

Currently, most providers have reached the conclusion that STN is the preferred site for DBS for treatment of PD and, as a result, few patients are recommended for GPi DBS. However, in actuality, only one small, randomized controlled trial of STN vs GPi DBS has been published *(25)*. This study did not find a difference in off-medication/on-stimulation motor scores by surgical target. The authors concluded that stimulation of either the GPi or the STN improves many of the symptoms of advanced PD and that it is premature to exclude GPi as an appropriate target for DBS in PD. All other published studies have been retrospective observational studies and most have involved very small sample sizes. A meta-analysis of patient outcomes following STN vs GPi DBS also found no statistically significant difference in motor or ADL functioning by target of DBS *(26)*.

There is also little comparative data on health-related quality of life and no comparisons of the relative cost-effectiveness of GPi and STN DBS in PD. Because of the higher stimulus frequency and pulse width usually required to stimulate the larger region of the globus pallidum, GPi patients are likely to require battery replacement more frequently than their STN counterparts. On the other hand, data suggest that neuropsychological complications that appear to be more frequent in the STN group may result in higher costs due to increased hospitalizations and psychiatric medications, not to mention the adverse impact of such complications on patient quality of life. Furthermore, we have only limited data on the long-term effects of DBS. Two recent studies suggest that motor function is sustained for at least 4 to 5 years after bilateral GPi implantation *(24, 36)*. Long-term effects on other outcomes is even less clear. In a 5-year follow-up study, Krack et al. *(36)* reported the appearance of midpoint motor deficits, akinesia, speech deficits, and dementia in patients who underwent bilateral STN DBS, which was felt to be due to progression of PD. Unfortunately, similar data are not available for GPi DBS. It should also be recognized that because most centers abandoned GPi as a target in favor of STN, it is likely that the technique had become less refined by that point, resulting in less than optimal outcomes *(37)*.

It is likely that both GPi and STN DBS are effective interventions for PD. Optimal target selection may be dependent on the most prominent PD symptoms experienced by patients (e.g., the possible use of GPi DBS for severe dyskinesias or dystonia). Outcomes of DBS may also be influenced by patient characteristics such as age, duration of illness, or age at diagnosis. Large randomized controlled trials, such as a multicenter U.S. Veterans Administration study that is currently near completion *(38)*, will allow a more rational match of patients and surgical interventions in order to promote the best possible patient outcomes.

## References

1. Krauss J, Grossman R (2002) Surgery for Parkinson's disease and hyperkinetic movement disorders. In: Jankovic J, Tolosa E, eds. Parkinson's Disease and Movement Disorders, fourth edition. Philadelphia: Lippincott Williams & Wilkins, pp. 640–662.
2. Follett K (2000) The surgical treatment of Parkinson's disease. Annu Rev Med 51:135–147.
3. Kumar R (2002) Deep brain stimulation. In: Jankovic J, Tolosa E, eds. Parkinson's Disease and Movement Disorders, fourth edition. Philadelphia: Lippincott Williams & Wilkins, pp. 674–689.
4. Bejjani B, Damier P, Arnulf I, et al (1997) Pallidal stimulation for Parkinson's disease: two targets? Neurology 49:1564–1569.

5. Krack P, Pollak P, Limousin P, et al (1998) Opposite motor effects of pallidal stimulation in Parkinson's disease. Ann Neurol 43:180–192.
6. Katayama Y, Kasai M, Oshima H, Fukaya C, Yamamoto T, Mizutani T (2001) Double blind evaluation of the effects of pallidal and subthalamic nucleus stimulation on daytime activity in advanced Parkinson's disease. Parkinsonism Relat Disord 7:35–40.
7. Pahwa R, Wilkinson S, Smith D, Lyons K, Miyawaki E, Koller WC (1997) High-frequency stimulation of the globus pallidus for the treatment of Parkinson's disease. Neurology 49:249–253.
8. Melvin K, Doan J, Pellis S, et al (2005) Pallidal deep brain stimulation and L-dopa do not improve qualitative aspects of skilled reaching in Parkinson's disease. Behav Brain Res 160:188–194.
9. Vingerhoets G, Lannoo E, van der Linden C, et al (1999) Changes in quality of life following unilateral pallidal stimulation in Parkinson's Disease. J Psychosomatic Res 46:247–255.
10. Loher T, Burgunder J, Weber S, Sommerhalder R, Krauss J (2002) Effect of chronic pallidal deep brain stimulation on off period dystonia and sensory symptoms in advanced Parkinson's disease. J Neurol Neurosurg Psychiatry 73:395–399.
11. Kumar R, Lang A, Rodriguez-Oroz M, et al (2000) Deep brain stimulation of the globus pallidus pars interna in advanced Parkinson's disease. Neurology 55:S34–S39.
12. Gross C, Rougier A, Guehl D, Boraud T, Julien J, Bioulac B (1997) High-frequency stimulation of the globus pallidus internalis in Parkinson's disease: a study of seven cases. J Neurosurg 87:491–498.
13. Visser-Vandewalle V, Van Der Linden C, Temel Y, et al (2003) Long-term motor effect of unilateral pallidal stimulation in 26 patients with advanced Parkinson disease. J Neurosurg 99:701–707.
14. Limousin P, Greene J, Pollak P, Rothwell J, Benabid AL, Frackowiak R (1997) Changes in cerebral activity pattern due to subthalamic nucleus or internal pallidum stimulation in Parkinson's disease. Ann Neurol 42:283–291.
15. Krack P, Pollak P, Limousin P, et al (1998) Subthalamic nucleus or internal pallidal stimulation in young onset Parkinson's disease. Brain 121:451–457.
16. Ghika J, Villemure J, Fankhauser H, Favre J, Assal G, Ghika-Schmid F (1998) Efficiency and safety of bilateral contemporaneous pallidal stimulation (deep brain stimulation) in levodopa-responsive patients with Parkinson's Disease with severe motor fluctuations: a 2 year follow-up. J Neurosurg 89:713–718.
17. Brown R, Limousin Dowsey P, Brown P, et al (1999) Impact of deep brain stimulation on upper limb akinesia in Parkinson's disease. Ann Neurol 45:473–488.
18. Durif F, Lemaire J, Debilly B, Dordain G (1999) Acute and chronic effects of anteromedial globus pallidus stimulation in Parkinson's disease. J Neurol Psychiatry 67:315–321.
19. Pillon B, Ardouin C, Damier MA, et al (2000) Neuropsychological changes between "off" and "on" STN or GPi stimulation in Parkinson's Disease. Neurology 55:411–418.
20. Krause M, Fogel W, Heck A, et al (2001) Deep brain stimulation for the treatment of Parkinson's disease: subthalamic nucleus versus globus pallidus internus. J Neurol Neurosurg Psychiatry 70:464–470.
21. Volkmann J, Allert N, Voges J, Weiss PH, Freund HJ, Sturm V (2001) Safety and efficacy of pallidal or subthalamic nucleus stimulation in advanced PD. Neurology 56:548–551.
22. Deep-Brain Stimulation for Parkinson's Disease Study Group (2001) Deep-brain stimulation of the subthalamic nucleus or the pars interna of the globus pallidus in Parkinson's disease. N Engl J Med 345:956–963.
23. Minguez-Castellanos A, Escamilla-Sevilla F, Katati M, et al (2005) Different patterns of medication change after subthalamic or pallidal stimulation for Parkinson's

disease: target related effect or selection bias? J Neurol Neurosurg Psychiatry 76:34–39.
24. Rodriguez-Oroz MC, Obeso JA, Lang AE, et al (2005) Bilateral deep brain stimulation in Parkinson's disease: a multicentre study with 4 years follow-up. Brain 128:2240–2249.
25. Anderson VC, Burchiel KJ, Hogarth P, et al (2005) Pallidal vs subthalamic nucleus deep brain stimulation in Parkinson disease. Arch Neurol 62(4):554–560.
26. Weaver F, Follett K, Hur K, Ippolito D, Stern M (2005) Deep brain stimulation in Parkinson disease: a metaanalysis of patient outcomes. J Neurosurg 103(6):956–967.
27. Vitek JL (2002) Deep brain stimulation for Parkinson's disease. A critical re-evaluation of STN versus GPi DBS. Stereotact Funct Neurosurg 78:119–131.
28. Burchiel KJ, Anderson VC, Favre J, et al (1999) Comparison of pallidal and subthalamic nucleus deep brain stimulation for advanced Parkinson's disease: results of a randomized, blinded pilot study. Neurosurgery 45(6):1375–1382.
29. Katzenschlager R, Hughes A, Evans A, et al (2005) Continuous subcutaneous apomorphine therapy improves dyskinesias in Parkinson's disease: aprospective study using single-dose challenges. Mov Disord 20:151–157.
30. Rajput A, Martin W, Saint-Hilaire M, et al (1998) Tolcapone improves motor function in parkinsonian patients with the "wearing-off" phenomenon: a double-blind, placebo-controlled, multicenter trial. Neurology 50:S54–S59.
31. Peto V, Jenkinson C, Fitzpatrick R (1998) PDQ-39: a review of the development, validation and application of a Parkinson's disease quality of life questionnaire and its associated measures. J Neurol 245(Suppl 1):S10–S14.
32. Troster A, Fields J, Wilkinson S, et al (1997) Unilateral pallidal stimulation for Parkinosn's disease: neurobehavioral functioning before and 3 months after electrode implantation. Neurology 49:1078–1083.
33. Hariz MI (2002) Complications of deep brain stimulation surgery. Mov Disord 17(Suppl 3):S162–S166.
34. Blomstedt P, Marwan H (2006) Are complications less common in deep brain stimulation than in ablative procedures for movement disorders? Stereotact Funct Neurosurg 84:72–81.
35. Voon V, Kubu C, Krack P, Houeto J, Troster A (2006) Deep brain stimulation: neuropsychological and neuropsychiatric issues. Mov Disord 21:S305–S327.
36. Krack P, Batir A, Van Blercom N, et al (2003) Five-year follow-up of bilateral stimulation of the subthalamic nucleus in advanced Parkinson's disease. N Engl J Med 349:1925–1934.
37. Skidmore F, Rodriguez R, Fernandez H, Goodman W, Foote K, Okun M (2006) Lessons learned in deep brain stimulation for movement and neuropsychiatric disorders. CNS Spectr 11:521–537.
38. Follett K, Weaver F, Stern M, et al VA Cooperative Study #468. A comparison of best medical therapy and deep brain stimulation of subthalamic nucleus and globus pallidus for the treatment of Parkinson's disease (in preparation).

# 14
# Deep Brain Stimulation of the Subthalamic Nucleus for the Treatment of Parkinson's Disease

Marcelo Merello

## Abstract

Levodopa remains the gold standard for the treatment of Parkinson's disease (PD). However, its chronic use is associated with motor and psychiatric complications causing significant disability. Thus, there is a need for alternative approaches including surgical treatment. Better understanding of basal ganglia circuitry and the availability of an experimental animal model of Parkinson's disease in the form of the 1-methyl-4-phenyl-1,2,3,6 tetrahydropyridine (MPTP)-treated monkey have made evident the crucial role of the subthalamic nucleus (STN) in basal ganglia function. Deep brain stimulation (DBS) has become an acceptable treatment option, improving quality of life (QOL) for PD patients with medically intractable symptoms. Good pre-operative levodopa responsiveness and younger age appear to be the best predictors of surgical success, particularly with respect to improvement in motor function. Although benefits in mobility are achieved, complications are not infrequent, and risk–benefit ratio should be assessed on an individual basis for each patient depending on personal preferences, socioeconomic status, and local disease demographics. In this chapter, a comprehensive review of the current literature on the topic is presented in addition to our own results with STN DBS for the treatment of PD.

**Keywords:** deep brain stimulation, subthalamic nucleus, Parkinson's disease, functional neurosurgery

## Rationale for the STN as Target for PD Treatment

With time, as complications and failures of levodopa therapy were revealed, interest in PD surgery and ablative lesional therapy re-emerged *(1)*. Hyperactivity in STN projections to the globus pallidus internus (GPi) had been established as a crucial feature of parkinsonism in animal models of PD *(2, 3)*. The role of increased STN activity in the development of parkinsonism was derived from experiments in the MPTP monkey where lesions experimentally introduced in the STN were associated with a dramatic reversal of parkinsonian motor signs *(3, 4)*. In the past decade, most centers using ablative therapy have switched to DBS because it presents advantages over ablation including reversibility, lower reintervention rates due to inadequate lesion volume, and lower morbidity *(4)*. Since its introduction, the administration of continuous high-frequency electrical stimulation to the STN through a surgically implanted stimulator has been shown to improve motor symptoms in patients with advanced PD *(5, 6)*. However, the fact that it is not curative makes this therapy acceptable only to patients in whom symptomatic benefits are greater than inherent surgical risks and in whom it is expected to reduce disease burden more effectively than optimal drug treatment. Rapid and important advances in our understanding of basal ganglia physiology and anatomy have led to controversy over the best target for DBS. The thalamic target has proven effective for tremor, but much less so for other cardinal PD symptoms and presently is rarely considered. The controversy over which target is best overall for PD has led to an important showdown between GPi DBS and STN DBS. To date, a number of studies have shown that bilateral stimulation of GPi *(7–9)* and STN *(10–13)* are both safe and effective for PD symptom management. It is for both practical and theoretical reasons that STN is considered by many to be the preferred target for DBS in patients with advanced disease *(14–16)*. However, comparative studies are limited *(17–19)*. In one representative prospective double-blind randomized study conducted by Andersen et al. *(20)*, 23 patients with idiopathic PD, levodopa-induced dyskinesia and response fluctuations were randomized to implantation of bilateral GPi or STN DBS and tested pre-operatively and after 12 months of DBS. The authors found that off-medication Unified Parkinson's Disease Rating Scale (UPDRS) motor scores were improved after 12 months of GPi and STN stimulation. Bradykinesia tended to improve more with stimulation of STN than GPi and no improvement of on-medication function was observed in either group. Levodopa dose was reduced only in STN-stimulated patients while dyskinesias were reduced after stimulation of both GPi and STN (89 vs 62%). Cognitive and behavioral complications were observed only following STN DBS. These results indicate that it remains premature to conclude that the STN is a superior target for DBS in patients with advanced PD and that further studies are warranted.

## Indications and Contraindications for the Procedure

Selection of the right patient has a large impact on surgical outcome. There is general agreement that idiopathic PD patients with symptoms responding to levodopa, who retain normal cognition and, if present, respond to medication for depression or mood disorders, are ideal candidates for any of the neurosurgical procedures currently available including STN DBS. The main surgical indications for STN or GPi DBS include bradykinesia, rigidity, tremor, gait impairment, motor fluctuations, levodopa-induced dyskinesias, and dystonia. Lang and coworkers *(21)* stated that the ideal surgical candidate is severely disabled in the off-drug condition and fully independent in the on-drug condition related to cardinal PD symptoms and excluding dyskinesia-related disabilities, and that severe disability generally appears at a UPDRS motor score of about 30/108. Patients with UPDRS motor scores under 30 in the off-drug condition are usually not considered sufficiently disabled to justify invasive therapy but individual considerations may influence this decision. Some authors also advocate the use of STN DBS for patients with isolated, medication refractory rest tremor, regardless of their UPDRS score *(22)*.

Because certain disease variables affect clinical outcome, it is important to take these under consideration during the candidate selection process *(23)*. Response to antiparkinson drug therapy, but not levodopa-related motor complication severity, is considered predictive of surgical benefit *(24–26)*. Age is also an important factor and, although patients of all ages may respond well to STN surgery, younger patients generally do better than older patients *(26–28)*. In the literature, mean age at time of STN DBS ranges between 40 and 60, with the youngest reported patient being 30 and the oldest 80. Some articles mention ages of 70 to 75 years as the upper limit but do not specify the rationale for this cut off *(29–42)*. Others indicate greater benefit in younger patients and a negative correlation between age and outcome *(33, 43–44)*. In practice, the patient's biologic age at the time of proposed surgery should be the main consideration, although there is not a clear age cutoff and surgical indications may be more dependent on the patient's medical condition and comorbidities.

Brain atrophy on MRI and postural instability merit special mention. Specific CT or MRI findings have not been shown to predict response to surgery, although adequate data are lacking. In patients being considered for STN DBS, pre-operative imaging is mandatory, preferably MRI. During MRI screening, structural lesions as well as features of atypical parkinsonism such as multiple system atrophy (MSA) should be sought. With the exception of obvious structural lesions or abnormal anatomical findings, which may contraindicate the surgical procedure, imaging results alone should not be relied on to rule out STN DBS. Bonneville et al. *(45)* found normalized brain parenchyma volume and frontal scores to be lower in older patients with longer disease duration but also noted that brain atrophy was not predictive of postoperative outcome and should therefore not be considered an exclusion criterion for neurosurgery. Nevertheless, the fact that a smaller normalized mesencephalon surface was associated with less beneficial effect for parkinsonian motor disability after STN DBS suggested that this could be explored as a possible predictive factor for postoperative outcome. While functional imaging studies with 18-F-dopa PET or DA-transporter SPECT may be helpful in confirming the clinical diagnosis of PD, there have been no studies using functional imaging to predict outcome after DBS.

Axial signs that respond poorly to levodopa, especially postural instability and ON freezing, also respond poorly to DBS *(33, 36, 39)*. Ghel et al. *(46)* found that axial symptom severity was a negative predictive factor of the effect of STN DBS for speech disturbance and postural instability. This suggests that patients should be carefully evaluated for levodopa-resistant axial symptoms before referring them for surgery. Welter et al. *(33)* and Charles et al. *(43)* also found that age and residual axial symptoms observed after levodopa intake before surgery are predictive of unfavorable motor outcome after bilateral STN stimulation.

Patients unresponsive to medical therapy, with signs of a parkinson-plus syndrome, or with significant cognitive impairment are less likely to have long-lasting improvement, and may be unable to cooperate with testing during surgery *(46–48)*. Beneficial achievements of surgery in these particular patients, if any, are rapidly overcome by motor or non-motor disease progression and they should not undergo the procedure *(49–51)*. Patients suffering other progressive disabling clinical conditions including unstable heart disease, active infection, marked subcortical arteriosclerotic encephalopathy, other cerebrovascular disease, comorbid malignancy with reduced life expectancy that would significantly limit DBS benefits, or with increased surgical risk from other causes should also be excluded.

Effects of STN DBS on PD non-motor symptoms or whether their presence or absence should be considered an indication or contraindication to the procedure has yet to be established. Anti-parkinson drug sensitivity associated with visual hallucinations, excessive daytime sleepiness, or pathological gambling that respond to lowering of drug doses, if present in the absence of significant cognitive impairment, may not necessarily be contraindications to STN DBS although further investigation on the subject is necessary.

## Effects on Motor Aspects of PD

Advantages to using the STN as the target for surgical treatment of PD motor symptoms are reflected in the highly favorable results reported by many groups following earlier publications by the French pioneers in this area *(5, 6, 52–58)*.

### UPDRS

STN DBS has been reported to produce significant and sustainable improvement of the UPDRS activities of daily living subscore in the off-medication condition, in a range varying from 17 *(54)* to 82% *(59)*. For the UPDRS motor subscore, reductions varying between 31 *(39)* and 72% have been reported *(59)*. Significant heterogeneity in changes in UPDRS scores has been reported across studies but, on average, UPDRS off-state motor scores improved by approximately 52% over baseline. Coinciding with other published results, our own series of patients undergoing STN DBS showed sustained improvement during 36 months of follow-up of approximately 58% (Figure 14.1).

Effectiveness of STN stimulation on the parkinsonian triad of rigidity, bradykinesia, and rest tremor has been confirmed by electrophysiological studies. STN DBS reduced amplitude, regularity, and tremor-EMG coherence *(60)*. For bradykinesia, Lopiano et al. *(61)* found a significant effect of STN DBS on movement time, a parameter strongly related to bradykinesia. STN DBS *(62)* also increased movement speed and the amplitude of the first agonist burst and burst duration, reduced the number of agonist bursts and cocontractions, increased the size of the antagonist EMG, and reduced antagonist EMG centroid time in the same manner as levodopa. However, movement speed was not restored to normal due to limitations in the amplitude and temporal scaling of the agonist and antagonist bursting patterns *(63)*. Figure 14.2 displays values of rigidity, tremor, and bradykinesia in our own series of 34 patients at 36 months follow-up.

### Levodopa Equivalent Dose (LDED)

STN DBS has been reported to allow reduction of LDED ranging from 19.5 *(30)* to 100% *(64)* with many patients able to function with DBS as monotherapy. Despite the observation that the therapeutic effect of STN DBS on motor

14 Deep Brain Stimulation of the Subthalamic Nucleus for the Treatment of Parkinson's Disease 257

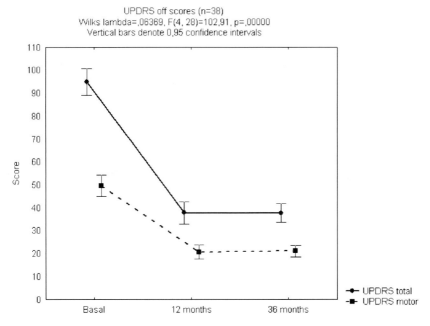

**Figure 14.1** Total and motor UPDRS III subscore in a group of 38 IPD patients who underwent bilateral STN DBS. Significant improvement was sustained at 36 months follow up

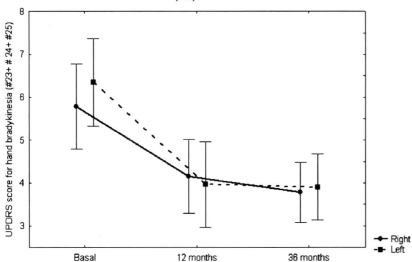

**Figure 14.2** UPDRS score for bradykinesia (A) rigidity (B) and rest tremor (C) in a group of 38 IPD patients underwent bilateral STN DBS. Significant improvement is sustained at 36 months follow-up

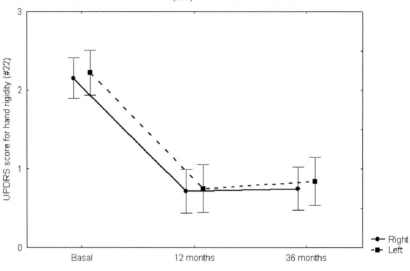

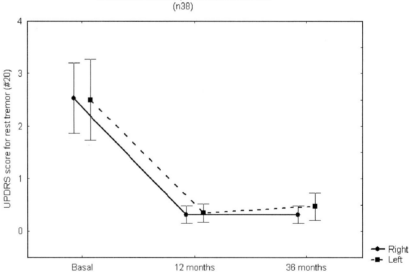

**Figure 14.2** (continued)

signs can be equivalent to that of levodopa, maintaining stimulation monotherapy is not an easy task and only a few patients can get along without medications for an extended period of time. Vingerhoets et al. reported that 50% of patients were able to stop all antiparkinson medications for up to 2 years *(65)*. Figure 14.3 displays LDED values obtained in our 34 patients previously described.

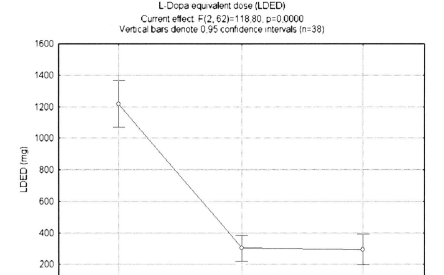

**Figure 14.3** L-DOPA equivalent dose in a group of 38 IPD patients who underwent bilateral STN DBS. Significant improvement was sustained al 38 months follow-up

## Dyskinesias

Dyskinesia reductions ranging from 39.6 *(66)* to 100% *(64)* have been reported after STN DBS. Variability of results is likely due to multiple causes including differences in length of follow-up and the dyskinesia rating scales which were used. Several mechanisms have been postulated as a possible explanation for dyskinesia reduction after STN DBS. These include a direct effect of STN DBS by activation of pallidofugal fibers running dorsal to STN and post-procedural levodopa dose reduction *(67, 68)*. We believe that the effect may also be due to continuous stimulation, which may interrupt or reverse downstream changes induced by pulsatile stimulation of the dopamine receptors. Both peak dose and diphasic dyskinesias are relieved after STN DBS. Interestingly, despite the apparently limited effect of STN DBS on primary dystonia *(69)*, its effect on levodopa-induced peak and off period dystonia is marked. Figure 14.4 displays effects on dyskinesia from our own series of 34 patients after 36 months.

## Motor Fluctuations

STN DBS has been reported to achieve a reduction of OFF time ranging from 17 *(54)* to 100% *(55)*. Evaluation of motor performance using UPDRS part IV and patient diaries showed a decrease in the severity and duration of immobility and a decrease in the duration and severity of dyskinesias among patients who underwent STN DBS *(70)*. STN DBS may compensate for the short-duration levodopa response *(71)* as a putative mechanism for the persistent mobility of patients receiving DBS monotherapy. Vallderiola et al. *(64)* found no significant

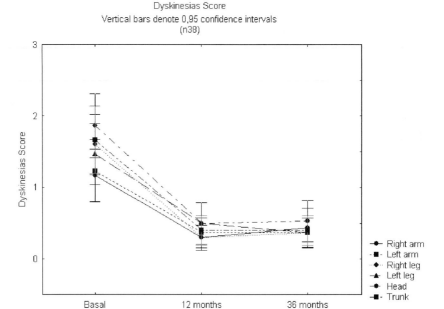

**Figure 14.4** Dyskinesia score in a group of 38 IPD patients who underwent bilateral STN DBS. Significant improvement is sustained at 36 months follow-up

differences in most clinical outcome measures when comparing patients who underwent STN DBS while still taking levodopa and dopamine agonists compared to patients receiving STN DBS as monotherapy. Several patients still taking anti-parkinson medication displayed mild dyskinesias and motor fluctuations while patients with STN DBS monotherapy did not, suggesting that its therapeutic effect on motor function may be equipotent to that of levodopa, with the added benefit of avoiding motor fluctuations and dyskinesias.

### Balance

Crenna et al. *(72)* have described beneficial effects of STN DBS on posture while standing including significant improvement of the vertical alignment of the trunk and shank, decreased hip joint moment, backward shift of the center of pressure, and reduction of abnormal tonic and/or rhythmic activity in the thigh and leg muscles. It would appear that STN DBS and levodopa may not act on the same neurological systems involved in postural regulation. The former could improve posture via effects on the pedunculopontine nucleus *(73)* known to be involved in postural regulation and by improving abnormal sensory aspects of postural instability and postural movement velocity. These are effects that medication does not modify. Neither STN DBS nor levodopa improve postural reaction time *(74)*. Vranken et al. *(75)* recently found that STN DBS improved postural control by reducing trunk sway during stance as well as duration of gait tasks, by increasing trunk pitch velocity while rising from a chair, and by improving roll stability. Coulnat-Coulboise et al. *(76)*

observed a decreased number of falls and more appropriate sensorimotor strategies after STN DBS in PD patients, together with improvement in equilibrium scores, suggesting that non-dopaminergic pathways may be involved in postural regulation and that STN DBS may influence the functioning of these pathways. Nonetheless, postural instability that is unresponsive to levodopa is unlikely to improve following STN DBS. In fact, worsening of balance was one of the most common side effects reported in a subgroup of patients receiving STN DBS, making equilibrium problems a point to carefully address prior to considering STN DBS in patients with this disability.

## Gait

STN DBS provides significant improvement in certain aspects of gait such as increased stride length and walking speed, increased range of motion of lower limb joints, greater physiologic mobility and postural attitude of the trunk, and an increased power production peak at push off. In most cases such improvements are similar to those associated with levodopa treatment. Effects on gait initiation include shortening of the imbalance phase, larger backward/lateral displacement of the center of pressure, and a more physiological expression of the underlying anticipatory muscular synergy *(72)*. Additional changes are shortening of the unloading phase, shortening of the first-swing phase and increase in the length of the first step. From a clinical point of view, several studies have shown that off-period freezing of gait is significantly improved with STN DBS while for on-period freezing no further improvement is registered *(77, 78)*. Figure 14.5 displays our data for postural instability and gait

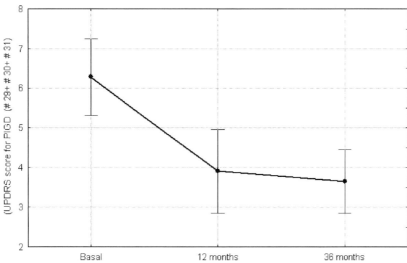

**Figure 14.5** Postural instability and gait disorders (PIGD; a composite score of UPDRS items 29–31) in a group of 38 IPD patients who underwent STN DBS. Significant improvement is sustained at 36 months follow-up

disorders as a composite score resulting from the combination of UPDRS items related to gait, posture, and balance in 34 patients 36 months after STN DBS, showing significant and persistant benefit while off medications.

## Effects on Nonmotor Aspects of PD

### Cognition

Studies on the cognitive effects of bilateral STN stimulation have shown inconsistent results *(78)*. Discrepancies are thought to be methodology-dependent and have varied according to DBS electrode localization *(79)* and the investigational tools used in each study. Morrison et al. *(80)* and Funkiewiez et al. *(81)* reported mild adverse effects on attention and verbal fluency. Ardouin et al. *(82)* and Alegret et al. *(83)* found little negative effect on cognition. Saint Cyr et al. *(84)* and Dujardin et al. *(85)* both found a decline in memory performance, mental speed, and fluency; the latter group also found STN stimulation induced overall cognitive decline and behavioral changes in some patients. In our series, STN DBS induced modest, albeit nonsignificant deterioration of attention, memory, verbal fluency, and visuospatial abilities at 1-year follow-up, without significant deterioration in Addenbroke's Cognitive Examination (ACE) scores. When patients were evaluated at 3 years follow-up however, ACE score deterioration had become significant (Figure 14.6). Whether these long-term changes are related to disease progression or to surgery-related effects is uncertain.

### Behavior

Effects of STN DBS on mood disorders is also a matter of some controversy. In a recent structured review by Takeshita *(86,87)*, average depression scale score improved or remained unchanged after STN DBS, in agreement with findings in our series where little effect on the Hamilton depression scale was observed during stimulation.

In our experience, apathy and irritability scores after STN DBS were significantly higher than preoperative scores. Mentation subscores in UPDRS part I also worsened after surgery. The ability of STN DBS to induce apathy has been a matter of controversy *(81, 88, 89)*, and a number of procedure-related psychiatric side effects are increasingly being reported, including a higher risk of suicide *(90)*. The core features of the apathy observed include motivational deficits and defective self-initiated response. It has been suggested that mesolimbic and nigrostriatal dopamine loss in PD may increase glutamate input signal in the ventral striatum (VS), which in turn, may produce disruption in the limbic ventropallidal system crucial for the translation of motivation into action *(91)*. We believe that stimulation in the motor STN region can, by current spread, affect areas outside the motor territories thereby producing nonmotor effects via its influence on neighboring limbic regions. There may also be potential disruption of the direct corticosubthalamic pathways or the indirect limbic corticostriatal circuits.

Dopamine dysregulation syndrome comprises a group of behaviors that may result from chronic use of dopaminergic drugs. These behaviors include "hedonistic homeostatic dysregulation," which is an excessive and pathological

14 Deep Brain Stimulation of the Subthalamic Nucleus for the Treatment of Parkinson's Disease    263

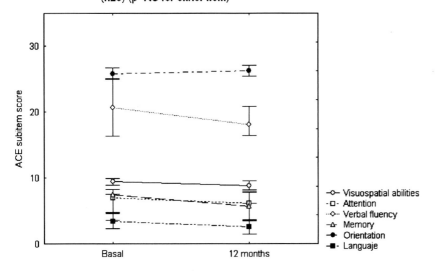

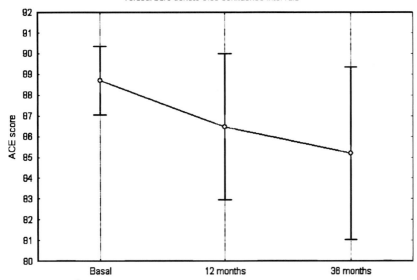

**Figure 14.6** Addenbroke's Cognitive Examination (ACE), a battery of tests evaluating six cognitive domains including attention, verbal fluency, memory, orientation, language, and visuo-spatial abilities in a group of 20 IPD patients who underwent bilateral STN DBS. A non-significant deterioration at 12 months follow-up in attention, memory, verbal fluency, and visuo-spatial abilities was observed. (B) Total ACE scores in the same group of patients. A non-significant deterioration was observed at 12 months follow-up. Differences became significant at 36 months follow-up when scores deteriorated in comparison with basal evaluations

use of dopaminergic medications for non-motor purposes as well as several compulsive behaviors such as hypersexuality and pathological gambling *(92)*. Witt et al. *(93)* suggested that depressive symptoms improve with levodopa and STN stimulation to the same extent. Nevertheless, several reports indicate that patients with preoperative levodopa "addiction" may have difficulty reducing dopaminergic medications postoperatively *(92, 94)*. Because it appears that hedonic tone improves with levodopa and not STN DBS there is apparently a dissociation of depressive symptoms and anhedonia in response to these treatments. Nevertheless, recently Bandini et al. *(91)* reported two patients with pathological gambling who improved dramatically after bilateral STN DBS and early postoperative withdrawal of dopaminergic therapy.

**Sexual Effects**

STN DBS appears to affect sexual function in a small but positive direction. Male patients with PD, especially when under age 60, reported improved sexual well-being over a short follow-up period after surgery. However, there are no case–control studies in the literature confirming this observation *(96)*.

**Sleep**

In advanced PD, chronic STN DBS is associated with subjective improvement in sleep quality, possibly through increased nocturnal mobility and reduction of sleep fragmentation *(97, 98)*. Lyons et al. *(99)* also found that bilateral STN DBS increased total sleep time and reduced patient-reported sleep problems and early morning focal dystonia for up to 24 months. These sleep changes were related to improvements in motor functioning, specifically those affected by bradykinesia. But, despite significant reductions in anti-parkinson medication, STN DBS did not reduce excessive daytime drowsiness *(99)*. Others have found that sleep quality and duration were improved, not only by the direct action on PD cardinal symptoms, but also by improving sleep architecture *(100)*. Recently, Driver-Dunckley et al. reported postoperative restless legs syndrome (RLS) improvement in six advanced PD patients. Despite a mean 56% decrease in their levodopa equivalents after surgery, RLS scores dropped by a mean of 84%, suggesting that bilateral STN DBS surgery may also improve RLS in patients with advanced PD *(101)*.

**Bladder Function**

Clinical studies have shown that STN DBS ameliorates urinary bladder dysfunction in PD by delaying the initial desire to void and increasing bladder capacity. This modulation may result from facilitated processing of afferent bladder information *(102)*.

## QOL

After STN DBS, patients on average perceive a general improvement in QOL of about 50%. However, when evaluated retrospectively, patient tend to overestimate their pre-operative functioning, therefore obscuring the true improvement achieved by surgery. Improvement in QOL following bilateral STN DBS appears to be maintained in the long term, and correlates strongly with improvements in motor function, primarily bradykinesia. By contrast, mental functions such as emotional well-being, social support, cognition, and communication showed milder improvement. A recent study by Deuschl et al. *(70)* demonstrated superior efficacy of neurostimulation over best medical management on quality of life measurements in patients with advanced PD and levodopa-related motor complications. In their study, neurostimulation was associated with a 25% improvement in the PDQ-39 summary index, consistent with 22% improvement in the SF-36, a generic QOL scale.

On the other hand, Schupbach et al. *(103)* stated that despite marked improvement in parkinsonian motor disability, the absence of significant changes in cognitive status indicated that social adjustment did not improve to the expected level. This may have been for several reasons including patient self-perception of body image, marital status, and patient profession.

## Side Effects and Complications of Chronic STN DBS

STN DBS is associated with several clinically significant adverse effects but, in properly selected patients, seems relatively safe from a cognitive standpoint. Current literature suggests that the risk of permanent complications is greatly exceeded by the beneficial effects offered by this treatment, with an overall cumulative incidence of adverse effects directly related to the surgical procedure of roughly 11% *(104)*. However, difficulty in identification of factors which underly some of the nonmotor aspects of the disease discussed earlier illustrates the need for careful patient selection to minimize side effects and complications. Despite good patient follow-up and detailed reporting of clinical outcomes, the true incidence of side effects and complications may not be reliably reported, and is probably underestimated *(104)*.

Many of the peri-operative side effects and complications of DBS STN, such as device-related infections, skin erosions over implanted hardware, cerebral infarct, subdural hematoma, air embolism, wound hematomas or seromas, peri-operative seizures, and postoperative confusion are not discussed here, as they are addressed elsewhere in this book. However, a serious complication that should be underscored is intracerebral bleeding. According to Bloomsted et al. *(105)*, hemorrhagic complications of DBS and ablative lesions for PD have been relatively uncommon and do not differ between the two procedures. Binder et al. *(106)* reported a relative risk of hematoma of 3.1% per lead implant and found brain targeting had a significant effect on the risk of hemorrhage. The incidence of hematoma by target site was 2.5% per lead for STN DBS, 6.7% for GPi DBS and 0% for VIM DBS and an overall risk of intra-operative or early postoperative symptomatic hemorrhage with microelectrode-guided DBS of 1.4% per lead implant. According to Benabid *(79)*, the risk of significant intracranial hemorrhage during subthalamic surgery is about 1.1%. At our center, with more than 200 procedures since 1994, a similar incidence of 0.95% has been observed. However, the only two hemorrhages which occurred were fatal because of rapid progression due to their large size and deep location. Currently, a prospective audit to evaluate bedside administration of recombinant activated factor VII in case of signs of bleeding during the surgical procedure is underway in our center *(107)*.

## Psychiatric Complications

Temel et al. *(108)*, in a review of the current literature, found a total of 1,398 reported patients who underwent bilateral STN DBS. Among them, cognitive problems occurred in 41%, depression in 8%, and hypomania or mania in 4%. Anxiety disorders were observed in less than 2% and personality changes, hypersexuality, apathy, anxiety, and aggressiveness occurred in less than 0.5%.

There have been an increasing number of reports of post-procedural psychiatric complications including depression, mania, aggression, and language deficits *(109)*. Among patients followed at our institution transient irritability, excitation, paranoia, severe insomnia, and severe apathy lasting for as much as 12 months were observed in several cases.

Okun et al. *(110)* reported a case of pseudobulbar crying with features of pseudobulbar palsy associated with STN DBS. Krack et al. *(111)* presented two PD patients in whom acute stimulation of an electrode located in the STN using stimulation parameters 50% above normal therapeutic range induced infectious laughter and hilarity whereas normal therapeutic parameters induced hypomanic behavior and marked improvement of akinesia.

Kulisevsky et al. *(112)* described three DBS patients with no prior psychiatric history who became manic after receiving stimulation at the most inferior contact of quadripolar electrodes implanted bilaterally in the STN. Symptoms developed within 48 hours after stimulation was begun, and satisfied DSM-IV criteria for mania due to a general medical condition. After stimulation was changed to more superior electrode contacts, manic symptoms resolved gradually over 2 weeks. It was suggested that the lower electrode contacts may have been stimulating neurons at the level of the midbrain, caudal to the subthalamic nucleus, where fibers from ventral tegmental areas or anterior cingulate cortical circuits may have been activated. Krack et al. *(113)* mentioned transient postoperative hypomania in 4 of 49 patients, none of whom had "major ongoing psychiatric illness." Houeto et al. *(11)* described a 61-year-old man with a history of depression who developed aggressiveness, irritability, exhibitionism, excessive gambling, and mood swings from depression to exaltation following subthalamic DBS. Because a hypomanic episode had occurred 10 years previously, it was thought that DBS had activated the patient's mood disorder. Mandat *(114)* described two patients who developed hypomania following STN DBS in whom adjustment of stimulation parameters resolved the hypomania while maintaining motor benefits. Although hypersexuality has been induced by DBS, in other circumstances DBS has also reduced levodopa-induced hypersexuality due to ability to reduce the levodopa dose *(115)*.

Suicide attempts and/or suicides have been documented in uncontrolled series ranging from 0.5 to 2.9%. *(109, 113, 116, 117)*. A multicenter study of 450 STN DBS patients reported a postoperative suicide rate of 0.5% *(109)*. In contrast, a study of 120 patients who underwent DBS (PD, dystonia, and essential tremor patients) documented a postoperative suicide rate of 2.9% in PD patients who had undergone STN DBS *(117)*. In this latter study, the authors suggested that young males with a history of multiple surgeries may be at greater risk of such outcomes. However, given the fact that the study was that of a small and uncontrolled retrospective cohort from a single center, conclusions made from this study must be very limited *(113, 116)*. In our own series, one patient committed suicide while waiting for battery replacement after the stimulator battery wore off, making loss of stimulation rather than stimulation itself a possible contributing factor.

**Dysarthria/Hypophonia and Weight Gain**

Dysarthria/hypophonia, weight gain, and postural instability have been the most frequent chronic long-term side effects reported with STN DBS. Guehl et al. *(46)* found that whereas dysarthria/hypophonia remained stable over time, weight gain and postural instability increased during the first year postoperatively.

Levodopa and STN DBS have been associated with both improvement and exacerbation of dysarthria in PD. It seems that, like other motor functions, motor subcomponents of speech can be improved, but that complex coordination of all speech-related anatomical substrates is not responsive to STN DBS *(118)*. In general, with normal settings, there was no significant difference between DBS in off or on modes, but in some patients intelligibility deteriorated with DBS on. Higher frequencies or amplitudes caused significant impairment of intelligibility, whereas changing the polarity between the separate electrode contacts did not *(119)*. Santens et al. *(120)* analyzed the effects of left and right STN DBS on different aspects of speech separately and found significant differences between left- and right-sided stimulation. It appears that selective left-sided stimulation has a profoundly negative effect on prosody, articulation, and intelligibility while right-sided stimulation does not. These differential effects were not found when bilateral DBS was compared with the DBS off condition *(120)*.

Patients with PD often lose weight, but weight gain has been observed after STN DBS associated with a reduction in energy expenditure without daily energy expenditure adjustment *(121)*. Magnitude of weight gain can be significant and DBS candidates should be given nutritional counselling before surgery to prevent rapid or excessive weight gain. Of patients undergoing STN DBS, 50% gain weight during the first 3 months after surgery while 30% continue to show weight gain at 1-year follow-up. In one study, mean weight gain was about 15% above body weight prior to surgery *(122)*.

**Dyskinesias**

Spontaneous dyskinesias may occur after STN DBS and although they can be common immediately after subthalamotomy, there are not many published reports on this issue following STN DBS. This may be due to their rapid reversibility after stimulation parameters are adjusted. We have reported on a patient who after bilateral STN DBS with a particular setting developed mild dyskinesias in the right foot, which became progressively more violent and severe and involved the entire limb *(123)*. When stimulator settings were returned to previous values, involuntary movements disappeared completely within ten minutes. Interestingly, and at variance with levodopa-induced dyskinesias, the involuntary movements observed in this case were unresponsive to amantadine *(123)*. Recently, Brodsky et al. published an interesting case of rebound dyskinesia in an off levodopa state after switching the stimulator off, generating still more controversy on the antidyskinetic effect of STN DBS *(124)*.

**Postural Instability**

As stated several times through the chapter, the response of postural instability to STN DBS remains an unresolved issue. Postural instability has been reported in many series as a frequent complication of STN DBS. This contrasts with the beneficial effect on postural instability observed when analyzed separately or within composite postural instability, gait disturbance (PIGD) scores where patients are taken as a group or when the beneficial effect was studied using laboratory kinematic analysis. Such discrepancies have raised the possibility that postural instability may not be related to STN DBS but either to electrode implantation or its trajectory through the thalamus. Further studies are necessary to clarify this point.

## Comparison of DBS to Subthalamotomy

A considerable body of evidence has suggested that the potential risk of hemiballismus subsequent to subthalamotomy *(125–127)* makes STN DBS preferable to surgical ablation. However, cost, need for regular hardware replacements, and side effects associated with STN DBS represent stimulation disadvantages, justifying the need to explore other therapeutic options. Given these circumstances, we recently conducted a prospective comparison on the efficacy and safety of both surgical STN approaches, in which a consecutive series of sixteen PD patients were randomized to receive either bilateral STN DBS, bilateral subthalamotomy, or unilateral subthalamotomy plus contralateral STN DBS implantation and were evaluated 1 year after surgery. Total UPDRS scores improved after each procedure at 12 months follow-up and no statistical differences were observed between the three groups. A deleterious effect of surgery was observed in UPDRS part I (mentation, behavior, and mood) in patients undergoing bilateral DBS. Significant beneficial effects were observed after surgery on UPDRS part II (activities of daily living) after all three procedures, as well as on UPDRS part III (motor examination) and UPDRS part IV (complications of therapy) in the medication-off condition (Figure 14.7). Significant beneficial effects were observed after each of the three procedures for bradykinesia, rigidity, tremor, dyskinesias, and on a composite score of postural instability and gait disorders (PIGD). No significant effect on mini-mental status examination score was observed after all three procedures, nor was any significant effect on ACE scores observed. ACE subitems, which showed statistically nonsignificant deterioration after surgery, were memory, verbal fluency and visuospatial abilities for bilateral DBS; attention, visuospatial abilities and language for bilateral subthalamotomy, and orientation in the combined group. Psychiatric evaluation showed significantly increased apathy and irritability scores and mood, mentation and behavioral deterioration after surgery in the bilateral DBS group as the only remarkable psychiatric side effects. One patient from the bilateral subthalamotomy group presented severe hemiballismus immediately after surgery that persisted for 3 months and requiring posteroventral pallidotomy for resolution. One patient from the combined technique group presented short-lived hemiballismus that resolved spontaneously. In summary, early motor performance improved significantly after all three surgical procedures without significant group differences with marked effects on cardinal motor symptoms as well as on drug-

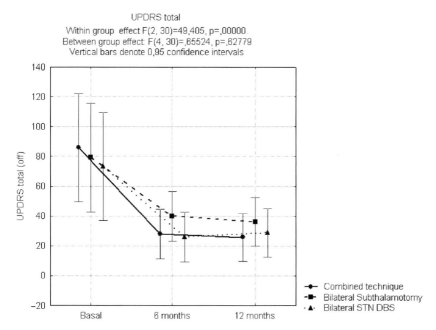

**Figure 14.7** Shows total UPDRS score of a group of 15 IPD patients randomized to Bilateral subthalamotomy ($n = 5$), bilateral STN DBS ($n = 5$), and a combination of unilateral subthalamotomy plus contralateral STN DBS ($n = 5$). A significant effect was observed after each procedure at 6 and 12 months follow-up but no differences between groups were observed

induced dyskinesias. There was levodopa dosage reduction at 1-year follow up in all three groups. The reduced frequency of psychiatric issues after ablative surgery is surprising and requires further clarification. Reduction of procedure-related costs and reduced risk of hardware related complications makes the combination of DBS plus contralateral ablation an option to be considered for bilateral STN interventions in appropriate cases.

## Conclusions: What Physician and Patient Should Expect

Beyond the known improvement of motor signs of PD, more evidence is needed to determine the impact of STN DBS on QOL, caregiver burden, social outcomes, non-motor and other non-dopaminergic symptoms. In addition, we also must address many methodological issues including the need for appropriate control groups and a mechanism by which difficulties in achieving blinding and randomization can be addressed before a definitive conclusion regarding STN DBS for the treatment of Parkinson's disease can be reached.

Currently, despite adequate patient selection, patients who have had an excellent motor response without major changes in cognition frequently feel vaguely unsatisfied after surgery. To address this issue five major points must be made explicitly clear for patients from the outset: (1) This is a non curative procedure. (2) It is applied in a progressive disease. (3) There is a risk of permanent complications. (4) There is a risk of cognitive side effects. (5) Lengthy and sometimes complex follow-up is required.

When pondering the degree of improvement the surgery may bring, abstract figures are difficult for patients to translate to real disabilities, which are not homogeneous. It is best is to imagine how patients feel, look and perform within their own social and working environment during their best moments of the day, even though this may be achieved only briefly, and to point out that the objective of surgery is to extend these moments to last the entire day together with significant reduction in anti-parkinson drug use.

Little information can be found in the literature concerning the percentage of PD patients who are suitable for STN DBS. Lopiano et al. *(128)* suggests that 30% of PD patients are suitable. In our unpublished experience this figure is lower. We believe that less than 10% of PD patients in a movement disorders clinic fulfill clinical criteria for STN DBS and are willing to accept the advantages and disadvantages of participating in a STN DBS program.

For the time being, in the absence of curative therapy, STN DBS, although far from ideal, represents a viable option in a relatively small group of patients with more advanced PD who fail to respond to best available medical treatment.

## References

1. Jankovic J (2005) Motor fluctuations and dyskinesias in Parkinson's disease: clinical manifestations. Mov Disord 20(Suppl 11):S11–S16.
2. Albin RL, Young AB, Penney JB (1989) The functional anatomy of basal ganglia disorders. Trends Neurosci 12:366–375.
3. Alexander GE, DeLong MR, Strick PL (1986) Parallel organization of functionally segregated circuits linking basal ganglia and cortex. Annu Rev Neurosci 9:357–381.
4. Obeso JA, Rodriguez-Oroz MC, Rodriguez M, Macias R, Alvarez L, Guridi J, Vitek J, DeLong MR (2000) Pathophysiologic basis of surgery for Parkinson's disease. Neurology 55(Suppl 6):S7–S12.
5. Benabid AL, Pollak P, Gross C, Hoffmann D, Benazzouz A, et al (1994) Acute and long-term effects of subthalamic nucleus stimulation in Parkinson's disease. Stereotact Funct Neurosurg 62:76–84.
6. Rodriguez-Oroz MC, Obeso JA, Lang AE, Houeto JL, Pollak P, et al (2005) Bilateral deep brain stimulation in Parkinson's disease: a multicentre study with 4 years follow-up. Brain 128:2240–2249.
7. Volkmann J, Sturm V, Weiss P, et al (1998) Bilateral high-frequency stimulation of the internal globus pallidus in advanced Parkinson's disease. Ann Neurol 44:953–961.
8. Ghika J, Villemure JG, Fankhauser H, Favre J, Assal G, Ghika-Schmid F (1998) Efficiency and safety of bilateral contemporaneous pallidal stimulation (deep brain stimulation) in levodopa-responsive patients with Parkinson's disease with severe motor fluctuations: a 2-year follow-up review. J Neurosurg 89:713–718.
9. Loher TJ, Burgunder JM, Weber S, Sommerhalder R, Krauss JK (2002) Effect of chronic pallidal deep brain stimulation on off period dystonia and sensory symptoms in advanced Parkinson's disease. J Neurol Neurosurg Psychiatry 73:395–399.
10. Thobois S, Mertens P, Guenot M, et al (2002) Subthalamic nucleus stimulation in Parkinson's disease: clinical evaluation of 18 patients. J Neurol 249:529–534.
11. Limousin P, Krack P, Pollak P, et al (1998) Electrical stimulation of the subthalamic nucleus in advanced Parkinson's disease. N Engl J Med 339:1105–1111.
12. Vesper J, Klostermann F, Stockhammer F, Funk T, Brock M (2002) Results of chronic subthalamic nucleus stimulation for Parkinson's disease: a 1-year follow-up study. Surg Neurol 57:306–313.

13. Kumar R, Lozano AM, Kim YJ, et al (1998) Double-blind evaluation of subthalamic nucleus deep brain stimulation in advanced Parkinson's disease. Neurology 51:850–855.
14. Krause M, Fogel W, Heck A, et al (2001) Deep brain stimulation for the treatment of Parkinson's disease: subthalamic nucleus versus globus pallidus internus. J Neurol Neurosurg Psychiatry 70:464–470.
15. Krack P, Limousin P, Benabid AL, Pollak P (1997) Chronic stimulation of subthalamic nucleus improves levodopa-induced dyskinesias in Parkinson's disease [letter]. Lancet 350:1676.
16. Brock M, Kern BC, Funk T, Afshar HF (1998) Pallidal or subthalamic stimulation. J Neurosurg 89:345–346.
17. Burchiel KJ, Anderson VC, Favre J, Hammerstad JP (1999) Comparison of pallidal and subthalamic nucleus deep brain stimulation for advanced Parkinson's disease: results of a randomized, blinded pilot study. Neurosurgery 45:1375–1382.
18. The Deep-Brain Stimulation for Parkinson's Disease Study Group (2001) Deep-brain stimulation of the subthalamic nucleus or the pars interna of the globus pallidus inParkinson's disease. N Engl J Med 345:956–963.
19. Esselink RA, de Bie RM, de Haan RJ, et al (2004) Unilateral pallidotomy versus bilateral subthalamic nucleus stimulation in PD: a randomized trial. Neurology 62:201–207.
20. Andersen VC, Burchiel KJ, Hogarth P, Favre J, Hammerstad JP (2005) Pallidal vs subthalamic nucleus deep brain stimulation in Parkinson disease. Arch Neurol 62(4):554–560.
21. Lang A, Houeto JL, Krack P, Kubu C, Lyons E, et al (2006) Deep Brain Stimulation: Preoperative Issues. Mov Disord 21:S171–S196.
22. Broggi G, Franzini A, Marras C, Romito L, Albanese A (2003) Surgery of Parkinson's disease: inclusion criteria and follow-up. Neurol Sci 24(Suppl 1):S38–S40.
23. Lopiano L, Rizzone M, Bergamasco B, et al (2002) Deep brain stimulation of the subthalamic nucleus in PD: an analysis of theexclusion causes. J Neurol Sci 195:167–170.
24. Pinter MM, Alesch F, Murg M, Helscher RJ, Binder H (1999) Apomorphine test: a predictor for motor responsiveness to deep brain stimulation of the subthalamic nucleus. J Neurol 246:907–913.
25. Krack P, Dowsey PL, Benabid AL, et al (2000) Ineffective subthalamic nucleus stimulation in levodopa-resistant postischemic parkinsonism. Neurology 54:2182–2184.
26. Welter ML, Houeto JL, Tezenas du Montcel S, et al (2002) Clinical predictive factors of subthalamic stimulation in Parkinson's disease. Brain 125:575–583.
27. Vitek JL, Bakay RA, Freeman A, et al (2003) Randomized trial of pallidotomy versus medical therapy for Parkinson's disease. Ann Neurol 53:558–569.
28. Baron MS, Vitek JL, Bakay RA, et al (1996) Treatment of advanced Parkinson's disease by posterior Gpi pallidotomy: 1-year results of a pilot study. Ann Neurol 40:355–366.
29. Deep-Brain Stimulation for Parkinson's Disease Study G (2001) Deep brain stimulation of the subthalamic nucleus or the pars interna of the globus pallidus in Parkinson's disease. N Engl J Med 345:956–963.
30. Ostergaard K, Sunde N, Dupont E (2002) Effects of bilateral stimulation of the subthalamic nucleus in patients with severe Parkinson's disease and motor fluctuations. Mov Disord 17:693–700.
31. Schroeder U, Kuehler A, Hennenlotter A, et al (2004) Facial expression recognition and subthalamic nucleus stimulation. J Neurol Neurosurg Psychiatry 75:648–650.
32. Krack P, Batir A, Van Blercom N, et al (2003) Five-year follow-up of bilateral stimulation of the subthalamic nucleus in advanced Parkinson's disease. N Engl J Med 349:1925–1934.

33. Capus L, Melatini A, Zorzon M, et al (2001) Chronic bilateral electrical stimulation of the subthalamic nucleus for the treatment of advanced Parkinson's disease. Neurol Sci 22:57–58.
34. Gironell A, Kulisevsky J, Rami L, Fortuny N, Garcia-Sanchez C, Pascual-Sedano B (2003) Effects of pallidotomy and bilateral subthalamic stimulation on cognitive function in Parkinson disease: a controlled comparative study. J Neurol 250:917–923.
35. Welter ML, Houeto JL, Tezenas du Montcel S, et al (2002) Clinical predictive factors of subthalamic stimulation in Parkinson's disease. Brain 125:575–583.
36. Landi A, Parolin M, Piolti R, et al (2003) Deep brain stimulation for the treatment of Parkinson's disease: the experience of the Neurosurgical Department in Monza. Neurol Sci 24(Suppl 1):S43–S44.
37. Broggi G, Franzini A, Ferroli P, et al (2001) Effect of bilateral subthalamic electrical stimulation in Parkinson's disease. Surg Neurol 56:89–94.
38. Limousin P, Pollak P, Benazzouz A, Hoffmann D, Broussolle E, et al (1995) Bilateral subthalamic nucleus stimulation for severe Parkinson's disease. Mov Disord 10:672–674.
39. Iansek R, Rosenfeld JV, Huxham FE (2002) Deep brain stimulation of the subthalamic nucleus in Parkinson's disease. Med J Aust 177:142–146.
40. Simuni T, Jaggi JL, Mulholland H, et al (2002) Bilateral stimulation of the subthalamic nucleus in patients with Parkinson disease: a study of efficacy and safety. J Neurosurg 96:666–672.
41. Molinuevo JL, Valldeoriola F, Tolosa E, et al (2000) Levodopa withdrawal after bilateral subthalamic nucleus stimulation in advanced Parkinson disease. Arch Neurol 57:983–988.
42. Martinez-Martin P, Valldeoriola F, Tolosa E, et al (2002) Bilateral subthalamic nucleus stimulation and quality of life in advanced Parkinson's disease. Mov Disord 17:372–377.
43. Charles PD, Van Blercom N, Krack P, et al (2002) Predictors of effective bilateral subthalamic nucleus stimulation for PD. Neurology 59:932–934.
44. Kleiner-Fisman G, Fisman DN, Sime E, Saint-Cyr JA, Lozano AM, Lang AE (2003) Long-term follow up of bilateral deep brain stimulation of the subthalamic nucleus in patients with advanced Parkinson disease. J Neurosurg 99:489–495.
45. Bonneville F, Welter ML, Elie C, du Montcel ST, Hasboun D, Menuel C, Houeto JL, Bonnet AM, Mesnage V, Pidoux B, Navarro S, Cornu P, Agid Y, Dormont D (2005) Parkinson disease, brain volumes, and subthalamic nucleus stimulation. Neurology 64:1598–1604.
46. Guehl D, Cuny E, Benazzouz A, Rougier A, Tison F, Machado S, Grabot D, Gross C, Bioulac B, Burbaud P (2006) Side-effects of subthalamic stimulation in Parkinson's disease: clinical evolution and predictive factors. Eur J Neurol 13:963–971.
47. Deuschl G, Bain P (2002) Deep brain stimulation for tremor: patient selection and evaluation. Mov Disord 17(Suppl 3):S102–S111.
48. Vitek JL, Bakay RA, Hashimoto T, et al (1998) Microelectrode-guided pallidotomy: technical approach and its application in medically intractable Parkinson's disease. J Neurosurg 88:1027–1043.
49. Talmant V, Esposito P, Stilhart B, Mohr M, Tranchant C (2006) Subthalamic stimulation in a patient with multiple system atrophy: a clinicopathological report. Rev Neurol (Paris) 162(3):363–370.
50. Miyasaki J, Lozano A, Duff J, Saint-Cyr J, Lang A (1994) The role of posteroventral pallidotomy in advanced Parkinson's disease (PD) and striatonigral degeneration (SND). Neurology 1994; 44 (suppl 2): A322–23.
51. Tarsy D, Apetauerova D, Ryan P, Norregaard T (2003) Adverse effects of subthalamic nucleus DBS in a patient with multiple system atrophy. Neurology 61(2):247–249.

52. Schupbach WM, Chastan N, Welter ML, Houeto JL, Mesnage V et al (2005) Stimulation of the subthalamic nucleus in Parkinson's disease: a 5 year follow up. J Neurol Neurosurg Psychiatry 76:1640–1644.
53. Ostergaard K, Sunde N, Dupont E (2002) Effects of bilateral stimulation of the subthalamic nucleus in patients with severe Parkinson's disease and motor fluctuations. Mov Disord 17:693–700.
54. Krause M, Fogel W, Mayer P, et al (2004) Chronic inhibition of the subthalamic nucleus in Parkinson's disease. J Neurol Sci 219:119–124.
55. Pahwa R, Wilkinson SB, Overman J, Lyons KE (2003) Bilateral subthalamic stimulation in patients with Parkinson disease: longterm follow up. J Neurosurg 99:71–77.
56. Thobois S, Mertens P, Guenot M, et al (2002) Subthalamic nucleus stimulation in Parkinson's disease: clinical evaluation of 18 patients. J Neurol 249:529–534.
57. Herzog J, Volkmann J, Krack P, et al (2003) Two-year follow-up of subthalamic deep brain stimulation in Parkinson's disease. Mov Disord 18:1332–1337.
58. Ford B, Winfield L, Pullman SL, et al (2004) Subthalamic nucleus stimulation in advanced Parkinson's disease: blinded assessments at one year follow up. J Neurol Neurosurg Psychiatry 75:1255–1259.
59. Tamma F, Rampini P, Egidi M, et al (2003) Deep brain stimulation for Parkinson's disease: the experience of the Policlinico–San Paolo Group in Milan. Neurol Sci 24(Suppl 1):S41–S42.
60. Sturman MM, Vaillancourt DE, Metman LV, Bakay RA, Corcos DM (2004) Related Effects of subthalamic nucleus stimulation and medication on resting and postural tremor in Parkinson's disease. Brain 127:2131–2143.
61. Lopiano L, Torre E, Benedetti F, Bergamasco B, Perozzo P, Pollo A, Rizzone M, Tavella A, Lanotte M (2003) Temporal changes in movement time during the switch of the stimulators in Parkinson's disease patients treated by subthalamic nucleus stimulation. Eur Neurol 50:94–99.
62. Lopiano L, Torre E, Benedetti F, et al (2003) Temporal changes in movement time during the switch of the stimulators in Parkinson's disease patients treated by subthalamic nucleus stimulation. Eur Neurol 50:94–99.
63. Vaillancourt DE, Prodoehl J, Verhagen Metman L, et al (2004) Effects of deep brain stimulation and medication on bradykinesia and muscle activation in Parkinson's disease. Brain 127:491–504.
64. Valldeoriola F, Pilleri M, Tolosa E, Molinuevo JL, Rumia J, Ferrer E (2002) Bilateral subthalamic stimulation monotherapy in advanced Parkinson's disease: long-term follow-up of patients. Mov Disord 17:125–132.
65. Vingerhoets FJ, Villemure JG, Temperli P, Pollo C, Pralong E, Ghika J Subthalamic DBS replaces levodopa in Parkinson's disease: two-year follow-up. Neurology 58(3):396–401.
66. Lagrange E, Krack P, Moro E, et al (2002) Bilateral subthalamic nucleus stimulation improves health-related quality of life in PD. Neurology 59:1976–1978.
67. Kumar R, Lozano AM, Montgomery E, Lang AE (1998) Pallidotomy and deep brain stimulation of the pallidum and subthalamic nucleus in advanced Parkinson's disease. Mov Disord 13(Suppl 1):73–82.
68. Herzog J, Pinsker M, Wasner M, Steigerwald F, Wailke S, Deuschl G, Volkmann J (2007) Stimulation of subthalamic fibre tracts reduces dyskinesias in STN DBS. Mov Disord 22(5):679–684.
69. Detante O, Vercueil L, Krack P, Chabardes S, Benabid AL, Pollak P (2004) Off-period dystonia in Parkinson's disease but not generalized dystonia is improved by high frequency stimulation of the subthalamic nucleus. Adv Neurol 94:309–314.
70. Deuschl G, Schade-Brittinger C, Krack P, Volkmann J, Schafer H, et al (2006) German Parkinson Study Group, Neurostimulation Section. A randomized trial of deep-brain stimulation for Parkinson's disease. N Engl J Med 355(9):896–908.

71. Wider C, Russmann H, Villemure JG, Robert B, Bogousslavsky J, Burkhard PR, Vingerhoets FJ (2006) Long-duration response to levodopa in patients with advanced Parkinson disease treated with subthalamic deep brain stimulation. Arch Neurol 63:951–955.
74. Shivitz N, Koop MM, Fahimi J, Heit G, Bronte-Stewart HM (2006) Bilateral subthalamic nucleus deep brain stimulation improves certain aspects of postural control in Parkinson's disease, whereas medication does not. Mov Disord
75. Vrancken AM, Allum JH, Peller M, Visser JE, Esselink RA, Speelman JD, Siebner HR, Bloem BR (2005) Effect of bilateral subthalamic nucleus stimulation on balance and finger control in Parkinson's disease. J Neurol 252:1487–1494.
76. Colnat-Coulbois S, Gauchard GC, Maillard L, Barroche G, Vespignani H, Auque J, Perrin J (2005) Bilateral subthalamic nucleus stimulation improves balance control in Parkinson's disease. Neurol Neurosurg Psychiatry 76:780–787.
72. Crenna P, Carpinella I, Rabuffetti M, Rizzone M, Lopiano L, Lanotte M, Ferrarin M (2006) Impact of subthalamic nucleus stimulation on the initiation of gait in Parkinson's disease. Exp Brain Res 172:519–532.
77. Davis JT, Lyons KE, Pahwa R (2006) Freezing of gait after bilateral subthalamic nucleus stimulation for Parkinson's disease. Clin Neurol Neurosurg 108:461–464.
78. Woods SP, Fields JA, Troster AI (2002) Neuropsychological sequelae of subthalamic nucleus deep brain stimulation in Parkinson's disease: a critical review. Neuropsychol Rev 12:111–126.
79. Benabid AL, Chabardes S, Seigneuret E (2005) Deep-brain stimulation in Parkinson's disease: long-term efficacy and safety. What happened this year? Curr Opin Neurol 18:623–630.
80. Morrison CE, Borod JC, Perrine K, et al (2004) Neuropsychological functioning following bilateral subthalamic nucleus stimulation in Parkinson's disease. Arch Clin Neuropsychol 19:165–181.
81. Funkiewiez A, Ardouin C, Caputo E, Krack P, Fraix V, Klinger H, Chabardes S, Foote K, Benabid A-L, Pollak P (2004) Long term effects of bilateral subthalamic nucleus stimulation on cognitive function, mood, and behaviour in Parkinson's disease. J Neurol Neurosurg Psychiatry 75:834–839.
82. Ardouin C, Pillon B, Peiffer E et al (1999) Bilateral subthalamic or pallidal stimulation for Parkinson's disease affects neither memory nor executive functions: a consecutive series of 62 patients. Ann Neurol 46:217–223.
83. Alegret M, Junque C, Valldeoriola F, et al (2001) Effects of bilateral subthalamic stimulation on cognitive function in Parkinson disease. Arch Neurol 58:1223–1227.
84. Saint-Cyr JA, Trepanier LL, Kumar R, Lozano AM, Lang AE (2000) Neuropsychological consequences of chronic bilateral stimulation of the subthalamic nucleus in Parkinson's disease. Brain 123:2091–2108.
85. Dujardin K, Defebvre L, Krystkowiak P, Blond S, Destee A (2001) Influence of chronic bilateral stimulation of the subthalamic nucleus on cognitive function in Parkinson's disease. J Neurol 248:603–611.
86. Takeshita S, Kurisu K, Trop L et al (2005) Effect of subthalamic stimulation on mood state in Parkinson's disease: evaluation of previous facts and problems. Neurosurg Rev 28:179–186.
87. Daniele A, Albanese A, Contarino MF, et al (2003) Cognitive and behavioural effects of chronic stimulation of the subthalamic nucleus in patients with Parkinson's disease. J Neurol Neurosurg Psychiatry 74:175–182.
88. Czernecki V, Pillon B, Houeto JL, et al (2005) Does bilateral stimulation of the subthalamic nucleus aggravate apathy in Parkinson's disease? J Neurol Neurosurg Psychiatry 76:775–779.
89. Biseul I, Sauleau P, Haegelen C, et al (2005) Fear recognition is impaired by subthalamic nucleus stimulation in Parkinson's disease. Neuropsychologia 43:1054–1059.

90. Doshi PK, Chhaya N, Bhatt MH (2002) Depression leading to attempted suicide after bilateral subthalamic nucleus stimulation for Parkinson's disease. Mov Disord 17:1084–1085.
91. Horvitz JC (2000) Mesolimbocortical and nigrostriatal dopamine responses to salient non-reward events. Neuroscience 96:651–656.
92. Giovannoni G, O'Sullivan JD, Turner K, Manson AJ, Lees AJ (2000) Hedonistic homeostatic dysregulation in patients with Parkinson's disease on dopamine replacement therapies. J Neurol Neurosurg Psychiatry 68:423–428.
94. Moro E, Scerrati M, Romito LM, Roselli R, Tonali P, Albanese A (1999) Chronic subthalamic nucleus stimulation reduces medication requirements in Parkinson's disease. Neurology 53:85–90.
93. Witt K, Daniels C, Herzog J, Lorenz D, Volkmann J, Reiff J, Mehdorn M, Deuschl G, Krack P (2006) Differential effects of L-dopa and subthalamic stimulation on depressive symptoms and hedonic tone in Parkinson's disease. J Neuropsychiatry Clin Neurosci 18:397–401.
95. Bandini F, Primavera A, Pizzorno M, Cocito L (2006) Using STN DBS and medication reduction as a strategy to treat pathological gambling in Parkinson's disease. Parkinsonism Relat Disord published online PMID 17049455.
96. Lanotte B, Bergamasco L, Lopiano L, Castelli P, Perozzo ML, Genesia E, Torre M, Pesare A, Cinquepalmi M (2004) Sexual well being after deep brain stimulation of the subthalamic nucleus. J Neurol Neurosurg Psychiatry 75;1260–1264.
97. Iranzo A, Valldeoriola F, Santamaria J, Tolosa E, Rumia J (2002) Sleep symptoms and polysomnographic architecture in advanced Parkinson's disease after chronic bilateral subthalamic stimulation J Neurol Neurosurg Psychiatry 72:661–664.
98. Antonini A, Landi A, Mariani C, DeNotaris R, Pezzoli G (2004) Deep brain stimulation and its effect on sleep in Parkinson's disease. Sleep Med 5(2):211–214.
99. Lyons KE, Pahwa R (2006) Effects of bilateral subthalamic nucleus stimulation on sleep, daytime sleepiness, and early morning dystonia in patients with Parkinson disease. J Neurosurg 104:502–505.
100. Cicolin A, Lopiano L, Zibetti M, Torre E, Tavella A, Guastamacchia G, Terreni A, Makrydakis G, Fattori E, Lanotte MM, Bergamasco B, Mutani R (2004) Effects of deep brain stimulation of the subthalamic nucleus on sleep architecture in parkinsonian patients. Sleep Med 5:207–210.
101. Driver-Dunckley E, Evidente VG, Adler CH, Hillman R, Hernandez J, Fletcher G, Lyons MK (2006) Restless legs syndrome in Parkinson's disease patients may improve with subthalamic stimulation. Mov Disord 21:1287–1289.
102. Herzog J, Weiss PH, Assmus A, Wefer B, Seif C, Braun PM, Herzog H, Volkmann J, Deuschl G, Fink GR (2006) Subthalamic stimulation modulates cortical control of urinary bladder in Parkinson's disease. Brain published online PMID 17077105.
103. Schupbach M, Gargiulo M, Welter ML, Mallet L, Behar C, Houeto JL, Maltete D, Mesnage V, Agid Y (2006) Neurosurgery in Parkinson disease: a distressed mind in a repaired body? Neurology 66:1811–1816.
104. Boucai L, Cerquetti D, Merello M (2004) Functional surgery for Parkinson's disease treatment: a structured analysis of a decade of published literature. Br J Neurosurg 18:213–222.
105. Blomstedt P, Hariz MI (2006) Are complications less common in deep brain stimulation than in ablative procedures for movement disorders? Stereotact Funct Neurosurg 84:72–81.
106. Binder DK, Rau G, Starr PA (2003) Hemorrhagic complications of microelectrode-guided deep brain stimulation. Stereotact Funct Neurosurg 80:28–31.
107. Mayer SA, Rincon F (2005) Treatment of intracerebral haemorrhage. Lancet Neurol 4:662–672.
108. Temel Y, Kessels A, Tan S, Topdag A, Boon P, Visser-Vandewalle V (2006) Behavioural changes after bilateral subthalamic stimulation in advanced Parkinson disease: a systematic review. Parkinsonism Relat Disord 12:265–272.

109. Voon V, Moro E, Saint-Cyr J, Lozano A, Lang A (2005) Psychiatric symptoms following surgery for Parkinson's disease with an emphasis on subthalamic stimulation. Adv Neurol 96:130–147.
110. Okun, MS, Raju DV, Walter BL, Juncos JL, DeLong MR, Heilman K, McDonald WM, Vitek JL (2004) Pseudobulbar crying induced by stimulation of the region of the subthalamic nucleus. J Neurol Neurosurg Psychiatry 75(6):921–923.
111. Krack P, Kumar R, Ardouin C, et al (2001) Mirthful laughter induced by subthalamic nucleus stimulation. Mov Disord 16:867–875.
112. Kulisevsky J, Berthier ML, Gironell A, et al (2002) Mania following deep brain stimulation for Parkinson's disease. Neurology 59:1421–1424.
113. Krack P, Batir A, Van Blercom N, et al (2003) Five years follow-up of bilateral stimulation of the subthalamic nucleus in advanced Parkinson's disease. N Engl J Med 349:1925–1934.
114. Mandat TS, Hurwitz T, Honey CR (2006) Hypomania as an adverse effect of subthalamic nucleus stimulation: report of two cases. Acta Neurochir (Wien) 148(8):895–897.
115. Romito LM, Raja M, Daniele A, et al (2002) Transient mania with hypersexuality after surgery for high-frequency stimulation of the subthalamic nucleus in Parkinson's disease. Mov Disord 17:1371–1374.
116. Houeto JL, Mesnage V, Mallet L, et al (2002) Behavioural disorders, Parkinson's disease and subthalamic stimulation. J Neurol Neurosurg Psychiatry 72:701–707.
117. Burkhard PR, Vingerhoets FJ, Berney A, Bogousslavsky J, Villemure JG, Ghika J (2004) Suicide after successful deep brain stimulation for movement disorders. Neurology 63:2170–2172.
118. Pinto S, Gentil M, Krack P, Sauleau P, Fraix V, Benabid AL, Pollak P (2005) Changes induced by levodopa and subthalamic nucleus stimulation on parkinsonian speech. Mov Disord 20(11):1507–1515.
119. Tornqvist AL, Schalen L, Rehncrona S (2005) Effects of different electrical parameter settings on the intelligibility of speech in patients with Parkinson's disease treated with subthalamic deep brain stimulation. Mov Disord 20:416–423.
120. Santens P, De Letter M, Van Borsel J, De Reuck J, Caemaert J (2003) Lateralized effects of subthalamic nucleus stimulation on different aspects of speech in Parkinson's disease. Brain Lang 87:253–258.
121. Macia F, Perlemoine C, Coman I, Guehl D, Burbaud P, Cuny E, Gin H, Rigalleau V, Tison F (2004) Parkinson's disease patients with bilateral subthalamic deep brain stimulation gain weight. Mov Disord 19:206–212.
122. Barichella M, Marczewska AM, Mariani C, Landi A, Vairo A, Pezzoli G (2003) Body weight gain rate in patients with Parkinson's disease and deep brain stimulation. Mov Disord 18:1337–1340.
123. Merello M, Perez-Lloret S, Antico J, Obeso JA (2006) Dyskinesias induced by subthalamotomy in Parkinson's disease are unresponsive to amantadine. J Neurol Neurosurg Psychiatry 77:172–174.
124. Brodsky MA, Hogarth P, Nutt JG (2006) OFF-off rebound dyskinesia in subthalamic nucleus deep brain stimulation of Parkinson's disease. Mov Disord 21(9):1487–1490.
125. Guridi J, Herrero MT, Luquin MR, et al (1996) Subthalamotomy in parkinsonian monkeys. Behavioural and biochemical analysis. Brain 119:1717–1727.
126. Guridi J, Obeso JA (2001) The subthalamic nucleus, hemiballismus and Parkinson's disease: reappraisal of a neurosurgical dogma. Brain 124:5–19.
127. Chen CC, Lee ST, Wu T, et al (2002) Hemiballism after subthalamotomy in patients with Parkinson's disease: report of 2 cases. Mov Disord 17:1367–1371.
128. Lopiano L (2004) Deep brain stimulation of the subthalamic nucleus in PD: an analysis of the exclusion causes. J Neurolog Sci 195:167.

# 15
# Deep Brain Stimulation of the Globus Pallidus Pars Interna and Subthalamic Nucleus in Parkinson's Disease: Pros and Cons

Jorge Guridi, Maria C. Rodriguez-Oroz, and Jose A. Obeso

## Abstract

Proper comparison of the therapeutic efficacy of subthalamic nucleus (STN) deep brain stimulation (DBS) vs globus pallidus internus (GPi) DBS is not possible with the information currently available. Multi-center randomized studies are in progress that may settle this point. Despite this, the choice of GPi as a surgical target has decreased enormously in practice and most recent studies concern data derived from patients treated with STN DBS. Why this has occurred cannot be entirely explained on scientific grounds. Perhaps the larger number of experimental studies demonstrating the impact of STN stimulation on parkinsonism as well as the anatomo-physiological data indicating the prominent capacity of the STN to modulate basal ganglia output created a scenario that has led specialists to prefer the STN. Finally, the ability to reduce or even discontinue levodopa and other antiparkinson treatments after STN DBS undoubtedly has had a major influence on its relative popularity.

**Keywords:** deep brain stimulation, DBS, globus pallidus internus, subthalamic nucleus, Parkinson's disease

## Introduction

The development and application of DBS for treatment of Parkinson's disease (PD) has been greatly influenced by pathophysiological concepts. During the 1980s, research studies in animal models of parkinsonism, particularly the 1-methyl, 4-phenyl-1,2,3,6 tetrahydropyridine (MPTP) monkey model, showed that dopamine depletion leads to increased neuronal activity of the STN and the output nuclei of the basal ganglia, i.e., the GPi and the substantia nigra pars reticulata (SNr; refs. *1–3*). In the 6-hydroxydopamine (6-OHDA) rat model, the subthalamic lesion was associated with a robust normalization of neuronal metabolic markers in the basal ganglia *(4)*. Subthalamotomy performed in MPTP monkeys induced a marked motor benefit and a concomitant reduction in neuronal activity in the GPi and SNr *(5–7)*. Initial experimental studies did not target the GPi. However, the fear of inducing severe hemichorea-ballism secondary to lesions of the STN precluded the application of these experimental results and concepts to PD surgery. In 1992, Laitinen et al. reported striking benefits derived from unilateral pallidotomy, which facilitated the resurgence of surgery for PD with GPi as the target *(8)*. Pallidotomy quickly became the surgical treatment of choice for PD patients in the mid-1990s. The clinical benefits were significant but occurred mainly contralateral to the lesion *(9)*, which limited the benefit of this approach, because the majority of patients requiring surgical treatment display generalized or bilateral motor manifestations. On the other hand, bilateral pallidotomy induced severe cognitive and speech deficits in a substantial proportion of patients *(10)*. Although cognitive deficits may have been associated with larger lesions that included nonmotor regions of GPi, even well placed smaller lesions were sometimes associated with speech deficits.

DBS mimicking the effect of ablative lesions was initially introduced in the surgical armamentarium to replace thalamotomy in patients with resting tremor *(11)*. The realization that thalamic DBS contributed a benefit against tremor similar to that of a lesion *(12)*, the need for bilateral surgery in the majority of candidates and studies in MPTP monkeys using high-frequency stimulation *(13, 14)* led the Grenoble group to introduce STN DBS for the treatment of advanced PD *(13)*. Coincidentally, Siegfried and Lippitz (1994) successfully applied DBS to the GPi seeking to mimic the effect of pallidotomy described by Laitinen *(15)*. Initial results were positive and set the stage for larger clinical experiences. A multi-center trial was begun in 1996 to assess the safety, viability, and short-term efficacy of DBS of either STN or GPi *(16)*. The trial was not randomized and no specific guidelines were issued for allocating patients to one target or the other. Both groups showed significant improvement induced by stimulation *(16)*. Over the years, many groups all over the world have applied DBS of the STN and GPi to treat PD (Tables 15.1 and 15.2) but publications properly comparing the therapeutic efficacy of the two targets were limited to only a single group *(17)*.

Nevertheless, STN DBS has become by and large the preferred procedure in most centers *(18)*. It is interesting to ask why this preference has prevailed. There appear to be three main reasons. First, after the initial clinical trial, there was the impression that clinical benefit for the cardinal features of PD obtained by STN DBS was greater than for GPi DBS, despite the absence of validated data. Second, from a surgical point of view, it appeared to be easier to define the sensorimotor region and surrounding structures of the STN physiologically than the GPi using microrecording and microstimulation. Finally, and perhaps the major distinction between the two procedures was that STN DBS allowed for a significant reduction in the daily dose of levodopa, which could not be achieved with GPi DBS. This was a very attractive clinical option, considering the profusion of motor (i.e., dyskinesias) and non-motor (i.e., psychiatric complications, sleep problems, etc.) adverse effects associated with chronic levodopa treatment. However, it should be noted that the ability to reduce levodopa dosage after STN DBS was discovered only after doses were reduced to deal with exacerbated dyskinesia. Because GPi DBS directly reduces levodopa-induced dyskinesia (LID) there may have been little motivation to lower levodopa dose after GPi DBS.

**Table 15.1** Clinical results of patients treated with DBS of the STN.

| | Follow-up (month) | Age at surgery | Mean H&Y (off) | Disease duration (years) | Pre-operative levodopa response (UPDRS III off/on: % change) | % change in UPDRS II score (post-op stim on/med off vs pre-op med off) | % change in UPDRS III score (post-op stim on/med off vs pre-op med off) | LED (% change) | Dyskinesia (% change) | % Change in duration of daily OFF |
|---|---|---|---|---|---|---|---|---|---|---|
| Herzog (n = 20; ref. 52) | 24.0 | 60.0 ± 6 | 3.7 | 15.0 ± 5 | 57.0 | 43.6 | 57.2 | 67.0 | 85.0 | NA |
| Krause (n = 24; ref. 58) | 29.8 ± 8.5 | 57.7 | 4.3 | 14.4 ± 5.8 | 65.0 | 17.0 | 38.3 | 30.0 | 70.0 | 16.0% |
| Rodriguez-Oroz (n = 10; ref. 47) | 48.0 | 62.0 (53–73) | NA | NA | 75.0 | 62.0 | 62.0 | 50.0 | 53 | NA |
| Kleiner-Fisman (n = 25; ref. 53) | 24.0 (12–52) | 57.2 ± 11.7 | NA | 13.4 ± 4.3 | 54.5 | 26.0 | 39.0 | 42.0 | 65.5 | 58% |
| Krack (n = 42; ref. 25) | 60.0 | 55.0 (34–68) | NA | 14.6 ± 5.0 | 74.3 | 49.0 | 54.0 | 63.0 | 67 | NA |
| Pahwa (n = 19; ref. 54) | 27.8 (22–42) | 56.4 (35–76) | 3.2 | 12.1 (3.9–27.2) | 36.6 | 27.0 | 27.7 | 57.0 | 42 | 61% |
| Romito (n = 33; ref. 56) | 25.7 ± 13.5 | 56.8 ± 7.1 | NA | 13.8 ± 5.5 | 59.4 | 68.5 | 51.6 | 56.2 | 83.9 | 94.2% |
| Rodriguez-Oroz (n = 49; ref. 20) | 36–48 | 59.8 ± 9.8 | 4.3 ± 0.8 | 15.4 ± 6.3 | 59.78 | 43 | 50 | 35 | 59 | 56% |
| Visser-vandewalle (n = 20; ref. 55) | 53.6 ± 2.6 | 60.9 ± 8.1 | NA | 15 ± 4.4 | NA | 59 | 42.8 | 47.2 | 79 | 78% |
| Ostergaard (n = 18; ref. 57) | 48 ± 2 | 63 ± 8 | 3.7 ± 0.8 | 19 ± 5 | 54.19 | 42 | 55 | 29 | 90 | 67% |
| Shupbach (n = 30; ref. 26) | 60 | 54.9 ± 9.1 | 5 | 15.2 ± 5.3 | 69 | NA | 49.51 | 54.56 | 79 | 67% |

LED, levodopa equivalent dose; n, effective sample size.
Data reported as mean ± SD/range

**Table 15.2** Clinical results of patients treated with DBS of the GPi.

| Citation | Follow-up (months) | Age at surgery | Mean H&Y (off) | Disease duration (years) | Pre-operative levodopa response (UPDRS III off/on: % change) | % change in UPDRS II score (post-op stim on/med off vs pre-op med off) | % change in UPDRS III score (post-op stim on/med off vs pre-op med off) | LED (% change) | Dyskinesia (% change) | % Change in duration of daily OFF |
|---|---|---|---|---|---|---|---|---|---|---|
| Obeso (n = 36; ref. 16) | 6 | 55.7 ± 9.8 | NR | 14.5 | NR | 36 | 33.3 | UCH | 67 | 35% |
| Rodriguez-Oroz (n = 20; ref. 20) | 46.8 | 55.8 ± 9.4 | NR | 15.4 | NR | 28 | 39 | UCH | 76 | 45% |
| Volkmann (n = 11; ref. 27) | 12; n = 10 | NR | NR | 11.2 ± 2.7 | 44 | 50 | 56 | UCH | 58 | NR |
|  | 36; n = 9 |  |  |  |  | 30 | 43 |  | 63 |  |
|  | 60; n = 5 |  |  |  |  | 10 | 24 |  | 64 |  |
| Rodrigues (n = 11; ref. 51) | 24.8 | 61.45 | 2.7 | 14.54 | 50 | NR | 46 | UCH | 76 | NR |
| Durif (n = 5; ref. 48) | 36 | 64 | 4.3 ± 0.2 | 15 ± 2 | 72 | 9 | 32 | UCH | 50 | 10% |
| Ghika (n = 6; ref. 29) | 24 | 55 | 4.2 | 15.5 | 33 minimum | >50 | >50 | UCH | 75 | >50% |
| Loher (n = 10; ref. 49) | 12 | 64.6 ± 9.9 | 4.4 ± 0.7 | 19.6 ± 7.9 | NR | 34 | 41 | UCH | 71 | NR |
| Kumar (n = 17; ref. 50) | 2 | 52.7 ± 8.5 | NR | 14.8 ± 6.1 | NR | 39 | 31 | UCH | 68 | NR |
| Anderson (n = 10; ref. 17) | 10 | 54 ± 12 | 4 | 10.3 ± 2 | 57 | 23 | 39 | 3 | 89 | NR |

n, effective sample size; NR, not reported; UCH, unchanged.
Data reported as mean ± SD/range
*Four patients with lack of efficacy, operated in the STN after 2 years (n = 2) and 3 years (n = 2).
#Worsening after 1 year in three patients with stimulation resistant gait ignition failure.

Overall, the issue of the advantages and disadvantages of either target have remained open to question *(18, 19)*. It is surprising to realize that critical questions such as relative efficacy and the incidence of adverse events and complications have remained unanswered for more than 10 years since the generalized application of DBS for PD began. To re-assess the pros and cons of these targets, this chapter reviews available published reports that have compared STN and GPi DBS carried out by the same group *(16, 17, 20–24)*.

## Clinical Results

The data available from different studies which describe the clinical results of STN and GPi DBS show an overall improvement of cardinal motor features and a significant reduction in the "off" Unified Parkinson's Disease Rating Scale (UPDRS) motor subscore (part III; Tables 15.1 and 15.2). This is accompanied by decreased time spent in the "off" state condition and increased number of "on" hours without disabling dyskinesias. Although not prospectively and systematically studied in controlled fashion, a reduction in the daily dose of levodopa has occurred after STN DBS and no change or a slight increase in levodopa dose has occurred after GPi DBS *(16, 17, 21)*. However, appropriate comparison of the therapeutic merits of either target would require a randomized study.

Most surgical groups have selected the basal ganglia target on the basis of the patient's predominant clinical characteristics and the biases and surgical experience of the group. For example, we initially chose to use STN DBS to treat patients with predominant gait and axial features and allocate to GPi DBS those with severe LIDs, particularly those with diphasic dyskinesias. It is also notable that most publications concerning GPi DBS have generally reported assessment over a relatively short follow-up compared with STN DBS for which several reports have followed up for 4 to 5 years after surgery *(20, 25, 26)*.

### Effect of DBS Against Cardinal Features of PD and "Off" Disability

Anderson et al. reported the only prospective and randomized comparative study of STN and GPi DBS with 12 months of follow-up evaluation in 20 patients (10 each group; ref. *17*). They showed that "off" medication and on stimulation improvement was 39% for GPi DBS patients and 48% for STN DBS patients. There was no improvement in on-medication function in either group (Table 15.3). Improvement of tremor, rigidity, and bradykinesia was not significantly different between the two treatment groups, although bradykinesia tended to improve more in the STN DBS group ($p < 0.06$). Improvement of axial symptoms was also not significantly different ($p < 0.12$; Table 15.3) and LIDs were reduced for both targets with no difference between groups. This reduction was 89% for GPi DBS and 68% for STN DBS. Levodopa was reduced only in the STN DBS group but it is unclear whether any attempt was made to reduce levodopa in the GPi DBS group. This prospective, randomized study therefore found no evidence of a substantially better response with STN DBS than GPi DBS.

Volkmann et al. retrospectively compared patients treated with STN DBS ($n = 16$) versus GPi DBS ($n = 11$) at 12 months postoperatively *(21)*.

**Table 15.3** Clinical Results of studied including DBS of the GPi and STN.

| Author | Baseline | 6 months | 12 months | 3 to 4 years | 3 to 4 years vs 1 year |
|---|---|---|---|---|---|
| Volkmann et al. 16 STN 11 GPi *(21)* | | | | | |
| UPDRS III STN/GPi | 56.4/52.5 | 18.6/22.9 | 22.4/16.7 | | |
| Bradykinesia | 2.5/2.5 | 1.1/1.3 | 1.3/1.3 | | |
| Rigidity | 2.4/2.2 | 0.5/1.1 | 0.6/1.1 | | |
| Tremor | 0.9/0.8 | 0.1/0.2 | 0.1/0.2 | | |
| Posture/Gait | 2.7/2.2 | 1.0/0.8 | 1.1/0.8 | | |
| Swallowing | 1.7/1.3 | 1.2/0.9 | 1.3/0.9 | | |
| Krack et al. 8 STN 5GPi *(23)* | | | | | |
| UPDRS III STN/Gpi | 57.3/53.6 | 17.1/32.5; $p < 0.05$ | | | |
| Tremor | 4.0/4.0 | 0.5/1.6 ns | | | |
| Rigidity | 13.8/13.9 | 4.5/6.8 ns | | | |
| Akinesia | 19.9/19.7 | 5.7/13.7; $p < 0.05$ | | | |
| Gait scores | 14.1/13.5 | 3.0/8.0; $p < 0.05$ | | | |
| Anderson et al. 10 STN 10 GPi *(17)* | | | | | |
| UPDRS III STN/GPi | 51/50 | | 27.0/30.0; $p < 0.40$ | | |
| Rigidity | 10.5/9.5 | | 5.0/5.0; $p < 0.18$ | | |
| Tremor | 9.0/7.0 | | 1.0/1.5; $p < 0.51$ | | |
| Bradykinesia | 18/15 | | 10/10; $p < 0.6$ | | |
| Axial scores | 8/7.5 | | 4.5/4.5; $p < 0.12$ | | |
| Rodriguez-Oroz et al. 49 STN 20 GPi *(20)* | | | | | |
| UPDRS III STN/GPi | 56.7/51.7 | | 24.6/29.2 | 28.6/31.7 | $p < 0.02$/ns |
| Tremor | 13.1/11.3 | | 2.3/2.7 | 1.7/1.7 | ns/ns |
| Rigidity | 10.8/10.9 | | 3.8/6.5 | 4.4/6.5 | ns/ns |
| Bradykinesia | 19.9/18.3 | | 10.7/10.9 | 11.3/12.9 | ns/ns |
| Postural stability | 2.6/2.3 | | 1.2/1.4 | 1.8/1.7 | $p < 0.001$/ns |
| Gait | 2.8/2.5 | | 1.4/1.5 | 1.7/1.8 | $p < 0.02$/ns |

ns, not significant.

Motor UPDRS was significantly reduced for both targets ($p < 0.005$; Table 15.3), but somewhat exceptionally, limb symptoms such as tremor, rigidity, and bradykinesia were only significantly reduced following STN DBS. Posture and gait also improved for both targets but only STN DBS reached a significant difference (Table 15.3). Dyskinesias were alleviated significantly for STN ($p < 0.001$) and GPi ($p < 0.005$). Reduction in levodopa dose reached a significant difference with respect to the pre-operative dose after STN (65.3%) but not GPi DBS (16%; ref. *21*).

A similar study was described by Krause et al. in a prospective non-randomized study in which six patients were treated with GPi DBS and 12 with STN DBS. They described a superior effect of STN DBS for most of the motor scores assessed. STN induced significant improvement in motor UPDRS, whereas GPi DBS had no significant effect. Motor fluctuations were reduced only by STN DBS *(22)*.

Krack et al. compared eight patients with bilateral STN DBS vs five patients with GPi DBS at 6 months postoperatively (Table 15.3; ref. 23). They reported that motor UPDRS was alleviated in both targets after surgery but this was significant only in the STN DBS group ($p < 0.05$). Tremor and rigidity showed similar degrees of improvement but akinesia was better alleviated with STN DBS ($p < 0.05$). Axial symptoms, such as gait scores, were significant reduced with STN DBS ($p < 0.05$) but not with GPi DBS *(23)*.

The most comprehensive study of STN DBS compared with GPi DBS in the largest number of patients assessed using the same methodology was conducted at 18 centers worldwide between 1995 and 1999 *(16)*. This comprised 134 patients with bilateral implantation (96 STN and 38 GPi). Initial results were reported in 2001. This prospective trial was not randomized for the surgical target but did include a randomized double-blind evaluation of the effect of DBS at 3 months. This study showed that either target significantly improved motor function in the "off" medication state. At 6 months (open evaluation), patients with STN DBS showed 74% ($p < 0.001$) improvement in "on" time without dyskinesias (27% baseline) while patients with GPi DBS a 64% ($p < 0.01$; 28% baseline) improvement *(16)*.

A follow-up study of patients in this multi-center study has been recently published 3 to 4 years postoperatively *(20)*. Patients treated with STN DBS ($n = 49$) outnumbered the GPi DBS treated group ($n = 20$). The analysis compared both targets at 3 to 4 years compared with the effects seen at baseline and 1 year postoperatively. Although the trial was not originally designed for direct comparison of target efficacy, the demographic characteristics of both groups were very similar, with the important exception (see later) of cognitive impairment. Thus, this study may be considered to be the most important data source available to compare the effect of GPi DBS vs STN DBS for cardinal features of PD after prolonged follow-up. UPDRS motor scores remained significantly improved after 3 to 4 years compared with baseline for both targets ($p < 0.0001$), but the STN DBS group showed worsening in UPDRS motor scores compared with the benefit obtained at 1 year ($p < 0.02$). By contrast, the GPi DBS group maintained the benefit observed at 1 year when re-evaluated 3 to 4 years later. In this study, cardinal features such as tremor, rigidity and bradykinesia were still improved after 3 to 4 years in both groups compared with the baseline and 1-year assessments. Postural stability showed no significant difference compared with baseline in the GPi DBS group while gait improved. Both postural stability and gait were improved at 3 to 4 years compared with baseline in the STN DBS group ($p < 0.0001$). However gait, postural instability, and speech all significantly declined in the STN DBS group while off medication between the 1-year and 3- to 4-year assessment but showed no change in the GPi DBS group. Dyskinesias also remained reduced for both targets at 3 to 4 years vs baseline ($p < 0.0001$) but were not significantly different compared with the 1-year evaluation. The study concluded that STN and GPi DBS both continue to produce improvement 3 to 4 years after surgery but that there is a decline in axial motor signs in the STN DBS group while off medication that was not evident in the GPi DBS group. The reason for the latter finding is uncertain but may relate to a number of factors such as possible residual long-duration effects of the larger dose of levodopa the GPi DBS patients were taking and other possible underlying differences in the two patient populations *(20)*. Superiority of GPi DBS over STN DBS cannot be concluded from this study but other commonly held assumptions that STN DBS may be superior to GPi DBS may also be unwarranted.

Some GPi DBS follow-up studies have reported failure of long-term relief of parkinsonian disability with some patients requiring a second operation to implant electrodes in the STN *(27, 28)*. Volkmann et al. reported on 11 patients with bilateral GPi DBS at long term follow-up (5 years) in whom initial alleviation of off-period motor symptoms and fluctuations declined after the first year. Four patients with waning efficacy were re-operated with STN DBS *(27)*. Other authors have described patients with motor improvement following GPi DBS, in whom efficacy at 2 years was markedly less than that at 1 year *(29)*. The reason for these late failures is uncertain but could possibly include suboptimal lead location, patient selection, and programming issues, none of which were adequately studied or discussed.

### Effects of DBS in the "On" Medication State

Assessment of the effect of stimulation in both targets has revealed that the "on" medication condition is not usually improved after surgery. This indicates that there is no additional DBS benefit over and above the levodopa effect *(17, 20, 21, 23)*. In the large multi-center study discussed earlier *(20)*, at 1 year the total motor UPDRS score on medication and on DBS was not significantly improved for either STN or GPi DBS and had significantly worsened at 3 to 4 years ($p < 0.01$ and 0.05 for STN and GPi). When the results at 1 vs 3 to 4 years were compared while on medication, gait and postural stability deteriorated in the STN DBS group but only gait and not postural instability deteriorated in the GPi DBS group. Similar to results off medication discussed above, these results are of uncertain significance and may have been affected by underlying differences in the two treatment groups.

All studies have found a marked reduction in levodopa dyskinesia with either GPi or STN DBS. Although the reduction of dyskinesia in STN DBS patients is statistically equivalent to GPi DBS, the pathophysiological mechanisms may be different. Daily levodopa equivalents were reduced in STN DBS patients but not GPi DBS patients at 1 and 3 to 4 years *(17, 20, 21, 23)*. Similar to effects of pallidotomy, GPi DBS may alleviate levodopa dyskinesia by disrupting or interfering with neuronal signals in the pallido-thalamic motor circuit. There is general agreement that STN DBS primarily reduces dyskinesia by an indirect effect mediated by reduction in daily levodopa dose *(30–32)*. On the other hand, a direct antidyskinetic effect of chronic STN DBS possibly mimicking the effects of continuous dopaminergic stimulation has been suggested by other authors *(33–35)*.

In summary, DBS of both targets alleviates the cardinal features of PD during the "off" condition at long-term follow-up. A major improvement in on-medication scores is not expected but dyskinesias are prominently attenuated, leading to a marked improvement in activities of daily living in the "on" condition. Comparisons of the effect of DBS in either target on specific motor features such as gait, postural stability, and speech is not possible due to lack of proper randomization in all studies. Although some authors have suggested that STN DBS may convey a more striking benefit than GPi DBS, this is not supported by the only randomized study published to this time *(17, 20)*. There may be theoretical reasons to favor STN over GPi DBS. It may be that the volume of tissue affected by stimulation in STN (about 160 mm$^3$) compared with GPi volume (about 460 mm$^3$; ref. *36*) could allow activation of a larger proportion of STN than GPi outflow. Another point may be that STN DBS could have an impact on both efferent systems of the basal ganglia, the GPi and SNr, and their projections to the brainstem as well as nigro-striatal fibers projecting over the STN. This effect on larger numbers of efferent circuits may possibly be an advantage over GPi DBS, but at this time has not been validated by results of randomized, controlled clinical trials.

## Adverse Events

Events related to hardware, such as lead fracture, infection, and skin erosions seem to be similar for both targets and are not considered here. Battery replacement has been more frequent in GPi DBS than STN DBS, likely related to the higher voltages and pulse widths used in GPi DBS *(20)*. We consider in this section the analysis of adverse events related to stimulation.

Two studies have reported that GPi DBS may induce different effects depending on electrode placement *(37, 38)*. The more dorsal contacts appear to induce dyskinetic movements and alleviate akinesia and are considered "prokinetic," whereas the most ventral ones may induce akinesia and are antidyskinetic. This suggests that parkinsonian and antidyskinetic responses to GPi DBS may be a reflection of at least two different anatomo-functional loops within GPi and possibly GPe *(37–39)*.

It is also noteworthy that very few psychiatric or mood disorders have been described after GPi DBS *(17, 20)*. On the contrary, STN DBS has been associated with depression, apathy, disinhibition, hallucinations and abulia *(20, 40–43)*. An important point to consider is that some patients may already have had psychiatric complications or cognitive deficits that were aggravated after surgery. In this context, Houeto et al. have described depression in patients who had depressive episodes prior to surgery *(44)*. Nevertheless, cognitive changes such as mood disorders or depression are reported more frequently after STN than GPi DBS and may be related to the spread of current to limbic or associative portions of the nucleus. However, cognitive and psychiatric disturbances are also frequently described in advanced PD patients treated chronically with levodopa *(45)*. In this context, it would therefore be necessary to distinguish between behavioral disturbances caused by DBS or progression of the disease itself. An analysis of the cohort of patients included in the 3 to 4 year multi-center study discussed above has shown that the occurrence of altered cognition and incidence of depression were more frequent in the STN group than the GPi group of patients *(20, 46)*.

## Conclusions

Proper comparison of the therapeutic efficacy of STN DBS versus GPi DBS is not possible with currently available information. Multi-center randomized studies are in progress, which may settle this point. Despite this, the choice of GPi as a surgical target has decreased enormously in practice and most recent studies concern data derived from patients treated with STN DBS. Why this has occurred cannot be entirely explained on scientific grounds *(19)*. Perhaps the larger number of experimental studies demonstrating the impact of STN stimulation as well as the anatomo-physiological data indicating the prominent capacity of the STN to modulate basal ganglia output, created a scenario that has led specialists to prefer the STN. Finally, the ability to reduce or even discontinue levodopa and other anti-parkinson treatments after STN DBS undoubtedly has had a major influence on its relative popularity.

Notwithstanding the above considerations, we generally agree with a preferential choice of STN DBS for surgical treatment of PD. Currently, patients are submitted to surgery for two major reasons: Problems derived from severe dopaminergic depletion leading to highly disabling and frequent "off" episodes and limited mobility during bed hours and problems related to the effects of dopaminergic drugs consisting of dyskinesias and psychiatric complications. The available data and our experience indicate that STN DBS significantly ameliorates "off" disability while simultaneously reducing daily levodopa requirements, so that drug-induced complications are immediately reduced. The potential to decrease the demand for dopaminergic drugs is a major long-term benefit of STN DBS. However, there are a few instances where we may prefer GPi DBS. This includes patients with unusually severe LIDs including severe and unmanageable diphasic dyskinesias. In such cases, GPi surgery will be immediately effective against dyskinesias and secure better overall clinical control. STN DBS may be less effective in this situation, especially when STN stimulation is not able to remove the need for levodopa treatment. Another clinical scenario where we may prefer GPi DBS is when the patient has a speech problem or cannot afford to suffer speech deterioration for professional or social reasons. All points considered, however, current data are not sufficient to state that one target is superior to another and the choice for target selection will continue to be made based on local preferences and interpretation of the data collected to date.

Curiously, more than 10 years after DBS was first initiated in several centers worldwide, simple questions such as the optimal target remain unclear. Data from long-term follow-up of patients treated with either approach is needed to allow a better definition of the benefit to risk ratio for either target. Fortunately, there are two prospective and randomized clinical trials currently under way in the United States, which will hopefully shed some light on this debate and provide a clinically based rationale for target selection for the treatment of PD in the future.

## References

1. Mitchell IJ, Clarke CE, Boyce S, Crossman AR (1989) Neural mechanisms underlying parkinsonian symptoms based upon regional uptake of 2-deoxyglucose in monkeys exposed to 1-methyl-4-phenyl-1,2,3,6 tetrahydropyridine. Neuroscience 32:213–226.
2. Bergman H, Wichmann T, Karmon B, DeLong MR (1994) The primate subthalamic nucleus.II. Neuronal activity in the MPTP model of parkinsonism. J Neurophysiol 72:507–519.
3. Vila M, Levy R, Herrero MT, Ruberg M, Facheux B, Obeso JA (1997) Consequences of nigrostriatal denervation on the functioning of the basal ganglia in human and nonhuman primates: an in situ hybridization study of cytocrome oxidase subunit 1 mRNA. J Neurosci 17:765–773.
4. Blandini F, García-Osuna M, Greenamyre JT (1997) Subthalamic ablation reverses changes in basal ganglia oxidative metabolism and motor response to apomorphine induced by nigrostriatal lesions in rats. Eur J Neurosci 9:1407–1413.

5. Bergman H, Wichmann T, DeLong MR (1990) Reversal of experimental parkinsonism by lesions of the subthalamic nucleus. Science 249:1436–1438.
6. Aziz TZ, Peggs D, Sambrook MA, Crossman AR (1991) Lesion of the subthalamic nucleus for the alleviation of MPTP-induced parkinsonism in the primate. Mov Disord 6:288–293.
7. Guridi J, Herrero MT, Luquin MR, Guillen J, Ruberg M, Laguna J, et al (1996) Subthalamotomy in parkinsonian monkeys. Behavioural and biochemical analysis. Brain 119:1717–1727.
8. Laitinen LV, Bergenheim AT, Hariz MI (1992) Leksell's posteroventral pallidotomy in the treatment of Parkinson's disease. J Neurosurg 76:53–61.
9. Lang AE, Lozano AM, Montgomery E, Duff J, Tasker RR, Hutchison W Posteroventral pallidotomy in advanced Parkinson's disease. N Engl J Med 337:1036–1042.
10. Merello M, Starkstein S, Nouzeilles MI, Kuzis G, Leiguarda R (2001) Bilateral pallidotomy for treatment of Parkinson's disease induced corticobulbar syndrome and psychic akinesia avoidable by globus pallidus lesion combined with contralateral stimulation. J Neurol Neurosurg Psychiatry 71:611–614.
11. Benabid AL, Pollak P, Hommel M, Gao JM, de Rougemont J, Perret T (1989) Traitement du tremblement parkinsonien par stimulation chronique du noyau ventral intermediére du thalamus. Rev Neurol (Paris) 145:320–323.
12. Benabid AL, Pollak P, Seigneuret E, Hoffmann D, Gay E, Perret J (1993) Chronic VIM thalamic stimulation in Parkinson's disease, essential tremor and extrapiramidal dyskinesias. Acta Neurochir (Wien) Suppl 58:39–44.
13. Pollak P, Benabid AL, Gross C, Gao DM, Laurent A, Benazzouz A, Hoffmann D, et al (1993) Effects of the stimulation of the subthalamic nucleus in Parkinson disease. Rev Neurol (Paris) 149:175–176.
14. Benazzouz A, Gross C, Feger J, Boraud T, Bioulac B (1993) Reversal of rigidity and improvement in motor pèrformance by subthalamic high-frequency stimulation in MPTP-treated monkeys. Eur J Neurosci 5:382–389.
15. Siegfried J, Lippitz B (1994) Bilateral chronic electrostimulation of ventroposterolateral pallidum: A new therapeutic approach for alleviating all parkinsonian symptoms. Neurosurgery 35:1126–1130.
16. Obeso JA, Guridi J, Rodriguez-Oroz MC, Agid Y, Bejjani P, Bonnet AM, Lang AM, Lozano AM, Kumar R, et al (2001) Deep-Brain stimulation of the subthalamic nucleus or the pars interna of tha globus pallidus in Parkinson's disease. N Engl J Med 345:956–963.
17. Anderson VC, Burchiel KJ, Hogarth P, Favre J, Hammerstad JP (2005) Pallidal vs subthalamic nucleus deep brain stimulation in Parkinson disease. Arch Neurol 62:554–560.
18. Vitek JL (2002) Deep brain stimulation for Parkinson's disease. Sterotact Funct Neurosurg 78:119–131.
19. Okun MS, Foote KD (2005) Subthalamic nucleus vs globus pallidus interna deep brain stimulation, the rematch. Arch Neurol 62:533–536.
20. Rodriguez-Oroz MC, Obeso JA, Lang AE, Houeto JL, Pollak P, Rehncrona S, Kulisevsky J, et al (2005) Bilateral deep brain stimulation in Parkinson's disease: a multicentre study with 4 years follow-up. Brain 128:2240–2249.
21. Volkmann J, Allert N, Voges J, Weiss PH, Freund H-J, Sturm V (2001) Safety and efficacy of pallidal or subthalamic nucleus stimulation in advanced PD. Neurology 56:548–551.
22. Krause M, Fogel W, Heck A, Hacke W, Bonsanto M, et al (2001) Deep brain stimulation for the treatment of Parkinson's disease: subthalamic nucleus versus globus pallidus internus. J Neurol Neurosurg Psychiatry 70:464–470.
23. Krack P, Pollak P, Limousin P, Hoffmann D, Xie J, et al (1998) Subthalamic nucleus or internal pallidal stimulation in young onset Parkinson's disease. Brain 121:451–457.

24. Katayama Y, Kasai M, Oshi,ma H, Fukaya C, Yamamoto T, Mizutani T (2001) Double blinded evaluation of the effects of pallidal and subthalamic nucleus stimulation on daytime activity in advanced Parkinson's disease. Parkinsonism Relat Disord 7:35–40.
25. Krack P, Batir A, Van Blercom N, Chabardes S, Fraix V, Ardouin C, et al (2003) Five-year follow-up of bilateral stimulation of the subthalamic nucleus in advanced Parkinson's disease. N Engl J Med 349:1925–1934.
26. Schüpbach WMM, Chastan N, Welter ML, Houeto JL, Masnage V, Bonnet AM, Czernecki V, Maltete D, Hartmann A, Mallet L, Pidoux B, Dormont D, Navarro S, Cornu P, Mallet A, Agid Y (2005) Stimulation of the subthalamic nucleus in Parkinson's disease: a 5 year follow up. J Neurol Neurosurg Psychiatry 76:1640–1644.
27. Volkmann J, Allert N, Voges J, Sturm V, Schnitzler A, et al (2004) Long-term results of bilateral pallidal stimulation in Parkinson's disease. Ann Neurol 55:871–875.
28. Houeto JL, Bejjani PB, Damier P (2000) Failure of long-term pallidal stimulation corrected by subthalamic stimulation in PD. Neurology 55:728–730.
29. Ghika J, Villemure J-G, Frankhauser H, Favre J, Assal G, et al (1998) Efficiency and safety of bilateral contempouraneous pallidal stimulation (deep brain stimulation) in levodopa-responsive patients with Parkinson's disease with severe motor fluctuations: a 2-year follow-up review. J Neurosurg 89:713–718.
30. Houeto JL, Damier P, Bejjani PB, Staedler C, Bonnet M, Arnulf I, Pidoux B, Dormont D, Cornu P, Agid Y (2000) Subthalamic stimulation in Parkinson's disease. A multidisciplinary Approach. Arch Neurol 57:461–465.
31. Molinuevo J, Valdeoriola F, Tolosa E, Rumia J, Vals-Sole J, Roldan H, Ferrer E (2000) Levodopa withdrawal after bilateral subthalamic nucleus stimulation in advanced Parkinson disease. Arch Neurol 57:983–988.
32. Vingerhoets FJG, Villemure JG, Temperli P, Pollo C, Pralong E, Ghika J (2002) Subthalamic DBS replaces levodopa in Parkinson's disease. Two year follow-up. Neurology 58:396–401.
33. Krack P, Pollak P, Limousin P, Bennazouz A, Deuschl G, Benabid AL (1999) From off-period dystonia to peak-dose chorea: the clinical spectrum of variying subthalamic nucleus activity. Brain 1133–1146.
34. Rodriguez-Oroz MC, Gorospe A, Guridi J, Ramos E, Linazasoro G, Rodriguez Palmero M, Obeso JA (2000) Bilateral deep brain stimulation of the subthalamic nucleus in Parkinson's disease. Neurology 55(Suppl):45–51.
35. Guridi J, Obeso JA, Rodriguez-Oroz MC, Lozano AM, Manrique M Levodopa induced dyskinesias and stereotactic surgery for Parkinson's disease. Neurosurgery (accepted for publication)
36. Yelnik J (1998) Functional anatomy of the basal ganglia. Mov Disord 13(Suppl 1): 73–82.
37. Bejjani BP, Damier P, Arnulf I, Papadopoulos S, Bonnet AM, Vidailhet M, Agid Y, et al (1998) Deep brain stimulation in Parkinson's disease: opposite affects of stimulation in the pallidum. Mov Disord 13:969–970.
38. Krack P, Pollak P, Limousin P, Hoffmann D, Benazzouz A, Le Bas JF, Koudsie A, Benabid AL (1998) Opposite motor effects of pallidal stimulation in Parkinson's disease. Ann Neurol 43:180–192.
39. Yelnik J, et al (2000) Functional mapping of the human globus pallidus: Contrasting effect of the stimulation in the internal and external pallidum in Parkinson's disease. Neuroscience 101:77–87.
40. Bejjani BP, Damier P, Arnulf I, Thivard L (1999) Transient acute depression induced by high-frequency deep-brain stimulation. N Engl J Med 340:1476–1480.
41. Saint-Cyr JA, Trepanier L, Kumar R, Lozano AM (2000) Neuropsychological consequences of chronic bilateral stimulation of the subthalamic nucleus in Parkinson's disease. Brain 123:2091–2108.
42. Doshi PK, Chaya N, Bhatt MH (2002) Depression leading to attempted suicide after bilateral subthalamic nucleus stimulation for Parkinson's disease. Mov Disord 17:1084–1085.

43. Herzog J, Reiff J, Krack P, Witt K (2003) Manic episode with psicotic symptoms induced by subthalamic nucleus stimulation in patients with Parkinson's disease. Mov Disord 18:1382–1384.
44. Houeto JL, Mallet L, Mesnage V, Tezenas du Montcel S, Behar C, Gargiulo M, Torny F, et al (2006) Subthalamic stimulation in Parkinson disease: behavior and social adaptation. Arch Neurol 63:1090–1095.
45. Lang AE, Obeso JA (2004) Challenges in Parkinson's disease: restoration of the nigrostriatal dopamine system is not enough. Lancet Neurol 3:309–316.
46. Hariz MI, Rehncrona S, Quinn N, Speelman JD, Wensing C and the Multi-center Advanced Parkinson's disease Deep Brain Stimulation Group Adverse events at 3–4 years follow-up in patients with parkinson's disease treated with deep brain stimulation in the globus pallidus interna or in the subthalamic nucleus. An independent assessment. Brain (submitted for publication).
47. Rodriguez-Oroz MC, Zamarbide I, Guridi J, Palmero M, Obeso JA (2004) Efficacy of deep brain stimulation of the subthalamic nucleus in Parkinson's disease 4 years after surgery: double blind and open evaluation. J Neurol Neurosurg Psychiatry 75:1382–1385.
48. Durif F, Lemaire JJ, Debilly D, Dordain G (1999) Acute and chronic effects of anteromedial globus pallidus stimulation in Parkinson's disease. J Neurol Neurosurg Psychiatry 67:315–321.
49. Loher T, Burgunder JM, Pohle T, Weber S, Sommerholder R, Krauss JK (2002) Long-term pallidal deep brain stimulation in patients with advanced Parkinson's disease: 1-year follow-up study. J Neurosurg 96:844–853.
50. Kumar R, Lang AE, Rodriguez-Oroz MC, Lozano AM, Limousin P, Pollak P, Benabid AL, Guridi J, Ramos E, el al (2000) Deep brain stimulation of the globus pallidus pars interna in advanced Parkinson's disease. Neurology 55(12 Suppl 6):34–39.
51. Rodrigues JP, Walters SE, Watson P, Stell R, Mastaglia FL (2007) Globus pallidus stimulation in advanced Parkinson's disease. J Clin Neurosci 14:208–215.
52. Herzog J, Volkmann J, Krack P, Kopper F, Potter M, Lorenz D, Steinbach M, Klebe S, Hamel W, Schrader B, et al (2003) Two-year follow-up of subthalamic deep brain stimulation in Parkinson's disease. Mov Disord 18:1332–1337.
53. Kleiner-Fisman S, Fisman D, Sime E, Saint-Cyr J, Lozano AM, Lang AE (2003) Long-term follow-up of bilateral deep brain stimulation of the subthalamic nucleus in patients with advanced Parkinson's disease. J Neurosurg 99:489–495.
54. Pahwa R, Wilkinson S, Overeman J, Lyons K (2003) Bilateral subthalamic stimulation in patients with Parkinson's disease. J Neurosurg 99:71–77.
55. Visser-Vanderwalle V, van der Linden C, Temel Y Celik H, Ackermans L, Spincemaille G, Caemaert J (2005) Long-term of bilateral subthalamic nucleus stimulation in advanced Parkinson's disease: a four year follow-up study. Parkinsonism Relat Disord 11:157–165.
56. Romito LM, Contarino MF, Ghezzi D, Franzini A, Garavaglia B, Albanese A (2005) High frequency stimulation of the subthalamic nucleus is efficacious in Parkin disease. J Neurol 252:208–211.
57. Ostergaard K, Aa Sunde N (2006) Evolution of Parkinson's disease during 4 years of bilateral deep brain stimulation of the subthalamic nucleus. Mov Disord 21:624–631.
58. Krause M, Fogel W, Mayer P, Kloss M, Tronnier V (2004) Chronic inhibition of the subthalamic nucleus in Parkinson's disease. J Neurol Sci 219:119–124.

# 16
# Deep Brain Stimulation in Atypical Parkinsonism

Ludy Shih and Daniel Tarsy

## Abstract

Deep brain stimulation (DBS) for Parkinson's disease (PD) has gained widespread acceptance for improving motor function and disability. Patients with features suggestive of atypical parkinsonism (AP) tend have a much poorer and less sustained response to levodopa and also a poorer prognosis overall. DBS experience with this group of patients is very limited and evidence is lacking with regard to its efficacy and adverse effects. In this chapter, we review the available published experience of DBS surgery in patients with multiple system atrophy and other forms of secondary parkinsonism. Based on the limited data reviewed here, DBS for patients with multiple system atrophy is not recommended.

**Keywords:** deep brain stimulation, DBS, atypical parkinsonism, parkinson plus syndrome, multiple system atrophy, radiation induced parkinsonism, hypoxic-ischemic parkinsonism

## Introduction

Subthalamic nucleus (STN) DBS provides effective treatment for properly selected patients with advanced PD. STN DBS improves the cardinal motor features of PD and reduces motor complications. It is the only surgical therapy for PD that allows the levodopa dose to be reduced, thereby ameliorating levodopa induced dyskinesia. DBS of the internal segment of globus pallidus (GPi) has also been used with good effect in both idiopathic PD and primary generalized and segmental dystonia *(1–4)*. By contrast with patients with idiopathic PD, it is believed that patients with AP experience little relief of symptoms and disability after DBS. However, evidence-based consensus statements concerning DBS for PD have been unable to properly address the role of DBS in AP due to a lack of published evidence in this area *(5–7)*. Here we examine the available literature describing outcomes of DBS for AP, including the specific syndromes for which they were treated, the anatomic sites selected for surgery, and whether future surgical targets can be identified for these diseases.

## Atypical Parkinsonism

Parkinsonism is a syndrome clinically defined by the presence of akinesia, rigidity, rest tremor, and postural instability. Many efforts have been made to distinguish idiopathic PD, the most common cause of parkinsonism, from AP, as the response to treatment and the prognosis of these diseases differ significantly *(8)*. Also known as parkinsonism-plus syndromes, they have received attention due to their poor response to anti-parkinson medications, such as dopamine agonists and levodopa, as well as their more rapid progression and generally poorer prognosis *(9)*.

The diagnosis of these syndromes is based on several clinical features that, when present, should alert clinicians to the possibility of AP. Several studies investigating the accuracy of clinical diagnosis as compared to the gold standard of post-mortem pathologic examination have placed accuracy of diagnosing PD as between 77 and 98%, depending on the patient population studied and the expertise of the physicians making the diagnosis *(10, 11)*. The most common misdiagnoses of idiopathic PD are made in patients found to have multiple system atrophy (MSA), progressive supranuclear palsy, dementia with Lewy bodies, Alzheimer's disease, and vascular pathology *(12)*. Clinical features that should suggest AP include early postural instability with falls, symmetric onset of motor findings, absence of rest tremor, rapid disease progression, poor or unsustained response to levodopa therapy, prominent and early autonomic features, oculomotor or cerebellar deficits, or early dementia (Table 16.1). In a recent study, 30 of 34 post-mortem proven cases of MSA

**Table 16.1** Features suggestive of an AP disorder (adapted from ref. *53*).

Motor

Rapid disease progression
   Early instability and falls
   Absent, poor, or not maintained response to levodopa therapy
   Myoclonus
   Pyramidal signs
   Cerebellar signs
   Early dysarthria and/or dysphagia
   Early dystonia/contractures (unrelated to treatment)

Autonomic features
   Impotence/decreased genital sensitivity in females
   Early orthostatic hypotension unrelated to treatment
   Early and/or severe urinary disturbances

Oculomotor
   Marked slowing of saccades
   Difficulty initiating saccades, gaze (oculomotor apraxia)
   Supranuclear gaze palsy
   Nystagmus

Cognitive and behavioral
   Early and severe frontal or cortical dementia
   Visual hallucinations not induced by treatment
   Ideomotor apraxia
   Sensory or visual neglect/cortical disturbances

who were evaluated by movement disorder specialists were correctly diagnosed (11). However, it should be emphasized that diagnostic accuracy is less in patients with early and milder symptoms and is also confounded by the fact that 10 to 20% of patients with MSA have features of asymmetry, levodopa responsiveness, dyskinesias, and motor fluctuations (13).

Because effective treatment options for AP are usually lacking, strategies normally reserved for patients with idiopathic PD have been used in patients with AP with variable success. Stereotactic surgical procedures are usually reserved for patients with levodopa-responsive idiopathic PD and disabling motor complications, but have also been carried out in patients with suspected AP. Prior to the era of DBS, posteroventral pallidotomy was carried out in a number of patients with levodopa unresponsive parkinsonism with very limited success (14), although improvement was reported in a small number of cases (15, 16). Thalamotomy for tremor was carried out in two MSA patients and was not beneficial (17). We do not review responses to ablative surgery here, limiting this review to the use of DBS in AP with the major emphasis on MSA (Table 16. 2).

## Multiple System Atrophy (MSA)

A consensus statement on the diagnosis of MSA (18) formalized previous criteria delineated by Quinn (19) for the diagnosis of MSA. There have been several attempts to identify factors that reliably differentiate MSA from PD (13, 20, 21). These include symmetric onset, absence of rest tremor, poor or unsustained response to levodopa, rapid progression, and autonomic signs. DBS has been carried out more frequently in MSA than other forms of atypical or secondary parkinsonism. This is due to the frequent close clinical resemblance of MSA to PD and the fact that 10 to 20% of patients with MSA may have features of asymmetry, levodopa responsiveness, dyskinesias, and motor fluctuations. Moreover, about 30% of patients with MSA initially respond to levodopa, although only about 13% retain this response after several years of treatment (22).

### *STN DBS in MSA Patients with Features of PD*

Berciano et al. reported the first pathologically proven patient with MSA who was treated with DBS (23). A 63-year-old man initially presented with bradykinesia and rest tremor in the left hand. He had a good initial response to levodopa 300 mg/day and was diagnosed with idiopathic PD. He subsequently developed significant motor fluctuations and axial, appendicular, and orofacial dyskinesias, which were only partially relieved by levodopa and pergolide. There were no autonomic signs and brain MRI was normal. He underwent bilateral STN DBS 6 years after presentation and showed initial improvement (UPDRS-III score off medication declined from 49 to 26) which allowed him to reduce his levodopa dose by 60%. However, postoperatively he developed hypomania, paranoia, impaired gait, fever, and a pleural effusion and died 3 weeks after surgery of a massive pulmonary embolism. DBS electrodes were properly placed within the subthalamic nuclei. There was severe loss of pigmented neurons in the substantia nigra and locus coeruleus without Lewy bodies. There was no cell loss or gliosis in the putamen, caudate, or subthalamic nuclei. There was mild to moderate neuronal loss with gliosis in basis pontis, inferior olivary nuclei, dentate nuclei, and cerebellar cortex. Numerous

**Table 16.2** Published case reports concerning DBS in patients with MSA.

| Author | Signs | Asymmetry | Motor fluctuations | Levodopa-responsive | MSA diagnosis | DBS site of stimulation | UPDRS-III change from off to on stimulation (off medication) | DBS response | Early adverse effects | Subsequent clinical course |
|---|---|---|---|---|---|---|---|---|---|---|
| Berciano et al. | Bradykinesia, rigidity, rest tremor | Yes | Wearing off, peak dose dyskinesia (axial, appendicular, orofacial) | Yes | Post-mortem | STN | 49 to 26 | Improved | Hypomania, paranoia, impaired gait, lethargy | Died 3 weeks after DBS |
| Tarsy et al. | Bradykinesia, rigidity, postural instability, hyperreflexia, extensor plantar responses, autonomic symptoms | Yes | Wearing off, peak dose dyskinesias (facial, axial) | Yes | Clinical, MRI | STN | 40 to 36 | Improved upper extremity bradykinesia; no midline improvement | Dysarthria, dysphagia, postural instability, bradykinesia | Stable after stimulators turned off |
| Leczano et al. | Akinesia, rest tremor, rigidity | Yes | Wearing off, peak dose cranial dyskinesia | Yes | Post-mortem | STN | 56 to 39 | Transient improvement | Compulsive gambling, paranoia | Progressive dysphagia, anarthria, and motor deterioration |
| Visser-Vandewalle et al.[*] | Akinesa, rigidity, ataxia, autonomic failure | No | None | No | Clinical, IBZM-SPECT | STN | Mean of 42 to 23.5 at 1 month; 53 to 41 at >2 yrs | Improved | None | Decline in UPDRS-III response at 12 months |

(continued)

**Table 16.2** (continued)

| | | | | | | | | | |
|---|---|---|---|---|---|---|---|---|---|
| Alterman et al.** | Postural instability, blepharospasm, leg cramps | ND | On/off phenomenon in 1 patient | Yes | Clinical, PET | STN | 29% improvement in 1 patient | One patient mildly improved | Dysarthria | Progressive worsening of gait |
| Chou et al. | Bradykinesia, rest tremor, rigidity, choking, bladder dysfunction | Yes | Wearing off, cervical dyskinesia | Yes | Post-mortem | STN | ND | Worsening bradykinesia and rigidity | Dysphagia, marked bradykinesia and rigidity | Died 12 weeks after DBS after repeated aspiration |
| Talmant et al. | Akinesia, rigidity, gait difficulty, hypophonia, bladder dysfunction | Yes | "motor fluctuations" | Yes | Post-mortem | STN | 53 to 29 at 12 months (35 at 18 months) | Transient improvement at 1 year | ND | Progressive axial signs with falls, increased dysarthria and dysphagia |
| Huang et al. | Bradykinesia, rigidity, falls, stridor, myoclonus | No | Wearing off, peak dose dyskinesia | Yes | Postmorten | GPi | Overall UPDRS score decreased by 26%, dyskinesias improved | Improved for 15 months | None | Maintained improvement for 15 months. Died 18 months after surgery. |
| Patrick et al. | Akinesia, rigidity, dysphagia, stridor, axial and cervical dystonia | Yes | No | No | Clinical | GPi | 61 to 77 | Markedly increased akinesia | Severe dysphagia | Severe akinesia, unable to walk, persistent dystonia. Died 7 months after surgery |

ND, not documented
*Four patients
**Two patients

glial cytoplasmic inclusions (GCI), the pathologic hallmark of MSA, were present throughout the hippocampi, subcortical white matter, globus pallidus, brainstem, cerebellum, and spinal cord. Therefore, despite a clinical picture indicative of PD, the pathological findings were diagnostic of MSA. The patient's response to levodopa was attributed to the preserved striatum in this case, which contains nigrostriatal dopaminergic receptors. A normal putamen is observed in approximately 10% of MSA patients examined at postmortem *(24, 25)* and there is a trend for levodopa response to inversely correlate with the degree of putaminal damage *(13, 26)*.

Lezcano et al. *(27)* reported a patient whose clinical presentation was indistinguishable from idiopathic PD who received bilateral STN DBS. This 57-year-old man presented with right-sided resting tremor, akinesia, and rigidity and had a good response to levodopa. He developed severe motor fluctuations and peak-dose cranial and orofacial dyskinesias 2 years after beginning levodopa. Brain MRI was normal. SPECT-IBZM revealed abnormal and asymmetric D2 receptor density in the putamen. He underwent bilateral STN DBS 6 years after onset of symptoms. Seven days following DBS initiation he developed compulsive gambling with paranoid delirium. Levodopa dose was reduced and olanzapine was added with remission of psychiatric symptoms. Akinesia and rigidity improved but he developed severe dysarthria and dysphagia requiring a nasogastric tube. Three months after surgery UPDRS motor score off medication improved during stimulation from 43 to 39. However, even on both medication and stimulation, UPDRS motor score was worse than on medication prior to surgery (31 vs 16). Six months after surgery he was evaluated off stimulation and off medication and had significant tremor, akinesia, and dysphagia. Twelve months after surgery, he was evaluated while on and off stimulation, with and without medication. Stimulation while off medication continued to provide a reduction of UPDRS motor score (56 vs 39) but this improvement was not as great as the effect of medication without stimulation (56 vs 35). Notably, being on stimulation and on medication made him worse than being on medication alone (44 vs 35). He died of aspiration pneumonia 1.5 years after surgery. Autopsy showed countless GCI, neuronal depletion, and gliosis in substantia nigra without Lewy bodies, only a small decrease of large neurons limited to dorsal putamen, and moderate Purkinje cell loss in cerebellum. Similar to Berciano et al. *(23)*, these authors attributed the temporary response to DBS to the limited neuronal loss found in the putamen *(27)*.

Chou et al. *(28)* reported a 54-year-old man who presented with tremor and impaired dexterity in left hand followed over the next several years by bradykinesia and rigidity involving left more than right side, bilateral arm tremor, unsteady gait, and choking. Levodopa produced a marked benefit until the appearance of motor fluctuations, and cervical dyskinesias. MRI showed mild brainstem and cerebellar atrophy. He underwent bilateral STN DBS 8 years after onset with a presumptive diagnosis of PD. There was no response to DBS with immediate postoperative confusion and marked worsening of bradykinesia, rigidity, and dysphagia. He died 12 weeks after surgery after repeated aspiration pneumonia. Post-mortem examination revealed multiple alpha-synuclein positive GCI in all brain regions, most abundant in cerebellum, brainstem, and striatum without Lewy bodies. There was profound neuronal loss with gliosis in substantia nigra and, to a lesser extent, in striatum and globus pallidus. The authors speculated that the poor response to DBS may have been due, at least in part, to the pathologic findings in striatum.

In contrast to the above cases, Tarsy et al. *(29)* reported the effects of bilateral STN DBS in a patient in whom MSA was suspected prior to surgery but who had displayed prominent levodopa-induced dyskinesias and wearing off effects. She was a 57-year-old woman who presented with right upper extremity bradykinesia and unsteady gait. Facial masking, hypophonia, asymmetric bradykinesia, and rigidity, and extensor plantar responses were evident within 2 years. After 4 years, she developed prominent autonomic features and mild cerebellar signs. Levodopa markedly improved bradykinesia, gait, and balance but was followed within a year by severe wearing off effects and limb, trunk, cervical, and facial dyskinesias followed by less responsive bradykinesia, gait disturbance, freezing, and hypophonia. Bilateral STN DBS was carried out 7 years after disease onset and produced improvement, which was limited to upper extremity bradykinesia with a decline in UPDRS motor score while off medication from 40 to 36. Gait, postural instability, and dysarthria failed to improve. Over the next 9 months, dysarthria, dysphagia, aspiration, gait difficulty, and freezing increased. Stimulators were turned off 11 months after surgery with improvement in swallowing, aspiration, and drooling but no change in gait or balance.

Talmant et al. *(30)* reported a 63-year-old patient with a 6-year history of levodopa-responsive parkinsonism who experienced a 45% decrease in UPDRS motor score after STN DBS. Although he experienced dysphagia, erectile dysfunction and obstructive urinary retention, he was diagnosed with idiopathic PD. Pyramidal or cerebellar involvement and orthostatic hypotension were not prominent. He then developed disabling fluctuations and midline motor signs, which lasted for 1 year before he underwent bilateral STN DBS. Postoperatively, UPDRS motor score improved by 45%. One year after surgery, he developed axial symptoms, recurrent falls, and increased dysarthria and dysphagia. He died suddenly following prostate surgery 2 years after DBS surgery. Autopsy disclosed severe neuronal depletion in substantia nigra without Lewy bodies and numerous GCI in basal ganglia, pontine nuclei, and cerebellar white matter. The authors concluded that although STN DBS may be temporarily beneficial in MSA, the procedure could not be recommended for patients with MSA because of the striatonigral degeneration characteristic of this disease.

Among case series of PD patients undergoing STN DBS, several cases of MSA have been mentioned in passing whose diagnosis became more apparent after DBS. Okun et al. *(31)* refer to four cases of AP in a series describing patients who experienced a suboptimal response to DBS. Out of 41 patients referred for DBS failure, five received revised diagnoses for conditions that DBS would not be expected to help, including two cases of MSA, and one case each of corticobasal degeneration, progressive supranuclear palsy, and myoclonus. In three of these cases, reprogramming was attempted but no improvement occurred except for one patient who experienced slight improvement in motor symptoms. Schupbach et al. *(32)* reported a case of a patient who died suddenly of probable cardiac arrest after DBS surgery and on autopsy was found to have MSA. There was no information published regarding her disease history or clinical features.

### STN DBS in Patients with Typical MSA

STN DBS has also been carried out in patients experiencing prominent motor symptoms, which were known to be poorly responsive to levodopa at the time of surgery. Pinter et al. *(33)* reported a 54-year-old woman with MSA who was unresponsive to levodopa or apomorphine. Nonetheless, she underwent bilateral STN DBS, which did not improve her symptoms.

Visser-Vandewalle *(34)* reported four patients with probable MSA who underwent bilateral STN DBS, three of whom experienced moderate benefit. Patients were selected specifically on the basis of having levodopa-unresponsive parkinsonism. All had severe akinetic-rigid syndromes, gait ataxia, absence of tremor, and autonomic failure and were not receiving anti-parkinson medications. IBZM-SPECT scanning showed significantly decreased postsynaptic striatal dopamine receptors in each patient. Four patients were assessed 1 month postoperatively and a second time 6, 28, 29, or 44 months after surgery. One patient died of pneumonia 6 months after implantation. At one month, median UPDRS motor scores decreased from a baseline of 45.5 to 23.5 ($p < 0.05$) with DBS. At the second evaluation, 6 to 44 months after surgery, median UPDRS motor scores decreased from 53 off stimulation to 41 ($p < 0.05$) on stimulation. Improvement in gait and postural instability was minor and less than the improvement in rigidity and akinesia. There was also significant improvement in UPDRS activities of daily living scores and Schwab and England functional scores at 1 month, which was no longer evident at 6 to 44 months. Gait ataxia did not change and bulbar symptoms were not mentioned. They emphasized the lack of alternative treatments for MSA and concluded that these results justified a larger, prospective controlled trial.

Alterman et al. reported in abstract form *(35)* two patients with MSA who underwent bilateral STN DBS. Both were levodopa-responsive, and one had motor fluctuations. There was mild, subjective improvement in parkinsonism at 3 and 12 months postoperatively. UPDRS motor scores improved by 29% in one patient. Postoperatively, both patients had worsening of dysarthria, and one had a progressively worsening gait. The authors concluded that DBS may be potentially effective in selected patients with AP who have had a beneficial response to levodopa.

### Globus Pallidus DBS for Patients with MSA

In one case of MSA with features typical for PD and in two cases in which prominent dyskinesias and dystonia were associated with MSA, medial globus pallidus (GPi) DBS was carried out with variable effects. Ghika et al. reported on seven patients who received GPi DBS for PD, one of whom developed autonomic symptoms, pyramidal signs and decreasing clinical improvement after DBS despite continued adjustments of settings *(36)*. Her UPDRS scores were excluded for analysis and therefore not published.

Huang et al. *(37)* reported a 49-year-old woman with autopsy proven MSA who underwent GPi DBS. She presented at age 35 with left leg bradykinesia and postural instability. Asymmetrical limb akinesia and rigidity evolved over several years and she subsequently developed dysarthria, postural hypotension, inspiratory stridor, and action myoclonus of the fingers. She was initially levodopa responsive and within 1 year developed severe motor fluctuations and peak-dose generalized axial dyskinesias. GPi DBS was carried out 14 years after onset of symptoms primarily to manage severe dyskinesias. There was striking improvement in dyskinesia, a 26% reduction in total UPDRS score, and improved gait and quality of life. It is not clear whether motor assessments were done on or off stimulation and medication. She died 18 months after surgery following an episode of inspiratory stridor followed by pneumonia. Post-mortem examination showed abundant GCI throughout the brain and neuronal loss limited to substantia nigra and locus coeruleus, consistent with "minimal-change" MSA *(38)*. Similar to other investigators reported earlier, the authors conclude that relative sparing of striatal neurons in relatively early stages of MSA may account for an initial response to levodopa and DBS.

Patrick et al. *(39)* reported a 57-year-old man with MSA with prominent dystonia who died 7 months after bilateral GPi DBS surgery. He initially presented with left-sided bradykinesia and pyramidal signs without tremor. He was unresponsive to levodopa and other anti-parkinson medications. He later developed blepharospasm, laryngeal stridor, and axial dystonia with anterocollis that did not abate with levodopa withdrawal or respond to tetrabenazine or botulinum toxin. GPi was targeted because of success of GPi DBS for primary generalized dystonia. Postoperatively he developed increased akinesia, anarthria, dysphagia, and inability to walk. There was only temporary improvement in axial dystonia. He died suddenly 7 months postoperatively due to suspected pulmonary embolism, but autopsy was not performed. Taken together with previous published cases, the authors concluded that MSA patients are unsuitable candidates for DBS.

### STN DBS in Other Forms of AP

Following a case report in which a patient with parkinsonism due to hypoxic encephalopathy showed improved motor signs after pallidotomy *(15)*, Krack et al. *(40)* reported a 63-year-old man who developed parkinsonism after cardiac arrest. Following recovery, cognition was relatively unaffected but the patient had severe akinesia, rigidity, hypophonia, dysphagia, gait disorder, and postural instability. Levodopa produced no improvement. Striatal PET measurements of dopa decarboxylase activity, postsynaptic D2 receptor binding, and metabolism were all decreased. Bilateral STN DBS was carried out 3 years after the cardiac arrest. He experienced subjective improvement in swallowing and gait but double-blind UPDRS motor assessments showed no change. The authors concluded that levodopa-unresponsiveness, striatal hypometabolism, or decreased striatal D2 receptor binding may be considered predictive of lack of response to bilateral STN stimulation.

Revilla et al. *(41)* reported a 20-year-old man who developed parkinsonism following whole brain radiation at age 7. At age 16, he developed rest tremor in both arms and dystonia in left hand and arm followed several months later by shuffling gait and postural instability. Following treatment with levodopa, UPDRS motor score declined from 79 to 47. $^{18}$F-dopa PET revealed reduced uptake in the striatum bilaterally. Following bilateral STN DBS, UPDRS motor score off medication improved from 70 off stimulation to 57 on stimulation, there was a 33% reduction in levodopa dose, and wearing off effects and levodopa induced dyskinesias were improved.

## Future Targets for DBS in AP Syndromes

Levodopa-responsiveness is the most robust predictor of the clinical response to STN DBS in patients with idiopathic PD *(42, 43)*. The question is whether the same is true for AP, especially MSA. As reviewed earlier, although several patients with AP who have undergone STN or GPi DBS were levodopa-responsive, there has usually been a limited or poor outcome following surgery. Although 10 of the 13 patients with MSA summarized in the table were reported to show some improvement this was often very limited, typically lasted for a year or less, and was accompanied by early adverse effects on motor or bulbar function and continued progression of disabling motor and bulbar signs following surgery. In addition, four deaths occurred within 18 months of surgery, two of these occurring within 3 months of surgery. One death occurring 7 months after surgery was precipitated by increasing bulbar dysfunction caused by active DBS.

It has been postulated that in MSA progressive postsynaptic striatal degeneration may account for whether DBS is either ineffective or lacks durable benefit. In MSA and other striatal degenerations, $^{18}$FDG PET imaging, a measure of regional cerebral glucose metabolism, shows decreased striatal metabolism thereby distinguishing such patients from those with PD in which pathology is limited to the substantia nigra *(44)*. In MSA, there is a preferential loss of striatal neurons containing D2 receptors as evidenced by studies using $^{11}$C raclopride, which specifically binds D2 receptors *(45, 46)* and by studies using $^{123}$I IBZM SPECT, a D2 receptor marker *(47)*. In idiopathic PD, dopamine deficiency causes disinhibition of D2 receptors in the striatum resulting in disinhibition of activity in the indirect striatopallidal pathway and excitation of STN activity. The benefit produced by dopaminergic therapy is due to reversal of this sequence of changes in striatopallidal activity. In MSA and other forms of AP, the limited response to STN DBS is likely due to degeneration of striatal output neurons and downstream striopallidal hypoactivity *(44)*.

Another issue is the different range of symptoms and disabilities that are prominent in AP. STN DBS is effective in treating tremor, bradykinesia, and rigidity but midline abnormalities such as gait disturbance, axial symptoms, postural instability, dysarthria and dysphagia may not be due to degeneration of striatonigral connections but rather to other brainstem nuclei degenerations, which are independent of the dopaminergic system *(48)*.

Recent attention has been paid to DBS of the pedunculopontine nucleus (PPN) for idiopathic PD. The PPN has extensive connections between the basal ganglia and corticospinal tracts and is thought to be a modulator of gait and postural stability *(49)*. In 1-methyl-4-phenyl-1,2,3,6-tetrahydropyridine (MPTP)-treated monkeys, low-frequency PPN stimulation improved akinesia. In patients with advanced PD gait disturbance, freezing of gait and postural instability are commonly not improved significantly following STN DBS. Three groups recently described the use of PPN DBS in PD patients. Two subjects reported by Plaha and Gill *(50)* experienced significant improvement in gait and postural instability after undergoing PPN DBS as well as a 57% reduction in UPDRS motor score and 18 to 47% reduction in their levodopa-equivalent dose. Mazzone et al. *(51)* also reported improvement in a limited UPDRS motor score assessment during intra-operative stimulation. Stefani et al. *(52)* reported improvement of gait and postural stability using DBS of both STN and PPN targets simultaneously in six advanced PD patients with prominent gait and postural instability. Although it is unclear what role the PPN may play in AP, it is thought to play an important role in gait and postural instability and therefore may be a more appropriate target in patients who have significant disability in this domain.

## Conclusions

:::DBS, while highly effective for alleviating symptoms and disability associated with idiopathic PD, has been largely ineffective for parkinsonism due to other etiologies. MSA represents the largest cohort of patients with AP who have undergone DBS and nearly all groups have reported poor outcomes with surgery, including functionally limiting dysphagia, dysarthria, and postural stability and death within several months after surgery in over a quarter of the patients. DBS target selection for treatment of midline symptoms which are poorly responsive to STN DBS may have an important future role to play as new targets for DBS therapy become available for consideration.

## References

1. Anderson VC, Burchiel KJ, Hogarth P, Favre J, Hammerstad JP (2005) Pallidal vs subthalamic nucleus deep brain stimulation in parkinson disease. Arch Neurol 62;554–560.
2. Kupsch A, Benecke R, Muller J, Trottenberg T, Schneider GH, Poewe W et al (2006) Pallidal deep-brain stimulation in primary generalized or segmental dystonia. N Engl J Med 355:1978–1990.
3. Vidailhet M, Pollak P (2005) Deep brain stimulation for dystonia: make the lame walk. Ann Neurol 57:613–614.
4. Deuschl G, Schade-Brittinger C, Krack P, Volkmann J, Schafer H, Botzel K et al (2006) A randomized trial of deep-brain stimulation for Parkinson's disease. N Engl J Med 355:896–908.
5. Goetz CG, Poewe W, Rascol O, Sampaio C (2005) Evidence-based medical review update: pharmacological and surgical treatments of Parkinson's disease: 2001 to 2004. Mov Disord 20:523–539.
6. Hallett M, Litvan I (2000) Scientific position paper of the Movement Disorder Society evaluation of surgery for Parkinson's disease. Task Force on Surgery for Parkinson's Disease of the American Academy of Neurology Therapeutic and Technology Assessment Committee. Mov Disord 15:436–438.
7. Kleiner-Fisman G, Herzog J, Fisman DN, Tamma F, Lyons KE, Pahwa R et al (2006) Subthalamic nucleus deep brain stimulation: summary and meta-analysis of outcomes. Mov Disord 21(Suppl 14):S290–S304.
8. Tarsy D (2005) Diagnostic criteria for Parkinson's disease. In: M Ebadi; R Pfeiffer, eds. Parkinson's Disease. Boca Raton: CRC Press, pp. 569–578.
9. Litvan I (1998) Parkinsonian features: When are they Parkinson disease? JAMA 280:1654–1655.
10. Hughes A, Ben-Shlomo Y, Daniel S, Lees A (1992) What features improve the accuracy of clinical diagnosis in Parkinson's disease: a clinicopathologic study. Neurology 57:S34–S38.
11. Hughes AJ, Daniel SE, Ben-Shlomo Y, Lees AJ (2002) The accuracy of diagnosis of parkinsonian syndromes in a specialist movement disorder service. Brain 125:861–870.
12. Hughes AJ, Daniel SE, Kilford L, Lees AJ (1992) Accuracy of clinical diagnosis of idiopathic Parkinson's disease: a clinico-pathological study of 100 cases. J Neurol Neurosurg Psychiatry 55:181–184.
13. Wenning GK, Ben-Shlomo Y, Hughes A, Daniel SE, Lees A, Quinn NP (2000) What clinical features are most useful to distinguish definite multiple system atrophy from Parkinson's disease? J Neurol Neurosurg Psychiatry 68:434–440.
14. Lang AE, Lozano A, Montgomery EB, Tasker RR, Hutchison WD (1999) Posteroventral Medial Pallidotomy in Advanced Parkinson's Disease. Adv Neurol 80:575–583.

15. Goto S, Kunitoku N, Soyama N, Yamada K, Okamura A, Yoshikawa M et al (1997) Posteroventral pallidotomy in a patient with parkinsonism caused by hypoxic encephalopathy. Neurology 49:707–710.
16. Krauss JK, Jankovic J, Lai EC, Rettig GM, Grossman RG (1997) Posteroventral Medial Pallidotomy in Levodopa-Unresponsive Parkinsonism. Arch Neurol 54:1026–1029.
17. Speelman JD, Schuurman R, de Bie RMA, Esselink RAJ, Bosch DA (2002) Stereotactic neurosurgery for tremor. Mov Disorders 17:S84–S88.
18. Gilman S, Low PA, Quinn N, Albanese A, Ben-Shlomo Y, Fowler CJ et al (1999) Consensus statement on the diagnosis of multiple system atrophy. J Neurol Sci 163:94–98.
19. Quinn N (1994) Multiple system atrophy. In: Marsden C, Fahn S, eds. Movement Disorders 3. London: Butterworths.
20. Colosimo C, Albanese A, Hughes AJ, de Bruin VM, Lees AJ (1995) Some specific clinical features differentiate multiple system atrophy (striatonigral variety) from Parkinson's disease. Arch Neurol 52:294–298.
21. Litvan I, Booth V, Wenning GK, Bartko JJ, Goetz CG, McKee A, et al (1998) Retrospective application of a set of clinical diagnostic criteria for the diagnosis of multiple system atrophy. J Neural Transm 105:217–227.
22. Wenning GK, Ben Shlomo Y, Magalhaes M, Daniel SE, Quinn NP (1994) Clinical features and natural history of multiple system atrophy. An analysis of 100 cases. Brain 117(Pt 4):835–845.
23. Berciano J, Valldeoriola F, Ferrer I, Rumia J, Pascual J, Marin C, et al (2002) Presynaptic parkinsonism in multiple system atrophy mimicking Parkinson's disease: a clinicopathological case study. Mov Disord 17:812–816.
24. Lantos PL (1998) The definition of multiple system atrophy: a review of recent developments. J Neuropathol Exp Neurol 57:1099–1111.
25. Wenning GK, Ben-Shlomo Y, Magalhaes M, Daniel SE, Quinn NP (1995) Clinicopathological study of 35 cases of multiple system atrophy. J Neurol Neurosurg Psychiatry 58:160–166.
26. Fearnley JM, Lees AJ (1990) Striatonigral degeneration. A clinicopathological study. Brain 113:1823–1842.
27. Lezcano E, Gomez-Esteban JC, Zarranz JJ, Alcaraz R, Atares B, Bilbao G et al (2004) Parkinson's disease-like presentation of multiple system atrophy with poor response to STN stimulation: a clinicopathological case report. Mov Disord 19:973–977.
28. Chou KL, Forman MS, Trojanowski JQ, Hurtig HI, Baltuch GH (2004) Subthalamic nucleus deep brain stimulation in a patient with levodopa-responsive multiple system atrophy. Case Report. J Neurosurg 100:553–556.
29. Tarsy D, Apetauerova D, Ryan P, Norregaard T (2003) Adverse effects of subthalamic nucleus DBS in a patient with multiple system atrophy. Neurology 61:247–249.
30. Talmant V, Esposito P, Stilhart B, Mohr M, Tranchant C (2006) Subthalamic stimulation in a patient with multiple system atrophy: a clinicopathological report. Rev Neurol (Paris) 162:363–370.
31. Okun MS, Tagliati M, Pourfar M, Fernandez HH, Rodriguez RL, Alterman RL, et al (2005) Management of referred deep brain stimulation failures: a retrospective analysis from 2 movement disorders centers. Arch Neurol 62:1250–1255.
32. Schupbach MW, Welter ML, Bonnet AM, Elbaz A, Grossardt BR, Mesnage V, et al (2006) Mortality in patients with Parkinson's disease treated by stimulation of the subthalamic nucleus. Mov Disord.
33. Pinter MM, Alesch F, Murg M, Helscher RJ, Binder H (1999) Apomorphine test: a predictor for motor responsiveness to deep brain stimulation of the subthalamic nucleus. J Neurol 246:907–913.
34. Visser-Vandewalle V, Temel Y, Colle H, van der Linden C (2003) Bilateral high-frequency stimulation of the subthalamic nucleus in patients with multiple system atrophy—parkinsonism. Report of four cases. J Neurosurg 98:882–887.

35. Alterman R, Tagliati M, Shils J, Rogers J (2005) Subthalamic nucleus deep brain stimulation in two cases of multiple system atrophy. Mov Disord 20:S129.
36. Ghika J, Villemure JG, Fankhauser H, Favre J, Assal G, Ghika-Schmid F (1998) Efficiency and safety of bilateral contemporaneous pallidal stimulation (deep brain stimulation) in levodopa-responsive patients with Parkinson's disease with severe motor fluctuations: a 2-year follow-up review. J Neurosurg 89:713–718.
37. Huang Y, Garrick R, Cook R, O'Sullivan D, Morris J, Halliday GM (2005) Pallidal stimulation reduces treatment-induced dyskinesias in "minimal-change" multiple system atrophy. Mov Disord 20:1042–1047.
38. Wenning GK, Seppi K, Tison F, Jellinger K (2002) A novel grading scale for striatonigral degeneration (multiple system atrophy). J Neural Transm 109:307–320.
39. Patrick S, Kristl V, Miet DL, Katya VD, Anne S, Jacques DR, et al (2006) Deep brain stimulation of the internal pallidum in multiple system atrophy. Parkinsonism Relat Disord 12:181–183.
40. Krack P, Dowsey PL, Benabid AL, Acarin N, Benazzouz A, Kunig G, et al (2000) Ineffective subthalamic nucleus stimulation in levodopa-resistant postischemic parkinsonism. Neurology 54:2182–2184.
41. Revilla F, Mink J, McGee-Minnich L, Antenor J, Leverich L, Moerlein S, et al (2002) Radiation-induced parkinsonism with good response to levodopa and bilateral subthalamic nuclei stimulation. Mov Disord 17:1113.
42. Welter ML, Houeto JL, Tezenas du Montcel S, Mesnage V, Bonnet AM, Pillon B, et al (2002) Clinical predictive factors of subthalamic stimulation in Parkinson's disease. Brain 125:575–583.
43. Kleiner-Fisman G, Fisman DN, Sime E, Saint-Cyr JA, Lozano AM, Lang AE (2003) Long-term follow up of bilateral deep brain stimulation of the subthalamic nucleus in patients with advanced parkinson disease. J Neurosurg 99:489–495.
44. Eidelberg D, Takikawa S, Moeller JR, Dhawan V, Redington K, Chaly T, et al (1993) Striatal hypometabolism distinguishes striatonigral degeneration from parkinson's Disease. Ann Neurol 33:518–527.
45. Antonini A, Leenders KL, Vontobel P, Maguire RP, Missimer J, Psylla M, et al (1997) Complementary pet studies of striatal neuronal function in the differential diagnosis between multiple system atrophy and Parkinson's disease. Brain 120:2187–2195.
46. Ghaemi M, Hilker R, Rudolf J, Sobesky J, Heiss WD (2002) Differentiating multiple system atrophy from Parkinson's disease: contribution of striatal and midbrain mri volumetry and multi-tracer pet imaging. J Neurol Neurosurg Psychiatry 73:517–523.
47. Kim YJ, Ichise M, Ballinger JR, Vines D, Erami SS, Tatschida T et al (2002) Combination of dopamine transporter and D2 receptor spect in the diagnostic evaluation of PD, MSA, and PSP. Mov Disord 17:303–312.
48. Lang AE, Obeso JA (2004) Challenges in Parkinson's disease: restoration of the nigrostriatal dopamine system is not enough. Lancet Neurol 3:309–316.
49. Pahapill PA, Lozano AM (2000) The pedunculopontine nucleus and Parkinson's disease. Brain 123(Pt 9):1767–1783.
50. Plaha P, Gill SS (2005) Bilateral deep brain stimulation of the pedunculopontine nucleus for Parkinson's disease. Neuroreport 16:1883–1887.
51. Mazzone P, Lozano A, Stanzione P, Galati S, Scarnati E, Peppe A, et al (2005) Implantation of human pedunculopontine nucleus: a safe and clinically relevant target in Parkinson's disease. Neuroreport 16:1877–1881.
52. Stefani A, Lozano Am, Peppe A, Stanzione P, Galati S, Tropepi D, et al (2007) Bilateral deep brain stimulation of the pedunculopontine and subthalamic nuclei in severe Parkinson's disease. Brain 130(pt 6):1596–1607.
53. Litvan I (2005) What is an atypical parkinsonian disorder? In: Litvan I, ed. Atypical Parkinsonian Disorders: Clinical and Research Aspects. Totowa, NJ: Humana Press, pp. 1–9.

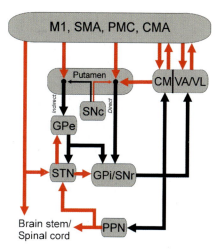

**Color Plate 1.** *Figure 1.1.* Anatomical structure of the basal ganglia circuitry. Red arrows denote excitatory (glutamatergic) connections, black arrows indicate inhibitory (GABAergic) connections. Abbreviations: GPe, external pallidal segment; STN, subthalamic nucleus; GPi, internal pallidal segment; SNr, substantia nigra pars reticulata; SNc, substantia nigra pars compacta; PPN, pedunculopontine nucleus; CM, centromedian nucleus of the thalamus; VA/VL, ventral anterior and ventrolateral nucleus of the thalamus; M1, primary motor cortex; SMA, supple mentary motor area; PMC, premotor cortex; CMA, cingulate motor area.

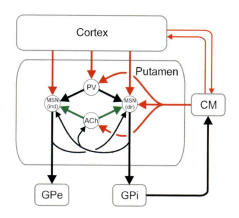

**Color Plate 2.** *Figure 1.2.* Intrinsic striatal circuitry. Red arrows denote excitatory (glutamatergic) connections, black arrows show inhibitory (GABAergic) projections, and green arrows symbolize cholinergic projections. Abbreviations: Ach, striatal cholinergic interneurons; GPe, external pallidal segment; GPi, internal pallidal segment; CM, centromedian nucleus of the thalamus; MSN (ind), striatal GABAergic medium spiny neurons, projecting to GPe as part of the indirect pathway; MSN (dir), striatal GABAergic medium spiny neurons, projecting to GPi as part of the direct pathway; PV striatal GABAergic interneurons containing parvalbumin.

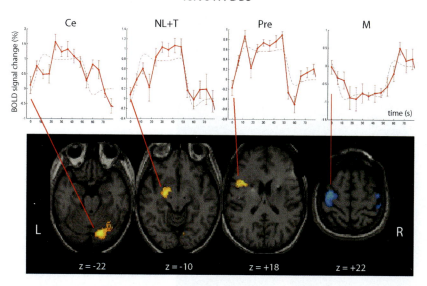

**Color Plate 3.** *Figure 9.1.* Manifestations of acute STN DBS in a 1.5 T fMRI scan of a PD patient (woman, 63 years, PD duration 12 years, UPDRS III: OFF = 53, ON = 30). Bipolar left-sided DBS was switched on and off every 48 seconds (130 Hz, 60 μs, 3.2 V) with right-sided DBS switched off throughout the procedure. The patient lay at rest with eyes closed. With DBS on, there was activation in the ipsilateral thalamus (T), nucleus lentiformis (NL), ipsilateral premotor cortex (Pre), and contralateral cerebellum (Ce), and simultaneous hypoactivation mainly affecting the ipsilateral primary motor cortex (M). $P < 0.05$, False Discovery Rate corrected.

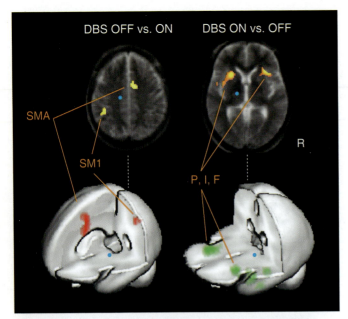

**Color Plate 4.** *Figure 9.2.* Effects of left-sided STN DBS on motion-related activity in eight patients with PD scanned with 1.5 T fMRI after overnight discontinuation of L-DOPA. During fMRI, patients executed sequential movements with the fingers of the right-hand (the motor and resting phases changed periodically every 48 seconds). With DBS on, motion-related activity decreased in the primary sensorimotor cortex (SM1) and supplementary motor area (SMA), and increased in the putamen, insula and inferolateral frontal cortex (P, I, F). $P < 0.001$, uncorrected.

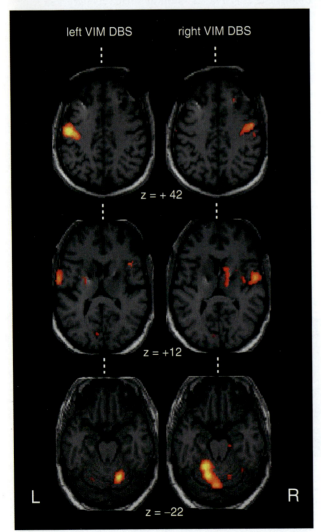

**Color Plate 5.** *Figure 9.3.* 1.5 T fMRI during acute VIM DBS in a patient with essential tremor (man, 58 years, tremor duration 20 years). Unilateral bipolar DBS was switched on and off every 48 seconds (130 Hz, 60 μs, 3V) while the patient lay at rest with eyes closed. Unilateral stimulation of the left and right VIM nucleus activated mirror subcortical and cortical areas. $P < 0.05$, False Discovery Rate corrected.

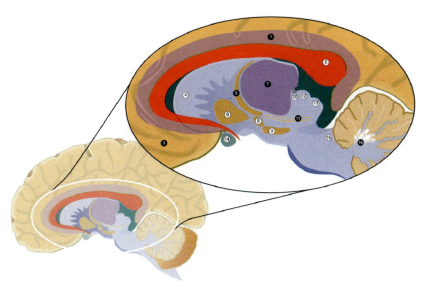

**Color Plate 6.** *Figure 18.1.* A schematic drawing of brain areas that have been targeted in surgery for Tourette's syndrome and other relevant neuroanatomical structures. The frontal lobe (3) was targeted during prefrontal lobotomy and bimedial leucotomy. In limbic leucotomy and anterior cingulotomy, the cingulate cortex (1) was lesioned. The thalamus (7) was targeted for lesioning of the midline, intralaminar, and ventrolateral thalamic nuclei and for DBS. Infrathalamic lesions were performed at the level of the H fields of Forel (11) and the zona incerta (5). Cerebellar surgery involved lesioning of the dentate nucleus (16). The surrounding brain areas include: (2) corpus callosum, (4) caudate-putamen complex, (6) globus pallidus, (8) subthalamic nucleus, (9) substantia nigra, (10) posterior commissure, (12) superior colliculus, (13) inferior colliculus, (15) superior cerebellar peduncle, and (14) optic chiasm.

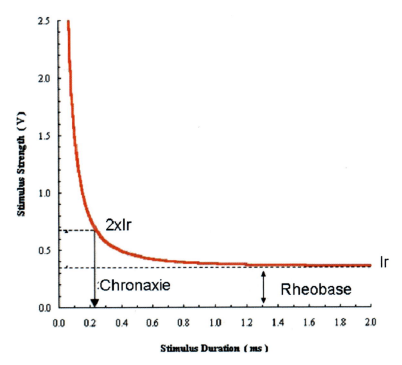

**Color Plate 7.** *Figure 20.1.* Strength-duration curve showing the inverse relationship between pulse width and voltage of stimulation. Chronaxie is the pulse duration equivalent to double the rheobase current, which is the minimal amount of current necessary to stimulate with a long pulse width.

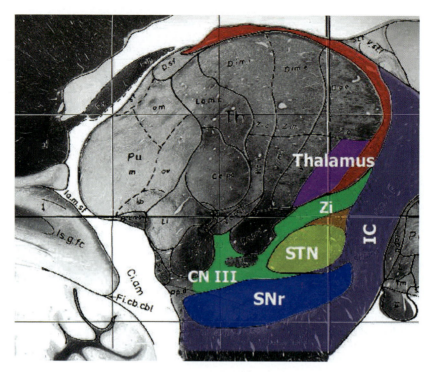

**Color Plate 8.** *Figure 20.7.* Sagittal view of the thalamic and subthalamic area at 12 mm from the midline, illustrating the anatomical relationships of the subthalamic nucleus (STN). CN III, oculomotor nerve fibers; IC, internal capsule; SNr, substantia nigra pars reticulata; Zi, zona incerta. (Courtesy of Dr. Jay Shils)

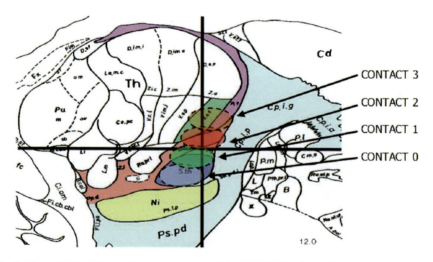

**Color Plate 9.** *Figure 20.8.* Schematic representation of the 3387 DBS electrode placement in the subthalamic area, illustrating the approximate anatomical areas that can be stimulated by the four contacts. Contact 2 and 3, when activated, cover an area dorsal to the STN, including the Zona incerta and possibly the anterior thalamus. (Courtesy of Dr. Jay Shils)

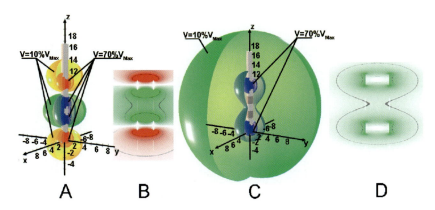

**Color Plate 10.** *Figure 23.8.* Graphical representations of an analytic solution to the voltage (A and C) and electric (B and D) fields generated by the Medtronic DBS lead. The hot colors (yellow and red) represent the anodal field while the cool colors (blue and green) represent the cathodal field.

# 17
# Deep Brain Stimulation in Dystonia

Marie Vidailhet, David Grabli, and Emmanuel Roze

## Abstract

Accumulating and more controlled data is providing strong evidence that bilateral pallidal deep brain stimulation (DBS) produces a marked beneficial effect in dystonia severity and disability in selected patients, with the greatest benefit found in primary generalized dystonia, some primary segmental dystonias, and tardive dystonia. To date, the preferred target for DBS is the internal pallidum but other targets such as thalamus or subthalamic nucleus (STN) may turn out to be an option in some forms of secondary dystonia or in patients who do not improve with pallidal stimulation. Successful treatment of patients with generalized dystonia related to birth injury remains a serious challenge for neurostimulation. Alleviating the burden of these disorders would potentially allow patients to enjoy a more normal social, affective, and professional life. Moreover, the alleviation of dystonia and restoration of normal motor control may help provide insights into mechanisms of cerebral plasticity and learning capabilities of the sensorimotor system.

**Keywords:** dystonia, deep brain stimulation, DBS, globus pallidus

## Introduction

Dystonia is characterized by twisting repetitive movements or abnormal postures that result from involuntary muscle contractions *(1)*. Despite this apparently straightforward definition, the complexity of dystonia appears, not only in term of clinical features and therapeutic approaches, but also in terms of its multiplicity of causes and potential progression of the syndrome.

The mainstay of treatment for focal and segmental dystonia (mainly primary dystonia) is the injection of botulinum toxin. When this approach fails, because too many muscles are involved or the movement pattern is too complex, the management of dystonia may become difficult as other pharmacological treatments usually have limited efficacy or are associated with unacceptable adverse effects. Alternatively, surgical approaches, such as DBS, have provided a favorable risk–benefit ratio in selected cases. DBS has recently demonstrated beneficial effects in primary dystonia in several open label studies *(2–6)* and more recently in two prospective controlled studies *(7, 8)*. Within the past few years, DBS has also been more frequently utilized to treat not only primary dystonia but also various forms of secondary dystonia. However, in most cases of secondary dystonia patients experience only partial benefit, although a few patients may experience clinical improvements similar to those observed in primary dystonia. By contrast, a mean 50% improvement of motor symptoms and disability may be obtained in primary dystonia (this may extend up to 90% improvement in select cases), whereas a small number of patients have unexpectedly had little improvement, without evident explanation. The appropriate selection of patients for DBS is a crucial issue for both neurologists and neurosurgeons. Moreover, several variables should be taken into consideration such as selection of the surgical target, accuracy of localization of therapeutic contacts, and patient management including use of appropriate DBS parameter settings, standardized evaluation of treatment efficacy, long-term beneficial effects, and evaluation of adverse events. Better knowledge concerning the pathophysiological mechanisms that underlie dystonia may help us to identify predictive factors for the best beneficial outcome.

## Clinical Results

Ablative surgery, mainly of the thalamus (Vim, Voa/Vop, VL, pulvinar; ref. *9*), and to a lesser extent the globus pallidus internus (GPi; refs. *10–12*) has been carried out in the past but now been almost abandoned. In select cases, a few patients have been treated with thalamic (VoA, VL; refs. *13* and *14*) or subthalamic region (STN, Forel's field, zona incerta) DBS *(15, 16)*. Although thalamic DBS inspired modern functional neurosurgery, bilateral GPi stimulation is currently the most popular surgical method for treatment of dystonia. Unilateral GPi DBS is sometimes used in patients with hemidystonia or those with generalized dystonia with markedly asymmetric signs. Overall, DBS targeting the internal globus pallidus is a reversible procedure with low morbidity.

## Evaluation of the Efficacy of Treatment

A standardized evaluation is mandatory in any surgical center that treats patients with dystonia. The most commonly used rating scale is the Burke–Fahn–Marsden (BFM) scale for dystonia *(17)*. This scale has two sections, a movement scale based on a motor examination, and a disability scale based on patient interview. The BFM scale has shown excellent internal consistency, validity, and inter-rater reliability *(17, 18)*. Although this scale has been designed for the assessment of generalized dystonia, it has also been used in segmental dystonia. The Toronto Western Spasmodic Torticollis Rating Scale (TWSTRS) rating score has also been used for pre- and postoperative assessment in patients with spasmodic torticollis *(19, 20)*. Evaluation of quality of life (SF-36; ref. *21*), neuropsychological performance, and mood are also an important part of the evaluation of safety and surgical outcomes.

# Primary Dystonia

**Generalized Dystonia**

Since the seminal description by Coubes of a dramatic improvement of dystonia by bilateral pallidal stimulation in a 8-year-old girl who had suffered since the age of 3 severe, progressive and disabling non-DYT1 generalized dystonia *(22)*, more than 50 papers have been published on the beneficial effect of DBS for dystonia. Case reports or small groups of patients with primary generalized dystonia (both DYT1-positive and -negative) were scattered or embedded in reports of heterogeneous groups of patients *(3, 6, 13, 20, 23–31)*, including those with secondary *(2, 6, 13, 25, 27, 32, 33)* or focal dystonia *(3, 20, 27)*. Most patients had a beneficial outcome with improvements of up to 90% on the BFM severity scale (average beneficial effect was about 50% improvement with some variability among patients, including several with little or no improvement). In early studies, results in patients with primary non-DYT1 dystonia appeared slightly inferior to those in patients with DYT1-positive dystonia. A large uncontrolled study demonstrated long-term efficacy and safety of bilateral GPi DBS in 31 adults and children with primary dystonia with 2 years of follow-up *(5)*. In this group, although dystonia severity scores on the BFM scale were slightly more improved in children than in adults, there was no significant difference in improved disability. Despite the earlier impression that DYT1 positive patients were better candidates for DBS with better outcomes, no significant difference was found according to genetic DYT status in this series. Overall, dystonia was improved by 79% and disability by 65%. Dystonic movements of the limbs and axial muscles were equally improved while oromandibular dystonia showed less improvement. Similar results have been obtained by other groups from Europe and North America and are outlined in Table 17.1.

In the first prospective, double-blind, video-controlled multi-center study in 22 patients with primary generalized dystonia with a follow-up of 12 months, the SPIDY Group reported a mean improvement of 51% at 1 year (BFM movement score; ref. *7*). Compared to baseline, the majority of movement subscores were improved at month 3 and remained stable until month 12. Twelve months postoperatively, axial and limb subscores improved by 68 and 52% respectively. Face and speech subscores were unchanged at follow-up assessments compared to pre-operative values. We observed that the patients with the greatest improvement were those with mobile or phasic dystonia, whereas patients with more severe tonic postures showed little improvement. Although this observation has also been found by other groups *(32, 34)*, it cannot be taken as a predictive factor for good outcome because currently there is limited ability to assess this factor due to a lack of standardized criteria for classifying patterns of dystonia. The global disability score was improved at 3 months and continued to be improved through 12 months (47% improvement). All rated items were improved (dressing, feeding, walking, hygiene, eating and swallowing, writing) except for speech. Although most patients were improved (some of them up to 90%), there was still some variability of results as has also been found in open label studies. Three patients showed little or no improvement. The improvement of quality of life (SF-36 scale), especially general health and physical functioning, paralleled the reduction of

**Table 17.1** Survey of the main studies that have addressed the question of pallidal DBS efficacy in dystonia.

| Author (year) | Study design | Patients ITD / SD (n) | Gen. / Seg. (n) | DYT 1 + (n) | Duration of DBS (Months) | Outcome Improvement of dystonia (%) |
|---|---|---|---|---|---|---|
| **Primary dystonia** | | | | | | |
| Kupsch et al. (2006) | Randomized / blinded | 20 / 0 | 12 / 8 | 2 | 3 | 39, 3 |
| Vidailhet et al. (2005) | Open | 22 / 0 | 22 / 0 | 7 | 12 | 51 (0–100) |
| Bittar et al. (2005) | Open | 12 / 0 | 6 / 6 | NA | 12 | 46, Gen ITD 59, Cervical dystonia |
| Eltahawy et al. (2004) | Open | 4 / 0 | 0 / 4 | NA | 15 | 73 (61–85) |
| Katayama et al. (2003) | Open | 5 / 0 | 5 / 0 | NA | 6 | 51–92 |
| Vesper et al. (2002) | Open | 2 / 0 | 2 / 0 | 1 | 6 | 80–95 |
| Bereznai et al. (2001) | Open | 6 / 0 | 1 / 5 | 1 | 3 | 72, 5 (50–100) |
| Krauss et al. (1999) | Open | 3 / 0 | 0 / 3 | NA | 3 | 44 (43–70) |
| **Tardive dyskinesia** | | | | | | |
| Trottenberg et al. (2005) | Open | 0 / 5 (Tar. Days.) | 5 / 0 | 0 | 12 | 87 |
| Franzini et al. (2005) | Open | 0 / 2 (Tar. Dys.) | 2 / 0 | NA | 12 | >90 |
| **Heterogenous population** | | | | | | |
| Cif et al. (2003), Coubes et al. (2004) | Open | 32 / 21 | 53 / 0 | 15 | 12 | 71, ITD DYT 1 + 74, ITD DYT 1 – 7, SD |
| Krause et al. (2004) | Open | 10 / 6 | NA | 4 | 12–48 | 56, ITD DYT 1 +) 35, ITD DYT 1 – 6–77, SD |
| Krauss et al. (2003) | Open | 2 / 4 | 6 / 0 | 0 | 24 | 70–78, ITD 23, SD |
| Yianni et al. (2003) | Open | 19 / 6 | 18 / 7 | NA | 12.3 (4–24) | 45, 8 (19–85), Gen ITD 59, 5 (44–84), Cervical dystonia 37,1 (0–73,9 ), SD |

Survey of the main studies that have addressed the question of pallidal DBS efficacy in dystonia. For each the study the main clinical characteristics of the patients together with the improvement of dystonia severity are given. According to the studies, the average and/or the range (between bracket) of improvement are provided. For studies that included primary and secondary dystonia, results for the different subgroups are given when available.

ITD, idiopathic torsion dystonia; SD, secondary dystonia; Tar. Dys., post-neuroleptic tardive dyskinesia; Gen, generalized; Seg, segmental dystonia, mainly cervical dystonia; NA, not available

disability due to dystonia. This quality of life finding was consistent with other studies, although sample sizes were small *(29, 35, 36)*. The beneficial effect of DBS was also demonstrated by double-blind video-controlled assessment at 3 months. In another multi-center study, patients were assigned to receive either neurostimulation or sham stimulation for 3 months in double-blind fashion *(8)*. Similar results were obtained with 39% improvement in dystonia severity, 38% improvement in disability, 30% improvement in quality of life (SF-36 scale) at 3 months, and 47% improvement of dystonia severity (open label) at 6 months.

Long-term beneficial effects have been reported in open-label studies *(5)*. This result was confirmed and expanded by the prospective 3-year follow-up of 22 generalized dystonia subjects *(37)*. The motor improvement observed at 1 year (51%) was maintained at 3 years (58%). Improved quality of life (SF-36 questionnaire) was similar to that observed at 1 year. Relative to baseline and to a 1-year evaluation, cognition, and mood were unchanged 3 years following surgery but slight improvements were noted in concept formation, reasoning, and executive functions. Bilateral pallidal stimulation was terminated in three patients (due to lack of improvement, technical dysfunction, and infection), and unilaterally in two patients (due to electrode breakage, stimulation-induced contracture). No permanent adverse effects were observed.

Overall, the main conclusions concerning DBS treatment of primary generalized dystonia may be summarized as follows: (A) A mean 50% improvement of dystonia severity and disability is expected with a wide range of results (from >90% in some patients to little or no improvement in a small number of other patients); (B) No definite predictive factors of good outcome have been identified including age, gender, disease duration, pre-operative BFM scores, DYT1 status, or specific electrode localization within the GPi. However, but this finding may be due to a lack of power in all studies, due to the relatively small number of studied patients. Importantly, however, several groups have had the clinical impression that mobile, phasic, and hyperkinetic patterns of dystonia appear to be good predictors of marked improvement, suggesting that the pattern and possibly the underlying pathophysiology of dystonia may play a role in the therapeutic response; (C) A parallel improvement in severity of dystonia, disability and quality of life was observed; (D) DBS carries a good risk–benefit ratio with no deleterious effects on mood or cognition; (E) Beneficial effects may be sustained over a period of at least 3–5 years; (F) Even in patients who have previously undergone thalamotomy or pallidotomy, GPi stimulation has provided a beneficial effect.

## Focal and Segmental Dystonia

Next to primary generalized dystonia, cervical dystonia has been the most frequently reported application of bilateral pallidal DBS. Operated patients have usually been poor responders to botulinum toxin injections. Some have had complex cervical dystonia with severe anterocollis, laterocollis, or retrocollis sometimes associated with head tremor, myoclonus, and cranial, brachial, or truncal dystonia. The initial reports by Krauss and colleagues in an open-label study demonstrated a symptomatic and functional improvement of 50 to 90% for up to 2.5 years *(38, 39)*. These results have since been confirmed by other groups *(3, 20, 30, 33, 35, 40–49)* with significant beneficial effects at 6 months and a sustained improvement at 2 to 3 year follow-up *(33, 35, 39, 50)*. Using a blinded assessment in a small number of patients, Kiss et al. found an improvement of 79% in the TWSTRS total score, improvement in pain, and 36% improved quality of life *(35)*. As in generalized dystonia, rare patients experienced limited effects or incomplete improvement *(33)*. Recently, long-term beneficial effects were reported after a mean follow-up of 32 months in 12 patients with cervical dystonia *(50)*. TWSTRS severity score improved by 55%, TWSTRS disability score improved by 59.1%, and TWSTRS pain score improved by 50% *(50)*. Other types of focal dystonia have been less frequently reported, either in the form of individual case reports or small series. Cranial dystonia including blepharospasm, Meige syndrome and oromandibular and lingual dystonia with severe tongue protrusion *(43, 51–54)* has been improved but swallowing difficulties were unchanged. One long-term follow-up of 2 years was reported with either recurrence of symptoms or arrest of stimulation with a rebound effect *(51)*. Reports concerning upper limb dystonia are rare. A beneficial effect of Vop pallidotomy has been reported in occupational dystonia in musicians and writer's cramp with a follow-up period of 13 months in 12 patients *(55, 56)*, suggesting a need to further explore pallidal DBS in limb dystonia.

General conclusions concerning focal and segmental dystonia must be limited to cervical and truncal dystonia in which only open-label data is available. Good improvement with sustained benefit over time (at least 3 years) has been reported in most patients.

**Dystonia-Plus Syndromes and Other Exceptional Cases**

Promising results have been reported in a small number of cases of myoclonic dystonia *(57)*, or myoclonus-dystonia *(58–60)*. Although this particular form of dystonia seems to have a good outcome after DBS, genetic status concerning mutation of the epsilon-sarcoglycan gene has not been predictive of outcome *(61)*. In one patient with paroxysmal nonkinesigenic dyskinesia and dystonia, a long-term beneficial effect was maintained over 4 years after thalamic ventral intermediate (Vim) stimulation *(62)*. In one patient with chorea-acanthocytosis with facial dystonia and severe trunk spasms, chorea and trunk spasms were improved by bilateral thalamic stimulation, which was maintained at 1-year follow-up *(63)*.

Rare forms of dystonia such as rapid onset-dystonia-parkinsonism *(64)* or post-traumatic fixed dystonia of the leg *(65)* have not been improved by bilateral pallidal stimulation. Status dystonicus is a life-threatening condition that sometimes occurs in primary dystonia, post-anoxic dystonia, or pantothenate kinase associated neurodegeneration (PANK2; ref. *66*). In rare cases, bilateral pallidal stimulation *(67–69)* or pallidotomy have been performed as emergency measures with moderate improvement *(70)*.

**Secondary Dystonia**

Results in secondary dystonia have been very variable. Among other things, this variability likely reflects the multiple causes of secondary dystonia *(71)*. Secondary dystonia due to brain injury has responded poorly *(72)*. Tardive dystonia, some cases of post-traumatic dystonia and some cases of PANK2 has shown a much better response. In tardive dystonia, the beneficial effects of bilateral pallidal stimulation are similar to those observed in primary dystonia *(73–77)*. Rapid improvement has been observed within 12 to 72 hours *(76)* to within a few days *(77)*. A substantial improvement (50 to 87%) has been obtained and in some cases dyskinesias have almost completely disappeared. However, failure of GPi stimulation has been reported in one case *(33)*. In a single case, symptoms of depression improved substantially in addition to a partial improvement of tardive dyskinesia *(78)*. In a group of 10 patients (STARDYS study), 6 months after pallidal DBS the Extrapyramidal Symptoms Rating Scale score decreased compared with baseline by more than 40% (mean improvement, 61%; range, 44–75%; ref. *74*). Treatment efficacy was confirmed by double-blind evaluation, with a mean improvement of 50% (range, 30–66%; ref. *74*).

In delayed onset post-traumatic dystonia (cervical dystonia and hemi-dystonia), a beneficial effect lasting 4 years has been obtained *(79, 80)*. These types of post-traumatic dystonia were related to brain injury in which patients usually develop delayed clinical features that resemble those of primary dystonia and are markedly different from the fixed postures that occur after peripheral trauma of the limb *(81)* and respond poorly to DBS.

In PANK2 patients, marked beneficial effect has been reported by some groups in open-label studies *(2, 82, 83)*, whereas others have observed only a mild beneficial effect *(16, 26)*, little effect on speech intelligibility, and no persistent improvement with secondary worsening of the disease at a 5 years follow-up *(33)*. These differences may possibly be related to the variable severity of the disease at the time of surgery, the variability of evolution of the disease among patients, and genetic status (presence of PANK2 mutations), although inconsistent results have also been observed in mutated patients *(16, 83)*.

In a group of secondary dystonias related to various miscellaneous causes including metabolic disorders, mitochondrial disorders, and basal ganglia lesions, the Montpellier group found a 31% improvement in severity of dystonia *(2)*. In well identified metabolic disorders such as GM1 gangliosidosis, little effect has been documented *(84)*.

In patients with post-anoxic birth injury who have severe disability with preservation of intellectual functions, the potential beneficial effects of DBS have created high expectations. To date, the Montpellier group has observed an improvement of 30% at 1 year, 40% at 3 years *(2, 85)*, and a 23% improvement at 2 years postoperatively *(6)*. A prospective, controlled study is ongoing (SPIDY 2).

Overall, in secondary dystonia, relatively few conclusions can be drawn: (A) Beneficial effects of bilateral pallidal stimulation are likely when the clinical features of dystonia are similar to those observed in primary dystonia and when total or partial integrity of the therapeutic pallidal or thalamic target is preserved; (B) Sustained benefit is dependent on the evolution of the disease (e.g., stable in tardive dystonia, worsening of symptoms in PANK2 or other genetic or metabolic disorders) and, possibly on the acquisition of normal motor control prior to the development of dystonia; (C) Most reports have been based on heterogeneous groups of patients in open-label studies. More selective studies in specific subgroups of disorders are necessary.

## Safety

Surgical procedures, targeting, and operative electrophysiological recording will not be discussed in this chapter. We will assume that the therapeutic contact is accurately positioned within the posteroventrolateral sensorimotor portion of the globus pallidus. Electrode implantation techniques and methods of target localization remain a source of debate. Generalized or local anaesthesia are performed in different centers and microelectrode recording results are partially influenced by on these conditions.

### Complications of DBS Therapy

The risks of intra-operative haemorrhage are in the range of 2 to 4%, but relatively few of these are symptomatic *(86)*. Hardware-related events such as lead fractures, skin erosions and infection have been described in up to 25% of patients undergoing functional neurosurgery *(87, 88)*. There has been a relatively high risk of lead fracture in dystonia, likely related to persistence of abnormal cervical and axial movements leading to mechanical stress on the lead connectors *(8, 89)*. Infections are nearly always local, either in the scalp or the stimulator pocket. Intracerebral infection has been extremely rare. In one prospective controlled study, two lead fractures and four infections occurred among 44 patients over 6 months *(8)*. In a second prospective study, implanted material was removed in one patient because of infection and two lead-breakages were observed among 22 patients over 3 years *(7)*. Although hardware failure in patients with dystonia may potentially be complicated by acute relapse with severe worsening of the patient's condition *(32)*, severe rebound phenomena have only rarely been observed.

Stimulation-related complications are reversible effects related to current spread to adjacent structures such as the internal capsule or optic tracts. The most frequent stimulation-related adverse event after pallidal DBS for dystonia has been worsening of voice intelligibility and freezing of speech *(8, 33, 37, 39, 48)*. This adverse effect, sometimes associated with stiffening of the dystonic arm, may limit the therapeutic efficacy of the procedure.

Overall, these various adverse events account for the 2 to 8% rate of complications reported for DBS and the overall rate of hardware-related complications of 4.3% per electrode-year *(89, 90)*. Close follow-up of dystonia patients is recommended, both for prevention and rapid treatment of complications.

### Neuropsychological Performances and Mood

Pallidal stimulation does not seem to adversely affect cognitive function in patients with dystonia *(7, 8, 91, 92)*. We found that after 3 years of follow-up cognitive test results were stable relative to those obtained at 1 year, while in a few cases some functions such as concept formation, reasoning, memory, and executive functions were mildly improved *(37)*. We speculate that these improvements may be related to a reallocation of cognitive resources previously invested in motor control but a test-learning phenomenon must also be considered. Overall, bilateral pallidal stimulation has had no noticeable deleterious effect on mood in any of the studies. As previously mentioned, in a single case of tardive dystonia, pre-operative symptoms of depression improved substantially after DBS *(78)*.

## Stimulation Arrest and Safety

A rebound exacerbation of dystonia has been reported after sudden arrest of stimulation *(20, 51)*, but this phenomenon appears to be rare. Acute relapse of dystonia might therefore be observed during replacement of the neurostimulator. However, no rebound phenomenon was observed during a 10-hour cessation of stimulation that occurred during a double-blind assessment of dystonia *(7)*. Moreover, in a prospective study we found that no rebound phenomenon occurred during 48 hours of stimulator arrest under carefully monitored conditions. We also observed that recurrence of dystonic symptoms took more than 24 hours to occur when the stimulator was turned off whereas is took only a few hours for patients to return to their usual level of improvement when the stimulator was turned on. Nevertheless, close observation of dystonia patients is recommended both for prevention of unexpected stimulator arrest and for monitoring of battery end-of-life.

## Patient selection, Management, and Practical Issues

### Patient Selection

To date, patient selection has been based on empirical and intuitive criteria but most neurologists and neurosurgeons who treat patients with dystonia have generally agreed on the guidelines they employ to evaluate the risk–benefit ratio for each patient. As mentioned earlier, there are no predictive factors of good surgical outcome but some rules of thumb are commonly used *(93)*. (A) Primary generalized dystonia and complex cervical or truncal dystonia unresponsive to medical treatment are suitable indications for DBS; (B) Young patients may have a better surgical outcome owing possibly to their potential for cerebral plasticity and relative absence of orthopaedic contractures and other deformations; (C) Hyperkinetic, phasic or mobile dystonic movements appear to be improve sooner and better than fixed dystonic postures; (D) Presence of normal motor and cognitive development prior to the onset of dystonia may be favourable indicators; (E) Normal brain MRI with integrity of the therapeutic targets within the basal ganglia is an important consideration; (F) Stable disease with relatively little progression is important but not absolutely necessary; and (G) DBS should be considered very carefully before being recommended for secondary dystonia. Based on current uncontrolled data, tardive dystonia, dystonia associated with PANK2, and some cases of dystonia due to brain injury may be suitable for consideration.

### Management and Practical Issues

#### Parameter Settings
The programming of DBS parameters differs among different centers. Although pulse width has varied from 90 to 450 μs, and rate has varied from 60–180 Hz, a pulse width of 210 μs and rate of 130 Hz are most commonly used. In our 3-year follow-up study *(37)*, persistent improvement in motor and cognitive performance was obtained with the same settings as those used at 1 year. Monopolar stimulation (one contact or two contiguous contacts) was used, mean voltage was $3.8 \pm 0.7$ V, mean pulse width was $127 \pm 107$ μs, and rate 130 to 185 Hz.

These parameter settings are close to those of most open-label studies and of the one other published controlled study at 6 months follow-up (mean voltage 3.2 ± 0.9 V, pulse width was 123 ± 37 μs and the rate 135 ± 37 Hz; ref. 8). Several reports on the management of cervical (39) or generalized dystonia (5) have shown little or no need for further programming after 6 to 9 months. Although careful observation of some patients is important, such as monitoring of battery life in severe dystonia, routine follow-up is usually simple and most patients need to be seen only yearly.

The role of different frequencies, pulse widths and total energy delivery remains a matter of some debate. It has been suggested that lower stimulation frequencies may be associated with better control of dystonia (94). A patient could not be treated with the usual stimulation parameters using ventral pallidal contacts because of adverse effects and had unsatisfactory results using dorsal contacts. By reducing stimulation frequency to 80 Hz, the patient experienced a dramatic improvement in function that persisted for 1 year. Although in this patient lowering stimulation frequency to 60 Hz resulted in a worsening of symptoms, 60 Hz stimulation frequency has reportedly resulted in improvement of dystonia in another group of patients (Tagliati, personal communication).

Analysis of differential effects of bilateral short (60–90 μs), medium (120–150 μs) and long (450 μs) pulse widths has shown that short-duration stimulus pulse widths are as effective as longer ones (Vercueil et al., personal communication). This is of potential interest as shorter pulse widths would be associated with fewer adverse events due to current spread and battery life would be longer.

The effects of ventral vs dorsal pallidal stimulation have also been studied (Houeto et al, personal communication). Bilateral ventral stimulation resulted in improvement of dystonia when stimulation contacts were located in the GPi or internal lamina. By contrast, stimulation of dorsal contacts, commonly located in GPe, had more variable clinical effects. Half of patients studied had little or no effect or dystonia was even aggravated compared to baseline.

## Conclusion

Accumulating and more controlled data is providing strong evidence that bilateral pallidal DBS produces a marked beneficial effect in dystonia severity and disability in selected patients, with the greatest benefit found in primary generalized dystonia, some primary segmental dystonias, and tardive dystonia. To date, the preferred target for DBS is the internal pallidum but other targets such as thalamus or subthalamic nucleus may turn out to be an option in some forms of secondary dystonia or in patients who do not improve with pallidal stimulation. Successful treatment of patients with generalized dystonia related to birth injury remains a serious challenge for neurostimulation. Alleviating the burden of these disorders would potentially allow patients to enjoy a more normal social, affective, and professional life. Moreover, the alleviation of dystonia and restoration of normal motor control may help provide insights into mechanisms of cerebral plasticity and learning capabilities of the sensorimotor system.

*Acknowledgements*: We are indebt to Pierre Pollak, Paul Krack, and Laurent Vercueil at the Department of Biological and Clinical Neurosciences University Hospital of Grenoble, Joseph-Fourier University in Grenoble, France, for their helpful discussions, sharing of knowledge, and close collaboration.

## References

1. Fahn S, Bressman SB, Marsden CD (1998) Classification of dystonia. Adv Neurol 78:1–10.
2. Cif L, El Fertit H, Vayssiere N, et al (2003) Treatment of dystonic syndromes by chronic electrical stimulation of the internal globus pallidus. J Neurosurg Sci 47:52–55.
3. Bereznai B, Steude U, Seelos K, Botzel K (2002) Chronic high-frequency globus pallidus internus stimulation in different types of dystonia: a clinical, video, and MRI report of six patients presenting with segmental, cervical, and generalized dystonia. Mov Disord 17:138–144.
4. Coubes P, Roubertie A, Vayssiere N, Hemm S, Echenne B (2000) Treatment of DYT1-generalised dystonia by stimulation of the internal globus pallidus. Lancet 355:2220–2221.
5. Coubes P, Cif L, El Fertit H, et al (2004) Electrical stimulation of the globus pallidus internus in patients with primary generalized dystonia: long-term results. J Neurosurg 101:189–194.
6. Krauss JK, Loher TJ, Weigel R, Capelle HH, Weber S, Burgunder JM (2003) Chronic stimulation of the globus pallidus internus for treatment of non-dYT1 generalized dystonia and choreoathetosis: 2-year follow up. J Neurosurg 98:785–792.
7. Vidailhet M, Vercueil L, Houeto JL, et al (2005) Bilateral deep-brain stimulation of the globus pallidus in primary generalized dystonia. N Engl J Med 352:459–467.
8. Kupsch A, Benecke R, Muller J, et al (2006) Pallidal deep-brain stimulation in primary generalized or segmental dystonia. N Engl J Med 355:1978–1990.
9. Andrew J, Fowler CJ, Harrison MJ (1983) Stereotaxic thalamotomy in 55 cases of dystonia. Brain 106(Pt 4):981–1000.
10. Ford B (2004) Pallidotomy for generalized dystonia. Adv Neurol 94:287–299.
11. Lozano AM, Kumar R, Gross RE, et al (1997) Globus pallidus internus pallidotomy for generalized dystonia. Mov Disord 12:865–870.
12. Vitek JL, Zhang J, Evatt M, et al (1998) GPi pallidotomy for dystonia: clinical outcome and neuronal activity. Adv Neurol 78:211–219.
13. Vercueil L, Pollak P, Fraix V, et al (2001) Deep brain stimulation in the treatment of severe dystonia. J Neurol 248:695–700.
14. Ghika J, Villemure JG, Miklossy J, et al (2002) Postanoxic generalized dystonia improved by bilateral Voa thalamic deep brain stimulation. Neurology 58:311–313.
15. Chou KL, Hurtig HI, Jaggi JL, Baltuch GH (2005) Bilateral subthalamic nucleus deep brain stimulation in a patient with cervical dystonia and essential tremor. Mov Disord 20:377–380.
16. Detante O, Vercueil L, Krack P, et al (2004) Off-period dystonia in Parkinson's disease but not generalized dystonia is improved by high-frequency stimulation of the subthalamic nucleus. Adv Neurol 94:309–314.
17. Burke RE, Fahn S, Marsden CD, Bressman SB, Moskowitz C, Friedman J (1985) Validity and reliability of a rating scale for the primary torsion dystonias. Neurology 35:73–77.
18. Krystkowiak P, du Montcel ST, Vercueil L, et al (2007) Reliability of the Burke-Fahn-Marsden scale in a multicenter trial for dystonia. Mov Disord
19. Comella CL, Stebbins GT, Goetz CG, Chmura TA, Bressman SB, Lang AE (1997) Teaching tape for the motor section of the Toronto Western Spasmodic Torticollis Scale. Mov Disord 12:570–575.

20. Bittar RG, Yianni J, Wang S, et al (2005) Deep brain stimulation for generalised dystonia and spasmodic torticollis. J Clin Neurosci 12:12–16.
21. Ware JE Jr, Sherbourne CD (1992) The MOS 36-item short-form health survey (SF-36). I. Conceptual framework and item selection. Med Care 30:473–483.
22. Coubes P, Echenne B, Roubertie A, et al (1999) Treatment of early-onset generalized dystonia by chronic bilateral stimulation of the internal globus pallidus. Apropos of a case. Neurochirurgie 45:139–144.
23. Kumar R, Dagher A, Hutchison WD, Lang AE, Lozano AM (1999) Globus pallidus deep brain stimulation for generalized dystonia: clinical and PET investigation. Neurology 53:871–874.
24. Vesper J, Klostermann F, Funk T, Stockhammer F, Brock M (2002) Deep brain stimulation of the globus pallidus internus (GPI) for torsion dystonia—a report of two cases. Acta Neurochir Suppl 79:83–88.
25. Tronnier VM, Fogel W (2000) Pallidal stimulation for generalized dystonia. Report of three cases. J Neurosurg 92:453–456.
26. Vercueil L, Krack P, Pollak P (2002) Results of deep brain stimulation for dystonia: a critical reappraisal. Mov Disord 17(Suppl 3):S89–S93.
27. Eltahawy HA, Saint-Cyr J, Giladi N, Lang AE, Lozano AM (2004) Primary dystonia is more responsive than secondary dystonia to pallidal interventions: outcome after pallidotomy or pallidal deep brain stimulation. Neurosurgery 54:613–619.
28. Katayama Y, Fukaya C, Kobayashi K, Oshima H, Yamamoto T (2003) Chronic stimulation of the globus pallidus internus for control of primary generalized dystonia. Acta Neurochir Suppl 87:125–128.
29. Kupsch A, Klaffke S, Kuhn AA, et al (2003) The effects of frequency in pallidal deep brain stimulation for primary dystonia. J Neurol 250:1201–1205.
30. Yianni J, Bain P, Giladi N, et al (2003) Globus pallidus internus deep brain stimulation for dystonic conditions: a prospective audit. Mov Disord 18:436–442.
31. Tisch S, Limousin P, Rothwell JC, et al (2006) Changes in forearm reciprocal inhibition following pallidal stimulation for dystonia. Neurology 66:1091–1093.
32. Tagliati M, Shils J, Sun C, Alterman R (2004) Deep brain stimulation for dystonia. Expert Rev Med Devices 1:33–41.
33. Krause M, Fogel W, Kloss M, Rasche D, Volkmann J, Tronnier V (2004) Pallidal stimulation for dystonia. Neurosurgery 55:1361–70.
34. Krauss JK, Kiss ZH, Doig K, et al (2002) Deep brain stimulation for dystonia in adults. Stereotact Funct Neurosurg 78:168–182.
35. Kiss ZH, Doig K, Eliasziw M, Ranawaya R, Suchowersky O (2004) The Canadian multicenter trial of pallidal deep brain stimulation for cervical dystonia: preliminary results in three patients. Neurosurg Focus 17:E5.
36. Diamond A, Jankovic J (2005) The effect of deep brain stimulation on quality of life in movement disorders. J Neurol Neurosurg Psychiatry 76:1188–1193.
37. Vidailhet M, Vercueil L, Houeto JL, et al (2007) Bilateral, pallidal, deep-brain stimulation in primary generalised dystonia: a prospective 3 year follow-up study. Lancet Neurol 6:223–229.
38. Krauss JK, Pohle T, Weber S, Ozdoba C, Burgunder JM (1999) Bilateral stimulation of globus pallidus internus for treatment of cervical dystonia. Lancet 354:837–838.
39. Krauss JK, Loher TJ, Pohle T, et al (2002) Pallidal deep brain stimulation in patients with cervical dystonia and severe cervical dyskinesias with cervical myelopathy. J Neurol Neurosurg Psychiatry 72:249–256.
40. Wohrle JC, Weigel R, Grips E, Blahak C, Capelle HH, Krauss JK (2003) Risperidone-responsive segmental dystonia and pallidal deep brain stimulation. Neurology 61:546–548.
41. Lozano AM, Abosch A (2004) Pallidal stimulation for dystonia. Adv Neurol 94:301–308.
42. Kulisevsky J, Lleo A, Gironell A, Molet J, Pascual-Sedano B, Pares P (2000) Bilateral pallidal stimulation for cervical dystonia: dissociated pain and motor improvement. Neurology 55:1754–1755.

43. Muta D, Goto S, Nishikawa S, et al (2001) Bilateral pallidal stimulation for idiopathic segmental axial dystonia advanced from Meige syndrome refractory to bilateral thalamotomy. Mov Disord 16:774–777.
44. Andaluz N, Taha JM, Dalvi A (2001) Bilateral pallidal deep brain stimulation for cervical and truncal dystonia. Neurology 57:557–558.
45. Parkin S, Aziz T, Gregory R, Bain P (2001) Bilateral internal globus pallidus stimulation for the treatment of spasmodic torticollis. Mov Disord 16:489–493.
46. Islekel S, Zileli M, Zileli B (1999) Unilateral pallidal stimulation in cervical dystonia. Stereotact Funct Neurosurg 72:248–252.
47. Coubes P, Vayssiere N, El Fertit H, et al (2002) Deep brain stimulation for dystonia. Surgical technique. Stereotact Funct Neurosurg 78:183–191.
48. Eltahawy HA, Saint-Cyr J, Poon YY, Moro E, Lang AE, Lozano AM (2004) Pallidal deep brain stimulation in cervical dystonia: clinical outcome in four cases. Can J Neurol Sci 31:328–332.
49. Loher TJ, Pohle T, Krauss JK (2004) Functional stereotactic surgery for treatment of cervical dystonia: review of the experience from the lesional era. Stereotact Funct Neurosurg 82:1–13.
50. Hung SW, Hamani C, Lozano AM, et al (2007) Long-term outcome of bilateral pallidal deep brain stimulation for primary cervical dystonia. Neurology 68:457–459.
51. Capelle HH, Weigel R, Krauss JK (2003) Bilateral pallidal stimulation for blepharospasm-oromandibular dystonia (Meige syndrome). Neurology 60:2017–2018.
52. Foote KD, Sanchez JC, Okun MS (2005) Staged deep brain stimulation for refractory craniofacial dystonia with blepharospasm: case report and physiology. Neurosurgery 56:E415; discussion E415.
53. Schneider SA, Aggarwal A, Bhatt M, et al (2006) Severe tongue protrusion dystonia: clinical syndromes and possible treatment. Neurology 67:940–943.
54. Houser M, Waltz T (2005) Meige syndrome and pallidal deep brain stimulation. Mov Disord 20:1203–1205.
55. Taira T, Hori T, Harashima S, et al (2003) Stereotactic ventrooralis thalamotomy for task-specific focal hand dystonia (writer's cramp). Stereotact Funct Neurosurg 80:88–91.
56. Shibata T, Hirashima Y, Ikeda H, et al (2005) Stereotactic Voa-Vop complex thalamotomy for writer's cramp. Eur Neurol 53:38–39.
57. Magarinos-Ascone CM, Regidor I, Martinez-Castrillo JC, et al (2005) Pallidal stimulation relieves myoclonus-dystonia syndrome. J Neurol Neurosurg Psychiatry 76:989–991.
58. Cif L, Valente EM, Hemm S, et al (2004) Deep brain stimulation in myoclonus-dystonia syndrome. Mov Disord 19:724–727.
59. Liu X, Griffin IC, Parkin SG, et al (2002) Involvement of the medial pallidum in focal myoclonic dystonia: A clinical and neurophysiological case study. Mov Disord 17:346–353.
60. Trottenberg T, Meissner W, Kabus C, et al (2001) Neurostimulation of the ventral intermediate thalamic nucleus in inherited myoclonus-dystonia syndrome. Mov Disord 16:769–771.
61. Tezenas du Montcel S, Clot F, Vidailhet M, et al (2006) Epsilon sarcoglycan mutations and phenotype in French patients with myoclonic syndromes. J Med Genet 43:394–400.
62. Loher TJ, Krauss JK, Burgunder JM, et al (2001) Chronic thalamic stimulation for treatment of dystonic paroxysmal nonkinesigenic dyskinesia. Neurology 56:268–270.
63. Burbaud P, Rougier A, Ferrer X, et al (2002) Improvement of severe trunk spasms by bilateral high-frequency stimulation of the motor thalamus in a patient with chorea-acanthocytosis. Mov Disord 17:204–207.
64. Deutschlander A, Asmus F, Gasser T, Steude U, Botzel K (2005) Sporadic rapid-onset dystonia-parkinsonism syndrome: failure of bilateral pallidal stimulation. Mov Disord 20:254–7.

65. Capelle HH, Grips E, Weigel R, et al (2006) Posttraumatic peripherally-induced dystonia and multifocal deep brain stimulation: case report. Neurosurgery 59:E702.
66. Manji H, Howard RS, Miller DH, et al (1998) Status dystonicus: the syndrome and its management. Brain 121(Pt 2):243–252.
67. Angelini L, Nardocci N, Estienne M, et al (2000) Life-threatening dystonia-dyskinesias in a child: successful treatment with bilateral pallidal stimulation. Mov Disord 15:1010–1012.
68. Teive HA, Munhoz RP, Souza MM, et al (2005) Status Dystonicus: study of five cases. Arq Neuropsiquiatr 63:26–29.
69. Zorzi G, Marras C, Nardocci N, et al (2005) Stimulation of the globus pallidus internus for childhood-onset dystonia. Mov Disord 20:1194–1200.
70. Balas I, Kovacs N, Hollody K (2006) Staged bilateral stereotactic pallidothalamotomy for life-threatening dystonia in a child with Hallervorden-Spatz disease. Mov Disord 21:82–85.
71. Marks WJ (2005) Deep brain stimulation for dystonia. Curr Treat Options Neurol 7:237–243.
72. Tarsy D (2007) Deep-brain stimulation for dystonia: new twists in assessment. Lancet Neurol 6:201–202.
73. Eltahawy HA, Feinstein A, Khan F, Saint-Cyr J, Lang AE, Lozano AM (2004) Bilateral globus pallidus internus deep brain stimulation in tardive dyskinesia: a case report. Mov Disord 19:969–972.
74. Damier P, Thobois S, Witjas T, et al (2007) Bilateral deep brain stimulation of the globus pallidus to treat tardive dyskinesia. Arch Gen Psychiatry 64:170–176.
75. Trottenberg T, Paul G, Meissner W, et al (2001) Pallidal and thalamic neurostimulation in severe tardive dystonia. J Neurol Neurosurg Psychiatry 70:557–559.
76. Trottenberg T, Volkmann J, Deuschl G, et al (2005) Treatment of severe tardive dystonia with pallidal deep brain stimulation. Neurology 64:344–346.
77. Franzini A, Marras C, Ferroli P, et al (2005) Long-term high-frequency bilateral pallidal stimulation for neuroleptic-induced tardive dystonia. Report of two cases. J Neurosurg 102:721–725.
78. Kosel M, Sturm V, Frick C, et al (2006) Mood improvement after deep brain stimulation of the internal globus pallidus for tardive dyskinesia in a patient suffering from major depression. J Psychiatr Res 73:588–590.
79. Chang JW, Choi JY, Lee BW, Kang UJ, Chung SS (2002) Unilateral globus pallidus internus stimulation improves delayed onset post-traumatic cervical dystonia with an ipsilateral focal basal ganglia lesion. J Neurol Neurosurg Psychiatry 73:588–590.
80. Loher TJ, Hasdemir MG, Burgunder JM, Krauss JK (2000) Long-term follow-up study of chronic globus pallidus internus stimulation for posttraumatic hemidystonia. J Neurosurg 92:457–460.
81. Jankovic J, Vercueil L, Krack P, et al (1994) Post-traumatic movement disorders: central and peripheral mechanisms. Neurology 44:2006–2014.
82. Umemura A, Jaggi JL, Dolinskas CA, Stern MB, Baltuch GH (2004) Pallidal deep brain stimulation for longstanding severe generalized dystonia in Hallervorden-Spatz syndrome. Case report. J Neurosurg 100:706–709.
83. Castelnau P, Cif L, Valente EM, et al (2005) Pallidal stimulation improves pantothenate kinase-associated neurodegeneration. Ann Neurol 57:738–741.
84. Roze E, Navarro S, Cornu P, et al (2006) Deep brain stimulation of the globus pallidus for generalized dystonia in GM1 Type 3 gangliosidosis: technical case report. Neurosurgery 59:E1340.
85. Gil-Robles S, Cif L, Biolsi B, et al (2006) Neurosurgical treatment in childhood dystonias and dyskinesias. Rev Neurol 43(Suppl 1):S169–S172.
86. Umemura A, Jaggi JL, Hurtig HI, et al (2003) Deep brain stimulation for movement disorders: morbidity and mortality in 109 patients. J Neurosurg 98:779–784.

87. Oh MY, Abosch A, Kim SH, Lang AE, Lozano AM (2002) Long-term hardware-related complications of deep brain stimulation. Neurosurgery 50:1268–1274; discussion 1274–1276.
88. Hariz MI (2002) Complications of deep brain stimulation surgery. Mov Disord 17(Suppl 3):S162–S166.
89. Yianni J, Nandi D, Shad A, Bain P, Gregory R, Aziz T (2004) Increased risk of lead fracture and migration in dystonia compared with other movement disorders following deep brain stimulation. J Clin Neurosci 11:243–245.
90. Blomstedt P, Hariz MI (2005) Hardware-related complications of deep brain stimulation: a ten year experience. Acta Neurochir (Wien) 147:1061–1064.
91. Halbig TD, Gruber D, Kopp UA, Schneider GH, Trottenberg T, Kupsch A (2005) Pallidal stimulation in dystonia: effects on cognition, mood, and quality of life. J Neurol Neurosurg Psychiatry 76:1713–1716.
92. Pillon B, Ardouin C, Dujardin K, et al (2006) Preservation of cognitive function in dystonia treated by pallidal stimulation. Neurology 66:1556–1558.
93. Volkmann J, Benecke R (2002) Deep brain stimulation for dystonia: patient selection and evaluation. Mov Disord 17(Suppl 3):S112–S115.
94. Alterman RL, Shils JL, Miravite J, et al (2007) Lower stimulation frequency can enhance tolerability and efficacy of pallidal deep brain stimulation for dystonia. Mov Disord 22:366–368.
95. Paluzzi A, Bain PG, Liu X, Yianni J, Kumarendran K, Aziz TZ (2006) Pregnancy in dystonic women with in situ deep brain stimulators. Mov Disord 21:695–698.

# 18

# Deep Brain Stimulation in Tourette's Syndrome

Linda Ackermans, Yasin Temel, and Veerle Visser-Vandewalle

## Abstract

Motivation to choose a specific target for deep brain stimulation (DBS) treatment of Tourette's syndrome (TS) has been based on the effects of the historical ablative surgical literature available for that target, as well as on the effects of DBS in that target for similar symptoms in other disorders such as dyskinesias and obsessive compulsive disorders. DBS in TS is still investigational and published experience is very limited. The best target remains to be determined and the effects of stimulation of currently used targets are not fully appreciated. The rationale for target selection, the results of available studies, and current guidelines for DBS treatment of TS are reviewed here.

**Keywords:** DBS, Tourette's syndrome, tics, tic disorders, obsessive–compulsive disorders

## Introduction

### Clinical Characteristics and Prevalence

Georges Gilles de la Tourette first described the syndrome that bears his name in 1885 as a nervous affection characterized by lack of motor coordination accompanied by echolalia and coprolalia. Later, Charcot named the condition Tourette's syndrome.

TS is a chronic complex neuropsychiatric disorder characterized most prominently by tics. Tics are sudden, rapid, recurrent, non-rhythmic, stereotyped muscle contractions (motor tics) or sounds produced by moving air through the nose, mouth, or throat (vocal tics; ref. *1*). They may be abrupt in onset, fast, and brief (clonic tics) or may be slow and sustained (dystonic or tonic tics; ref. *2*). The motor patterns of tics may involve individual muscles or small groups of muscles with discrete contractions (simple tics) like eye blinking, nose twitching, sniffing, or grunting. Complex tics involve a larger number of muscles acting in a coordinated pattern to produce complicated

From: *Current Clinical Neurology: Deep Brain Stimulation in Neurological and Psychiatric Disorders*
Edited by: D. Tarsy, J.L. Vitek, P.A. Starr, and M.S. Okun © Humana Press, Totowa, NJ

movements that may resemble purposeful voluntary movements *(1)*. Complex tics include head shaking, scratching, throwing, touching, or uttering short phrases. Uttering obscene words (coprolalia) occurs in only 10% or less of patients. Tics increase with stress and decrease with relaxation or when the individual is engaged in acts that require selective attention. Tics may in some cases be temporarily suppressed by an effort of will or concentration, but typically rebound in severity afterwards *(3)*.

The onset of tics in TS most commonly occurs in early childhood, with a mean age of 7 years *(2)*. Severity of tics typically increases during the pre-pubescent years, and often declines in frequency and intensity by the beginning of adulthood. Ninety percent of TS patients will experience substantial remission and more than 40% will be symptom-free by age 18. According to the Diagnostic and Statistical Manual of Mental Disorders (DSM-IV TR; ref. *4*), TS is defined by the presence of both multiple motor tics and one or more vocal tics throughout a period of more than 1 year, during which time there is absence of a tic-free period of more than 3 consecutive months *(5)*. The tic repertoire of an individual with TS includes fluctuations in type of tic, body location, and the impairment it produces *(1)*.

An important feature of TS is its association with a wide range of co-morbid behavioral abnormalities that, in some patients, are far more disabling than the tics themselves *(5)*. Attention deficit hyperactivity disorder (ADHD), obsessive–compulsive behavior (OCB), and self-injurious behavior (SIB) are strongly linked to TS and are probably an integral part of the syndrome. The occurrence of ADHD in TS patients ranges from 21 to 90% *(2)*. Symptoms include inattention and distractibility with or without behavioral hyperactivity. OCB may occur in up to 50% of TS patients. More severe obsessions in TS may involve sexual, violent, religious, aggressive, and symmetrical themes; the compulsions may manifest with symptoms such as checking, counting, forced touching, and self-damage. Like tics, OCB symptoms often wax and wane during the course of the illness. Robertson et al. *(2)* reported that more than one-third of TS patients carried out SIB. The most frequent type of SIB was head banging.

Although once thought to be rare, TS is now recognized as a relatively common disorder with an estimated worldwide prevalence of 4 to 5/10,000, which occurs three to four times more commonly in males *(6)*. There is considerable variation among studies reporting on prevalence of TS, which is most likely due to variations in sex, age, diagnostic criteria, and methods of assessment *(7)*.

## Treatment of TS

For many patients, especially those with mild symptoms, psychobehavioral strategies provide sufficient treatment. Pharmacological treatment may be considered when symptoms interfere with social interactions, academic or job performance, or with activities of daily living. The most commonly prescribed medications for more severe TS are dopamine antagonists such as tetrabenazine and dopamine-blocking agents such as haloperidol or other antipsychotic drugs *(2)*. Clonidine, clonazepam, and injections with botulinum toxin are also widely used. Selective serotonin reuptake inhibitors are recommended for treating OCB but are not helpful for tics. Psychostimulants, such as methylphenidate, are the treatment of choice for ADHD *(8)*.

For patients who are refractory to any behavioral and medical treatment, surgery may be considered as a treatment of last resort. Although no precise numbers are available, this likely represents a very small percentage of patients with TS.

## History of Neurosurgical Treatment of TS

In the past, several attempts were made to treat these patients through neurosurgical ablative procedures (Figure 18.1; ref. 9). The target sites have been diverse and have included the frontal lobe (prefrontal lobotomy and bimedial frontal leucotomy), the limbic system (limbic leucotomy and anterior cingulotomy), the thalamus, and the cerebellum. Combined approaches have also been tried such as anterior cingulotomy plus infrathalamic lesions. The results have often been unsatisfactory and major side effects have occurred such as hemiplegia or dystonia.

DBS was first introduced as a new surgical technique for the treatment of intractable TS in 1999 *(10)*. Vandewalle et al. *(10)* performed chronic bilateral stimulation of the medial part of the thalamus, in the centromedian-parafascicular complex and voi. This target was chosen on the basis of the favorable results of thalamotomy in this location previously described by Hassler in 1970

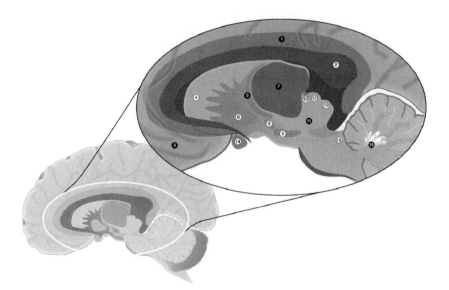

**Figure 18.1** A schematic drawing of brain areas that have been targeted in surgery for Tourette's syndrome and other relevant neuroanatomical structures. The frontal lobe (3) was targeted during prefrontal lobotomy and bimedial leucotomy. In limbic leucotomy and anterior cingulotomy, the cingulate cortex (1) was lesioned. The thalamus (7) was targeted for lesioning of the midline, intralaminar, and ventrolateral thalamic nuclei and for DBS. Infrathalamic lesions were performed at the level of the H fields of Forel (11) and the zona incerta (5). Cerebellar surgery involved lesioning of the dentate nucleus (16). The surrounding brain areas include: (2) corpus callosum, (4) caudate-putamen complex, (6) globus pallidus, (8) subthalamic nucleus, (9) substantia nigra, (10) posterior commissure, (12) superior colliculus, (13) inferior colliculus, (15) superior cerebellar peduncle, and (14) optic chiasm. (To view this figure in color, see insert)

*(11)*. The same group described the promising effects of bilateral thalamic DBS in three patients in greater detail in 2003 *(12)*. With follow-up periods of 5 years, 1 year and 8 months respectively, there was an improvement in both tics (tic reduction of 90, 72, and 83% respectively with stimulation on compared with stimulation off) and in associated behavioral disorders. Stimulation induced side effects consisted of drowsiness and changes in sexual functioning *(12, 13)*.

## Targets

After the initiation of thalamic DBS as a potential treatment for patients with refractory TS, several other targets have been used (Table 18.1). Published reports are sparse *(10, 12, 14–20)* and the low number of cases may reflect the very small group of potential candidates for surgery. Up until now, six targets have been used for DBS for TS in 33 patients: (A) medial portion of thalamus, at the cross point of CM-Spv-Voi *(10, 12, 14–16)*; (B) medial portion of thalamus, CM-Pf *(17)*; (C) the globus pallidus internus (GPi); posteroventrolateral part *(18, 19)*; (D) GPi, anteromedial part *(17)*; (E) nucleus accumbens (NAC); and (F) anterior limb of internal capsule (IC; ref. *20*). Servello et al. *(15)* reported on the beneficial effects of DBS of the same target described by Vandewalle in 18 patients with TS, with a follow up of 3 to 17 months. In this report there was an improved response of motor tics when compared to phonic tics due to thalamic DBS. These authors also reported positive effects on behavioral disorders.

The effects of bilateral DBS in the posteroventral (motor) portion of the GPi in a single patient were described by Van der Linden et al. in 2002 *(18)*. This choice of target was based on the beneficial effects of DBS in the same brain region on hyperkinetic movements induced by levodopa in patients with Parkinson's disease (PD). At 6 months follow-up, a tic reduction of 95% was observed. In 2004, Diederich et al. described the beneficial effects of chronic stimulation of the same target in another patient, with a follow-up period of 14 months *(19)*. However, there was no change in the patient's "very mild compulsive tendencies."

Houeto et al. described the effects of bilateral pallidal and thalamic stimulation in one patient *(17)*. The pallidal target was located in the anteromedial (limbic) part of the GPi. In this patient, both thalamic and pallidal stimulation had similar effects on tics, but thalamic stimulation was superior for treatment of the associated behavior disturbance.

Flaherty et al. *(20)* described the effects of bilateral stimulation of the anterior portion of the internal capsule in a single patient with TS who suffered from severe tics without associated behavioral disorders. After 18 months, there was a 25% reduction in tics. In this patient, the lowest electrode contacts produced mild depression while the highest contacts caused hypomania. Finally, DBS of the NAC has been performed in three patients with TS with a 75% reduction in tics and a beneficial effect on behavior. These patients were included in a group of patients with OC disorder (OCD; Sturm, personal communication).

Except for a small hematoma around the tip of one electrode, no serious surgical complications have been reported to date in the published literature.

**Table 18.1** Reports on deep brain stimulation in patients with Tourette's syndrome.

| First author, year | Target | No. of patients | Follow-up period | Tic reduction | Effect on behavioral disorders | Side effects | Complications |
|---|---|---|---|---|---|---|---|
| Vandewalle, 1999 | Thal (med.) | 1 | 4 monhs | 90–100% | n.m. | n.m. | None |
| van der Linden, 2002 | Thal (med.)/ Gpi vpl | 1 | immediately postoperatively/6 months | 80%/95% | n.m. | None | None |
| Visser-Vandewalle, 2003 | Thal (med.) | 3 | 5 year, 1 year, 8 months | 90%, 72%, 83% | Very good | Drowsiness, changes in sexual behavior (two patients) | None |
| Diederich, 2005 | Gpi vpl | 1 | 14 months | 66% | No effect on compulsions | Impairment of left rapidly alternating movements | Small H around right electrode tip |
| Houeto, 2005 | Thal (CM-Pf)/ Gpi am | 1 | 24 months | 70% (both) | Very good (both) | With Gpi DBS more depressed | None |
| Egidi, 2005 | Thal (med.) | 1 | 6 months | 78% | n.m. | Mild dysarthria | None |
| Servello, submitted | Thal (med.) | 18 | 3–17 months | Good | Good | Reduced energy | Wound dehiscence, abdominal subcutaneous hematoma. |
| Lenartz, 2005 | NAC | 3 | 2 years, 4 months, 4 months | 75% (average) | Very good | None | None |
| Flaherty, 2005 | Internal capsule | 1 | 18 months | 25% | — | Hypomania and depression | None |

Thal, thalamus; med., medial part (CM-Spv-Voi); CM, centromedian nucleus; Spv, substantia periventricularis; Voi, nucleus ventro-oralis internus; Pf, Parafascicular nucleus; Gpi, globus pallidus internus; vpl, ventroposterolateral part; am, anteromedial part; NAC, nucleus accumbens; H, hematoma; n.m., not mentioned.

However, unexpected stimulation-induced side effects such as drowsiness, reduced energy, changes in sexual behavior, and mild dysarthria, seem to be emerging in the majority of reported cases *(9, 12, 13, 15)*. One patient treated with bilateral thalamic and bilateral anteromedial GPi DBS appeared to be more depressed with pallidal stimulation *(17)*. The stimulation-dependent changes in the execution of movements in one case with posteroventrolateral pallidal stimulation probably had to do with the small haematoma *(19)*.

## Neuroanatomical Basis for DBS in TS

The pathophysiology of TS remains poorly understood. It is widely believed that abnormalities in dopamine neurotransmission play a fundamental role in the pathogenesis of TS. This hypothesis arises from the clinical observation that dopamine D2 receptor blocking drugs and presynaptic dopamine depletors successfully suppress tics in many cases, whereas potentiation of dopamine transmission with stimulant medications often increases the number and severity of tics (1). Moreover, a number of functional neuroimaging studies have revealed abnormalities in dopamine transporter and dopamine receptor binding in the striatum of TS patients (21). Dopamine has a strong regulatory function on striatal activity. Within the brain, there are anatomically segregated, parallel circuits representing different functions (motor, oculomotor, cognitive, and limbic). These basal ganglia circuits traverse the cortex, striatum, globus pallidus, and thalamus. Each circuit includes a direct and an indirect pathway. Dopaminergic hyperactivity in TS is hypothesized to inhibit the indirect pathway, leading to an overactivity of thalamocortical drive. Other cortical-subcortical loops may also be implicated in TS pathophysiology. The excitatory feedback loop from the thalamus back towards the striatum, which originates from the centromedian-parafascicular complex (CM-Pf), and the midline thalamic nuclei (substantia periventricularis [Spv]) is a circuit that may be affected in TS and explain the action of DBS in this location. CM strongly projects to the sensorimotor region of the putamen, Pf projects to the associative regions of both caudate nucleus and putamen, and Spv projects to limbic related parts of the striatum. Several studies have suggested that both the sensorimotor and the limbic-innervated parts of the basal ganglia, including the dorsal and ventral striatum, are involved in the pathophysiology of TS (23–26). This may also explain both motor and non-motor symptoms. Dopaminergic hyperactivity in TS may dysregulate sensorimotor and limbic circuits within the basal ganglia, leading to thalamic hyperactivity. This thalamic hyperactivity would lead to excessive stimulation of the cortex, and maintain itself through a feedback loop including the striatum, which may be inappropriately modulated by an excess of dopamine.

### Rationale for Targeting the Medial Portion of the Thalamus

In 1970, Hassler and Diekman reported on the beneficial effects of lesioning the intralaminar and midline thalamic nuclei in patients suffering from TS and, in patients with facial tics, also included the Voi nucleus (ventro-oralis internus of the thalamus; ref. 11).

High-frequency stimulation of a nucleus has similar clinical effects on symptoms as an ablative lesion but has the advantages of being programmable and reversible (27). Thus, it was attractive to postulate that DBS of the intralaminar and midline thalamic nuclei and Voi might have a beneficial effect on symptoms in TS. The difficulty in interpretation of the historical data is that Hassler performed up to ten coagulations in each hemisphere. Therefore a strategic "nodal" point had to be found in order that as many of the nuclei targeted by Hassler could be stimulated using a single electrode. This strategic locus was found, using the Schaltenbrand-Wahren atlas (28), on a coronary slice 4 mm posterior to the midpoint of a line connecting the anterior commissure

(AC) with the posterior commissure (PC) and 5 mm lateral to the AC-PC line. In line with the hypotheses discussed earlier, high-frequency stimulation of the thalamus and more specifically of the nuclei projecting to cortex on one side and back to striatum on the other would decrease cortical drive and interrupt the circuit responsible for enhanced thalamic hyperactivity. The Voi projects directly to the premotor cortex. The CM projects back to the dorsal (motor) striatum, and Spv projects back to the ventral (limbic) striatum. Thus, DBS of the medial part of the thalamus was hypothesized to have a good effect on motor and limbic symptoms in patients with intractable TS. This was then confirmed in three patients *(12)*.

## Rationale for Targeting the Globus Pallidus

The GPi is a large nucleus in which the posteriorly located motor portion is relatively far from the anterior limbic portion. "Relatively far" means too far to be reached by a single electrode. In other words, one has to choose whether the motor or limbic part of the GPi will be targeted. This stands in contrast to the thalamus, in which motor and limbic-related nuclei are located close together *(12)*.

### *Posterolateral and Anterior Portions of the GPi*
Prior to the era of subthalamic DBS treatment for PD, DBS of the posteroventrolateral part of the GPi was performed in patients with advanced PD. There were improvements in PD symptoms as well as an anti-dyskinesia effect *(29)*. More recently, GPi DBS has been widely performed in patients suffering from dystonia *(30, 31)*. The good results obtained are not so much a consequence of effects on continuous muscular hypertonia as on the associated hyperkinetic movements. According to this and reasoning that tics may also be regarded as hyperkinesias, clinicians have decided to target the motor (posteroventrolateral) part of the GPi *(18, 19)*. While Van der Linden et al. have targeted the motor part of the GPi *(18)*, other authors have reported good results of DBS in the anterior, limbic-related, part of the GPi *(17)*.

## Rationale for Targeting the Nucleus Accumbens

TS and OCD share many clinical similarities and show strong co-morbidity. A recent study with event-related brain potentials indicated that frontal inhibitory mechanisms may be similarly altered in TS and OCD *(32)*. DBS of the NAC has been performed in patients suffering from OCD *(33)*. In an unpublished study, it was shown that patients suffering from TS, included in a study of NAC DBS in OCD patients, also showed improvement in tics (Sturm, personal communication).

It has been hypothesized that a neuropathological model based on NAC mechanisms may be central to the pathology and physiology of TS. This model assumes that external and internal events occurring during the development of the nervous system induce modular changes in the NAC *(34)*. Considering this, it is possible that the reported mild effects of IC stimulation in a single patient with TS *(20)* might be explained by spread of current to the nearby NAC region, since the electrode in this case was located in the vicinity of the NAC.

## Clinical and Surgical Evaluation

### Patient Selection

As mentioned in the first section, in most cases TS symptoms wane before or at the onset of adolescence. Not all patients require therapy and, of those who do, only a minority fail to respond to medical treatment. TS patients considered for DBS should comprise only very severe cases who have received careful trials of standard therapies without adequate benefit. The Dutch-Flemish Tourette Surgery Study Group has established guidelines for DBS in TS *(35)*, and recently the Movement Disorders Society published a position statement concerning this issue *(36)*. These statements include the following selection criteria.

*Inclusion of Patients*
1. The patient has definite TS, established by two independent clinicians. The diagnosis is established according to DSM-IV-TR criteria *(4)* and with the aid of the Diagnostic Confidence Index (DCI; ref. *37*).
2. The patient has severe and incapacitating tics as his primary problem.
3. The patient is treatment refractory. This means that the patient either has not or very partially responded to three different medication regimes, each for at least 12 weeks, and in adequate doses, or has been proven not to tolerate medications due to side effects. Three different groups of neuroleptics should have been tried:

   i) "Classic" Dopamine-2 antagonists (haloperidol, pimozide or clonidine)
   ii) Modern antipsychotic medications (e.g., risperidone, olanzapine, clozapine, sulpiride, aripiprazole)
   iii) Experimental drugs (e.g., pergolide)

   Finally, a trial of at least 10 sessions of behavioral therapy for tics, such as habit reversal or exposure in vivo, may be attempted.

4. The patient should be over 25 years of age.

*Exclusion of Patients*
Patients should be excluded from neurosurgical treatment if they have a tic disorder other than TS, severe psychiatric co-morbid conditions (other than associated behavioral disorders), or mental deficiency. Contraindications for surgical treatment for DBS in TS are severe cardiovascular, pulmonary or haematological disorders, structural MRI-abnormalities, and active suicidal ideation. Together with the Tourette Syndrome Association, a group of investigators has published guidelines for groups interested in implanting TS, which are slightly different than the Dutch Flemish group *(36)*.

### Surgical Procedure

The technique of DBS applied to TS is similar to that used for more classical indications. Targets for TS such as the nuclei of the medial portion of the thalamus, are not visible with current imaging techniques. Moreover, TS patients may pull themselves out of the stereotactic frame because of frequent motor tics that occur in the head region. One solution is to operate under general anaesthesia *(17, 19)*. Because of the uncertainty of the ideal target and the importance of intra-operative findings, it is preferable if the patient is awake and cooperative during surgery. To avoid general anaesthesia, patients may be sedated with a combination of lormetazepam and clonidine *(12)* or with Propofol Target Controlled Infusion *(18)*, which reduce tics sufficiently to improve safety and efficacy of the stereotactic procedure. With the patient awake the symptoms can be assessed so that acute negative stimulation-induced side effects can be detected and the position of the electrode adjusted as needed.

**Peri-operative Evaluation**

It is of paramount importance that in TS patients treated with DBS the exact location of the electrode and position of the stimulating contact is precisely determined and all effects are meticulously described. A more comprehensive survey of guidelines for the peri-operative assessment of the effects of DBS in TS is available *(36)*.

**Post-operative Evaluation**

For the assessment of clinical effects, a careful and detailed description of the effects of DBS on tics and associated behavioral disorders and stimulation-induced side effects are mandatory. The most commonly used scale for tic rating is the Yale Global Tic Severity Scale (YGTSS; ref. *38*). The Rush Videotape scale is also commonly used. For a more objective evaluation, the patient should also be video-recorded with and without stimulation. The tics should be rated on video by two independent investigators. Ideally, the patient and investigator should be blinded to the status of the stimulation. Careful psychiatric and neuropsychological evaluations should be performed at regular intervals. Clinical effects should be correlated to the exact position of the electrode. The most prudent approach may be to perform a CT scan postoperatively and fuse these images with pre-operative MR images, although many centers successful employ other imaging approaches (Figure 18.2). Only if these prerequisites are fulfilled and a maximum amount of data is exchanged between centers, can the yet to be determined optimal target be established.

**Programming**

According to our experience with DBS in the medial portion of the thalamus, the best effect in the majority of patients is obtained with a frequency between 75 and 100 Hz and a pulse width of 210 μsec. From day 1 postoperatively bipolar stimulation is started (to obtain the most selective effect), with each pole made active during four consecutive days (e.g., day 1: pole 0 −, pole 1 +; day 2: pole 1 −, pole 2 +, etc). During programming, the voltage is progressively increased until unwanted side effects occur. Thereafter, the combination of electrodes may be altered (e.g., two electrodes negative), or monopolar stimulation may be chosen, as suggested by clinical effects. As for other DBS indications, programming is a matter of "trial and error," as directed by the best clinical effects of bipolar stimulation and fewest adverse effects.

## Other Considerations

The motivation to choose a specific target for DBS treatment of TS has so far been based on the effects of the historical ablative surgical literature available for that target or on the effects of DBS in that target on similar symptoms in other disorders. DBS in TS is still investigational and the best target has yet to

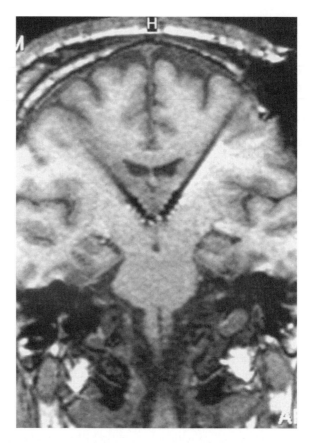

**Figure 18.2** Postoperative MRI-scan (coronary slide) of a patient with TS, after implantation of two electrodes in the medial part of the thalamus

be determined. The effects of stimulation of the currently used targets are not fully appreciated. Surgery with the patient sufficiently awake to be cooperative during test stimulation makes the intra-operative detection of acute stimulation- induced side effects possible, so that the position of the electrode can be changed before its final fixation. However, negative effects may sometimes become prominent later in the course of postoperative follow-up such as, for example, changes in sexual behavior. Patients should be carefully informed about this before surgery. DBS in TS can be a safe procedure if it remains in the hands of experienced neurosurgeons who are working with a multidisciplinary team and approval has bee obtained from an investigational review board. Because so few cases have been published, timely exchange and on-going assessment of clinical experience will be important to guide the field toward safer and more efficacious approaches.

## References

1. Mink JW (2001) Basal ganglia dysfunction in Tourette's syndrome: a new hypothesis. Pediatric Neurology 25:190–198.
2. Robertson MM (2000) Tourette syndrome, associated conditions and the complexities of treatment. Brain 123:425–462.

3. Berardelli A, Curra A, Fabbrini G, Gilio F, Manfredi M (2003) Pathophysiology of tics and Tourette syndrome. J Neurol 250:781–787.
4. American Psychiatric Association (2000) Diagnostic and statistical manual of mental disorders, fourth edition text revision. Washington, DC: American Psychiatric Association.
5. Hoekstra PJ, Anderson GM, Limburg PC, Korf J, Kallenberg CG, Minderaa RB (2004) Neurobiology and neuroimmunology of Tourette's syndrome: an update. Cell Mol Life Sci 61:886–898.
6. Riederer F, Stamenkovic M, Schindler SD, Kasper S (2002) Tourette's syndrome—a review. Nervenarzt 73:805–819.
7. Leckman JF (2002) Tourette's syndrome. Lancet 360:1577–1586.
8. Silay YS, Jankovic J (2005) Emerging drugs in Tourette syndrome. Expert Opin Emerg Drugs 10:365–380.
9. Temel Y, Visser-Vandewalle V (2004) Surgery in Tourette syndrome. Mov Disord 19:3–14.
10. Vandewalle V, van der Linden C, Groenewegen HJ, Caemaert J (1999) Stereotactic treatment of Gilles de la Tourette syndrome by high frequency stimulation of thalamus. Lancet 353:724.
11. Hassler R, Dieckmann G (1970) Traitement stereotaxique des tics et cris inarticulés ou coprolaliques considérés comme phénomène d'obsession motrice au cours de la maladie de Gilles de la Tourette. Rev Neurol Paris 123:89–100.
12. Visser-Vandewalle V, Temel Y, Boon P, Vreeling F, Colle H, Hoogland G, Groenewegen H, van der Linden CH (2003) Chronic bilateral thalamic stimulation: a new therapeutic approach in intractable Tourette syndrome. J Neurosurg 99:1094–1100.
13. Temel Y, van Lankveld JJ, Boon P, Spincemaille GH, van der Linden C, Visser-Vandewalle V (2004) Deep brain stimulation of the thalamus can influence penile erection. Int J Impot Res 16:91–94.
14. Servello D, Sassi M, Geremia L and Porta M (2005) Bilateral thalamic stimulation for intractable Tourette syndrome. Proceedings of the 14th meeting of the WSSFN, Rome, Italy, June 13–17.
15. Servello D, Porta M, Sassi M, Brambilla A, Robertson MM (in press) Deep brain stimulation in 18 patients with severe Gilles de la Tourette Syndrome refractory to treatment; the surgery and stimulation J Neurol Neurosurg Psychiatry
16. Egidi M, Carrabba G, Priori A, Rampini P, Locatelli M, Bossi B, Cogiamanian F, Mrakic-Sposta S, Prada F, Tamma F, Caputo E, Gaini SM (2005) Thalamic DBS in Tourette's syndrome: Case report. Proceedings of the 14th meeting of the WSSFN, Rome, Italy, June 13–17.
17. Houeto JL, Karachi C, Mallet L, Pillon B, Yelnik J, Mesnage V, Welter ML, Navarro S, Pelissolo A, Damier P, Pidoux B, Dormont D, Cornu P, Agid Y (2005) Tourette's syndrome and deep brain stimulation. J Neurol Neurosurg Psychiatry 76:904
18. Van der Linden C, Colle H, Vandewalle V, Alessi G, Rijckaert D, De Waele L (2002) Successful treatment of tics with bilateral internal pallidum (GPi) stimulation in a 27-year-old male patient with Gilles de la Tourette's syndrome. Mov Disord 17;S341.
19. Diederich NJ, Bumb A, Mertens E, Kalteis K, Stamenkovic M, Alesch F (2004) Efficient internal segment pallidal stimulation in Gilles de la Tourette syndrome: A case report. Mov Disord 19:S440.
20. Flaherty AW, Williams ZM, Amimovin R, Kasper E, Rauch SL, Cosgrove SL, Eskander EN (2005) Deep brain stimulation of the internal capsule for the treatment of Tourette syndrome: technical case report. Neurosurgery 57:E403.
21. Singer HS, Szymanski S, Giuliano J, Yokoi F, Dogan AS, Brasic JR, Zhou Y, Grace AA, Wong DF (2002) Elevated intrasynaptic dopamine release in Tourette's syndrome measured by PET. Am J Psychiatry 159:1329–1336.

22. Graybiel AM (2000) The basal ganglia. Curr Biol 10:R509–511.
23. Groenewegen HJ, van den Heuvel OA, Cath DC, Voorn P, Veltman DJ (2003) Does an imbalance between the dorsal and ventral striatopallidal systems play a role in Tourette's syndrome? A neuronal circuit approach. Brain Dev 25:S3–14.
24. Peterson BS, Skudlarski P, Anderson AW, Zhang H, Gatenby JC, Lacadie CM, Leckman JF, Gore JC (1998) A functional magnetic resonance imaging study of tic suppression in Tourette syndrome. Arch Gen Psychiatry 55:326–333.
25. Peterson BS, Thomas P, Kane MJ, Scahill L, Zhang H, Bronen R, King RA, Leckman JF, Staib L (2003) Basal ganglia volumes in patients with Gilles de la Tourette syndrome. Arch Gen Psychiatry 60:415–424.
26. Stern E, Silbersweig DA, Chee KY, Holmes A, Robertson MM, Trimble M, Frith CD, Frackowiak RS, Dolan RJ (2000) A functional neuroanatomy of tics in Tourette syndrome. Arch Gen Psychiatry 57:741–748.
27. Lozano AM, Mahant N (2004) Deep brain stimulation surgery for Parkinson's disease: mechanisms and consequences. Parkinsonism Relat Disord 10:S49–S57.
28. Schaltenbrand G, Wahren W (1977) Atlas for Stereotaxy of the Human Brain, second edition. Stuttgart, Thieme.
29. Follett KA (2004) Comparison of pallidal and subthalamic deep brain stimulation for the treatment of levodopa-induced dyskinesias. Neurosurg Focus 17:E3.
30. Krause M, Fogel W, Kloss M, Rasche D, Volkmann J, Tronnier V (2004) Pallidal stimulation for dystonia. Neurosurgery 55:1361–1368; discussion 1368–1370.
31. Vidailhet M, Vercueil L, Houeto JL, Krystkowiak P, Benabid AL, Cornu P, Lagrange C, Tezenas du Montcel S, Dormont D, Grand S, Blond S, Detante O, Pillon B, Ardouin C, Agid Y, Destee A, Pollak P; French Stimulation du Pallidum Interne dans la Dystonie (SPIDY) Study Group (2005) Bilateral deep-brain stimulation of the globus pallidus in primary generalized dystonia. N Engl J Med 352:459–467.
32. Johannes S, Wieringa BM, Nager W, Rada D, Muller-Vahl KR, Emrich HM, Dengler R, Munte TF, Dietrich D (2003) Tourette syndrome and obsessive-compulsive disorder: event-related brain potentials show similar mechanisms [correction of mechanisms] of frontal inhibition but dissimilar target evaluation processes. Behav Neurol 14:9–17.
33. Sturm V, Lenartz D, Koulousakis A, Treuer H, Herholz K, Klein JC, Klosterkotter J (2003) The nucleus accumbens: a target for deep brain stimulation in obsessive-compulsive- and anxiety-disorders J Chem Neuroanat 26:293–299.
34. Brito GN (1997) A neurobiological model for Tourette syndrome centered on the nucleus accumbens. Med Hypotheses 49:133–142.
35. Visser-Vandewalle V, Van der Linden Ch, Ackermans L, Temel Y, Tijssen MA, Schruers K, Nederveen P, Kleijers M, Boon P (2006) Deep brain stimulation in Gilles de la Tourette's syndrome. Guidelines of the Dutch-Flemish Tourette Surgery Study Group. Neurosurgery 58:E590.
36. Mink JW, Walkup J, Frey KA, Como P, Cath D, DeLong MR, Erenberg G, Juncos J, Leckman JF, Swerdlow N, Visser-Vandewalle V, Vitek JL for the Tourette Syndrome Association, Inc (2006) Recommended Guidelines for Deep Brain Stimulation in Tourette Syndrome. Mov Disord 21(11):1831–1838.
37. Robertson MM, Banerjee S, Kurlan R, Cohen DJ, Leckma JF, McMahon W, Pauls DL, Sandor P, van de Wetering BJ (1999) The Tourette syndrome diagnostic confidence index: development and clinical associations. Neurology 53:2108–2112.
38. Leckman JF, Riddle MA, Hardin MT, Ort SI, Swartz KL, Stevenson J, Cohen DJ (1989) The Yale Global Tic Severity Scale: initial testing of a clinician-rated scale of tic severity. J Am Acad Child Adolesc Psychiatry 28:566–573.

# 19

# The Role of Deep Brain Stimulation (DBS) in the Treatment of Postural Instability and Gait Disorders of Parkinson's Disease

Helen Bronte-Stewart

## Abstract

Postural instability and gait disorders are movement abnormalities commonly associated with advanced Parkinson's disease (PD) that lead to loss of independence. Although the available literature varies in methodology and design, there appears to be consensus among many studies concerning the effect of subthalamic nucleus (STN) or globus pallidus internus (GPi) deep brain stimulation (DBS) on postural stability and gait disorders in PD. In the short term, DBS improves all postural and gait subscores of the UPDRS including freezing in the off-medication state.

Quantitative studies have revealed considerable detail concerning the effect of DBS on postural instability and gait disorders. This is especially the case in the area of postural stability, where medication and DBS both reduce postural tremor as well as the resonant behavior seen in postural sway in quiet stance. However, in both quiet stance and on unstable surfaces medication worsens, whereas STN DBS improves postural sway velocity and the area over which the body sways. Concerning voluntary postural movement, medication and DBS both improve postural bradykinesia, although this has only been only significant for DBS and DBS plus medication. Neither DBS nor medication improve righting responses to external perturbations. From the available data, this may be due to a lack of improvement in postural reaction times and automatic postural reflexes.

By contrast, medication and DBS appear to have similar effects on most aspects of gait. Gait initiation and gait velocity improve on DBS while off medication, mostly due to improvement in stride length. The irregularity in gait parameters and time spent in double stance also improve. Very few studies have examined the effect of DBS on freezing of gait (FOG) but there is consensus that both STN and GPi DBS improve FOG in the off-medication but not the on-medication state. Studies of long-term STN DBS in PD support continued benefit for retropulsion and gait in the off-medication state after 4 to 5 years. In the on medication state, there was worsening of axial scores and

FOG after 5 years. Preliminary experience with pedunculopontine nucleus (PPN) DBS indicates a significant short-term benefit of PPN DBS alone on posture and gait scores compared to pre-operative on-medication scores.

This is an exciting time for research and development of new therapies in gait and balance disorders. These previously incapacitating disorders may eventually be treatable in PD and in other forms of parkinsonism, in which gait and postural instability are especially prominent features.

**Keywords:** postural control, postural instability, gait, Parkinson's disease, deep brain stimulation, freezing of gait

## Introduction

This chapter aims to summarize the current literature concerning the effect of DBS on postural instability and gait disorders in PD. Studies of the effect of DBS on postural control and gait disorders in PD are variable in many respects: the number of subjects studied, whether control subjects were included, and whether outcomes were compared to pre-operative off or on medication baselines or to post-operative off medication/OFF DBS baselines. In the latter set of studies the duration for OFF DBS has varied greatly. Measures of postural control and gait varied from purely qualitative assessments to clinical rating scales to quantitative measures such as 3-D motion analysis and posturography. The chapter follows the process of standing and walking of a human subject.

Many of the studies to be reviewed use similar technology that may be unfamiliar to the reader. Section 19.3 is a methods section covering most of the assessment and measurement technology used in studies of the effect of DBS on gait and postural control in PD. As postural stability is the foundation for a biped such as a human to maintain a vertical structure (the body) over a base of support, Section 19.4 covers postural instability, followed by sections on changing posture, gait initiation, walking, FOG, and long-term outcomes of STN and GPi DBS. Section 19.5 covers the data known to date concerning the effect of PPN DBS on gait and postural control in PD.

## Methods: Clinical Assessments and Quantitative Measures

Postural control is a complex task and a single measurement cannot describe the many facets of postural control. Functional measures employed in rehabilitative settings, such as functional reach and external perturbation tasks serve an important purpose but are less suited to numerical outcome data *(1)*. A wide variety of clinical and quantitative measures of postural control have been used in the literature concerning the role of DBS in postural stability. These are summarized in the following section.

### Clinical Assessments

Clinical balance scales used in the studies reported in this section include the Tinnetti mobility scale which assesses posture and postural sway in everyday actions such as sitting, standing, arising, turning, and being "nudged" while standing. It also assesses gait initiation and maintenance. The examiner has two or three integers to choose from, the lower the score the more the subject is unstable and likely to fall (maximum of 16 on the balance section and 12 on the gait section; a combined score of <19 indicates a high risk of falling; ref. *2*). The activities-specific balance confidence (ABC) scale is a questionnaire that asks the subject to rate their level of confidence carrying out various everyday activities such as bending to pick up an object, walking on various surfaces, reaching and standing on their toes, etc. (0–100% for each item; ref. *3*). The ABC scale has been reliable and valid when compared to the Falls Efficacy Scale and more suitable for high-functioning seniors. Clinical assessments of postural control in PD are also derived from items in standardized clinical rating scales such as the Unified Parkinson's Disease Rating Scale (UPDRS; ref. *4*). The UPDRS is a comprehensive clinical rating scale encompassing cognition, mood, activities of daily living, motor function, and complications of therapy. It allows the choice of an integer between 0 and 4 for each item; the higher the score, the worse the function. Some studies have used the commonly accepted subscore postural instability and gait disorder (PIGD) of the UPDRS activities of daily living (part II) and motor disability (part III) scales. This approach comprises historical questions relating to falling, walking, freezing, and objective ratings of the patient's ability to change posture, walk, and maintain equilibrium during a retropulsive or propulsive pull *(5)*. The tests that comprise the PIGD score are performed under normal sensory conditions and therefore may weight more heavily the motor adjustment component of postural control. This score also includes and may over-weight gait assessment. Other studies have used different items of the PIGD subscore.

Clinical assessment of the act of walking using the UPDRS combines the patient's assessment of walking speed, their degree of freezing, and the frequency of falls with an examiner's assessment of their walking. An additional timed walking test is sometimes employed in which the time is measured for the patient to get up from a chair, walk a certain distance, and then sit again.

**Quantitative Measures of Postural Control**

*Posturography*
Posturography is the study of postural movement while standing and is calculated from the forces exerted through the feet. Subjects stand in prescribed places on non-movable (static) or movable (dynamic) single or dual force plates. Their feet are carefully aligned over defined axes on the force plates, which are referenced to load cells or force transducers mounted underneath. Some force plates only measure vertical forces imposed by the upright subject (Smartequitest, Neurocom Int, Clackamas Oregon), whereas others have additional force transducers and can also measure shear forces (medial/lateral [ML] direction, anterior/posterior forces [AP direction]), and 3-D moment measurements about the center of the platform (Kistler platform, Winterthur, Switzerland). A variable that is widely used to measure postural instability is the center of pressure (CoP; refs. *6–8*). As the subject stands on the platform, the forces are not distributed equally about the sole of the foot. Some parts of the sole will have more force due to the activity and/or the anatomy of the foot. When all the forces over every part of the sole are averaged together, the resultant force can be represented by a single vector acting through one point

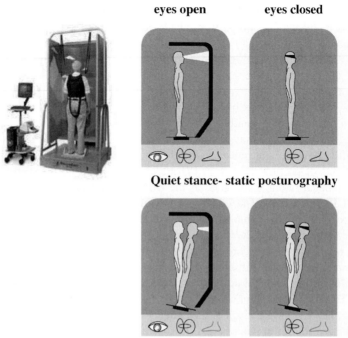

**Figure 19.1** Computerized dynamic posturography. The Smart Equitest, Neurocom Int Clackamas Oregon and the outline of the subject orientation for static and dynamic posturography

on the planar surface of the force platform under the person's foot. This point is called the CoP. If the position of the patient's foot on the platform is known, the CoP can then be translated from the platform's coordinate system to the patient's anatomical coordinate system. A correlation between the CoP and the body's center of mass (CoM) has been established which consequently provides a mechanism to track the body's CoM in reference to its base of support, the feet *(9)*. If the height and the weight of the patient are also used, then the CoM or center of gravity (CoG) angle can be calculated. The change in the CoG angle is measured in real time and is called CoG sway (angular velocity).

Several studies have used static posturography to measure the effect of DBS on certain aspects of postural control in PD. In these studies the subjects stand on a still platform with eyes open or closed (Figure 19.1). Extracted measures include the mean CoP position, the CoP displacement from the mean, the CoP sway or velocity in AP and ML directions, the area subtended by the spontaneous sway, and the frequency, below which occurs 95% of the power of CoP sway *(10–14)*.

*Voluntary Postural Movement*
Measures of the subject's voluntary movement can be made if there is also a visual representation of their CoG or CoM as an icon on a screen they are viewing. When prompted by a target they are instructed to move from the ankles such that they move the icon towards the target as fast as possible. Their

postural reaction time, movement velocity, ability to lean away from their base of support, and trajectory can be measured from the sway path of the CoP or CoM (CoG; ref. *15*). The platform remains stationary.

### *Dynamic Posturography*
The addition of dynamic posturography expands the repertoire of measures of postural control. Moveable force plates can be programmed to deliver unexpected but reproducible perturbations to the subject such as ramps (toes up or down), translations (forward or backward), and/or sinusoidal oscillations. These tests measure the subject's ability to react to external perturbations such as one might encounter on an irregular or moving surface and/or to being pushed. The force plates can also be programmed to move in direct relation to the subject's spontaneous sway but in an incongruent direction (sway referenced conditions). For instance, if the subject sways forward the force plates move downwards with the same velocity and amplitude. This effectively minimizes proprioceptive feedback from the feet, as there is very little or no rotation about the ankle joint (Figure 19.1). The sway-referenced movement can be tested with eyes open and eyes closed. This type of dynamic posturography has been used to examine the sensory organisational process in PD *(6, 14–19)*. It mimics real life conditions such as getting out of bed or a chair in dim light and standing on thick carpeting or sand.

### *Kinematics-3-D Motion Analysis*
Quantitative measures of the process of walking include gait velocity (speed of walking a certain distance), cadence (number of steps per second), stride length (distance between successive (same) heel strikes or the length of two consecutive steps), leg swing velocity and duration, the percent of stride time spent with both feet on the ground (double stance duration), and/or the percent of time that the leg is in the swing phase. Temporal aspects such as the regularity of the gait velocity, stride length, and cadence may be measured, along with measures of the symmetry of spatiotemporal gait parameters between legs.

Technology employed to obtain these measures includes shoes with pressure sensors in the soles and a microcomputer backpack (Ultraflex system, Infrotonic, Tubbergen, The Netherlands, or B and L engineering, Santa Fe Springs, CA). Another common method for measuring postural control and quantitative gait analysis is 3-D motion analysis: the use of a 3-D infra-red movement analysis system in which infra-red cameras monitor the movement of markers attached to specific parts of the feet, legs, pelvis, and trunk while the patient walks (ELITE system, BTS, Garbanate Italy, 3-D Motion Analysis). This can be done across a floor or on a treadmill. This also allows measurement of the range of amplitude of the hip, knee, and ankle joint angles, all joint moments and powers, pelvic orientation, trunk lateral flexion, and trunk torsion with respect to the pelvis. Other studies have used optoelectronic (Optotrak, Waterloo Canada) or angular velocity transducers (Swaystar system, Balance International Innovations, GmbH, Switzerland). Ground reaction force information may be gathered by the use of static forceplates, over which the patient walks. Three-D motion analysis systems have also been used to measure trunk and limb kinematics during spontaneous or perturbed postural sway on force plates, although these are more commonly used for gait studies.

# The Effect of DBS on Postural Instability

Balance or postural stability results from the interaction of many physiological systems with a goal to maintain the body's CoM within the boundaries of the body's base of support while seated, standing, walking, or changing posture *(20)*. Postural stability is required to keep the body oriented appropriately while performing voluntary movements, during external perturbations, and when the support surface or environment changes.

Components of the system include posture itself (the orientation of the head and neck on the trunk, the trunk on the pelvis, and the pelvis on the legs), the orientation senses (proprioception, vision, and vestibular sensation), the tone of the postural musculature, and the central nervous system (CNS). The role of the CNS is to integrate incoming sensory information and execute coordinated and properly scaled motor commands such that the trunk and pelvis can respond to changes in the base of support and/or environment with sufficient speed and accuracy. It has been proposed that the orientation senses listed preivously are integrated within the CNS based on an adaptive hierarchal system called the sensory organizational process *(21)*. This system functions on two levels *(22)*. The first level is considered to be the bottom up approach (lower level), where inputs from the orientation senses are weighted and directly affect the activity of the postural muscles. In the second level, the top-down organization, higher level, vestibular inputs provide the orientation reference, against which conflicts in support surface and visual orientation are identified and the combination of inputs are adapted to the task conditions. For postural stability, information from the lower level must be coherent with the inertial-gravitational reference of the higher level and any conflicting orientation inputs must be quickly suppressed in favor of those congruent with the internal reference. Thus, the sensory organizational process is context specific due to the rapid weighting and re-weighting of sensory inputs to/from the lower level by the higher level adaptive process *(21, 23)*.

**Postural Instability in PD**

Postural instability is one of the cardinal motor manifestations of PD and usually occurs in the middle to late stages of the disease *(24)*. It is usually reported in the context of falling or of fear of falling rather than in the context of ataxia. Imbalance or postural instability in PD is noted during walking or upon arising from a seated or lying position and even while standing still. The cardinal motor manifestations of PD such as akinesia, bradykinesia, and rigidity may contribute to postural instability due to an inability to adjust the CoG quickly enough to account for perturbations in the environment. Patients with PD report increased imbalance in conditions where there is limited sensory feedback such as in a dimly lit room or on an uneven surface.

**Measures of Postural Instability in PD**

*Clinical Assessment*

The main determination of postural instability contained in the UPDRS is when the patient takes several steps backward after a retropulsive pull about the shoulders and/or when they report falling. Thus the clinical assessment of postural instability is determined from a perturbation of the CoM off the base of support. Bloem et al. compared the retropulsion test to a quantitative external perturbation of rapid toe up tilt and found moderate correlation in the off medication state and no correlation in the on medication state. They suggested that by itself the retropulsion test does not measure postural instability in PD *(25)*. The PIGD score combines gait and postural scores and is abnormal in almost all patients with moderate to advanced PD *(5, 6, 15, 26, 27)*. The Tinetti mobility and ABC scales were also abnormal in PD *(28)*.

*Posturography and 3-D Motion Analysis*
Findings from studies using computerized posturography and 3-D motion analysis have greatly expanded our understanding of postural instability in PD.

*Quiet Stance:* Using static posturography and 3-D motion analysis several studies have shown that there are increased CoP excursions from the mean position in PD patients off therapy compared to controls during quiet stance. The increased excursions are only of the order of 3 mm in the AP and ML directions. However, the movement had a higher mean velocity *(10, 12)*. The CoP velocity power spectral density plots contained higher frequencies than controls with peaks in the 0.7 to 1.1 Hz and 5 Hz, even when patients with known tremor were excluded. The mean CoP position was displaced posteriorly *(14)* and the area subtended by CoP movement tended to increase in the AP direction *(10)*. Maurer et al. also showed increased upper and lower body coupling, which they interpreted to reflect increased axial stiffness *(12)*.

*Altered Sensory Feedback*: Studies using dynamic posturography where proprioceptive feedback is minimized or altered with or without visual feedback have shown that patients with PD sway more in the AP and ML directions in sway referenced conditions eyes open or closed *(6, 13–15, 28, 29)*. These results support the patients' reports that they are more unstable in conditions of limited proprioceptive and visual feedback.

*External Perturbations*: Maurer et al. showed that there was an abnormally large excursion of the upper body during a platform tilt that went with the platform direction and did not correct back to a normal position *(12)*. Impaired righting responses to more rapid external translational or tilt perturbations have been reported in PD in several studies *(12, 13, 30, 31)* and appear to be partly related to an abnormally enhanced destabilizing medium latency long loop reflex along with a posteriorly displaced CoP and delayed corrective action of the long latency long loop reflexes. Recently it has been shown that postural reaction times are prolonged and postural movement velocity is reduced in PD patients, which also contributes to difficulty responding appropriately to external perturbations *(15)*.

**The Effect of Medication on Postural Stability in PD**

*Clinical Assessment*
Most studies have shown that medication improves the PIGD score and other combinations of axial scores from the UPDRS, although many of these reflect the performance of gait more than postural instability *(5, 6, 30, 32–34)*.

### Quiet Stance

Dopaminergic medication has been shown to decrease the mean CoP velocity and the high frequencies in the CoP velocity power spectrum towards control values. However, medication increased the CoP excursions and the sway area and shifts its axis to the ML direction *(10–12, 14)*. Thus medication tends to increase the amplitude and area of spontaneous CoP movement but at lower frequencies compared to controls and to PD patients off therapy. The amplitude of upper and lower body sway increased but the tight coupling of upper and lower body movements (axial stiffness) was reduced. Thus in quiet stance medication lowers the axial stiffness but promotes larger sway amplitudes especially in the ML direction.

### Altered Sensory Feedback

On medication, patients with PD have increased CoP excursion and ML sway area along with increased sway velocities on an unstable surfaces, especially when proprioception and vision are minimized *(6, 14)*. Thus, while on medication, patients with PD appear to have even more difficulty maintaining an upright stance when they do not have adequate environmental sensory feedback.

### External Perturbations

Different studies have shown that the righting response to external perturbations is not improved with medication, partly due to the abnormal upper body excursion and partly due to only partial correction of the early (medium latency) and no improvement of the stabilizing (long latency) automatic reflexes *(30, 31)*. The abnormal CoP displacement and excursions also were not corrected on medication *(10–12, 14)*. Although voluntary postural movement velocities tended to increase on medication, this was not significant when corrected for multiple comparisons. Additionally, the delayed postural reaction times did not improve on medication *(15)*.

## Effect of DBS on Postural Instability in PD

### Clinical Assessments

Studies using the PIGD subscore or axial components of the UPDRS have shown improvements ranging from 40 to 60% from DBS compared to preoperative off medication scores *(14, 15, 32–34)*. Many of these included gait outcomes as well as postural scores and some studies did not observe improvement in the retropulsion score of UPDRS, part III by STN DBS or medication *(25, 28, 35)*. A recent randomized controlled study of STN DBS in PD revealed that patients reported better mobility on DBS than on medication *(36)*. Thus, although there is some consistency in these outcomes and patients may report better mobility and balance after DBS, there is very little information about changes in the various components of postural control either in quiet stance, or during different environmental sensory conditions. The components that contribute to the ability to recover from a perturbation such as retropulsion, such as postural reaction time and postural bradykinesia are not assessed clinically. Thus, using only clinical assessments of postural stability leaves many questions unanswered concerning the role of DBS in the treatment of postural instability in PD.

## Quantitative Measures

The studies using quantitative measures to examine the effect of DBS on postural control are summarized in Table 19.1.

To be noted are the different durations after surgery at the time of testing, and the fact that most studies used as their baseline the off medication/OFF DBS state, and most had only turned off the stimulators for 20 to 30 minutes. One study showed that UPDRS assessed axial scores may take at least 3 to 4 hours to reach baseline after DBS has been turned OFF *(37)*. Thus studies using the post-operative off/OFF state as a baseline may have underestimated the improvement from DBS compared to pre-operative values.

## Quiet Stance

During quiet stance, the effect of GPi and STN DBS was a reduction in abnormally large CoP sway velocity and high frequency oscillations *(10–12, 14)*. The sway area decreased to approximately or slightly less than control values, which was a marked difference from the effect of medication, which increased sway area especially in the ML direction. The tight coupling between the upper and lower body measures improved with DBS toward control values.

## Altered Sensory Feedback

Under dynamic conditions and compared to pre-operative off medication values, Shivitz et al. *(14)* and Guehl et al. *(15)* showed that STN DBS improved the increased sway, which occurred in sensory-deprived conditions and when the support was unstable. Of note, several studies have shown that medications increased sway under these conditions. Colnat-Coubois *(13)* and Shivitz *(15)* showed that the combination of DBS plus medication improved the abnormal sway seen on best medical therapy pre-operatively. Thus STN DBS alone and DBS plus medication improve the postural instability in sensory altered states seen either off or on medication pre-operatively. Vrancken et al. *(28)* used reflective markers on the trunk and measured trunk sway post-operatively (time post DBS not given) on medication, when patients were standing on an unstable surface. They compared their performance ON versus OFF DBS (OFF for 30 minutes) and showed that DBS reduced the 5 Hz oscillations (postural tremor) seen in the AP (pitch) and ML (roll) trunk sway.

## External Perturbations

Few studies have examined the effect of DBS on the righting response to external perturbations. Maurer et al. *(12)* did not report any improvement from STN DBS in the abnormal upper body excursion during an external perturbation of platform tilt even though it corrected back to normal position after the tilt, which was not seen off therapy and on medication/ON DBS. Several studies showed no improvement after a retropulsive pull from clinical assessments (see previous section). Colnat-Coubois et al. *(13)* showed no change in automatic reflexes on DBS and medication compared to on medication pre-operatively when subjects were subjected to a sudden toe-up rapid ramp of the platform. However, there appeared to be less postural sway postoperatively during rapid unexpected ramp perturbations. Shivitz et al. *(15)* showed that STN DBS failed to improve postural reaction times during a voluntary postural movement task. However, STN DBS improved postural voluntary movement velocity, the effect being significant compared to pre-operative values for STN DBS alone and STN DBS plus medication.

Table 19.1 Studies specifically examining the effect of DBS on postural instability in PD.

| Author/year | No. of subjects/site of DBS | Mean age (years) | No. of control subjects | Type of measurement* | Comparison-medication/DBS | Duration OFF DBS |
|---|---|---|---|---|---|---|
| Rocchi/2002 | 6/3 STN, 3 GPi | 61 | 10 | Static posturography | No pre-op 6 months post-op off/OFF, off/ON, on/OFF, off/OFF | 20 minutes |
| Maurer/2003 | 8/STN (young onset) | 48.1 | 10 | Static and dynamic posturography | No pre-op 15.4 (± 10.6) months post-op off/OFF, off/ON, on/OFF, off/OFF | 30 minutes |
| Rocchi/2004 | 9/5 STN, 4 GPi (6 same as 2002) | 60.5 | 10 | Static posturography | No pre-op 6 months post-op off/OFF, off/ON, on/OFF, off/OFF | "Approximately 30 minutes" |
| Vrancken/2005 | 14/STN (11 young onset) | 50 | 20 | Trunk angular velocity sensors Tinetti Mobility index, ABC scale | No pre-op Post-op (time not given) on/OFF, on/ON | 2 hours |
| Colnat-Coubois/2005 | 12/STN | 58.5 | None | Static and dynamic posturography | Pre-op on 6 months post-op on/ON | N/A |
| Guehl/2006 | 7/STN | 57.3 | None | Static and dynamic posturography UPDRS | Pre-op off (meds×12 hours), on 3 months post-op off/OFF, off/ON, on/OFF, off/OFF | 30 minutes |
| Shivitz/2006 | 28/STN | 58.4 | 123 (Smart Equitest manual) | Static and dynamic posturography UPDRS | Pre-op off (meds×12 hours), on 6 months post-op off/OFF, off/ON, on/OFF, off/OFF | 17–23 hours |

*All studies except Colnat-Coubois et al. reported UPDRS scores in general; papers that reported the UPDRS III gait and posture subscores separately are listed in measurement column.

## Does DBS Exert Long-Term or Adaptive Changes on Postural Instability in PD?

Very few studies have examined whether DBS exerts a long-term effect on postural systems; i.e., do the improvements persist after DBS is turned OFF. Temperli et al. *(37)* studied the return of motor signs using the UPDRS immediately and up to 4 hours after the stimulators were turned off. Patients ($N = 30$) were studied off medication and after a mean duration of 6.7 months of DBS. The axial subscore using items from the UPDRS, part III (arising from a chair, posture, gait, and response to a retropulsive pull) took 3 to 4 hours to return to the pre-operative off medication value. Of note, this score included gait assessment and the only objective assessment of postural stability was an external perturbation. Much of the work was not directly related to postural stability in the standing position. Shivitz et al. *(15)* studied 21 patients with static and dynamic posturography, 17 to 23 hours OFF DBS (off medication for 36–48 hours, 6–12 months post DBS onset) and showed that the improvements in postural sway in sensory deprived conditions (seen ON DBS compared to pre-op off or to on medication values) persisted. However, the improvement in postural bradykinesia did not persist and the postural movement velocity and reaction time off all therapy were not different from pre-operative off medication values. Thus there appears to be long-term changes in the sensory aspects of postural control, but not in postural bradykinesia or delayed reaction time.

## Underlying Pathophysiology of Postural Instability in PD and Theories for the Effect of DBS

One explanation proposed for the faster postural sway at higher frequencies measured in PD patients during quiet stance while off therapy was that the body axis in PD behaves like a passive system with high stiffness. Such a system would tend to sway faster at higher frequencies. Although DBS improves rigidity including axial stiffness, which would support this hypothesis, this system should also show reduced sway amplitude. This would tend to move the lower body together with the platform with external tilting, and thus produce large lower body excursions rather than the smaller lower body excursions reported by Maurer et al. *(10–12)*. Another concept based on control theory assumes that rigidity is centrally produced and proposes that adding a delay and changing the relative gains of the viscous versus elastic components of the system would produce resonance at higher frequencies and increased sway velocities *(12, 38, 39)*. Maurer et al. proposed that the abnormalities of spontaneous sway in quiet stance in PD may reflect a resonance behavior in the sensorimotor control loop for postural control. DBS appears to reduce this resonance behavior and eliminates the approximately 5 Hz postural tremor seen in quiet stance and on unstable surfaces *(39)*.

Alternatively, Rocchi et al. suggested that the increased spontaneous sway velocity was due to a deficit in the use of sensory information by the CNS in PD, which may lead to poor fine-tuning of movement *(10)*. Studies using dynamic posturography have also suggested that in PD there is a deficit in the ability of the CNS to maintain postural stability in the absence of coincident, congruent proprioceptive and visual feedback and/or when the surface is unstable *(6, 14, 15, 29)*. STN DBS appeared to restore this function to within normal range, consistent with the theory that STN DBS restores the passage of sensorimotor information through basal ganglia circuitry by reducing the electrical "noise" *(15, 40)*.

In contrast, medication can make sensory aspects of postural control worse as well as increasing spontaneous ML sway and sway velocity *(6, 10–15)*. Most studies have hypothesized that the increased sway with dopaminergic replacement therapy is due to reduced stiffness of the system without improvement in the patient's use of sensory or internally generated signals for postural control. Thus medication can result in reduced postural control, especially in the ML direction, in addition to a loss of stability caused by medication-induced involuntary movements (dyskinesia). In the few studies examining the effect of DBS on external perturbations there are mixed results. This area needs further research with particular attention to dynamic posturography. One of the reasons that medication and possibly DBS as well may not fully correct the righting response to external perturbations is that the delayed postural reaction time is not sensitive to either. This, along with a posterior displacement of the mean CoP that is only partially corrected with DBS, would contribute to difficulty reacting quickly enough with a large enough corrective move to counteract a retropulsive pull and/or platform tilt.

**Summary of the Effects of DBS on Postural Instability in PD**

In summary, DBS improves (reduces) postural sway in quiet stance and in conditions of limited sensory feedback where medication may make postural sway worse. DBS reduces the high-frequency resonant behavior and postural tremor seen in postural movement during quiet stance, which may contribute to similar improvements in dynamic conditions such as unstable surfaces or external perturbations. DBS does not improve postural reaction time but does improve postural bradykinesia. From the limited available data DBS does not appear to correct the abnormalities seen in automatic posture stabilizing reflexes nor on the trunk's righting response to external perturbations.

There is, therefore, enough evidence for neurologists to recommend STN DBS for certain aspects of postural instability. In contrast to some assertions in the literature, it may be precisely those patients who are more unstable on medication who can derive the most benefit from STN DBS with regard to certain aspects of postural control. Importantly, it is not possible to predict this using only the UPDRS for assessment.

## The Effect of DBS on the Gait Disorder of PD

Walking is a learned motor program that usually progresses from crawling, to attempts to stand unassisted, to unassisted walking that is wide based with side to side as well as AP sway. Normally, the act of walking progresses to become a fluid repetitive process that starts with a change of posture (most commonly sitting to standing) and is followed by initiation of gait and alternating leg swing, heel strike, foot stance, and toe-off movements all executed with little side-to-side sway.

## The Act of Sit-to-Stand

Difficulty in arising from a seated position is often one of the early signs of PD. This will be mentioned only briefly as there are no studies specifically examining the effect of DBS on the sit-to-stand task. The task involves anticipatory postural control that programs postural adjustments to move the CoM over the base of support before and as the body rises *(43)*. For instance, when standing up from a seated position the CoM has to move forward with enough horizontal velocity such that the CoM comes within the new base of support as the legs straighten. Studies have shown that patients with PD perform the sit-to-stand act more slowly than controls and have reduced horizontal velocity, peak hip flexion, and torques of ankle dorsiflexion. It is hypothesized that a major deficit for PD patients, which underlies the reduced kinematics, is the loss of ability to switch directions from hip flexion to hip extension *(44)*. Patients tend to exaggerate the hip flexion strategy possibly to compensate for an inability to generate adequate lower limb strength, and also because this reduces balance demands. The reduction in balance demands is accomplished by increasing the time that the CoM stays within the base of support as the upper body is over the feet *(41, 43, 44)*.

## Gait Initiation

Gait initiation is defined as the act that takes the body from a motionless standing position to the completion of the first stride. In normal subjects and normal situations there is a very stereotypical preparation to initiate a step called the anticipatory postural adjustment (APA). This consists of a shift of body weight to the swing leg with a simultaneous decrease of weight on the standing leg. The weight then shifts to the standing leg with a shift backward and then forward to create forward momentum. The time at which the vertical force simultaneously increases in the swing leg and decreases in the standing leg is defined as the onset of the APA. The amplitude of the APA is the peak vertical force exerted on the swing leg, which is needed to generate a propulsive force on the swing foot before the foot lifts off the ground *(45)*. The AP ground shear force has been shown to be the most accurate index of the horizontal propulsive force that helps to initiate the first step. The amplitude of the APA (a vertical force) is strongly correlated with the anterior horizontal force in the swing foot, which represents the friction force between the foot and the floor *(45, 46)*. The movement execution (ME) phase is defined as the time between movement onset (swing foot lifts off the ground) and the end of the first stride.

### *Gait Initiation in PD*

Patients with PD show a significantly longer APA period, although the ME period appears to be normal *(47)*. The APA is abnormal in PD with reduced lateral shift forces and reduced APA amplitude and forward propulsive forces and a delay in the foot-lifting phase *(49)*.

### *Measures of Gait Initiation*

Measurements of gait initiation include displacement of the CoP and/or CoM, ground reactive forces, 3-D motion analysis, electromyographic data, and the duration of the APA and ME phases.

### The Effect of DBS on Gait Initiation

Very few studies have examined the effect of DBS on gait initiation and none have used pre-operative data as a baseline. Three studies have studied the effect of DBS, using the off medication/OFF DBS state as the baseline (Table 19.2).

Robertson et al. *(46)* and Liu et al. *(48)* showed that DBS resulted in an improvement in the amplitude of the APA and the latency to foot lift off of the swing foot. The increase in the amplitude of the APA corresponds to an improved forward propulsion force for gait initiation. The lateral displacement of the CoP was also increased (improved). The overall result was an improvement in gait initiation time. Crenna et al. *(49)* studied the effect of STN DBS on gait initiation in 10 patients using a single force plate. They studied the displacement of the CoP as a measure of APA, body kinematics, and EMG data. Compared to the off medication, OFF DBS state there was improvement in standing posture prior to gait initiation, a larger lateral and backward displacement of the CoP (corresponding to improved lateral postural control and forward propulsive force), and an increased length of the first step.

## Walking

Walking is defined as rhythmical alternating stepping for the maintenance of gait. For forward walking, one foot strikes the ground with the heel and begins the stance phase as the other is pushing off the hallux and beginning the swing phase. The CoM must stay over the base of support and thus move forward without more lateral sway than the width of the stride (how far apart the feet are). Thus for fluid walking a certain amount of CoM AP and ML sway over the base of support is needed. For normal subjects walking is described as an automatic motor act, even though all the systems involved in postural control are constantly adapting to the act of walking up or downhill, on rough terrain or moving surfaces, climbing over obstacles, going up and down stairs, and moving through restricted spaces such as doorways.

### Gait Disorder in PD

Walking is impaired in PD and is one of the cardinal motor abnormalities. Early in the disease process, patients may perceive this problem as a dragging of one leg and/or an overall slowing of walking velocity. As the disease progresses the patient and/or family members may notice that they walk slowly, steps are shorter, that their posture is stooped, and that they don't allow the trunk to sway much when walking. This creates the appearance of a shuffle. This same tendency causes the patient to turn with minimal truncal sway. The body appears to turn in one unit ("tourne en bloc") often through a pivoting action around one leg or with many, very short rotational movements of the feet. The knees and pelvis are flexed, the upper thorax is pitched forward, and the arms are flexed at the elbows beside or in front of the torso. The act of walking may be interrupted suddenly and/or when going through barriers such as doors, which leads to rapid short forward steps (festination), stepping in place, and even a complete halt to the walking process (freezing). As the disease progresses, postural instability, akinesia, bradykinesia, freezing, and slower reaction times limit the act of walking until independent walking is impossible without falling and the patient becomes wheelchair bound.

Table 19.2 Studies specifically examining the effect of DBS on gait initiation in PD.

| Author/year | No. of subjects/ site of DBS | Mean age (years) | No. of control subjects | Type of measurement* | Comparison- medication/DBS | Duration OFF DBS |
|---|---|---|---|---|---|---|
| Robertson LT/2001 | 6/3 STN, 3 GPi | 51.5 | 10 | Static posturography UPDRS | No pre-op 6 months post-op off/OFF, off/ON, off/OFF | 30 minutes |
| Liu/2006 | 11/STN | 53.7 | None | Static posturography | No pre-op 16.2 (6–32) months post-op off/OFF, off/ON, on/OFF, off/OFF | 30 minutes |
| Crenna/2006 | 10/STN | 60.2 | 10 | Optoelectronic markers Single platform static posturography Surface EMG | No pre-op 10.4 (± 7) months post-op off/OFF, off/ON, on/OFF, off/OFF | 1 hour |

## Measurement of Gait

*Clinical Assessment*: In general, UPDRS gait scores may be normal in very early stage PD but quantitative studies of very early stage untreated PD show reduced gait velocity, reduced swing times, and marked inconsistencies of the timing of gait *(50)*. The description of gait abnormalities in the UPDRS is broad and the clinical assessment of gait may lead to under-reporting of small reductions in step size and gait velocity in early stages of the disease. UPDRS gait scores are always abnormal in more advanced stages of disease but provide only a broad description of the abnormality.

*Quantitative Measures*: Quantitative gait studies have shown that decreased stride length and the inability to regulate stride length are characteristic abnormalities of walking in PD that worsen as the disease progresses *(51)*. Morris et al. also showed that stride length can be improved by visual and attention cueing, leading them to hypothesize that stride length abnormalities in PD are a result of problems in the motor set of the walking motor sequence rather than due to a deficit of internal cueing for successive submovements of a motor sequence *(51)*. Gait velocity is slow but cadence is usually increased to compensate for reduced stride length, often resulting in a higher cadence than in normal controls *(52, 53)*. Other studies have shown that the parkinsonian gait also includes reduced swing velocity (velocity of the leg during the swing phase of walking) and an increased percentage of the gait cycle in double stance rather than in the swing phase *(51–53)*. The variability of all gait parameters is increased in PD while off therapy. During walking, the range of motion of the hip, knees, and ankle joints are restricted when compared to normal subjects *(53, 54)*.

## Effect of DBS on Walking in PD

At least 13 studies have specifically examined the effect of DBS on the act of walking Seven groups studied pre- and post-DBS gait parameters while the rest studied only post-DBS, with durations after DBS from 3 months to 3 years (Table 19.3; refs. *52–64*).

One group studied patients 3 to 6 months after unilateral GPi or STN DBS. A subset were also studied 3 to 4 years after bilateral DBS *(62)*. These authors were the only group to withhold stimulation for 12 hours for the OFF DBS evaluation. In other studies, patients were usually OFF DBS for 30 to 60 minutes (one for 10 minutes, one subset for 8 hours). Medication was usually stopped for at least 12 hours *(64)*.

*Clinical Assessment*: Studies that have specifically looked at the effect of bilateral GPi and/or STN DBS on gait scores from the UPDRS, both from the patients' report (gait items from the UPDRS part II) and from the examiner's assessment (lower extremity and gait items from the UPDRS part III) have shown improvement ranging from 36 to 68% from DBS alone *(14, 15, 33, 34, 52, 56, 57, 61, 64)*. Additional improvement was noted with DBS and medication in some studies *(14, 33, 34, 60, 64)*.

*Quantitative Measurements*: Using quantitative analysis, significant increases in gait velocity after DBS have been a uniform finding in all the studies listed in Table 19.3. Most have shown that this was mainly due to significant

Table 19.3 Studies examining the effect of DBS on gait.

| Author/year | No. of subjects/site of DBS | Mean age (years) | No. of control subjects | Type of measurement* | Comparison-medication/DBS | Duration OFF DBS |
|---|---|---|---|---|---|---|
| Allert/2001 | 18/10 GPi, 8 STN | 55.2 (GPi) 57.4 (STN) | None | UPDRS* Pressure sensors in shoes | Pre-op off/on 3 months post-op off/OFF, off/ON, on/OFF, off/OFF | 1 hour |
| Xie/2001 | 10/STN | 55.8 | None | Stand-walk-sit test Pressure sensors in shoes | No pre-op 6 (3–36) months post-op off/OFF, off/ON, on/OFF, off/OFF | 10 minutes |
| Stolze/2001 | 9/STN 7-LD responsive gait disorder, 2 freezing on meds | 56 | 10 | UPDRS Infrared markers, treadmill | Pre-op off/on 3 months post-op off/OFF, off/ON, on/OFF, off/OFF | Not given |
| Faist/2001 | 8/STN (young onset) | 48.1 | 12 | Treadmill with force-plates, Special shoes Infrared markers Tinetti gait score | Pre-op off/on 15.4 (± 10.6) months post-op off/OFF, off/ON, on/OFF, off/OFF | 1 hour |
| Defebvre/2002 | 7/GPi | 58 | None | Static posturography Infrared markers UPDRS | Pre-op off/on 3 months post-op off/ON, on/ON | ON DBS |
| Rizzone/2002 | 9/STN | 59.3 | 9 | Optoelectronic markers and dynamometric force platform | No pre-op >3 months post-op off/OFF, off/ON | Not given |
| Ferrarin/2002 | 4/STN | 59.5 | 4 | Optoelectronic markers and dynamometric force platform | No pre-op 10.8 (± 3.2) months post-op off/OFF, off/ON | 1 hour |
| Krystkowiak/2003 | 10/STN | 57 | None | Infrared markers UPDRS gait score | Pre-op off/on 3 months post-op off/ON, on/ON | ON DBS |
| Bastian/2003 | 6/STN | 53.5 | Number not given | UPDRS Infrared markers | No pre-op 6 months post-op off/OFF off/ON (unilat and bilat DBS) | 3: DBS OFF for 8 hours, 3: DBS OFF for 30 minutes |

(continued)

Table 19.3 (continued)

| Author/year | No. of subjects/ site of DBS | Mean age (years) | No. of control subjects | Type of measurement* | Comparison-medication/DBS | Duration OFF DBS |
|---|---|---|---|---|---|---|
| Ferrarin/2005 | 10/STN | 52–68 | 10 | Optoelectronic markers and dynamometric force platform | No pre-op 10.4 (± 7) months off/OFF, off/ON, on/OFF, off/OFF | 1 hour |
| Piper/2005 | 21/10 STN, 11 GPi | 59.5 | None | Optoelectronic markers and dynamometric force platform | Pre-op off/on 3–6 months post-op-unilat DBS 3–4 years post-op with bilat DBS | 12 hours |
| Liu/2005 | 11/STN (same patients as in gait initiation table) | 53.7 | None | Optoelectronic markers and dynamometric force platform | No pre-op 16 (6–32) months post-op off/OFF, off/ON, on/OFF, off/OFF | 30 minutes |
| Lubik/2006 | 11/STN (patients picked for good overall response to DBS and meds) | 62.2 | None | UPDRS Pressure sensors in shoes | No pre-op 22.7 (± 12.5) months post-op off/OFF, off/ON, on/OFF, off/OFF | 30 minutes (long-acting medication stopped for 24 hours) |

*Papers that reported the UPDRS II and/or III gait and posture subscores separately are listed in measurement column.

increases in stride length with no change in cadence although some studies have also shown increased cadence *(54, 60, 62)*. Morris et al. *(51)* showed that the cardinal abnormality of gait in PD is a shortened and irregular stride length. Healthy subjects can increase gait velocity by increasing either stride length or cadence to a certain point after which walking becomes a run. Morris et al. *(65)* have also shown that PD patients display a similar relationship between stride length and cadence but that stride length is "set" lower such that it reaches its maximum at a lower cadence *(65)*. After that cadence usually increases as a compensatory mechanism to increase gait velocity. In addition the gait velocity was still low enough that both could effectively be used to increase gait velocity. Another explanation for the different results concerning cadence proposed by Ferrarin et al. was that some studies were performed on a treadmill and others over ground *(54)*. Walking on a treadmill alters some joint kinematics and postural control due to differences in the support surface and static environment. Other noted improvements were that less time was spent in double stance and the variability of gait parameters decreased (see references in Table 19.3). In many studies, certain patients who could not walk unassisted pre-operatively were able to walk postoperatively. In the studies that compared GPi to STN DBS there was no significant superiority of one site over the other for unilateral or bilateral stimulation *(52, 62)*. One study compared unilateral to bilateral STN DBS 6 months after DBS and found that bilateral DBS was superior for improving gait velocity and stride length *(61)*.

**The Effect of DBS on FOG**

FOG has become one of the most difficult aspects of PD to treat. FOG is defined as a sudden interruption of the process of walking and/or turning. It may be accompanied by very rapid, short steps at high cadences termed "festination." Difficulty initiating gait ("gait hesitation") is also common. FOG may be triggered by a loss of far vision of the gait trajectory, such as when one attempts to walk through doorways or in crowds and when attention is diverted. FOG can occur either off or on medication, during the wearing off phase, or completely at random. It has been hypothesized to be an underlying aspect of PD that is resistant to dopaminergic medication *(66)*, although others have suggested that on-medication FOG has a similar pathophysiology to dyskinesias *(67)*. FOG may be a failure of communication between the basal ganglia and supplementary motor cortex that usually runs each part of an automatic motor sequence in a timely (fluid) manner *(68)* and has also been shown to occur in other repetitive movements such as repetitive alternating finger tapping *(69)*.

*The Effect of DBS on FOG*

Very few studies have specifically studied the effect of DBS on FOG, although there is a growing clinical impression that FOG that occurs while on medication is also not very responsive to DBS. Stolze et al. *(56)* attempted to examine this in their study of the effects of DBS on gait. Two of nine patients had FOG both on and off medication and the other seven patients had FOG only off medication. All off-medication FOG was eliminated with STN DBS but the on-medication freezing persisted. Yokuchi et al. *(70)* studied the effect of STN DBS in eight patients who had FOG "mainly in the off phase and also in the on phase." Unfortunately, no quantitative data was provided and the only result given for the group was the UPDRS, part III. Davis et al. *(71)* used the freezing item of the UPDRS, part II, and examined the effect of STN DBS on FOG in 67 patients at 1 year and 32 patients at 2 years after DBS *(71)*. Off-medication freezing was significantly improved ON DBS 1 and 2 years after surgery but on-medication freezing was not. It has been hypothesized that FOG and other aspects of postural instability that are resistant to medication may be produced by circuits through the PPN, which is known to exhibit similar degeneration and pathophysiological changes to other nuclei of the basal ganglia in PD. The PPN has become another potential target for DBS and is addressed in the next section.

## DBS of the PPN for the Treatment of Postural Instability and Gait Disorders in PD

The PPN is part of the ventral mesencephalic locomotor area of the brainstem that has been studied extensively in cats and is integral to postural control and locomotion in animals *(72–74)*. The PPN appears to be part of a parallel basal ganglia-brainstem-thalamo-cortical pathway with dense connections with the STN, GPi, and thalamus and may play an important role in conditioned sensorimotor performance *(75)*. It appears to be involved in PD, showing neuronal degeneration and overactive irregular neuronal firing patterns. Bilateral lesions of the PPN region cause severe akinesia *(76)* but stimulation of the ventral mesencephalic region in the cat at low frequencies results in stepping *(77)*. Nandi et al. first reported implanting a unilateral DBS electrode into the PPN of a normal non-human primate *(78)*. Stimulation at frequencies above 45 Hz caused more akinesia and loss of postural control than stimulation at lower frequencies. Stimulation at low frequencies produced a contralateral 5 Hz tremor.

Until recently, it was thought to be too dangerous a site to approach with the current DBS linear tetrode (Medtronic 3389 or 3387, Medtronic Inc). It is surrounded by the cerebellar peduncles, the medial lemniscus, nucleus cuneiformis, and other important descending and ascending fiber bundles. However, in 2005 two groups reported safe implantation of DBS electrodes into the PPN of two patients in each study *(79, 80)*. Mazzone et al. demonstrated the surgical approach and electrophysiology of the region but did not include outcomes. Plaha et al. showed that PPN DBS alone improved off and on medication freezing (as reported in UPDRS, part II) after 42 and 16 days of DBS respectively. The retropulsion score was also improved. The optimal response was seen at frequencies of 20 to 25 Hz. Stimulation at frequencies of 185 Hz and higher resulted in a worse motor outcome. Recently, in an open label study, Steffani et al. *(81)* reported a series of six patients with PD and medication resistant gait disorder and postural instability who consented to bilateral STN and PPN DBS *(81)*. Patients were studied using the UPDRS 2 to 6 months after surgery both OFF and ON stimulation and off and on medication. Stimulation at each site independently produced improvement in UPDRS, part III scores. PPN DBS lost some overall effectiveness over 3 months (54% at onset down to a steady state of 32% at 3 months). STN DBS remained effective with 54% improvement. However PPN DBS was very effective for posture and gait items of the UPDRS and stimulation with both sites was significantly better than either site alone when the patients were in an on-medication state. UPDRS, part II scores also improved but the authors did not report effects on the item referring to freezing. The authors proposed that combined DBS of both PPN and STN may be beneficial for medication responsive signs of PD and also for the more resistant postural instability and gait disorder. This interesting preliminary data will require further research using quantitative measures of postural control and gait.

## Long-Term Effects of STN and GPi DBS on Postural Control and Gait in PD

As DBS has become an accepted standard therapy for advanced PD with motor complications, one of the first questions asked by patients contemplating the procedure is, "How long will this last?" This question is particularly germane to the subject of this chapter because there is a strong clinical impression that midline improvements of gait and balance do not "last" as long as other signs such as appendicular signs of tremor, bradykinesia, and rigidity. Two studies have examined large cohorts of patients for up to 4 and 5 years after DBS surgery *(33, 34)*. Another study examined quantitative gait outcomes 3 to 4 years after DBS, although because each side had been staged by 6 to 12 months, it is unclear how long the patients had bilateral STN or GPi DBS *(62)*. Krack et al. *(33)* studied the first 49 patients who had undergone bilateral STN DBS at the University of Grenoble, after 5 years of DBS. Overall UPDRS, part III scores off medication still showed a 54% improvement to their pre-operative value. The retropulsion, gait, and freezing scores from UPDRS, part II and III were significantly better off medication. However, all three scores were worse on medication and significantly worse than after 1 year of DBS. Rodriquez-Oroz et al. *(34)* studied 69 patients after 3 to 4 years of DBS, 49 with bilateral STN DBS and 20 with bilateral GPi DBS *(34)*. Both STN and GPi DBS still had significant positive effects on UPDRS III scores while off medication after 3 to 4 years (50% improvement with STN, 39% with GPi). STN DBS showed significant improvement in gait and retropulsion scores 3 to 4 years off medication but showed significant worsening of both scores on medication after 3 to 4 years. GPi DBS showed no significant effect on gait or retropulsion scores off medication. On medication there was no worsening but only the gait score was improved after 3 to 4 years. Piper et al. *(62)* studied 15 patients 3 to 4 years after bilateral DBS (eight STN, seven GPi) with 3-D motion analysis and showed that the gait velocity, cadence, and stride length were still significantly better than pre-operative scores with STN or GPi DBS alone. Of great interest, but not commented on, was their data showing dramatic improvement in the off medication/OFF DBS state compared to baseline 3 to 4 years prior *(62)*. In the on-medication state they reported no significant change from pre-operative baseline.

## References

1. Smithson F, Morris ME, Iansek R (1998) Performance on clinical tests of balance in Parkinson's disease. Physical Therapy 78:577–592.
2. Tinetti MS (1986) Performance oriented assessment of mobility problems in elderly patients. Am J Geriatr Soc 34:119–126.
3. Powell LE, Meyers AM (1995) The activities-specific balance confidence (ABC) scale. J Gerontol Med Sci 50A:M28–M34.

4. Fahn S, Elton RL, members of the UPDRS Development Committee, Unified Parkinson's Disease Rating Scale (1987) In Fahn S, et al., eds. Recent Developments in Parkinson's Disease. Florham Park, NJ: MacMillan Healthcare Information, pp. 153–163.
5. Lozano AM, Lang AE, Galvez-Jimenez N, Miyasaki J, Duff J, Hutchinson WD, Dostrovsky JO (1995) Effect of GPi pallidotomy on motor function in Parkinson's disease. Lancet 346:1383–1387.
6. Bronte-Stewart HM, Yuriko Minn A, Rodrigues K, Buckley EL, Nashner LM (2002) Postural instabilityin idiopathic Parkinson's disease: the role of medication and unilateral pallidotomy. Brain 125:2100–2114.
7. Faist M, Xie J, Kurz D, Berger W, Maurer C, Pollak P, Lucking CH (2001) Effect of bilateral subthalamic nucleus stimulation on gait in Parkinson's disease. Brain 124:1590–1600.
8. Morris ME, Huxham, F, McGinley J, Dodd K, Iansek R (2001) The biomechanics and motor control of gait in Parkinson disease. Clin Biomech 16:459–470.
9. Nashner LM (1993) Computerized dynamic posturogrpahy. In: Jacbson G, Newman C, Kartush J, eds. Handbook of Balance Function Testing. Chicago: Mosby-Year Book, pp. 280–307.
10. Rocchi L, Chiari L, Horak FB (2002) Effects of deep brain stimulation and levodopa on postural sway in Parkinson's disease. J Neurol Neurosurg Psychiatry 73(3):267–274.
11. Rocchi L, Chiari L, Cappello A, Gross A, Horak FB (2004) Comparison between subthalamic nucleus and globus pallidus internus stimulation for postural performance in Parkinson's disease. Gait and Posture 19(2):172–183.
12. Maurer C, Mergner T, Xie J, Faist M, Pollak P, Lucking CH (2003) Effect of chronic bilateral subthalamic nucleus (STN) stimulation on postural control in Parkinson's disease. Brain 126:1146–1163.
13. Colnat-Coulbois S, Gauchard GC, Maillard L, Barroche G, Vespignani H, Auque J, Perrin PhP (2005) Bilateral subthalamic nucleus stimulation improves balance control in Parkinson's disease. J Neurol Neurosurg Psychiatry 76(6):780–787.
14. Guehl D, Dehail P, de Seze MP, Cuny E, Faux P, Tison F, Barat M, Bioulac B, Burbaud P (2006) Evolution of postural stability after subthalamic nucleus stimulation in Parkinson's disease: a combined clinical and posturometric study. Exp Brain Res 170:206–215.
15. Shivitz N, Miller Koop M, Fahimi J, Heit G, Bronte-Stewart HM (2006) Bilateral subthalamic nucleus Deep Brain Stimulation improves certain aspects of postural control in Parkinson's disease, where medication does not. Mov Disord 21(8):1088–1097.
16. Bronstein AM, Hood JD, Gresty MA, Panagi C (1990) Visual control of balance in cerebellar and parkinsonian syndromes. Brain 113:767–779.
17. Waterston JA, Hawken MB, Tanyeri S, Jaantti P, Kennard (1993) Influence of sensory manipulation on postural control in Parkinson's disease. J Neurol Neurosurg Psychiatry 56:1276–1281.
18. Toole T, Park S, Hirsch MA, Lehman DA, Maitland CG (1996) The multicomponent nature of equilibrium in persons with parkinsonism: A regression approach. J Neural Transmission 103:561–580.
19. Trenkwalder C, Paulus W, Krafezyk S, Hawken M, Oertel WH (1995) Postural stability differentiates "lower body" from idiopathic parkinsonism. Acta Neurologica Scandinavica 91:444–452.
20. Blaszczyk JW (1994) Dynamic balance control during minimum reach movements in elderly and young adults. Gait & Posture 2:11–17.
21. Nashner LM, Black FO, Wall CD (1982) Adaptation to altered support and visual conditions during stance: patients with vestibular deficits. J Neurosci 2:536–544.

22. Horak FB, Macpherson JM (1996) Postural orientation and equilibrium. In: Rowell LB, Shepherd JT, eds. Handbook of Physiology, Sect. 12: Exercise Regulation and Integration of Multiple Systems. New York: Oxford University Press, pp. 255–292.
23. Wollacott MH, Shumway-Cook A, Nashner LM (1986) Aging and posture control: changes in sensory organization and muscular coordination. Int J Aging Human Dev 23:97–114.
24. Koller WC, Glatt S, Betere-Overfiled S, Hassanein R (1989) Falls and Parkinson's disease. Clin Neuropharmacol 12:98–105.
25. Bloem BR, Beckley DJ, van Hilten BJ, Roos RA (1998) Clinimetrics of postural instability in Parkinson's disease. J Neurol 245:669–673.
26. Lang AE, Lozano AM, Montgomery E, Duff J, Tasker R, Huchinson W (1997) Posteroventral medial pallidotomy in advanced Parkinson's disease. N Engl J Med 337:1036–1042.
27. Fine J, Duff J, Chen R, Chir B, Hutchison W, Lozano AM, Lang AE (2000) Long-term follow-up of unilateral pallidotomy in advanced Parkinson's disease. N Engl J Med 342:1708–1714.
28. Vrancken AMPM, Allum JHJ, Peller M, Visser JE, Esselink RAJ, Speelman JD, Siebner HR, Bloem BR (2005) Effect of bilateral subthalamic nucleus stimulation on balance and finger control in Parkinson's disease. J Neurol 252(12): 1487–1494.
29. Horak FB, Nutt JG, Nashner LM (1992) Postural inflexibility in parkinsonian subjects. J Neurolog Sci 111:46–58.
30. Bloem BR, Beckley DJ, van Dijk JG, Zwinderman AH, Remler MP, Roos RA (1996) Influence of dopaminergic medication on automatic postural responses and balance impairment in Parkinson's disease. Mov Disord 11:509–521.
31. Beckley DJ, Bloem BR, Remler MP (1993) Impaired scaling of long latency postural in patients with Parkinson's disease. Electroencephalogr Clin Neurophysiol 98:22–28.
32. Ostergaard K, Sunde N, Dupont E (2002) Effects of bilateral stimulation of the subthalamic nucleus in patients with severe Parkinson's disease and motor fluctuations Mov Disord 17:693–700.
33. Krack P, Blair A, Van Blercom N et al (2003) Five year follow-up of bilateral stimulation of the subthalamic nucleus in advanced Parkinson's disease. N Engl J Med 349:1925–1934.
34. Rodriguez-Oroz MC, Obeso J, Lang AE, et al (2005) Bilateral deep brain stimulation in patients with severe Parkinson's disease; a multicentre study with 4 years follow-up. Brain 128:2240–2249.
35. Krause M, Fogel W, Mayer P, et al (2004) Chronic inhibition of the subthalamic nucleus in Parkinson's disease. J Neurol Sci 219:119–124.
36. Deuschl G, Schade-Brittinger C, Krack P, et al (2006) A randomized trail of deep brain stimulation for Parkinson's disease. N Engl J Med 355:896–908.
37. Temperli P, Ghika J, Villemure J-G, Burkhard PR, Bogousslavsky J, Vingerhoets FJG (2003) How do parkinsonian signs return after discontinuation of subthalamic deep brain stimulation? Neurology 60:78–81.
38. Lee HM, Huang YZ, Chen JJ, Hwang IS (2002) Quantitative anlaysis of the velocity related pathophysiology of spasticity and rigidity in elbow flexors. J Neurol Neurosurg Psychiatry 72:621–629.
39. Maurer C, Mergner T, Peterka RJ (2004) Abnormal resonance behavior of the postural control loop in Parkinson's disease. Exp Brain Res 157:369–376.
40. Wingeier B, Tcheng T, Koop MM, Hill BC, Heit G, Bronte-Stewart HM (2006) Intra-operative STN DBS attenuates the prominent beta rhythm in the STN in Parkinson's disease. Exp Neurol 197(1):244–251.

41. Inkster LM, Eng JJ (2004) Postural control during a sit-to-stand task in individuals with mild Parkinson's disease Exp Brain Res 154(1):33–38.
42. Mak MK, Hui-Chan CW (2002) Switching of movement direction is central to parkinsonian bradykinesias in sit-to-stand. Mov Disord 17(6):1188–1195.
43. Schultz AB, Alexander NB, Ashton-Miller JA (1992) Biomechanical analyses of rising from a chair. J Biomech 12:1383–1391.
44. Coghlin SS, McFayden BJ (1994) Transfer strategies used to rise from a chair in normal and low back pain subjects. Clin Biomech 9:85–92.
45. Elbe RJ, Moody C, Leffler K, Sinha R (1994) The initiation of normal walking. Mov Disord 9:139–146.
46. Liu W, McIntire K, Kim SH, Zhang J, Dascalos S, Lyons KE, Pahwa R (2006) Bilateral subthalamic stimulation improves gait initiation in patients with Parkinson's disease. Gait & Posture 23(4):492–498.
47. Rosin R, Topka H, Dichgans J (1997) Gait initiaton in Parkinson's disease. Mov Disord 12(5):682–690.
48. Robertson LT, Horak FB, Anderson VC, Burchiel KJ, Hammerstad JP (2001) Assessments of axial motor control during deep brain stimulation in parkinsonian patients. Neurosurgery 48(3):544–552.
49. Crenna P, Carpinella I, Rabuffetti M, Rizzone M, Lopiano L, Lanotte M, Ferrarin M (2006) Impact of subthalamic nucleus stimulation on the initiation of gait in Parkinson's disease. Exp Brain Res 172(4):519–532.
50. Baltadjieva R, Giladi N, Greundlinger L, Peretz C, Hausdorff JM (2006) Marked alterations in the gait timing and rhythmicity of patients with de novo Parkinson's disease. Eur J Neurosci 24(6):1815–1820.
51. Morris ME, Iansek R, Matyas T, Summers JJ (1996) Stride length regulation in Parkinson's disease. Normalization strategies and underlying mechanisms. Brain 119:551–568.
52. Allert N, Volkmann J, Dotse S, Hefter H, Sturm V, Freund HJ (2001) Effects of bilateral pallidal or subthalamic stimulation on gait in advanced Parkinson's disease. Mo Disord 16(6):1076–1085.
53. Faist M, Xie J, Kurz D, Berger W, Maurer C, Pollak P, Lucking CH (2001) Effect of bilateral subthalamic nucleus stimulation on gain in Parkinson's disease. Brain 124:1590–1600.
54. Ferrarin M, Rizzone M, Bergamasco B, Lanotte M, Recalcati M, Pedotti A, Lopiano L (2005) Effects of bilateral subthalamic stimulation on gait kinematics and kinetics in Parkinson's disease. Exp Brain Res 160(4):517–527.
55. Xie J, Krack P, Benabid AL, Pollak P (2001) Effect of bilateral subthalamic nucleus stimulation on parkinsonian gait. J Neurol 248:1068–1072.
56. Stolze H, Klebe S, Poepping M, Lorenz D, Herzog J, Hamel W, Schrader B, Raethjen J, Wenzelburger R, Mehdorn HM, Deuschl G, Krack P (2001) Effects of bilateral subthalamic nucleus stimulation on parkinsonian gait. Neurology 57:144–146.
57. Defebvre LJP, Krystkowiak P, Blatt JL, Duhamel A, Bourriez JL, Perina M, Blond S, Guieu JD, Destee A (2002) Influence of pallidal stimulation and levodopa on gait and preparatory postural adjustments in Parkinson's disease. Mov Disord 17(1):76–83
58. Rizzone M, Ferrarin M, Pedotti A, Bergamasco B, Bosticco E, Lanotte M, Perozzo P, Tavella A, Torre E, Recalcati M, Melcarne A, Lopiano L (2002) High-frequency electrical stimulation of the subthalamic nucleus in Parkinson's disease: kinetic and kinematic gait analysis. Neurol Sci 23:S103–S104.
59. Ferrarin M, Lopiano L, Rizzone M, Lanotte M, Bergamasco B, Recalcati M, Pedotti A (2002) Quantitative analysis of gait in Parkinson's disease: a pilot study on the effects of bilateral sub-thalamic stimulation. Gait and Posture 16:135–148.

60. Krystkowiak P, Blatt JL, Bourriez JL, Duhamel A, Perina M, Blond S, Guieu JD, Destee A, Defebvre L (2003) Effects of subthalamic nucleus stimulation and levodopa treatment on gait abnormalities in Parkinson disease. Arch Neurol 60:80–84.
61. Bastian AJ, Kelly VE, Revilla FJ, Perlmutter JS, Mink JW (2003) Different effects of unilateral versus bilateral subthalamic nucleus stimulation on walking and reaching in Parkinson's disease. Mov Disord 18(9):1000–1007.
62. Piper M, Abrams GM, Marks Jr WJ (2005) Deep brain stimulation for the treatment of Parkinson's disease: Overview and impact on gait and mobility. NeuroRehabilitation 20(3):223–232.
63. Liu W, McIntire K, Kim SH, Zhang J, Dascalos S, Lyons KE, Pahwa R (2005) Quantitative assessments of the effect of bilateral subthalamic stimulation on multiple aspects of sensorimotor function for patients with Parkinson's disease. Parkinsonism Related Disord 11(8):503–508.
64. Lubik S, Fogel W, Tronnier V, Krause M, Konig J, Jost WH (2006) Gait analysis in patients with advanced Parkinson disease: different or additive effects on gait induced by levodopa and chronic STN stimulation. J Neural Transm 113(2): 163–173.
65. Morris ME, Iansek R, Matyas T, Summers JJ (1998) Abnormalities in the stride length-cadence relation in parkinsonian gait. Mov Disord 13:61–69.
66. Marsden CD, Parkes JD, Quinn N (1981) Fluctuations of disability in Parkinson's disease: clinical aspects. In: Marsdec CD, Fahn S, eds. Movement Disorders. London: Butterworth Scientific, pp. 96–122.
67. Giladi N, Treves TA, Simon ES, et al (2001) Freezing of gait in patients with advanced Parkinson's disease. J Neural Transm 108:53–61.
68. Iansek R, Huxham F, McGinley J (2006) The sequence effect and gait festination in Parkinson disease: contributors to freezing of gait? Mov Disord 21(9):1419–1424.
69. Brontë-Stewart HM, Ding L, Moore GP (2000) Quantitative Digitography (QDG)—a sensitive measure of motor control in Idiopathic Parkinson's Disease. Mov Disord 15(1):36–47.
70. Yokochi F (2006) Effect of deep brain stimulation on FOG. Parkinsonism Related Disords 12(Suppl 2):S67–S69.
71. Davis JT, Lyons KE, Pahwa R (2006) Freezing of gait after bilateral subthalamic nucleus stimulation for Parkinson's disease. Clin Neurol Neurosurg 108(5): 461–464.
72. Garcia-Rill E (1986) The basal ganglia and the locomotor regions. Brain Res 396:47–63.
73. Garcia-Rill E (1991) The pedunculopontine nucleus. Progress Neurobiol 36: 363–389.
74. Conde H, Dormont JF, Farin D (1998) The role of the pedunculopontine tegmental nucleus in relation to conditioned motor performance in the cat. II. Effects of reversible inactivation by intracerebral microinjections. Exp Brain Res 121: 411–418.
75. Dormont JF, Conde H, Farin D (1998) The role of the pedunculopontine tegmental nucleus in relation to conditioned motor performance in the cat. I. Context-dependent and reinforcement-related single unit activity. Exp Brain Res 121:401–410.
76. Aziz TZ, Davies L, Stein J, France S (1998) The role of descending basal ganglia connections to the brainstem in parkinsonian akinesia. Br J Neurosurg 12: 245–249.
77. Garcia-Rill E, Skinner RD (1988) Modulation of rhythmic function in the posterior brainstem. Neuroscience 27:639–654.
78. Nandi D, Liu X, Winter J, Aziz TZ, Stein JF (2002) Deep brain stimulation of the pedunculopontine region in the normal non-human primate. J Clin Neurosci 9(2):170–174.

79. Mazzone P, Lozano A, Stanzione P, Galati S, Scarnati E, Peppe A, Stefani A (2005) Implantation of human pedunculopontine nucleus: a safe and clinically relevant target in Parkinson's disease. Neuroreport 16(17):1877–1881.
80. Plaha P, Gill SS (2005) Bilateral deep brain stimulation of the pedunculopontine nucleus for Parkinson's disease. Neuroreport 16(17):1883–1887.
81. Stefani A, Lozano AM, Peppe A, Stanzione P, Galati S, Tropepi D, Pierantozzi M, Brusa L, Scarnati E, Mazzone P (2007) Bilateral deep brain stimulation of the pedunculopontine and subthalamic nuclei in severe Parkinson's disease. Brain 1–12.

# Part III

# Postoperative Management in Patients Undergoing Deep Brain Stimulation

# 20
# Deep Brain Stimulation Programming for Movement Disorders

Ioannis U. Isaias and Michele Tagliati

## Abstract

The clinical success of deep brain stimulation (DBS) for treating advanced movement disorders is crucially dependent on the quality of postoperative neurological management. A well-implanted lead in an appropriately selected patient is useless without the application of proper stimulation settings. DBS therapy introduces in many cases a delicate balance of electrical and pharmacological treatment that requires a critical understanding of the principles of pulse generator programming. While the countless number of possible setting combinations seems to make programming a complicated and time-consuming endeavor, a systematic approach can prove invaluable in optimizing DBS therapy. This chapter outlines the general principles of stimulation, including the parameters that may be modulated to optimize therapy. We also review the common steps required to select optimal DBS contacts independent of the anatomical target and general troubleshooting guidelines. Programming issues relative to individual brain targets are addressed, which include the elements of anatomy, contact selection, medication adjustment (when appropriate), and specific stimulation-related side effects.

**Keywords:** deep brain stimulation, DBS, programming parameters, thalamus, subthalamic nucleus, globus pallidum, Parkinson's disease, dystonia, tremor

## Introduction

As outlined in several chapters of this book, successful DBS therapy depends on the proper implementation of a series of interrelated procedures, including: (A) accurate candidate selection, (B) precise lead placement, (C) proficient electrode programming, (D) expert medication adjustments, (E) management of side effects, and (F) patient education and support. DBS therapy introduces a delicate balance of electrical and medical treatment that requires a critical understanding of the principles of pulse generator programming. Successful postoperative management of DBS patients requires a detailed knowledge of the anatomy and physiology of the target area, expertise in the pharmacological treatment of movement disorders, and familiarity with the protocols for setting optimal stimulation parameters.

In particular, competent programming of the implanted device is essential to optimize DBS therapy. A well-implanted lead in an appropriately selected patient is useless without the application of proper stimulation settings. More than one-third of patients referred to two specialized movement disorder centers for "DBS failures" were not properly programmed *(1)*. It is important to consider that even after long-term stable DBS, a movement disorders and DBS specialist who is directly responsible for stimulation programming, and simultaneous drug adjustments can still provide significant additional clinical benefits to patients with advanced Parkinson's disease (PD) treated with DBS *(2)*. Challenges to proficient programming include multiple anatomical targets with distinct response to stimulation; thousands of theoretical parameter setting combinations, numerous electrode contact configurations; unknown mechanisms of action, and multiple time-dependent effects of stimulation. A systematic, multi-step approach to pulse generator programming can aid in achieving the basic goals of DBS, mainly maximizing symptom suppression, and minimizing adverse effects.

In this chapter, we review the general principles of stimulation, including the parameters that may be modulated to optimize therapy. We also review the common steps required to select optimal DBS contacts independent of the anatomical target and general troubleshooting guidelines. Programming issues relative to individual brain targets are addressed, which include the elements of anatomy, contact selection, medication adjustment (when appropriate), and specific stimulation-related side effects.

## Stimulation Parameters

The main goal of DBS is to deliver electricity to the brain target of interest while minimizing stimulation or spread of this current to surrounding structures. Therefore, the ability to control the electrical field size is key to providing effective DBS. Stimulation parameters that can be modulated in order to achieve this result include electrode location and polarity, voltage (V), pulse width (PW), and frequency (F) of stimulation. DBS programmable variables (V, PW, and F) are mutually dependent in producing the energy of stimulation, according to a simple formula *(3)*:

$$\text{TEED}_{1sec} = \frac{voltage^2 \bullet frequency \bullet pulsewidth}{impedance} \bullet 1 second$$

In order to properly set therapeutic DBS parameters, it is necessary to be familiar with the basic physiology of electrical stimulation in neural tissues. Electrical stimulation of the brain can evoke behavioral effects by exciting, or possibly inhibiting, neural cells. These effects depend on the anatomical location of the stimulating electrode, the stimulation parameters that determine the electrical field spread, and the electrical properties of the surrounding tissue. For example, large myelinated fibers are more likely to be excited than small fibers or cell bodies, while fibers oriented parallel to the stimulating electrode will be more readily activated compared to those running perpendicular *(4)*. While it is not possible to control the biological properties of the tissue surrounding the electrode, the programmer can manipulate those stimulation parameters that will determine the recruitment of neural elements into the target area.

The currently available DBS electrodes consist of a quadripolar lead with four 1.5 mm contacts separated by a distance of 1.5 mm (Medtronic model 3387) or 0.5 mm (Medtronic model 3389). The electrode spans 7.5 to 10.5 mm into the target area, and can potentially stimulate different anatomical structures with each of four contacts. Telemetric control of stimulation parameters is made possible by the implementation of an external programmer (Medtronic model 7432 or Envision). Patients may also verify the status of the neurostimulator and turn it off or on with a handheld controller (Medtronic Access). With one particular neurostimulator (Medtronic Kinetra), patients may use their devices to manipulate basic stimulator parameters within limits set by the physician.

When utilized for the treatment of movement disorders, DBS is currently routinely targeted to three areas of the brain: the ventral intermediate nucleus of the thalamus (VIM), the globus pallidus internus (GPi), and the subthalamic nucleus (STN). An understanding of the local anatomy surrounding the implanted lead is key to optimizing the clinical response to DBS and to elements of regional anatomy. We further describe these important points in the paragraphs dedicated to stimulation of specific brain targets. Most importantly, effective control of stimulation parameters can enable the programmer to change the shape and influence the diffusion of the electrical field, thereby directing it to as much as possible of the therapeutic target.

**Amplitude**

Amplitude is the amount of voltage fluctuation of an electrical signal, measured in volts (V). With increasing amplitude of stimulation, neural elements located at gradually increasing distance from the electrode can be recruited. Therefore, by controlling the voltage it is possible to control the volume of tissue affected by stimulation. Classical neurophysiological data predict that a monopolar cathodic pulse of 200 μsec duration and current amplitude of 1 mA could excite neural elements up to a distance of 2 mm from the active contact *(4)*. These data are, however, a rough approximation of the real current-distance relation of available DBS systems. This is as a result of the critical impact of electrode design and biophysical properties as well as the impedance of the neural elements mediating the behavioral effect.

Currently available neurostimulators (Medtronic models Soletra and Kinetra) provide constant *voltage* stimulation and allow voltage variations in 0.05 to 0.1 V increments between 0 and 10.5 V. For accurately implanted leads, therapeutic amplitudes normally range between 1 and 3.5 V at a pulse width between 60 and 450 μsec (depending largely on the different stereotactic targets; refs. *5, 6*). DBS systems delivering constant *current* of stimulation are currently being tested for clinical use.

When certain neurostimulators (Medtronic Itrel II or Soletra) are used, the amplitude should not be pushed above 3.6 V, in order to avoid the so-called "circuit doubling" effect. The Itrel II and Soletra internal pulse generators (IPGs) draw on a 3.7-volt battery to operate their circuitry. To provide output amplitudes greater than or equal to 3.7 V the devices are equipped with voltage multiplier circuits. Though effective, these circuits increase battery drain in excess of the voltage gain and profoundly shorten battery life. Therefore, rather than increasing the amplitude above 3.6 V, the pulse width should be increased in order to deliver the necessary energy (see below). These reference values do not apply to the Kinetra system, which does not use a voltage multiplier circuit.

**Pulse Width**

PW is defined as the duration of the electrical pulse used to stimulate the target area. The current required to stimulate a neural element decreases as the pulse width increases. This nonlinear relation is described by an inverse exponential function (Figure 20.1) and the empirical equation $I = Ir(1 - C/t)$, where I is the current (or voltage), Ir is the rheobase current, t is time, and C is chronaxie *(4, 7)*. Chronaxie is a measure of the excitability of neural elements and has been defined as the pulse duration equivalent to the double rheobase current, which is the minimal amount of current necessary to stimulate with a long pulse width. Chronaxie for DBS effects has been estimated to be around 65 µs for thalamic and around 75 µs for pallidal stimulation *(8, 9)*.

In practical terms, modulating the pulse width will determine which neuronal elements are activated: axons have lower chronaxie than neuronal cell bodies *(4)* and can be activated by smaller pulse widths. Therefore, while voltage modulation can control the volume of neural tissue stimulated, modulating

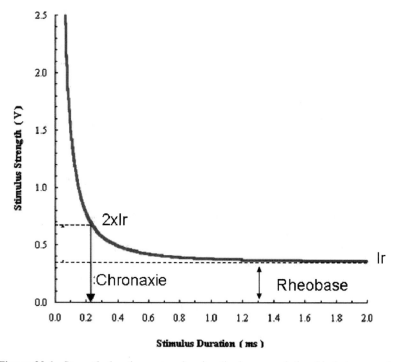

**Figure 20.1.** Strength-duration curve showing the inverse relationship between pulse width and voltage of stimulation. Chronaxie is the pulse duration equivalent to double the rheobase current, which is the minimal amount of current necessary to stimulate with a long pulse width. (To view this figure in color, see insert)

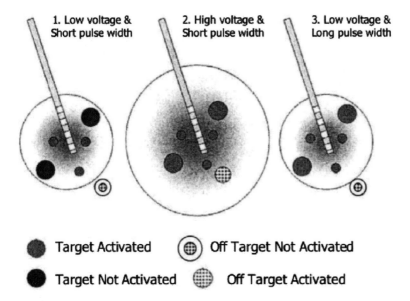

**Figure 20.2.** Changes in stimulated volume of neural tissue with variations of voltage and pulse width values (adapted from Montgomery [16])

PW can determine which neuronal elements are stimulated within that volume (Figure 20.2).

**Frequency**

Frequency (F) is defined by the number of electrical pulses delivered per second, in hertz (Hz). Pulse frequency plays a key role in the therapeutic effect of DBS. The amplitude-frequency relationship has been studied systematically for thalamic *(10, 11)* and subthalamic stimulation *(5)*. Low-frequency stimulation (<10 Hz) either has no effect or may aggravate tremor and parkinsonism *(5, 10)*, while higher frequencies (>50 Hz) improve symptoms at progressively lower stimulation intensity. The benefit increases linearly with F up to 130 Hz, followed by a smaller nonlinear increase in efficacy until a plateau is reached around 200 Hz. A further increase from 200 up to 10,000 Hz, using an external stimulator, does not further improve the anti-tremor effect of thalamic DBS *(10)*. The use of higher frequencies of stimulation was also supported in dystonia by the results of a study showing a superior response of dystonic symptoms to pallidal DBS as stimulation F was increased from 50 to 250 Hz *(12)*. However, other clinical reports have documented a response of dystonia at lower F of stimulation *(13–15)*, suggesting that the therapeutic role of F in dystonia may be more complex. These concepts will be further developed in the sections dedicated to pallidal stimulation.

The mechanism whereby a specific DBS frequency improves movement disorders is not known. The therapeutic effect of DBS on essential tremor (ET) and PD symptoms is only observed at frequencies above 100 Hz with a sharp threshold *(10)*. This nonlinear frequency dependency differs from the usual encoding of signal magnitude by neuronal firing rate. It has been suggested that high frequencies of stimulation can increase synaptic efficiency by taking advantage of temporal summation of post-synaptic excitatory potentials (EPSPs) through an additive effect *(16)*. Another possible mechanism may be related to a resonance effect, whereby the DBS pulse sets up a reentrant oscillation through a closed loop (basal ganglia-thalamic-cortical) to return to the original site of action and thereby effectively adds to a second pulse *(17)*.

**Electrode Configuration**

According to basic neurophysiologic principles, a negative (cathodal) stimulus applied outside a neuron may depolarize the cell and induce an action potential. Each of the four contacts of the quadripolar DBS lead can be programmed as a cathode and can be considered the "active" site of stimulation. The active contact can be used in a monopolar configuration with the neurostimulator case referenced as the anode. Alternatively, each contact can be activated as anode or cathode in a bipolar or tripolar configuration. Monopolar stimulation is associated with a radial electrical field, covering an approximately spherical space around the stimulating electrode assuming tissue impedance remains constant *(4)*. In reality, computerized models of STN stimulation predict that the electrical field generated by clinically effective monopolar stimulation spreads well beyond the borders of the target area and is dependent on the anisotropy of the internal capsule and the zona incerta *(18)*. Bipolar or tripolar configurations provide a narrower, more focused electrical field with a presumed maximal effect near the cathode *(4, 7, 19)*.

The ability to shape the electrical field and avoid side effects created by diffusion into neighboring neural structures is fundamental for successful DBS programming. Usually a monopolar configuration is tried first, as it requires lower stimulation intensity than bipolar stimulation to achieve approximately the same clinical benefit. However, when electrodes are not perfectly placed and the voltage needed to activate the target neuronal elements produces a field so large that it stimulates unintended elements, the use of different electrode configurations can be clinically significant. It is important to note that stimulation voltage decreases with the radius of the distance from the cathode ($V \propto 1/r$) using monopolar configurations, with the square radius ($V \propto 1/r^2$) using bipolar and with the cube of the radius ($V \propto 1/r^3$) using tripolar configurations (Figure 20.3). Therefore, monopolar configurations provide maximum voltage spread and tripolar configurations provide minimum voltage spread. This relationship can be successfully exploited to avoid unwanted side effects *(16)*.

In addition, the distance between cathode and anode in bipolar configuration affects the electrical field spread, because the voltage generated by the stimulating electrode increases with the square distance of the anode from the cathode ($V \propto d^2/r^2$). Therefore, the wider spaced DBS lead (Medtronic model 3387) can generate higher voltages with less battery drain and should be generally preferred *(16)*. In summary, impressive flexibility is provided by the knowledgeable manipulation of electrode configuration and stimulation parameters, which can be used to generate "custom-made" therapeutic electrical fields for each patient. Unfortunately, many of these combinations may need to be tried before the proper DBS settings are discovered. Experience and knowledge of regional anatomy usually help in determining which set of variations to undertake.

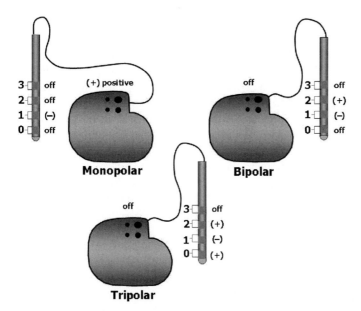

**Figure 20.3.** Electrode configurations. Monopolar configurations are obtained referring one (or more) active contacts to the case. They produce a rather large, radial electrical field. Bipolar configurations use one of the contacts as the reference and provide a narrower electrical field. Tripolar configurations further focus the field near the cathode using the two adjacent contacts as references (anode)

Finally, electrode configuration affects impedance and therefore the amount of electrical charge delivered to the brain. This issue is relevant because the safety threshold for the amount of stimulation that can be delivered to the brain depends on the electrode impedance, in addition to the voltage and PW of stimulation (16). In general, using multiple active electrodes will decrease impedance and modify the safety threshold, which is normally provided by the manufacturer.

## Basic Approach to DBS Programming

### Pre-programming Data

The primary goals of DBS are to maximize symptom suppression while minimizing adverse effects. Minimizing battery drain and maximizing medication reductions are significant secondary goals. To achieve these goals, one must take a systematic, multi-step approach to DBS programming. These steps include the acquisition of pertinent surgical and neurological data, the selection of the optimal contact, and the selection of appropriate stimulation parameters. Additionally, when indicated, the adjustment of CNS active medications and the management of medication-related side effects need to be addressed.

### *Surgical Information*

Before programming begins, it is important to obtain information regarding the patient's medical history and details of the surgical procedure. Communication with the implanting surgeon is critical in order to gain the necessary data regarding electrode type (model 3387 or 3389) and location in the basal ganglia, as well as the surgeon's assessment of the optimal therapeutic contact(s), which are established by intra-operative physiology and clinical testing (if it is performed). It is also essential to know whether a single (Soletra®) or double (Kinetra®) pulse generator was implanted. Finally, it is important to view the postoperative MRI to confirm that the lead is properly positioned.

As already mentioned, two DBS lead types are currently available: the Medtronic model 3387 with widely-spaced electrodes, spanning 10.5 mm and the Medtronic model 3389, which has closely spaced contacts with a span of 7.5 mm. Knowing the anatomical span of the stimulating electrode is fundamental to correctly evaluate the benefits and side effects related to stimulation. An overall span of 7.5 mm is appropriate given that the size of the efficient target region in most basal ganglia targets is less than 7.5 mm. However, a longer lead affords the ability to stimulate a greater region and possibly compensate a suboptimally placed lead. No data exist to recommend one type of lead over another *(20, 21)*.

Two types of neurostimulator are currently available: Soletra® and Kinetra® (Medtronic, Inc., Minneapolis, MN). The Soletra® neurostimulator accomodates one extension/lead. Therefore, two Soletra neurostimulators are required for bilateral therapy. The Kinetra® accommodates two extensions/leads and thus provides bilateral neurostimulation from a single neurostimulator. Most of the programming principles have been developed using the Soletra system, but can be applied, with some notable exceptions, to the Kinetra system. For example, individual contacts in the Kinetra system are labeled 0, 1, 2, and 3 on one side and 4, 5, 6, and 7 on the other. Infections of the Kinetra device may require removal of both leads (as compared to the Soletra), and the Kinetra is thicker which may impact individuals with small chests.

It is valuable to obtain the surgeon's assessment of electrode placement and optimal electrode(s) as established with microelectrode recordings and DBS testing in the operating room. This information can be used to guide optimal programming and aid in the eventual troubleshooting process. In this regard, we advocate routine postoperative MRI to confirm lead position.

*Neurological Information*

To determine the most troublesome symptoms to address for each patient, it is crucial to obtain documentation of the patient's pre-operative neurological status and medication regimen. The treating neurologist and the programmer may not be the same person, and may not even practice in close proximity to one another. Systematic evaluation tools like the Unified Parkinson Disease Rating Scale (UPDRS; ref. 22), timed tests and videotaping are strongly encouraged in order to quantify the results obtained with each contact and establish the best stimulator settings. Specific protocols for the evaluation of surgical patients have been validated and published *(23)*.

**Initial Programming**

The initial programming session is essential to assess each of the implanted contacts for beneficial and adverse effects and to determine therapeutic settings. In the experience of our group and others, initial programming is usually carried out about 2 to 4 weeks following surgery in order to allow for tissue healing and for resolution of microlesioning effects (i.e., transient improvement of parkinsonian symptoms often observed after electrode implantation). The patient should be scheduled for a morning visit, when possible, with medication withheld overnight or longer to place him in the OFF-drug condition.

The initial step involves the assessment and recording of the impedance and current drain for each contact. Baseline impedance is a critical piece of information, because it indicates the integrity of the electrical system and provides a reference for future troubleshooting. Each contact should be checked in monopolar mode using a consistent pulse width (210 μsec), rate (30 Hz) and amplitude. Normally, the impedance should range between 600 and 1300 Ω with a current drain of 10 to 30 μAmp. Impedance >2000 Ω with a current drain of <7 μAmp indicates an open circuit, while impedance <250 Ω with a current drain of >500 μAmp suggests the presence of a short circuit in the system. In addition, the same impedance in adjacent contacts may suggest a short circuit. These reference values are valid for the Itrel and Soletra systems. The Kinetra system can read impedances up to 4000 Ω; however, impedance and current drain data may not be reliably used to establish the presence of short or open circuits, unless higher testing voltages are used.

The most important step during initial programming is to determine the amplitude threshold for clinical benefits and adverse effects. A systematic approach should be used to minimize all of the many variables. The first step in DBS programming is to determine the "therapeutic window" for each contact, i.e., the voltage range between the initial observation of reliable antiparkinson effects and the threshold for adverse events.

Starting with contact 0 in monopolar configuration (i.e., case set to positive), the voltage is slowly titrated upward from 0 V in 0.1 to 0.2 V increments until beneficial effects are noted or the patient reports a nontransient side effect. This procedure is repeated for each of the four contacts. The voltage level at which benefits and adverse events for each contact are observed should be documented to create a database that will prove useful for future adjustments and troubleshooting. The contact that yields the greatest benefit and/or exhibits the greatest therapeutic window should be selected for chronic stimulation. The lowest effective voltage should be employed initially. When programming bilaterally, the contralateral side should be assessed independently, using the same protocol. However, the additive effects of bilateral stimulation may have to be assessed and adjusted further after both devices are activated.

If a single contact fails to provide satisfactory results, it may be useful to add an adjacent contact in monopolar configuration in order to broaden the effective field of stimulation. On the other hand, if unwanted adverse events are observed at the voltage needed to obtain a therapeutic effect, bipolar or tripolar settings can be used in order to achieve a more focused field of stimulation (see "Electrode configuration"). To do so, the contact with the best therapeutic window should be set as the active electrode (cathode) with the furthest contact set as the anode. Alternatively, the best contact can be referred to the second best in rank, or the best and second best as cathodes can be referred to the third as the anode (24). If no significant improvement is observed or stimulation-induced adverse events predominate at low voltages of stimulation, correct electrode position should be verified and technical troubleshooting initiated (7). Figure 20.4 illustrates an algorithm summarizing the general steps involved in initial DBS programming of the STN.

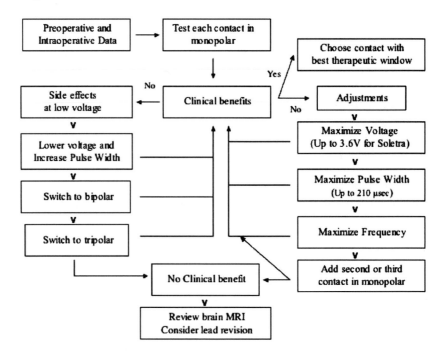

**Figure 20.4.** Programming algorithm

The *time course* of stimulation response can vary among targets and symptoms. For example, tremor suppression with effective stimulation of the VIM and STN is almost immediate, allowing effective amplitudes to be programmed during the first few sessions. Similar rapid responses can be expected for dyskinesias following GPi (and sometimes STN) DBS in PD. On the other hand, GPi DBS in patients with dystonia commonly results in delayed and gradual improvement over days to several months. Expected time courses of beneficial and adverse responses to DBS will be further developed in the paragraphs dedicated to specific brain targets.

**Follow-Up Programming**

Follow-up programming visits should be scheduled at short intervals until optimal stimulation is achieved (i.e., tremor suppression or clinical effect comparable to levodopa therapy in PD), and later may become more spaced out. Ultimately, follow-up visits should become less frequent than during the pre-surgical period, which was complicated by motor fluctuations and medication failures. Similar to initial programming, follow-up visits should also follow a systematic approach. An initial review of interim changes, including symptom response, medication changes and adverse events should be followed by device interrogation and analysis of whether the stimulation parameters are within the therapeutic range established during the initial programming visit. Based on this clinical evaluation, a management plan can be formulated to provide stimulation and/or medication adjustments or alternatively no changes may be required.

The complex syndromic nature of PD usually presents the greatest challenge. In general, we have empirically learned that "chasing" short-term PD exacerbations with stimulation adjustments should be avoided, as DBS parameters may drift from optimal settings. Patient diaries can be helpful, especially in the first few months of DBS therapy. It is always worth remembering that every PD patient is different, particularly during advanced stages of disease, and there may not be a single formula to solve diverse clinical problems. Clinical problems during the follow-up programming period are usually the result of a complex interaction of medication and stimulation. However, some tolerance (necessity to increase voltage) and rebound effect (symptoms much worse when the stimulation is switched off) can also occur. Sudden switching OFF the stimulation should be avoided in patients with dystonia because of the possibility of the acute onset of severe dystonic symptoms. In PD patients or patients with tremor, DBS can be switched OFF to assess disease progression and severity.

**Troubleshooting**

There are several reasons that may lead to a suboptimal response to DBS therapy, which range from poorly selected patients (unresponsive disease) to inaccurate lead placement and inadequate programming or medication adjustments. Poorly managed expectations can also generate a subjective perception of failure even when clinical results are objectively apparent. Finally, initial benefit may give way to symptom exacerbations in the presence of technical failures or device malfunctions. In most cases, DBS failures are preventable with proper screening, implanting, and programming approaches *(1)*. Common troubleshooting methods for DBS failures in movement disorders patients are reviewed.

*Unresponsive Disease*

The most important predictor of the success or failure of DBS therapy is appropriate patient selection. DBS consistently provides significant benefit in the treatment of idiopathic PD, ET, and dystonia *(6, 25, 26)*. Five out of 41 "non-responders" in one series had parkinsonian disorders that would not be expected to respond to DBS, and eight other (20%) had symptoms of dementia, which normally represents an exclusionary criteria for DBS *(1)*. Patients with levodopa-responsive idiopathic PD, medication-refractory primary dystonia and ET are considered prime candidates, but there are currently no formal guidelines for DBS screening. In practice, the original diagnosis and eligibility for DBS therapy should be re-evaluated if the patient is not responding despite a well-functioning device, appropriate lead locations, and optimized stimulation parameters and medication therapy.

*Imperfect Lead Location*

Different techniques can be used effectively for DBS implantation, with or without the use of microelectrode recording. However, regardless of the implantation technique, appropriate electrode placement is absolutely necessary to achieve optimal results. No amount of expert DBS programming can compensate for a poorly placed electrode. In the previously quoted series of "DBS failures," 46% of patients had a misplaced DBS electrode *(1)*. The assessment of thresholds for adverse effects and benefits at each electrode contact helps to identify and later to potentially correct electrode misplacements.

**Table 20.1** Localizing value of adverse effects signaling an inadequate lead location.

**VIM**

| Adverse event | DBS lead is likely | Structure stimulated |
|---|---|---|
| Persistent paresthesias | Too posterior | Ventral caudal nucleus |
| Tonic muscle contractions | Too lateral or ventral | Corticospinal fibers |
| Dysarthria | Too lateral or ventral | Corticobulbar fibers |
| Ataxia | Too medial and ventral | Cerebellar fibers |

**STN**

| Adverse event | DBS lead is likely | Structure stimulated |
|---|---|---|
| Dysarthria/dysphagia | Too anterior and lateral | Corticobulbar fibers |
| Tonic muscle contractions | Too lateral or anterior | Corticospinal fibers |
| Diplopia/eye deviations | Too medial and ventral | Oculomotor fibers |
| Ataxia | Too medial and ventral | Cerebellar fibers |
| Persistent dysesthesias | Too posterior and medial | Medial lemniscus |
| Acute depression | Too ventral | Substantia nigra |
| Dyskinesias | On target | STN |

**GPi**

| Adverse event | DBS lead is likely | Structure stimulated |
|---|---|---|
| Dysarthria | Too posteromedial | Corticobulbar fibers |
| Tonic muscle contractions | Too posteromedial | Corticospinal fibers |
| Visual phenomena | Too close to optic tract[*] | Optic tract |
| No effect at high voltage | Too superior, anterior, or lateral | — |
| Relief of dyskinesia and rigidity but worse akinesia | Too inferior | Ventral GPi |
| Relief of akinesia but no relief of dyskinesias | Too superior | Dorsal GPi |

While some location-specific adverse effects can always be elicited at moderate or high voltages (see below for details), poorly placed leads normally result in unacceptable adverse effects at low voltages, or produce no effects with test stimulation at high voltage and pulse width. The nature and localizing value of adverse effects that signal an inadequate lead location vary with the intended target and are summarized in Table 20.1. Imaging studies should be obtained in these cases in order to determine as accurately as possible the location of the DBS electrode and for planning eventual revision.

### *Inadequate Programming Parameters*

Appropriate access to adequate programming is an important determinant of the success or failure of DBS. Access can be hindered by a paucity of trained physicians available to program devices. Ideally, patients treated with DBS should receive programming at the same institution by the same team that implanted their devices. This provides continuity of care and immediate access to information concerning initial programming and electrode placement from the operating room. Inadequate programming accounted for 37% of ineffective stimulations in one series *(1)*. When suboptimal programming parameters are the suspected cause of DBS failure, the history of programming sessions and responses should be reviewed in detail. If this information is not available, a systematic approach such as recommended during initial programming should be followed. Strategies for optimizing benefits and reducing side effects are discussed in other chapters in this book reviewing programming issues relative to specific therapeutic targets.

*Suboptimal Medication Regimen*
Patients with movement disorders, with and without DBS, require frequent medication adjustments. In our published experience, 30 of 41 patients (73%) with inadequate response to DBS required medication changes, with some improving markedly from medication changes alone, and the majority after a combination of re-programming and medication changes *(1)*. Clearly, for PD patients in particular, surgery does not replace appropriate medical management. Simultaneous adjustment of medications and stimulation parameters can be complicated, but is usually rewarding. A detailed knowledge of the desired and unwanted effects of stimulation and medications is required to properly troubleshoot problems arising from inadequate medication adjustments. When postoperative care is personally managed by a DBS trained neurologist who is an expert in movement disorders further improvement can be achieved in the majority of patients, even following long-term stable stimulation *(2)*. Available strategies for medication adjustment following DBS are reviewed in other chapters in this book discussing programming issues relative to specific brain targets.

*Device-Related Issues or Malfunction*
Adverse events related to the implanted hardware have been reported with frequencies varying widely from 2.7 to 50% of patients *(21, 27–29)*. We reported a 15.3% incidence of hardware-related complications in our initial 131 cases *(30)*. Hardware-related complications include electrode fracture, extension wire failure, lead migration, skin erosion, foreign body reaction, granuloma and seroma formation, IPG malfunction, and pain over the pulse generator *(21)*. The literature regarding diagnosis, prevention, and treatment of hardware-related complications is very limited *(21, 31)*.

Currently available neurostimulators provide features that may help the programmer in distinguishing device-related problems from other forms of therapeutic failure. These include impedance measurement, battery status control, activation counters and stimulation time. Lack of response to stimulation during initial programming, a sudden loss of stimulation efficacy following previous stable symptom control, as well as intermittent side effects all suggest a device-related problem.

There are many possible causes of sudden IPG failure, including electromagnetic interferences, device malfunction, and battery end of life (EOL). The most frequent cause is an accidental turning off of one or both neurostimulators, which can be easily diagnosed when reviewing the stimulation parameters. The IPG can be tracked for unusually high numbers of activations by examining the neurostimulator log. Therefore, it is important to routinely reset the magnet activation counter at the end of each follow-up visit *(7, 32)*. Sources of electromagnetic interference that may switch neurostimulators off include household devices (<10 cm proximity). Magnetic refrigerator door strips, electric shavers and toothbrushes, microwaves, electric drills, and other power tools have been anecdotally reported to affect IPG function, as well as metal detectors, anti-theft devices in department stores, and static magnetic fields generated by large loudspeakers *(7, 32)*. A detailed patient history and an assessment of the time elapsed from the moment the IPG was switched off (as estimated by the usage function) can help while investigating the source of electromagnetic interference. Battery EOL should be suspected if the programming device does not connect telemetrically with the IPG. This occurs most often with high levels of stimulation (especially in some patients with dystonia) or after prolonged use, normally 3 to 5 years. Patients should routinely be educated on how to check their neurostimulation status using the Access Review device. In addition, the Kinetra neurostimulator can be programmed to a disabled setting to avoid electromagnetic interference.

If an accidental turning off of the neurostimulator is excluded, a system malfunction should be suspected. The detection of an open circuit (high impedance and low current drain) suggests the presence of an extension wire break or lead dislodgement. Damage to the insulation can be causative and gentle tapping along the wire may elicit tingling pain or dysesthesias. Ultimately, plain X-rays of the implanted system components (lead, extension wire and neurostimulator) will document the damage (Figure 20.5) and help localize the

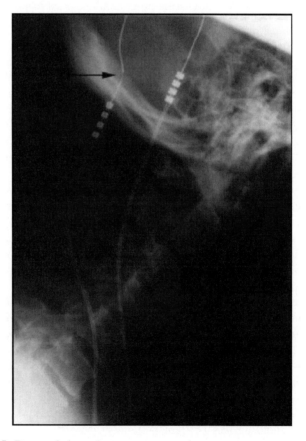

**Figure 20.5.** Damaged electrode

**Table 20.2** Most common device-related issues and their troubleshooting.

| Problem | Diagnosis | Treatment | Comments |
|---|---|---|---|
| IPG OFF | Interrogate with physician programmer | Switch IPG back to ON; identify problem's source(s) | Magnetic forces in the patient's environment may turn IPG OFF:<br>• refrigerator door strips<br>• electric shavers and toothbrushes<br>• microwaves<br>• electric drills and other power tools<br>• metal detectors and anti-theft devices |
| IPG intermittently OFF | Activation counter usually less than 99–100% use | Verify or program IPG to ON; reset activation counter for future assessment and identify source | As above |
| Short circuit | Check impedances: low impedance, high current; palpate device; X-ray for lead fracture | Surgical replacement of defective component | Failure may apply to only some contacts or may be intermittent |
| Open circuit | Check impedances: high impedance, very low current; palpate device; X-ray for lead fracture | Surgical replacement of defective component | Failure may apply to only some contacts or may be intermittent |
| Battery end of life | Check battery status | Replace IPG | Suspect with high levels of stimulation or long use |

problem. If troubleshooting procedures suggest a device-related complication affecting all electrodes or if the remaining intact electrodes cannot provide symptom relief, surgical revision may be necessary *(7)*. Table 20.2 summarizes some of the most common device-related issues and troubleshooting strategies.

**Patient Education**

Patient education and expectation management is of paramount importance to maximize DBS benefits. DBS is not a cure and probably does not slow or halt disease progression. Optimal results from DBS may take several months to achieve and may be different for each patient. DBS settings and medications need to be adjusted concurrently, with a concerted goal toward maximum benefit rather than the achievement of a state requiring no medication. Adjunctive therapies including physical therapy, occupational therapy, and speech therapy are often indicated to complement the effects of stimulation.

# Programming Issues Relative to Specific Brain Targets

DBS for movement disorders currently targets three areas of the brain: the VIM for the treatment of tremor, the GPi for the treatment of PD and dystonia, and the STN for the treatment of PD. An understanding of the local anatomy surrounding the implanted lead is key to optimizing the clinical response to DBS, and to allow for recognition of side effects caused by the diffusion of the electrical field to neighboring structures. Therefore, in the next few paragraphs we review essential elements of anatomy for each of the three main targets of DBS. In addition, specific strategies for optimal contact selection, medication adjustment (when indicated), and minimizing side effects are presented according to the literature and our own clinical experience.

## Thalamus

### Anatomy

Neuroanatomical studies in the monkey have provided information about organization, neuronal projection relationships, and local circuits of the ventral lateral nucleus of the thalamus (VL). According to Hassler, this area includes ventro-oralis posterior (Vop) and VIM nuclei, although some investigators believe that Vop is also associated with the pallidothalamic pathway *(33)*. The major subcortical afferent input to the VL is derived from all of the deep cerebellar nuclei with the bulk of fibers originating in the dentate nucleus. Another subcortical input to the VL derives from the spinal cord in the form of terminals from spinothalamic fibers *(34)*. In addition, cortical afferents to the VL in primates originate from primary motor cortex (area 4), the premotor cortex, and area 7 of posterior parietal cortex *(35–37)*. The regional anatomy of VIM is clinically important for the DBS programmer and includes three key neighboring structures: (1) the sensory relay nuclei in the ventral caudal nucleus (Vc) situated posterior to the VIM; (2) the Vop, which lies anterior to the VIM and receives pallidal outflow; and (3) the internal capsule, positioned laterally and ventrally to the VIM (Figure 20.6).

### Optimal Contact Selection

Thalamic DBS is indicated for the treatment of medically refractory tremors, including ET, PD tremor, and other types of cerebellar outflow tremors (e.g., multiple sclerosis, post-anoxic tremor, post-traumatic tremor; refs. *10, 38–42*).

Initial programming for VIM DBS electrodes follows the same principles previously reviewed. The thalamotomy-like microlesion effect commonly observed immediately after surgery usually requires waiting for 2 or 3 weeks before exploring electrode function. Using monopolar stimulation, therapeutic windows can be explored for each of the four contacts while keeping a constant pulse width of 60 to 90 μsec and frequency of 130 to 185 Hz. Voltage should be increased progressively, assessing both the effects on tremor and side effects. If a single contact fails to provide tremor suppression, it may be useful to add an adjacent contact to broaden the field of stimulation. If unwanted adverse events are observed at low voltages, increasing PW can be tested to increase current density without further spread of the electrical field. Finally, bipolar or tripolar settings can be used, with the most effective contact referred to the contact that is furthest away in space.

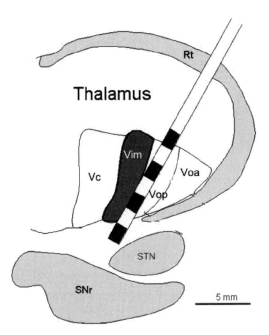

**Figure 20.6.** Schematic representation of DBS electrode placement in the VIM nucleus of the thalamus, illustrating the anatomical relationship with other thalamic areas and deep brain nuclei. Rt, Reticular thalamus; SNr, Substantia nigra pars reticulata; STN, subthalamic nucleus; Vc, ventral caudal nucleus; VIM, nucleus ventralis intermedius; Voa, nucleus ventro-oralis anterior; Vop, nucleus ventro-oralis posterior (courtesy of Dr. Philip Starr)

The effect of thalamic stimulation in ET patients is usually assessed for limb tremor, either postural or kinetic, while resting tremor is the therapeutic index used in PD. Tremor should be addressed under different levels of stress and during the movements of other parts of the body. Breakthrough tremor that occurs under stress usually needs additional current to be controlled. It is important to know in which limb position and during which movement the tremor of the patient worsens. Objective tests such as drawing a spiral, pouring water from one glass to another or finger-to-nose testing can be helpful in documenting effects. A useful videotape is available for assessment of ET *(43)*. Voice tremor can be assessed by asking the patient to speak or hold a tone and head tremor by observation *(44)*. Some investigators use a tremor rating scale *(43, 45)*.

### *Medication Adjustments*
When VIM DBS is used to control PD resting tremor, anti-parkinson drugs are either unchanged *(39)* or slightly reduced in a minority of patients *(46, 47)*. For ET and other types of tremor, medications can often be reduced *(40)*, but sometimes patients may need a combination of stimulation and medications to optimize tremor control.

### *Stimulation-Related Adverse Events*
The most frequent side effect of VIM stimulation is paresthesia involving the contralateral limbs or the face *(44, 48)*. This is usually caused by diffusion

**Table 20.3** Stimulation parameters used in largest studies of VIM DBS.

| Author and year | N | PW (sec) | Frequency (Hz) | Amp. (V) | Active Contacts used |||| 
|---|---|---|---|---|---|---|---|---|
| | | | | | 0 | 1 | 2 | 3 |
| Hubble et al., 1997 *(121)* | 19* 10** | 116.9 ± 86.1 | 161.9 ± 29.1 | 3.01 ± 1.05 | | N/A | | |
| Limousin et al., 1999 *(40)* | 44* 78** | 83.86 ± 31.42* 81.92 ± 30.45** | 163.64 ± 24.42* 162.95 ± 28.42** | 2.40 ± 0.77* 2.51 ± 0.93** | | +/−/OFF +/−/OFF | | |
| Schuurman et al., 2000 *(47)* | 7* 22** | N/A N/A | N/A N/A | N/A N/A | | N/A N/A | | |
| Koller et al., 2001 *(122)* | 25* | 55–145* | 135–185* | 2.3–4.9* | | N/A | | |
| Vaillancourt et al., 2003 *(123)* | 6* | 60–120 (75)* | 185* | 2.2–6.0 (2.2)* | − | N/A | +/− | +/− |
| Rehncrona et al., 2003 *(124)* | 14* 12** | 90.0 ± 39.0* 90.4 ± 32.6** | 181.4 ± 9.1* 160 ± 37.4** | 2.3 ± 1.0* 2.2 ± 0.9** | | N/A | | |
| Ushe et al., 2004 *(125)* | 16* | 60* | 185* | 2.8–4.4 (3.5)* | +/− | − | +/− | +/− |
| Lee et al., 2005 *(126)* | 19* | 90* | 170–185* | 0–3* | | N/A | | |
| Kuncel et al., 2006 *(127)* | 9* | 60–210 (90)* | 130–185 (145)* | 1–3.5 (3)* | − | +/− | +/− | + |
| Pahwa et al., 2006 *(25)* | 26* 19** | 111–129* 133–138** | 153–158* 143–166** | 1.4–5.9* 1.5–5.8** | | N/A N/A | | |

*mean or mean range for ET
**mean or mean range for PD

of the electrical field into Vc or to the lemniscal fibers entering the thalamus *(49)*. Paresthesias usually appear when the stimulation is switched on or the amplitude of stimulation is rapidly increased. When paresthesias rapidly habituate they are of no concern but if they persist *(50, 51)*, alternative contacts or configurations should be explored. Paresthesias are usually induced by the most ventral contacts or when the lead is posteriorly placed and can usually be avoided by activating more dorsal contacts. However, if the DBS lead is inserted with an excessive anterior-posterior angle, dorsal contacts may stimulate Vop and fail to control tremor *(16)*. In these cases, bipolar settings may help to stimulate the therapeutic target thereby avoiding sensory side effects. When paresthesias are elicited at low stimulation voltages, posterior placement of the lead should be suspected (see Section 20.4.4.2 and Table 20.1).

Tonic muscle contractions may be observed when the DBS lead is placed either too laterally or ventrally. In this case, the electrical field is affecting the internal capsule and activating the corticobulbar and corticospinal tracts. If the lead is too ventral, deep contacts will also produce sensory symptoms that are usually reversible with stimulation parameter changes, such as moving to a more dorsal contact or reverting to bipolar configuration. If all programming measures fail to avoid the side effects produced by a too ventrally placed lead, it can be physically withdrawn under fluoroscopic guidance.

Speech dysfunction (dysarthria) is a frequent complication of thalamic DBS, occurring with a prevalence ranging from 5 to 25%, and up to 75% when stimulation is applied bilaterally *(25)*. The nature of speech abnormalities observed during VIM DBS is not clear. Involvement of cerebellar output to the cortex and/or unwanted spread of the electrical field to corticobulbar fibers are potential underlying mechanisms. In the second case, similar to what can be observed for tonic muscle contractions, moving to a more dorsal active contact or to a bipolar configuration may relieve speech difficulties. A subcortical type of aphasia with word finding difficulty and dysfluency has been reported *(52)*, suggesting mechanisms related to the disruption of thalamic circuitry *(53)*.

Gait ataxia with postural instability may also be induced by thalamic stimulation. Balance problems have been reported in 3 to 7.5% of cases *(47, 48, 50, 54, 56, 57)* with an incidence of more than 50% with bilateral stimulation *(25, 40, 46)*. Similar to dysarthria, the nature of balance abnormalities during thalamic DBS has not been well elucidated, although interference with cerebellar afferents is suggested by the negative effects of varying PW *(7)* and internal capsule involvement may underpin other gait problems.

Very few studies have addressed the neuropsychological consequences of VIM DBS, which appears to have no significant effect on the cognitive abilities of PD patients *(58)* (Table 20.3).

## STN

### *Anatomy*

The STN is a small ovoid-shaped nucleus lying on the dorsomedial surface of the internal capsule. Like the substantia nigra (SN), the STN is a midbrain structure that is functionally included in the circuitry of the basal ganglia. The STN receives excitatory input from motor and premotor cortices, and inhibitory input from the GPe. The glutamatergic output of the STN projects to both segments of the GP and to the SN pars reticulata. The STN is divided into three components with the dorsolateral portion representing the sensorimotor region, which is the primary target of STN DBS.

Detailed knowledge of the spatial relationship of the neural structures in the subthalamic area (see Figure 20.7) is of critical importance in understanding the clinical side effects of STN DBS. Posterior-medial and dorsal to the STN is the large thalamic nuclear mass. The internal capsule is lateral and anterior. Ventral to the STN is the SN, and dorsal are the zona incerta and the H2 Field of Forel. If placed too medially and ventrally, the DBS electrode may stimulate fibers of the oculomotor nucleus. If posteromedially placed, the electrode may stimulate the red nucleus. The medial and ventral regions project to the regions involved in cognitive and emotional behaviors and stimulation of these regions can produce profound mood changes such as depression or hypomania.

### *Optimal Contact Selection*

Similar to programming of other targets, a standardized and systematic approach should be utilized. To this end, for STN DBS an initial pulse width of 60 µsec and a frequency of 130 to 185 Hz are customarily used *(5, 7, 32)*. The effects of stimulation at each contact are assessed as voltage is slowly increased. When assessing the effects of STN stimulation in PD patients, it is useful to use objective rating scales (e.g., UPDRS subscores, finger tapping,

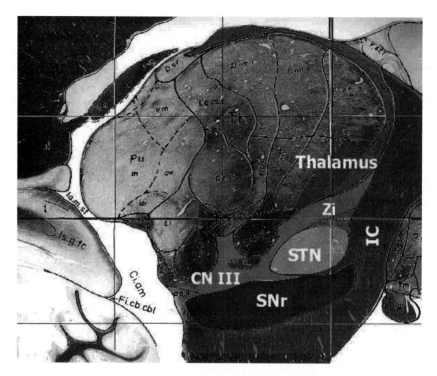

**Figure 20.7.** Sagittal view of the thalamic and subthalamic area at 12 mm from the midline, illustrating the anatomical relationships of the subthalamic nucleus (STN). CN III, oculomotor nerve fibers; IC, internal capsule; SNr, substantia nigra pars reticulata; Zi, zona incerta. (courtesy of Dr. Jay Shils) (To view this figure in color, see insert)

timed gait) and to remember a few key concepts relative to the response of PD symptoms to DBS:

1. Rigidity is considered the most reliable symptom to evaluate *(24)* because it has a short response time (20–30 seconds), is assessed with little patient cooperation and is relatively stable as compared to tremor and bradykinesia. Contralateral mirror maneuvers can be used to activate or stabilize rigidity *(59)*.
2. Tremor is also a very good target symptom, particularly in tremor-predominant PD. The latency of response is usually only a few seconds. However, resting tremor can fluctuate and is often greatly influenced by the emotional state of the patient.
3. Bradykinesia generally has the slowest latency of improvement and may occur after several hours or days. For this reason, it is typically the least useful symptom to monitor for initial programming. Moreover, bradykinesia is very sensitive to fatigue and motivation and can show a remarkable placebo effect during the expectation-laden first programming visit.
4. When present, off-medication dystonia is also relieved by STN DBS *(60)*.
5. Levodopa-induced dyskinesias can also be markedly improved by STN stimulation and can be among the most consistent results observed in successful DBS *(60)*. However, this symptom is not available at the initial

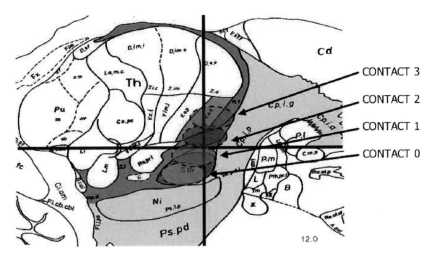

**Figure 20.8.** Schematic representation of the 3387 DBS electrode placement in the subthalamic area, illustrating the approximate anatomical areas that can be stimulated by the four contacts. Contact 2 and 3, when activated, cover an area dorsal to the STN, including the Zona incerta and possibly the anterior thalamus (courtesy of Dr. Jay Shils). (To view this figure in color, see insert)

programming session because patients are off medications and can be initially made worse when patients take their first dose of medication. The beneficial effect of STN DBS on dyskinesias is usually considered to be a byproduct of reduced levodopa requirements (61), but it may also be an immediate effect of stimulation, usually with the activation of the two most dorsal electrodes (62, 63).

In our experience, using the model 3387 DBS lead, the response to different PD symptoms and signs in STN DBS may be anatomically discrete (64). In a retrospective analysis of clinical data derived from the initial DBS programming sessions of 17 PD patients, we found that 11 of 13 (85%) patients with tremor responded best to stimulation of deeper contacts (0 and 1), while seven out of nine patients (78%) with rigidity and 11 of 17 (65%) patients with bradykinesia responded preferentially to stimulation of more dorsal contacts (1 and 2). As previously mentioned, dyskinesias responded to the activation of most dorsal electrodes (2 and 3). The pathophysiological relevance of this data needs to be elucidated, especially with regard to lead location, but it suggests that the entire STN region rather than only the STN itself may be a target of successful stimulation in PD (Figure 20.8).

*Medication Adjustments*
In STN DBS, increasing stimulation parameters are usually accompanied by a reduction in medication. With properly placed electrodes and accurate programming, the anti-parkinson effect of STN DBS should ultimately approximate or even match the benefits of levodopa therapy while eliminating or greatly reducing the associated motor fluctuations. STN DBS initiation is more complex than that of GPi or VIM, mainly due to the need to balance

**Table 20.4** Stimulation parameters used in largest studies of STN DBS.

| Author and year | N | PW (sec) | Frequency (Hz) | Amp. (V) | Active Contacts used 0 | 1 | 2 | 3 |
|---|---|---|---|---|---|---|---|---|
| Limousin, 1998 (59) | 24 | 60–450 | 2–185 | 0–10.5 | N/A | | | |
| Burchiel et al., 1999 (107) | 10 | 190 ± 76 | 185, one patient with 30 Hz | 3.0 ± 1.0 | N/A | | | |
| DBS Study Group, 2001 (67) | 91 | 60–450 (82) | 90–185 (152) | 0.8–8.0 (3.0) | N/A | | | |
| Volkmann et al., 2001 (78) | 16 | N/A | N/A | N/A | N/A | | | |
| Ostergaard et al., 2002 (128) | 26 | 60* | 130–200 | 3.1 ± 0.4 | N/A | | | |
| Romito et al., 2002 (129) | 22 | N/A | N/A | 2.92 ± 0.35 | N/A | | | |
| Vingerhoets et al., 2002 (130) | 19 | 73.5 ± 26.7** | 156.8 ± 44.4** | 2.75 ± 0.85** | N/A | | | |
| | | 76.5 ± 26.7*** | 160.5 ± 30.6*** | 2.80 ± 0.60*** | N/A | | | |
| Kleiner-Fisman, 2003 (131) | 25 | N/A | N/A | N/A | N/A | | | |
| Krack et al., 2003 (132) | 49 | 64 ± 12 | 145 ± 19 | 3.1 ± 0.4 | N/A | | | |
| Pahwa et al., 2003 (133) | 33 | 86 ± 20 | 165 ± 15 | 3 ± 0.5 | N/A | | | |
| Herzog et al., 2003 (134) | 48 | 62 ± 9 | 134 ± 12 | 2.9 ± 0.6 | N/A | | | |
| Funkiewiez et al., 2004 (70) | 77 | 60–90 | 130–185 | 2.4–3.6 (2.9) | N/A | N/A | N/A | – |
| Rodriguez-Oroz, 2005 (135) | 49 | 60–150 (72) | 90–185 (151) | 2.2–4 (3.1) | N/A | | | |
| Anderson et al., 2005 (136) | 10 | N/A | 130 or 185 | N/A | N/A | | | |
| Törnqvist et al., 2005 (137) | 10 | 60 | 130 | 2.5 | N/A | | | |
| Schupbach et al., 2005 | 37† | 64 ± 10 ** | 150 ± 27** | 2.8 ± 0.4 ** | N/A | | | |
| | | 62 ± 8 *** | 148 ± 26 *** | 2.9 ± 0.4*** | N/A | | | |
| Limousin et al., 2006 | 24 | 60–450 | 2–185 | 0–10.5 | N/A | | | |
| Fraix et al., 2006 (138) | 95 | N/A | N/A | N/A | N/A | | | |
| Moro et al., 2006 (2) | 44 | 60 | 130 | Below SE threshold or below 3.6 V | Off /+/– | Off /+/– | Off /+/– | Off /+/– |
| Deuschl et al., 2006 (26) | 78 | 63 ± 7.7 | 139 ± 18 | 2.9 ± 0.6 | N/A | | | |

*One patient received 60 μsec on one side and 90 μsec on the other; another received 90 μsec bilaterally.
**Right stimulator
***Left stimulator
†30 patients at 60 month follow-up

medication reduction with increasing stimulation intensity (31, 65–67). As the beneficial effects of DBS relate to all the cardinal symptoms and signs of PD, dopaminergic medication can usually be reduced after surgery. However, there is little agreement on exactly how to reduce medications. Some groups immediately discontinue levodopa after programming, while others take a slower and more conservative approach. There is no direct evidence as to whether it is best to decrease levodopa vs other dopaminergic drugs first or whether to reduce dose or dose frequency first.

On average, levodopa and other dopaminergic agents are reduced by 40 to 50% with bilateral DBS (60, 65, 68) and only rarely are patients able to discontinue their pharmacological therapy *(69)*. In other cases, and in particular when levodopa doses were kept to a minimum because of severe dyskinesias, levodopa dosage may sometimes be increased after surgery. Once a steady state has been achieved, medication adjustments should be carried out with extreme caution to avoid upsetting the equilibrium that has been achieved. This will also avoid potentially harmful consequences of discontinuing medications too quickly in patients treated for many years with high doses of dopaminergic drugs. In general, discontinuation of dopaminergic medications should never be set as a primary goal of STN DBS. However, failure to decrease dopaminergic medications sufficiently during chronic STN DBS may predispose the patient to sedation, excessive daytime sleepiness and mild confusional states. These side effects are well described in association with dopaminergic drugs *(70)* and are nearly always reversible with proper medication adjustment.

On the other hand, overly aggressive or rushed medication reductions can lead to unwanted re-emergence of either motor or nonmotor symptoms typical of low dopaminergic states. Temporary worsening of motor symptoms, particularly akinesia and freezing of gait, may be observed in these circumstances *(24)*. Similarly, depressive symptoms or apathy may be indications of excessive reduction of anti-parkinson medications *(24)*. Increased apathy appears to be the single most frequent psychiatric symptom in patients following STN DBS surgery *(71)*, in particular when large doses of levodopa are drastically reduced *(72)*. Patients who received very high doses of levodopa for many years (i.e., >1500 mg/day) usually will not tolerate quick dose reductions. The dopamine dysregulation syndrome is controversial but well described *(73, 74)* and needs to be taken into account in these cases. Apathy can be an independent symptom of PD, a symptom of dopaminergic "withdrawal," or seen in combination with a depressive syndrome.

Depression is frequently associated with PD, with figures ranging between 2.7 and 70% according to a recent review *(75)*. Depressive symptoms generally improve after STN DBS *(76, 77)*. However, a minority of patients may develop severe postoperative depression and occasional suicides have been reported *(24, 77)*. Increased dopaminergic stimulation generally improves depression, but it should be remembered that acute depression may result from stimulation of the subthalamic area as well. Finally, we and others have observed occasional symptoms of restless legs, likely related to an excessive decrease of dopaminergic therapy, which seems to respond to small doses of a dopamine agonist *(78)*.

### Stimulation-Related Adverse Events

Stimulation-related adverse events can be categorized as side effects that are specific to stimulation of the intended surgical target (STN), as well as side effects related to current diffusion into adjacent areas of the central nervous system.

### Target-Specific Adverse Events

The stereotypical target-related adverse event for STN is the development of dyskinesias, which are clinically similar to levodopa-induced dyskinesias, and may, in fact, be worsened by levodopa therapy. Stimulation-induced dyskinesias develop slowly over a period of minutes to hours *(24)*. The appearance of dyskinesias should be initially addressed by medication changes and not by reduction in STN parameters. However, if medication reduction is not effective or poorly tolerated, the use of more dorsal active contacts may also relieve dyskinesias.

A particularly troublesome adverse event related to target stimulation is hypotonia. Successful resolution of rigidity can predispose to rapid loss of tone of the antigravity muscles of the lower limbs, with resulting impairment of gait and postural instability. A complaint of "jelly legs" or falls that were not experienced before the surgery is not uncommon in the first few weeks of DBS therapy. Usually, these symptoms are exacerbated by levodopa and should be managed with a reduction in either levodopa dose or stimulation voltage. In addition, we find that specific gait rehabilitation with strengthening of antigravity muscles can further stabilize these symptoms. It is also important to consider that postural instability may be a consequence of spread of current into cerebello-thalamic fibers.

Apraxia of eyelid opening (AEO) is a rare condition in which patients have difficulty opening their eyelids. It is commonly associated with blepharospasm and neurodegenerative disorders such as PD and progressive supranuclear palsy. It has also occasionally been described after STN DBS *(60, 79)*. The specific cause or control center for both blepharospasm and AEO is poorly understood, as is the mechanism by which DBS causes or aggravates this problem. The fact that AEO is generally associated with good motor responses has led some authors to think that it may be a direct consequence of STN stimulation, possibly secondary to the involvement of the oculomotor loop *(24)*. Interestingly, AEO was also described as a side effect of campotomy, a neuroablative procedure from the pre-levodopa era *(80)*, suggesting that stimulation of the area dorsal to the STN may contribute to the pathogenesis of this rare adverse effect. A case report implicated electrical current spread to the dorsal trigeminothalamic tract, which is located just caudal and medial to the STN *(81)*. When functionally disabling, AEO can be treated either using more dorsal contacts or with pretarsal botulinum toxin injections.

A wide range of neuropsychiatric complications of STN DBS has been reported, including acute transient depressive and euphoric mood states, as well as the subacute onset of major depression, mania, anxiety, and substance abuse *(82, 83)*. Behavioral changes observed during programming are usually considered a consequence of an interaction with dopaminergic medications or secondary to stimulation of an unintended target (see below). However, additional factors independent of stimulation may contribute to profound mood changes, including implantation procedures with multiple electrode passes through the frontal lobes and the psychosocial consequences of an outstanding response, with forced normalization and loss of the sick role *(82)*.

Deterioration of cognitive function is a potentially devastating complication of movement disorder surgery, but one that can be avoided in most cases with appropriate candidate selection. The most frequently reported cognitive side effect appears to be a decline in verbal fluency *(58, 65, 71, 76, 77, 84–87)*. Older age and moderate cognitive impairment prior to surgery is associated with a greater risk of developing cognitive deficits *(83–85, 88, 89)*, although this has not been unequivocally demonstrated *(58)*. In addition, since dementia was an exclusion criterion in most DBS studies, there is virtually no data available on the potential effect of STN DBS on the cognitive function of patients with dementia prior to surgery. In general, there is no need to adapt stimulation parameters to these changes when present, although alternative settings with equal benefit on motor features may be considered (Table 20.4).

Weight gain may appear with variable incidence and has been up to 96% in some series *(90, 91)*. However, its cause remains unclear. This unintended effect of STN DBS may not be a direct effect of stimulation but may be at least partially related to decreased energy expenditure due to the resolution of involuntary movements in the absence of an adjustment of food intake *(91)*. Alternative hypotheses include an unproven regional effect of STN DBS on the satiety hypothalamic centers, and the possible effect of dopaminergic drug dosage reduction following STN DBS on hypothalamic homeostasis in PD *(91)*.

*Adverse Events Related to Current Diffusion to Adjacent Neural Areas:* Speech abnormalities are probably the single most frequent adverse events interfering with successful STN DBS in PD. Speech problems frequently occur in patients with PD, including hypophonia; monotonic pitch; hoarse, breathy, or tremulous voice; dysarthria; and hesitating or hyperkinetic speech. Therefore, it may be difficult to differentiate an adverse event related to stimulation from an unresolved or progressive symptom of the disease. In fact, as they are relatively resistant to levodopa therapy, speech abnormalities are usually unimproved by STN DBS *(60)*. Nevertheless, specific impairment of speech is frequently encountered during programming and is likely related to unwanted stimulation of corticobulbar fibers adjacent to the STN. Corticobulbar fibers pass directly anterior and lateral to the STN and are particularly affected when using the most ventral contacts, 0 and 1. Speech impairment secondary to stimulation is characterized subjectively by an increased effort in talking and objectively by hypophonia, hesitation, slurring of words and rapid fatigue *(24)*. As there is no habituation to this effect, the patient is sometimes faced with the dilemma of choosing between improved motor symptoms and more normal speech. However, careful adjustments of stimulation settings, including lowering amplitude and switching to more dorsal contacts and/or bipolar configuration will prevent severe speech impairment in the vast majority of cases. In our experience, using the 3387 lead, unless tremor represents the major PD symptom requiring treatment (see Section 20.3), speech problems can often be avoided using contacts 2 and 3. Speech therapy and particularly the Lee Silverman Voice Treatment technique may provide further improvement in these cases *(92)*.

Occasionally, we have encountered patients complaining of dysphagia after successful STN programming. Similar to speech abnormalities, dysphagia can be a symptom of untreated PD and only the temporal association with STN stimulation may suggest a pathogenetic correlation. The pathogenesis of dysphagia after STN DBS may be similar to dysarthria. Swallowing abnormalities may result from unwanted interference with corticobulbar fibers to the swallowing muscles. Indeed, we have observed significant improvement of dysphagia after applying the same approach described for speech abnormalities, i.e., lowering stimulation amplitude, switching to more dorsal contacts and/or switching to a bipolar configuration.

Activation of the corticobulbar and corticospinal tracts coursing in the internal capsule can produce tonic muscle contractionsof the contralateral face, hand, and more rarely arm and leg. The internal capsule borders the STN laterally, anteriorly, and medially. It can be determined if the electrode has been placed too anteriorly, laterally, or ventrally by the threshold voltage necessary to produce tonic contractions using different active contacts in monopolar configuration. The threshold to tonic contraction through the ventral contact will be very low for an STN DBS lead placed too ventrally and laterally.

Tonic contractions need to be clinically differentiated from off-medication dystonia in patients with PD. One way to accomplish this is to set the frequency to less than 10 Hz and observe the occurrence of single contractions caused by stimulation of the pyramidal fibers. In fact, tonic contractions time-locked with the activation of DBS contacts suggest current diffusion to corticospinal fibers, which run anterior and lateral to the STN. Reduction of amplitude and switching to another clinically effective contact are usually effective in preventing the unwanted activation of the pyramidal system. If these adjustments provide little relief, lead revision should be considered.

Diplopia, blurred vision, and abnormal eye movements may occur in patients with STN DBS. These are not symptoms usually seen in PD and clearly suggest current diffusion beyond the therapeutic target toward the fibers of the oculomotor nerve, which sweeps medially, ventrally and posteriorly to the STN. When stimulation affects the oculomotor nerve, adduction or downward movement of the ipsilateral eye can be seen. Deviation of the eyes is less common and is usually transient. It is possible that the electrical field of a DBS lead placed too laterally could activate the fronto-pontine tract in the internal capsule en route to brainstem nuclei to result in conjugate horizontal eye movements. However, the exact mechanism for conjugate deviation is not known. In these cases, it is imperative to switch to a more dorsal contact and eventually lower the amplitude or change the configuration to bipolar (field shaping). If abnormal eye movements are observed at unusually low voltages, lead revision should be considered.

Postural instability is another symptom frequently encountered in patients with PD that may occasionally worsen or present for the first time after STN DBS. Preexisting postural instability is generally improved by STN DBS *(93)*, unless it had not responded to levodopa therapy before surgery. In some cases, postural instability may derive from hypotonia caused by the additive effects of successful stimulation and levodopa therapy. In other cases, the patient complains of a more distinct truncal ataxia, with feeling of retropulsion and near falling. In these instances, the current is likely spreading to the cerebello-rubro-thalamic fibers medial to the STN or to the red nucleus positioned medially and ventrally *(24)*. Decreasing amplitude and PW, moving to more dorsal contacts and/or to a bipolar configuration may improve balance.

Transient contralateral "tingling" or sensation of "electrical current" are usually predictive of good location and positive stimulation outcome. However, if medial lemniscus fibers are activated, the patient will report persistent paresthesia. In most cases, programming adjustments like decreasing the amplitude and focusing the field with bipolar stimulation will relieve sensory symptoms. If the patient reports persistent dysesthesias at unusually low voltages, lead revision should be considered.

Transient acute depression has been reported during STN DBS and may be related to stimulation of the SN *(94)*. The SN is routinely mapped during neurophysiological targeting and some groups still implant the lowest contact of the DBS lead into the SN. Even after placing the most distal electrode at the ventral border of the STN *(95)* we have observed the acute emergence of unusual emotional lability with easy crying during the stimulation of contact 0 in one of our patients, likely caused by current diffusion to the SN. It is speculated that the pathogenesis of depression and mood liability with stimulation of the SN may be related to its anatomical connections with the amygdala and the limbic system *(94)*. In these cases, using more dorsal contacts will avoid this rare but dramatic adverse event.

## GP

### Anatomy

The GP is a large cellular mass with a triangular shape in its vertical diameter that appears elongated in its horizontal diameter. The anatomy and functional organization of the GP are well studied and provide potentially important information for the programmer. The GP is divided into internal (GPi) and external (GPe) sections by the internal medullary lamina (Figure 20.9). The anterior border of the GP is adjacent to the anterior commissure. The external medullary lamina separates the GP from the putamen. At the base of the GPi is the optic tract, and medial and posterior to the GPi is the internal capsule. With regard to complications, both of these regions are very relevant for DBS programming.

The GP is composed mainly of large multipolar cells, giving rise to efferent axons that form the main output of the basal ganglia. The afferent connections of the GP comprise the striatopallidal, thalamopallidal, nigropallidal, and corticopallidal fibers. Striatopallidal efferents are segregated in parallel systems associated with sensorimotor, associative, and limbic information. The posteroventral GPi is most prominently occupied by the sensorimotor area, while the associative territory is more dorsal, and the limbic area ventromedial *(96)*. The main efferent fibers from the GPi form the pallidothalamic system, which runs to the anterior nucleus of the thalamus in the fasciculus lenticularis and the ansa

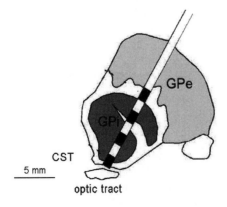

**Figure 20.9.** Schematic representation of DBS electrode placement in the globus pallidum, illustrating its anatomical relationships. GPe, globus pallidum pars externa; GPi, globus pallidum pars interna; CST, cortico-spinal tract (courtesy of Dr. Philip Starr)

lenticularis. Interestingly, these two pathways overlap in the posteroventral GPi *(97)*, making this area a particularly convenient target for modulating GPi output.

*Optimal Contact Selection*
GPi DBS can be performed for the treatment of advanced medication-refractory PD and severe dystonia. Contact selection and programming follow somewhat different principles for these two conditions and are addressed separately.

*PD*: There appear to be two different functional zones within the GPi: dorsal and posteroventral. Stimulation of the dorsal GPi (upper contacts) significantly improves gait, akinesia, and rigidity and may induce dyskinesia (similar to STN stimulation). It is debated whether this may actually be due to stimulation of the GPe when patients are in the "OFF" state. Stimulation in the posteroventral GPi (lower contacts) may significantly worsen gait and akinesia, block the beneficial effects of levodopa, while improving rigidity and markedly suppressing dyskinesias *(98, 99)*.

Initial programming for GPi DBS electrodes in PD patients follows the same principles reviewed for VIM and STN. To avoid a possible confounding microlesioning-like effect, 2 to 4 weeks should elapse before exploring electrode function. Using monopolar stimulation, therapeutic windows are explored for each of the four contacts keeping a constant pulse width of 90 to 120 μsec and frequency of 130 to 185 Hz *(100)*. Voltage should be increased progressively while assessing both therapeutic and side effects. If a single contact fails to provide expected benefits, it may be useful to add an adjacent contact to broaden the field of stimulation. If unwanted adverse events are observed at low voltages, further increases in PW should be tested to increase current density without further spread of the electrical field. Finally, bipolar or tripolar settings can be used, with the most effective contact referred to the contact that is furthest away in space.

*Dystonia*: GPi DBS can be very effective for disabling generalized dystonia that fails to respond to medical therapy *(6, 101, 102)*. Although a microlesion effect is usually not seen after GPi DBS in dystonia, it is still advisable to wait 2 to 3 weeks before initial programming. The main challenge of programming DBS for dystonia is the usual lack of beneficial effects observed during the programming session. Therefore, initial programming is mostly focused on mapping side effects following the same principles previously reviewed for PD patients. It is currently uncertain how long a delayed response should be awaited before considering changing contact configurations or parameters of stimulation.

Although a specific pattern of clinical effects correlating with stimulation in different parts of the GPi has not been described in patients with dystonia, many groups begin empirically with stimulation in the ventral part of the GPi just above the optic tract, as stimulation in this region has been shown to produce antidyskinetic effects in PD. The initial parameters used in programming for dystonia are less consistent among different groups than those observed in PD (Table 20.5). With very few exceptions *(103)*, most groups use monopolar configurations. Some begin by applying a very long PW, high frequency, and amplitude just below that which produces adverse effects *(104, 105)*. Others

**Table 20.5** Stimulation parameters used in largest studies of GPi DBS for dystonia.

|  | N | PW (μsec) | Freq. (Hz) | Amp. (V) | Active contacts |
|---|---|---|---|---|---|
| Bereznai et al., 2002 *(139)* | 6 | 120–180 | 130 | 1.8–3.5 | 1 (0 and 2) |
| Krauss et al., 2003 *(140)* | 6 | 210 | 130–145 | 2.2–4.5 | 1 and 2 |
| Yianni et al., 2003 *(102)* | 25 | 150–240 | 130–180 | 4.0–7.0 | Deepest available (bipolar) |
| Coubes et al., 2004 *(141)* | 31 | 450 | 130 | 0.8–1.6 | 1 (2) |
| Krause et al., 2004 *(142)* | 17 | 210 | 130–180 | N/A | One above phosphenes |
| Starr et al., 2004 *(143)* | 23 | 210 | 185 | 2.5–3.6 | 2 |
| Vidailhet et al., 2005 *(100)* | 22 | 120–150 | 100–185 | 3.7 ± 1.0 | N/A |
| Kupsch et al., 2006 *(101)* | 40 | 120 | 130 | 3.2 ± 1.1 | One above phosphenes |
| Alterman et al., 2007 *(106)* | 15 | 150–270 | 60 | 2.5–3.5 | 0, 1, 2 (3) |

use parameters more consistent with those used for pallidal stimulation in PD patients *(100, 101)*. We have recently found that a lower frequency of stimulation (60–80 Hz) can be as effective as higher frequencies while providing the additional benefit of saving battery life *(15, 106)*.

*Medication Adjustments*
Different from STN DBS, pallidal DBS does not usually permit substantial reductions in anti-parkinson medication dose *(20, 68, 99, 107–109)*. Available experience shows that PD medications are unchanged *(108, 110)*, slightly increased *(99)*, or slightly decreased *(111)*.

On the other hand, most patients with dystonia are able to substantially decrease their medications, which usually have been relatively ineffective, once the beneficial effect of stimulation is established, although this may take weeks or months to occur *(6, 101, 102, 104, 106)*.

*Stimulation-Related Adverse Events*
Current spread ventrally to the optic tract causes phosphenes (bright lights or scintillating visual illusions) and occasionally nausea. Visual side effects can be easily avoided by using more dorsal contacts or reducing the amplitude of stimulation.

Electrical current spreading medially or posteriorly into the internal capsule may evoke tonic muscle contraction of contralateral muscles, often associated with paresthesias or dysarthria *(100)*. In such cases, voltage can be reduced or alternative contacts used. If unwanted adverse events are observed at low voltages, further increases in PW should be tested in order to increase current density without further spread of the electrical field. Finally, bipolar or tripolar settings can be used.

Impairment of axial symptoms such as freezing *(99, 111)*, transient impairment of balance *(108)*, falling *(79)*, and persistent gait akinesia *(107)* have been also reported as a specific adverse effect of GPi stimulation, but the responsible lead location in these cases is uncertain. On average however, most studies report that axial symptoms improve following GPi DBS compared to the preoperative state *(68, 79, 99, 107, 108, 111–113)*.

Similar to STN DBS, the majority of studies addressing neuropsychological changes following GPi DBS have failed to reveal significant cognitive decline *(58)*. Mild declines in semantic word fluency *(109, 114)* and visuoconstruction scores *(114)* have been reported, while significant, but partially reversible, executive dysfunction was described in one report following bilateral pallidal stimulation *(115)*. Whether GPi stimulation is cognitively safer than STN stimulation is currently debated *(58, 116)*.

## Future Directions

Despite encouraging progress in genetic research and molecular biology, no cure for PD and dystonia is in sight. Therefore, it is realistic to expect that increasing knowledge and expertise in patient selection, electrode implantation, and post-surgical management will make DBS the treatment of choice for advanced movement disorders in the near future. In addition to the evaluation of its long-term efficacy and safety and the exploration of other deep targets such as the pedunculopontine nucleus *(117)*, future developments for DBS will necessarily include a better understanding of its mechanisms of actions and the optimization of stimulation parameters. In particular, the role of stimulation frequency will need further attention. Recent studies reported that lower stimulation frequencies may be effective on dystonia *(106)*, chorea *(118, 119)*, and parkinsonian gait *(120)*. These somewhat unexpected results seem to suggest that specific frequencies may differentially affect a variety of neurological symptoms. The study of these and other theoretical models (e.g., constant current vs constant voltage, asymmetrical pulses) will likely improve our ability to deliver safe and effective electrical therapy to human brains affected by basal ganglia disorders.

## References

1. Okun MS, Tagliati M, Pourfar M, et al (2005) Management of referred deep brain stimulation failures: a retrospective analysis from 2 movement disorders centers. Arch Neurol 2:1250–1255.
2. Moro E, Poon YY, Lozano AM, Saint-Cyr JA, Lang AE (2006) Subthalamic nucleus stimulation: improvements in outcome with reprogramming. Arch Neurol 63:1266–1272.
3. Koss AM, Alterman RL, Tagliati M, Shils JL (2005) Calculating total electrical energy delivered by deep brain stimulation systems. Ann Neurol 58:168–169.
4. Ranck JB Jr (1975) Which elements are excited in electrical stimulation of mammalian central nervous system: a review. Brain Res 98:417–440.
5. Moro E, Esselink RJ, Xie J, Hommel M, Benabid AL, Pollak P (2002) The impact on Parkinson's disease of electrical parameter settings in STN stimulation. Neurology 59:706–713.
6. Tagliati M, Shils J, Sun C, Alterman R (2004) Deep brain stimulation for dystonia. Expert Rev Med Devices 1:33–41.
7. Volkmann J, Herzog J, Kopper F, Deuschl G (2002) Introduction to the programming of deep brain stimulators. Mov Disord 17(Suppl 3):181–187.
8. Holsheimer J, Demeulemeester H, Nuttin B, de Sutter P (2000) Identification of the target neuronal elements in electrical deep brain stimulation. Eur J Neurosci 12:4573–4577.
9. Holsheimer J, Dijkstra EA, Demeulemeester H, Nuttin B (2000) Chronaxie calculated from current-duration and voltage-duration data. J Neurosci Methods 97:45–50.
10. Benabid AL, Pollak P, Gervason C, Hoffmann D, Gao DM, Hommel M, Perret JE, de Rougemont J (1991) Long-term suppression of tremor by chronic stimulation of the ventral intermediate thalamic nucleus. Lancet 337:403–406.

11. O'Suilleabhain PE, Frawley W, Giller C, Dewey RB Jr (2003) Tremor response to polarity, voltage, pulsewidth and frequency of thalamic stimulation. Neurology 60:786–790.
12. Kupsch A, Klaffke S, Kuhn AA, et al (2003) The effects of frequency in pallidal deep brain stimulation for primary dystonia. J Neurol 250:1201–1205.
13. Kumar R, Dagher A, Hutchison WD, Lang AE, Lozano AM (1999) Globus pallidus deep brain stimulation for generalized dystonia: clinical and PET investigation. Neurology 53:871–874.
14. Goto S, Mita S, Ushio Y (2002) Bilateral pallidal stimulation for cervical dystonia. An optimal paradigm from our experiences. Stereotact Funct Neurosurg 79: 221–227.
15. Alterman RL, Shils J, Miravite J, Tagliati M (2007) A lower stimulation frequency can enhance tolerability and efficacy of pallidal deep brain stimulation for dystonia. Mov Disord 22:366–368.
16. Montgomery EB Jr (2007) Deep brain stimulation. In Bakay RA, ed. Movement Disorder Surgery—The Essentials. New York: Thieme.
17. Baker KB, Montgomery EB Jr, Rezai AR, Burgess R, Luders HO (2002) Subthalamic nucleus deep brain stimulus evoked potentials: physiological and therapeutic implications. Mov Disord 17:969–983.
18. McIntyre CC, Mori S, Sherman DL, Thakor NV, Vitek JL (2004) Electric field and stimulating influence generated by deep brain stimulation of the subthalamic nucleus. Clin Neurophysiol 115:589–595.
19. McIntyre CC, Savasta M, Kerkerian-Le Goff L, Vitek JL (2004) Uncovering the mechanism(s) of action of deep brain stimulation: activation, inhibition, or both. Clin Neurophysiol 115:1239–1248.
20. Lang AE, Houeto JL, Krack, P, et al (2006) Deep brain stimulation: preoperative issues. Mov Disord 21(Suppl 14):171–196.
21. Rezai AR, Kopell BH, Gross RE, et al (2006) Deep brain stimulation for Parkinson's disease: surgical issues. Mov Disord 21(Suppl 14):197–218.
22. Fahn S, Elton R, Committee M. o. t. U. D (1987) In: Fahn S, Marsden C, Calne D, MG, eds. Recent Developments in Parkinson's Disease. Florham Park, NJ: Macmillan Health Care Information. 2:153–163, 293–304.
23. Defer GL, Widner H, Marie RM, Remy P, Levivier M (1999) Core assessment program for surgical interventional therapies in Parkinson's disease (CAPSIT-PD). Mov Disord 14:572–584.
24. Krack P, Fraix V, Mendes A, Benabid AL, Pollak P (2002) Postoperative management of subthalamic nucleus stimulation for Parkinson's disease. Mov Disord 17(Suppl 3):188–197.
25. Pahwa R, Lyons KE, Wilkinson SB, et al (2006) Long-term evaluation of deep brain stimulation of the thalamus. J Neurosurg 104:506–512.
26. Deuschl G, Schade-Brittinger C, Krack P, et al (2006) A randomized trial of deep-brain stimulation for Parkinson's disease. N Engl J Med 355:896–908.
27. Beric A, Kelly PJ, Rezai A, et al (2001) Complications of deep brain stimulation surgery. Stereotact Funct Neurosurg 77:73–78.
28. Hariz MI (2002) Complications of deep brain stimulation surgery. Mov Disord 17(Suppl 3):162–166.
29. Oh MY, Abosch A, Kim SH, Lang AE, Lozano AM (2002) Long-term hardware-related complications of deep brain stimulation. Neurosurgery 50:1268–1276.
30. Poulad D, Shils J, Tagliati M, Sullivan, Alterman R (2003) Proceedings of the Quadriennal Meeting of the ASSFN, New York.
31. Deuschl G, Herzog J, Kleiner-Fisman G, et al (2006) Deep brain stimulation: postoperative issues. Mov Disord 21(Suppl 14):219–237.
32. Volkmann J, Moro E, Pahwa R (2006) Basic algorithms for the programming of deep brain stimulation in Parkinson's disease. Mov Disord 21(Suppl 14):284–289.

33. Ilinsky IA, Kultas-Ilinsky K (2002) Motor thalamic circuits in primates with emphasis on the area targeted in treatment of movement disorders. Mov Disord 17(Suppl 3):9–14.
34. Mackel R (2001) Physiological evidence for spinal cord input to the motor thalamus. In: Ilinsky IA, Kultas-Ilinsky K, eds. Basal Ganglia and Thalamus in Health and Movement Disorders. New York: Kluwer/Academic/Plenum Publishers, pp. 105–116.
35. Ilinsky IA, Kultas-Ilinsky K (2001) Neuroanatomical organization and connections of the motor thalamus in primates. In: Ilinsky IA, Kultas-Ilinsky K, eds. Basal Ganglia and Thalamus in Health and Movement Disorders. New York: Kluwer/Academic/Plenum Publishers, pp. 77–91.
36. Kultas-Ilinsky K, Sivan-Loukianova E, Ilinsky IA (2003) Reevaluation of the primary motor cortex connections with the thalamus in primates. J Comp Neurol 457:133–158.
37. Taktakishvili O, Sivan-Loukianova E, Kultas-Ilinsky K, Ilinsky IA (2002) Posterior parietal cortex projections to the ventral lateral and some association thalamic nuclei in Macaca mulatta. Brain Res Bull 59:135–150.
38. Pollak P, Benabid AL, Limousin P Benazzouz A (1997) Chronic intracerebral stimulation in Parkinson's disease. Adv Neurol 74:213–220.
39. Koller W, Pahwa R, Busenbark K, et al (1997) High-frequency unilateral thalamic stimulation in the treatment of essential and parkinsonian tremor. Ann Neurol 42:292–299.
40. Limousin P, Speelman JD, Gielen F, Janssens M (1999) Multicentre European study of thalamic stimulation in parkinsonian and essential tremor. J Neurol Neurosurg Psychiatry 66:289–296.
41. Hariz MI, Shamsgovara P, Johansson F, Hariz G, Fodstad H (1999) Tolerance and tremor rebound following long-term chronic thalamic stimulation for Parkinsonian and essential tremor. Stereotact Funct Neurosurg 72:208–218.
42. Montgomery EB Jr, Baker KB, Kinkel RP, Barnett G (1999) Chronic thalamic stimulation for the tremor of multiple sclerosis. Neurology 53:625–628.
43. Louis ED, Barnes L, Wendt KJ, et al (2001) A teaching videotape for the assessment of essential tremor. Mov Disord 16:89–93.
44. Dowsey-Limousin P (2002) Postoperative management of VIM DBS for tremor. Mov Disord 17(Suppl 3)208–211.
45. Fahn S, Tolosa E, Marin C (1988) Clinical rating scale for tremor. In: Jankovic J, Tolosa E, eds. Parkinson's Disease and Movement Disorders. Baltimore, Munich: Urban & Schwarzenberg.
46. Benabid AL, Pollak P, Gao D, et al (1996) Chronic electrical stimulation of the ventralis intermedius nucleus of the thalamus as a treatment of movement disorders. J Neurosurg 84:203–214.
47. Albanese A, Nordera GP, Caraceni T, Moro E (1999) Long-term ventralis intermedius thalamic stimulation for parkinsonian tremor. Italian Registry for Neuromodulation in Movement Disorders. Adv Neurol 80:631–634.
48. Schuurman PR, Bosch DA, Bossuyt PM, et al (2000) A comparison of continuous thalamic stimulation and thalamotomy for suppression of severe tremor. N Engl J Med 342:461–468.
49. Kiss ZH, Anderson T, Hansen T, Kirstein D, Suchowersky O, Hu B (2003) Neural substrates of microstimulation-evoked tingling: a chronaxie study in human somatosensory thalamus. Eur J Neurosci 18:728–732.
50. Alesch F, Pinter MM, Helscher RJ, Fertl L, Benabid AL, Koos WT (1995) Stimulation of the ventral intermediate thalamic nucleus in tremor dominated Parkinson's disease and essential tremor. Acta Neurochir 136:75–81.
51. Deuschl G, Fogel W, Hahne, M, et al (2002) Deep-brain stimulation for Parkinson's disease. J Neurol 249(Suppl 3):36–39.

52. Pahwa R, Lyons KE, Wilkinson SB, Troster AI, Overman J, Kieltyka J, Koller WC (2001) Comparison of thalamotomy to deep brain stimulation of the thalamus in essential tremor. Mov Disord 16:140–143.
53. Bruyn RP (1989) Thalamic aphasia. A conceptional critique. J Neurol 236:21–25.
54. Caparros-Lefebvre D, Blond S, Vermersch P, Pecheux N, Guieu JD, Petit H (1993) Chronic thalamic stimulation improves tremor and levodopa induced dyskinesias in Parkinson's disease. J Neurol Neurosurg Psychiatry 56:268–273.
55. Kumar K, Kelly M, Toth C (1999) Deep brain stimulation of the ventral intermediate nucleus of the thalamus for control of tremors in Parkinson's disease and essential tremor. Stereotact Funct Neurosurg 72:47–61.
56. Lyons KE, Koller WC, Wilkinson SB, Pahwa R (2001) Long term safety and efficacy of unilateral deep brain stimulation of the thalamus for parkinsonian tremor. J Neurol Neurosurg Psychiatry 71:682–684.
57. Obwegeser AA, Uitti RJ, Witte RJ, Lucas JA, Turk MF, Wharen RE Jr (2001) Quantitative and qualitative outcome measures after thalamic deep brain stimulation to treat disabling tremors. Neurosurgery 48:274–284.
58. Voon V, Kubu C, Krack P, Houeto JL, Troster AI (2006) Deep brain stimulation: neuropsychological and neuropsychiatric issues. Mov Disord 21(Suppl 14): 305–327.
59. Tagliati M, Alterman R (2001) Guidelines for patient selection for ablative and deep brain stimulation surgery. Seminars Neurosurgery 17:193.
60. Limousin P, Krack P, Pollak P, Benazzouz A, Ardouin C, Hoffmann D, Benabid AL (1998) Electrical stimulation of the subthalamic nucleus in advanced Parkinson's disease. N Engl J Med 339:1105–1111.
61. Krack P, Pollak P, Limousin P, Benazzouz A, Deuschl G, Benabid AL (1999) From off-period dystonia to peak-dose chorea. The clinical spectrum of varying subthalamic nucleus activity. Brain 122:1133–1146.
62. Figueiras-Mendez R, Marin-Zarza F, Antonio Molina J, et al (1999) Subthalamic nucleus stimulation improves directly levodopa induced dyskinesias in Parkinson's disease. J Neurol Neurosurg Psychiatry 66:549–550.
63. Tagliati M, Huang N, Shils J (2002) Immediate relief of levodopa-induced dyskinesias after deep brain stimulation of the subthalamic nucleus in Parkinson's disease. Mov Disord 17:S199.
64. Shils J, Tagliati M, Miravite J (2002) Differential response of PD symptoms in the subthalamic nucleus during deep brain stimulation. Mov Disord 193.
65. Moro E, Scerrati M, Romito LM, Roselli R, Tonali P. Albanese A (1999) Chronic subthalamic nucleus stimulation reduces medication requirements in Parkinson's disease. Neurology 53:85–90.
66. Byrd DL, Marks WJ Jr, Starr PA (2000) Deep brain stimulation for advanced Parkinson's disease. Aorn J 72:387–390, 393–408; quiz 409–414, 416–418.
67. Thobois S, Corvaisier S, Mertens P, et al (2003) The timing of anti-parkinsonian treatment reduction after subthalamic nucleus stimulation. Eur Neurol 49:59–63.
68. (2001) Deep-brain stimulation for Parkinson's Disease Study Group. Deep-brain stimulation of the subthalamic nucleus or the pars interna of the globus pallidus in Parkinson's disease. N Engl J Med 345:956–963.
69. Molinuevo JL, Valldeoriola F, Tolosa E, Rumia J, Valls-Sole J, Roldan H, Ferrer E (2000) Levodopa withdrawal after bilateral subthalamic nucleus stimulation in advanced Parkinson disease. Arch Neurol 57:983–988.
70. O'Suilleabhain PE, Dewey RB Jr (2002) Contributions of dopaminergic drugs and disease severity to daytime sleepiness in Parkinson disease. Arch Neurol 59: 986–989.
71. Funkiewiez A, Ardouin C, Caputo E, et al (2004) Long term effects of bilateral subthalamic nucleus stimulation on cognitive function, mood, and behaviour in Parkinson's disease. J Neurol Neurosurg Psychiatry 75:834–839.

72. Krack P, Pollak P, Limousin P, Hoffmann D, Xie J, Benazzouz A, Benabid AL (1998) Subthalamic nucleus or internal pallidal stimulation in young onset Parkinson's disease. Brain 121:451–457.
73. Gschwandtner U, Aston J, Renaud S, Fuhr P (2001) Pathologic gambling in patients with Parkinson's disease. Clin Neuropharmacol 24:170–172.
74. Sanchez-Ramos J (2002) The straight dope on addiction to dopamimetic drugs. Mov Disord 17:223–225.
75. Burn DJ (2002) Beyond the iron mask: towards better recognition and treatment of depression associated with Parkinson's disease. Mov Disord 17:445–454.
76. Ardouin C, Pillon B, Peiffer E, et al (1999) Bilateral subthalamic or pallidal stimulation for Parkinson's disease affects neither memory nor executive functions: a consecutive series of 62 patients. Ann Neurol 46:217–223.
77. Berney A, Vingerhoets F, Perrin A, et al (2002) Effect on mood of subthalamic DBS for Parkinson's disease: a consecutive series of 24 patients. Neurology 59:1427–1429.
78. Kedia S, Moro E, Tagliati M, Lang AE, Kumar R (2004) Emergence of restless legs syndrome during subthalamic stimulation for Parkinson disease. Neurology 63:2410–2412.
79. Volkmann J, Allert N, Voges J, Weiss PH, Freund HJ, Sturm V (2001) Safety and efficacy of pallidal or subthalamic nucleus stimulation in advanced PD. Neurology 56:548–551.
80. Wycis Hat Spiegel EA (1969) Campotomy in myoclonia. J Neurosurg 30:708–713.
81. Shields DC, Lam S, Gorgulho A, Emerson J, Krahl SE, Malkasian D, DeSalles AA (2006) Eyelid apraxia associated with subthalamic nucleus deep brain stimulation. Neurology 66:1451–1452.
82. Mayberg HS, Lozano AM (2002) Penfield revisited? Understanding and modifying behavior by deep brain stimulation for PD. Neurology 59:1298–1299.
83. Houeto JL, Mesnage V, Mallet L, et al (2002) Behavioural disorders, Parkinson's disease and subthalamic stimulation. J Neurol Neurosurg Psychiatry 72:701–707.
84. Saint-Cyr JA, Trepanier LL, Kumar R, Lozano AM, Lang AE (2000) Neuropsychological consequences of chronic bilateral stimulation of the subthalamic nucleus in Parkinson's disease. Brain 123:2091–2108.
85. Alegret M, Junque C, Valldeoriola F, Vendrell P, Pilleri M, Rumia J, Tolosa E (2001) Effects of bilateral subthalamic stimulation on cognitive function in Parkinson disease. Arch Neurol 58:1223–1227.
86. Daniele A, Albanese A, Contarino MF, et al (2003) Cognitive and behavioural effects of chronic stimulation of the subthalamic nucleus in patients with Parkinson's disease. J Neurol Neurosurg Psychiatry 74:175–182.
87. Morrison CE, Borod JC, Perrine K, et al (2004) Neuropsychological functioning following bilateral subthalamic nucleus stimulation in Parkinson's disease. Arch Clin Neuropsychol 19:165–181.
88. Hariz MI, Johansson F, Shamsgovara P, Johansson E, Hariz GM, Fagerlund M (2000) Bilateral subthalamic nucleus stimulation in a parkinsonian patient with preoperative deficits in speech and cognition: persistent improvement in mobility but increased dependency: a case study. Mov Disord 15:136–139.
89. Dujardin K, Defebvre L, Krystkowiak P, Blond S, Destee A (2001) Influence of chronic bilateral stimulation of the subthalamic nucleus on cognitive function in Parkinson's disease. J Neurol 248:603–611.
90. Gironell A, Pascual-Sedano B, Otermin P, Kulisevsky J (2002) Weight gain after functional surgery for Parkinsons disease. Neurologia 17:310–316.
91. Macia F, Perlemoine C, Coman I, et al (2004) Parkinson's disease patients with bilateral subthalamic deep brain stimulation gain weight. Mov Disord 19:206–212.

92. Ramig LO, Sapir S, Fox C, Countryman S (2001) Changes in vocal loudness following intensive voice treatment (LSVT) in individuals with Parkinson's disease: a comparison with untreated patients and normal age-matched controls. Mov Disord 16:79–83.
93. Bronte-Stewart HM, Minn AY, Rodrigues K, Buckley EL, Nashner LM (2002) Postural instability in idiopathic Parkinson's disease: the role of medication and unilateral pallidotomy. Brain 125:2100–2114.
94. Bejjani BP, Damier P, Arnulf I, et al (1999) Transient acute depression induced by high-frequency deep-brain stimulation. N Engl J Med 340:1476–1480.
95. Shils J, Tagliati M, Alterman R (2002) In: Deletis V, Shils J, eds. Neurophysiology in Neurosurgery. Neurophysiological monitoring during neurosurgery for movement disorders. San Diego: Academic Press, pp. 393–436.
96. Parent A, Hazrati LN (1995) Functional anatomy of the basal ganglia. The cortico-basal ganglia-thalamo-cortical loop. Brain Res Brain Res Rev 20:91–127.
97. Patil AA, Hahn F, Sierra-Rodriguez J, Traverse J, Wang S (1998) Anatomical structures in the Leksell pallidotomy target. Stereotact Funct Neurosurg 70: 32–37.
98. Bejjani B, Damier P, Arnulf I, et al (1997) Pallidal stimulation for Parkinson's disease. Two targets? Neurology 49:1564–1569.
99. Krack P, Pollak P, Limousin P, et al (1998) Opposite motor effects of pallidal stimulation in Parkinson's disease. Ann Neurol 43:180–192.
100. Kumar R (2002) Methods for programming and patient management with deep brain stimulation of the globus pallidus for the treatment of advanced Parkinson's disease and dystonia. Mov Disord 17(Suppl 3)198–207.
101. Vidailhet M, Vercueil L, Houeto JL, et al (2005) Bilateral deep-brain stimulation of the globus pallidus in primary generalized dystonia. N Engl J Med 352:459–467.
102. Kupsch A, Benecke R, Muller J, et al (2006) Pallidal deep-brain stimulation in primary generalized or segmental dystonia. N Engl J Med 355:1978–1990.
103. Yianni J, Bain P, Giladi N, et al (2003) Globus pallidus internus deep brain stimulation for dystonic conditions: a prospective audit. Mov Disord 18:436–442.
104. Cif L, El Fertit H, Vayssiere N, et al (2003) Treatment of dystonic syndromes by chronic electrical stimulation of the internal globus pallidus. J Neurosurg Sci 47:52–55.
105. Coubes P, Roubertie A, Vayssiere N, Hemm S, Echenne B (2000) Treatment of DYT1-generalised dystonia by stimulation of the internal globus pallidus. Lancet 355:2220–2221.
106. Alterman RL, Miravite J, Weisz D, Shils JL, Bressman S and Tagliati M (2007) 60 Hertz pallidal DBS for primary torsion dystonia. Neurology 69:681–688.
107. Ghika J, Villemure JG, Fankhauser H, Favre J, Assal G, Ghika-Schmid F (1998) Efficiency and safety of bilateral contemporaneous pallidal stimulation (deep brain stimulation) in levodopa-responsive patients with Parkinson's disease with severe motor fluctuations: a 2-year follow-up review. J Neurosurg 89:713–718.
108. Burchiel KJ, Anderson VC, Favre J, Hammerstad JP (1999) Comparison of pallidal and subthalamic nucleus deep brain stimulation for advanced Parkinson's disease: results of a randomized, blinded pilot study. Neurosurgery 45:1375–1374.
109. Volkmann J, Allert N, Voges J, Sturm V, Schnitzler A, Freund HJ (2004) Long-term results of bilateral pallidal stimulation in Parkinson's disease. Ann Neurol 55:871–875.
110. Galvez-Jimenez, N, Lozano A, Tasker R, Duff J, Hutchison W, Lang AE (1998) Pallidal stimulation in Parkinson's disease patients with a prior unilateral pallidotomy. Can J Neurol Sci 25:300–305.
111. Volkmann J, Sturm V, Weiss P, et al (1998) Bilateral high-frequency stimulation of the internal globus pallidus in advanced Parkinson's disease. Ann Neurol 44:953–961.

112. Defebvre LJ, Krystkowiak P, Blatt JL, et al (2002) Influence of pallidal stimulation and levodopa on gait and preparatory postural adjustments in Parkinson's disease. Mov Disord 17:76–83.
113. Loher TJ, Burgunder JM, Pohle T, Weber S, Sommerhalder R, Krauss JK (2002) Long-term pallidal deep brain stimulation in patients with advanced Parkinson disease: 1-year follow-up study. J Neurosurg 96:844–853.
114. Troster AI, Fields JA, Wilkinson SB, Pahwa R, Miyawaki E, Lyons KE, Koller WC (1997) Unilateral pallidal stimulation for Parkinson's disease: neurobehavioral functioning before and 3 months after electrode implantation. Neurology 49:1078–1083.
115. Dujardin K, Krystkowiak P, Defebvre L, Blond S, Destee A (2000) A case of severe dysexecutive syndrome consecutive to chronic bilateral pallidal stimulation. Neuropsychologia 38:1305–1315.
116. Okun MS, Foote KD (2005) Subthalamic nucleus vs globus pallidus interna deep brain stimulation, the rematch: will pallidal deep brain stimulation make a triumphant return? Arch Neurol 62:533–536.
117. Stefani A, Lozano AM, Peppe A, et al (2007) Bilateral deep brain stimulation of the pedunculopontine and subthalamic nuclei in severe Parkinson's disease. Brain 130:1596–1607.
118. Moro E, Lang AE, Strafella AP, et al (2004) Bilateral globus pallidus stimulation for Huntington's disease. Ann Neurol 56:290–294.
119. Guehl D, Cuny E, Tison F, et al (2007) Deep brain pallidal stimulation for movement disorders in neuroacanthocytosis. Neurology 68:160–161.
120. Moreau C, Defevbre L, Krystkowiak P, et al (2007) Gait improvement by 60 hertz stimulation of the subthalamic nucleus in advanced parkinson's disease: A double blind clinical study. Neurology 68(Suppl.1):A101.
121. Hubble JP, Busenbark KL, Wilkinson S, Pahwa R, Paulson GW, Lyons K, Koller WC (1997) Effects of thalamic deep brain stimulation based on tremor type and diagnosis. Mov Disord 12:337–341.
122. Koller WC, Lyons KE, Wilkinson SB, Troster AI, Pahwa R (2001) Long-term safety and efficacy of unilateral deep brain stimulation of the thalamus in essential tremor. Mov Disord 16:464–468.
123. Vaillancourt DE, Sturman MM, Verhagen Metman L, Bakay RA, Corcos DM (2003) Deep brain stimulation of the VIM thalamic nucleus modifies several features of essential tremor. Neurology 61:919–925.
124. Rehncrona S, Johnels B, Widner H, Tornqvist AL, Hariz M, Sydow O (2003) Long-term efficacy of thalamic deep brain stimulation for tremor: double-blind assessments. Mov Disord 18:163–170.
125. Ushe M, Mink JW, Revilla FJ, et al (2004) Effect of stimulation frequency on tremor suppression in essential tremor. Mov Disord 19:1163–1168.
126. Lee JY, Kondziolka D (2005) Thalamic deep brain stimulation for management of essential tremor. J Neurosurg 103:400–403.
127. Kuncel AM, Cooper SE, Wolgamuth BR, et al (2006) Clinical response to varying the stimulus parameters in deep brain stimulation for essential tremor. Mov Disord 21:1920–1928.
128. Ostergaard K, Sunde N, Dupont E (2002) Effects of bilateral stimulation of the subthalamic nucleus in patients with severe Parkinson's disease and motor fluctuations. Mov Disord 17:693–700.
129. Romito LM, Scerrati M, Contarino MF, Bentivoglio AR, Tonali P, Albanese A (2002) Long-term follow up of subthalamic nucleus stimulation in Parkinson's disease. Neurology 58:1546–1550.
130. Vingerhoets FJ, Villemure JG, Temperli P, Pollo C, Pralong E, Ghika J (2002) Subthalamic DBS replaces levodopa in Parkinson's disease: two-year follow-up. Neurology 58:396–401.

131. Kleiner-Fisman G, Fisman DN, Sime E, Saint-Cyr JA, Lozano AM, Lang AE (2003) Long-term follow up of bilateral deep brain stimulation of the subthalamic nucleus in patients with advanced Parkinson disease. J Neurosurg 99:489–495.
132. Krack P, Batir A, Van Blercom N, et al (2003) Five-year follow-up of bilateral stimulation of the subthalamic nucleus in advanced Parkinson's disease. N Engl J Med 349:1925–1934.
133. Pahwa R, Wilkinson SB, Overman J, Lyons KE (2003) Bilateral subthalamic stimulation in patients with Parkinson disease: long-term follow up. J Neurosurg 99:71–77.
134. Herzog J, Volkmann J, Krack P, et al (2003) Two-year follow-up of subthalamic deep brain stimulation in Parkinson's disease. Mov Disord 18:1332–1337.
135. Rodriguez-Oroz MC, Obeso JA, Lang AE, et al (2005) Bilateral deep brain stimulation in Parkinson's disease: a multicentre study with 4 years follow-up. Brain 128:2240–2249.
136. Anderson VC, Burchiel KJ, Hogarth P, Favre J, Hammerstad JP (2005) Pallidal vs subthalamic nucleus deep brain stimulation in Parkinson disease. Arch Neurol 62:554–560.
137. Tornqvist AL, Schalen L, Rehncrona S (2005) Effects of different electrical parameter settings on the intelligibility of speech in patients with Parkinson's disease treated with subthalamic deep brain stimulation. Mov Disord 20:416–423.
138. Fraix V, Houeto JL, Lagrange C, et al (2006) Clinical and economic results of bilateral subthalamic nucleus stimulation in Parkinson's disease. J Neurol Neurosurg Psychiatry 77:443–449.
139. Bereznai B, Steude U, Seelos K, Botzel K (2002) Chronic high-frequency globus pallidus internus stimulation in different types of dystonia: a clinical, video, and MRI report of six patients presenting with segmental, cervical, and generalized dystonia. Mov Disord 17:138–144.
140. Krauss JK, Loher TJ, Weigel R, Capelle HH, Weber S, Burgunder JM (2003) Chronic stimulation of the globus pallidus internus for treatment of non-dYT1 generalized dystonia and choreoathetosis: 2-year follow up. J Neurosurg 98: 785–792.
141. Coubes P, Cif L, El Fertit H, et al (2004) Electrical stimulation of the globus pallidus internus in patients with primary generalized dystonia: long-term results. J Neurosurg 101:189–194.
142. Krause M, Fogel W, Kloss M, Rasche D, Volkmann J, Tronnier V (2004) Pallidal stimulation for dystonia. Neurosurgery 55:1361–1370.
143. Starr PA, Turner RS, Rau G, et al (2004) Microelectrode-guided implantation of deep brain stimulators into the globus pallidus internus for dystonia: techniques, electrode locations, and outcomes. Neurosurg Focus 17:E4.

# 21

# Neuropsychological Issues in Deep Brain Stimulation of Neurological and Psychiatric Disorders

Alexander I. Tröster, April B. McTaggart, and Ines A. Heber

**Abstract**

The past decade has seen an explosion in the number of medically refractory conditions and neuroanatomical structures targeted for DBS treatment. While a review of the literature and meta-analyses indicate DBS for movement disorders to be safe from a neurobehavioral standpoint it is also clear that a small subset of patients have experienced moderate or severe neurobehavioral morbidity. If one combines the various cognitive and psychiatric morbidities reported across studies, approximately 10% of patients with PD undergoing DBS have experienced one or another neurobehavioral adverse events. Furthermore, several small studies have indicated that improvements in motor symptoms and quality of life (QOL) may not necessarily translate into social readjustment. A greater role for ancillary health services, such as speech therapy, occupational and physical therapy, neuropsychology, and psychotherapy needs to be contemplated. Health care providers should not rely on subjective impression or spontaneous patient report to identify neurobehavioral and psychosocial issues. Recent consensus statements on patient selection, treatment, and outcome evaluation should facilitate greater uniformity in outcome reporting and identification of neurobehavioral risk.

What has proved elusive is the identification of reliable predictors and risk factors for such neurobehavioral changes. Ethical concerns and methodological limitations hinder the initiation of more sophisticated, controlled, blinded, comparative trials with large numbers of subjects needed to isolate predictors of neurobehavioral and QOL outcomes. Similarly, it is difficult to conclude at present that stimulation alone is associated with neurobehavioral morbidity, though in some cases, there are replicable effects on mood and cognition when stimulation is turned on and off. In the case of PD, and likely many of the disorders for which DBS is beginning to be investigated, outcomes may be related to an interaction of the surgical procedure and stimulation as well as subsequent changes in medications, psychosocial factors and pre-operative vulnerability. Conclusions that DBS is neuropsychologically safe in conditions such as dystonia, depression, obsessive compulsive diorder (OCD), Tourette syndrome (TS), epilepsy, multiple sclerosis (MS) and others must be considered highly preliminary until adequate controlled trials are completed. The emergence of cognitive and social neuroscience studies of DBS, particularly when accompanied by functional neuroimaging, are encouraging signs that DBS may be used as a vehicle to better understand the cognitive and behavioral roles of the basal ganglia.

**Keywords:** neuropsychology, cognition mood, quality of life, deep brain stimulation, Parkinson's disease, tremor, dystonia, epilepsy

## Introduction and Historical Overview

Neurosurgical interventions carried out during the 1950s and 1960s for movement disorders and psychiatric disorders almost entirely gave way to new medications by the early 1970s, while the neurosurgical treatment of intractable, chronic pain and epilepsy continued to evolve. Manifold factors underlie the divergent paths of functional neurosurgery for these various conditions, including the effectiveness, safety and availability of drug and other non-surgical therapies, ethical concerns, and the cost–benefit ratios associated with surgical procedures for different conditions. Disappointed by the limitations of pharmacotherapy and emboldened by technological advances in surgery, radiology, and a more refined understanding of pathophysiology, physicians and scientists charted the course of a renaissance of movement disorders surgery in the 1980s. Because even modern ablative neurosurgery, especially when carried out bilaterally, was associated with morbidity *(1, 2)*, a safer alternative was desired.

Based on the understanding of the pathophysiology of Parkinson's disease (PD), and observations that intra-operative electrical stimulation used for target identification could alleviate abnormal movements *(3, 4)*, chronic electrical stimulation of thalamus and basal ganglia (deep brain stimulation [DBS]) using fully implantable systems began to be explored *(5–7)*. Use of a similar, fully implantable DBS system came to be applied to epilepsy and psychiatric disorders in the late 1990s and 2000s. The reasons for this extension of DBS to other conditions probably parallel those spurring use of DBS in movement disorders: a need for safer surgical alternatives in patients deemed at risk for cognitive morbidity, such as persons with epilepsy and memory impairment *(8)*, a better understanding of the pathophysiology of corticostriatal-thalamic systems involved in neuropsychiatric disorders, and the intractability of some conditions to medication in a subset of patients. In addition, experience with DBS in movement disorders, observations about the cognitive and behavioral effects associated with DBS procedures in movement disorders, and availability of animal models facilitated extension of DBS to novel indications *(9–12)*.

A full historical review of surgical treatments for epilepsy, pain, movement disorders, and psychiatric conditions is beyond the scope of this chapter. Several reviews of the history of movement disorders surgery are available to the interested reader *(13–19)*, as are recent reviews of the history of functional neurosurgery in general *(20)*, psychosurgery *(21, 22)*, DBS for pain *(23, 24)*, and epilepsy *(25)*. It must be pointed out that electrical stimulation of various brain structures for neurological and psychiatric conditions is not a new endeavor. Acute electrical stimulation of the brain had been studied experimentally in humans as early as 1874 and for the localization of structure and/or function during neurosurgical operations on cortex *(26)*, and on deep brain structures *(27)*, and for relief of psychiatric illness prior to 1950 *(28)*. However, Delgado was the first to publish a peer-reviewed paper on the experimental use of chronically implanted electrodes in human brains *(29)*, and this report was followed shortly thereafter by those of Heath *(30, 31)* and Pool *(28)*. While chronically implanted electrodes connected to externalized bundles of wires began to be used for intermittent therapeutic stimulation in movement disorders in the 1960s *(32, 33)*, it was not until the late 1970s that a fully implantable system was used to treat movement disorders *(34)*.

Whereas early ablative studies tended to ignore neurobehavioral outcomes *(35)*, more attention has been paid to such outcomes in later studies and these findings have been reviewed in detail elsewhere *(36–38)*. Given the concern about the potential neurobehavioral morbidity associated with bilateral and ablative surgery for movement disorders, it is important to address neurobehavioral functioning and QOL outcomes of DBS. Similar evaluations of neurobehavioral and QOL outcomes have been conducted for some time for epilepsy surgery, and detailed neuropsychological evaluations are of particular importance in DBS for psychiatric conditions given the controversy and ethical issues surrounding psychosurgery and functional neurosurgery *(39–42)*. Some of the approved and investigational uses of DBS and the availability of neuropsychological outcome data relevant to various conditions and anatomical targets are listed in Table 21.1.

Consistent with the clinical focus of this volume, this chapter does not delve into the role that DBS might have in testing current models of brain–behavior relationships. Instead, the chapter focuses on neuropsychological evaluation and outcomes in neurosurgery for PD, and briefly explores the more limited literature pertaining to DBS for other movement disorders (essential tremor [ET] and dystonia) and other neurological and psychiatric conditions (epilepsy, multiple sclerosis [MS], cluster headache, Tourette's syndrome [TS], obsessive–compulsive disorder [OCD], depression, and aggression). Ablative neurosurgery has been used in China and Russia to treat opiate addiction *(43)* and, though DBS might be contemplated for such treatment, this practice faced considerable criticism and reportedly has ceased *(44, 45)*.

## Neuropsychological Evaluation: Purposes, Methods, and Interpretative Issues

The purposes, methods, and limitations of neuropsychological evaluation of patients with different conditions amenable or potentially amenable to DBS treatment overlap considerably. Some differences in the neurobehavioral domains assessed and tests used will emerge based upon empirical evidence concerning test sensitivity to the condition and treatment in question, known brain–behavior relationships and the pathophysiology of a given condition, the cognitive, motor, and sensory limitations of patients that might affect their ability to meet standardized test instruction comprehension and response requirements, and the local availability and relevance of tests.

Neuropsychological evaluation is a necessary component of the work-up of surgical candidates with PD, a fact highlighted by recent position and guideline papers *(46–49)*. A neuropsychological test battery has been recommended

**Table 21.1** Some established and current and past investigational indications for deep brain stimulation, targets (with sample reference), and availability of neuropsychological outcome data.

| Condition | Target | Established or Investigational | Availability of Published Neuropsychological Data |
|---|---|---|---|
| Parkinson's disease | STN *(5)*, GPi *(383)*, PPN *(384, 385)*, zona incerta *(386)*, motor cortex *(385)* | STN and GPi established | Moderate for STN and GPi |
| Tremor (ET, MS, Holmes, post-traumatic) | Ventral intermediate thalamic nucleus *(196, 387, 388)*, zona incerta *(389)* | VIM established | Limited for ET, very limited or absent for others |
| Dystonia | GPi *(390, 391)*, thalamus *(392)*, STN *(393)* | GPi established | Very limited |
| Tardive dystonia/dyskinesia | GPi *(394, 395)* | Investigational | Very limited or absent |
| Huntington's disease | GPi *(375, 396)* | Investigational | Absent |
| Multiple system atrophy (MSA) | GPi *(397)*, STN *(374)* | Investigational | Absent |
| Neuroacanthocytosis movement disorders | Thalamic *(398)*, GPi *(399)* | Investigational | Absent |
| Epilepsy | STN *(10)*, anterior thalamic nucleus *(350)*, centromedian thalamic nucleus *(352)*, caudate *(400)*, hippocampus *(8)*, cerebellum *(401)*, mammillary bodies and mammillothalamic tract *(354)* | Investigational | Very limited or absent |
| Pain | ventrocaudal (sensory) thalamus, periaqueductal grey, internal capsule, periventricular grey *(373, 402, 403)* | Investigational | Very limited or absent |
| Cluster headache | Hypothalamus *(371)* | Investigational | Absent |
| Depression | Subgenual cingulate *(11)*, thalamic peduncle *(359)*, caudate *(28)* | Investigational | Very limited or absent |
| Obsessive-compulsive disorder | Anterior limb of internal capsule *(12)*, nucleus accumbens *(363)*, caudate *(362)* | Investigational | Very limited or absent |
| Tourette's syndrome | Intralaminar thalamic nuclei *(404)*, GPi *(366, 368, 369)*, anterior limb of internal capsule *(405)* | Investigational | Very limited or absent |
| "Impulsive and violent behavior" | Posterior hypothalamus *(372)* | Investigational | Absent |

ET, essential tremor; MS, multiple sclerosis; GPi, globus pallidus internus, STN, subthalamic nucleus; PPN, pedunculopontine nucleus.

for evaluation of DBS candidates with TS *(50)*, and several suggestions have been made concerning screening and more extensive neuropsychological evaluation in movement disorders surgery *(47, 49, 51, 52)*. Similar recommendations have not been made for DBS for epilepsy, depression, or OCD. In the case of epilepsy, neuropsychological evaluation is an integral part of the evaluation of adult and pediatric surgical candidates *(53, 54)*. There is ample literature concerning ablative and vagus nerve stimulation procedures' neurobehavioral effects *(55–61)* that might guide test selection in epilepsy. Similarly, the literature on capsulotomy for OCD and other anxiety disorders *(62–67)* and on the effects of electroconvulsive therapy (ECT), repetitive

**Table 21.2** Purposes of neuropsychological evaluation for deep brain stimulation.

Pre-operative
- evaluate presence of surgery contraindications
- baseline for postoperative comparison
- differential diagnosis
- capacity to consent to treatment
- ability to cooperate and cope with pre-, peri- and postoperative care demands
- in some condition, to facilitate lateralization and localization of neuropathology

Postoperative
- documentation of surgical outcome
- rehabilitation planning
- detection of neurobehavioral effects of disease progression, seizures, medication, stimulation, mood disturbance, and external factors

transcranial magnetic stimulation (rTMS) and vagus nerve stimulation for depression *(59–61, 68–71)* might facilitate neuropsychological evaluation considerations in those conditions. Neuropsychological evaluation for DBS has different purposes, depending on whether the evaluation is carried out before or after surgery (Table 21.2).

**Purposes of Pre-Operative Neuropsychological Evaluation**

Pre-operative evaluation is typically carried out to determine whether selection and/or exclusion criteria for surgical intervention are met. In the case of PD, patients with executive dysfunction are at greater risk of developing dementia in the absence of surgical treatment *(72, 73)*, and prone to protracted confusional states after DBS *(74)*. Thus, even though not exclusionary, executive dysfunction needs to be considered in deciding whether or not to proceed with DBS. Despite absence of adequate empirical data, dementia is considered a relative contraindication and DBS in patients with dementia should only be carried out in exceptional medical and humanitarian circumstances after careful discussion and documentation of the issues and circumstances *(49)*. Older age may also be associated with poorer neurobehavioral outcomes but is not exclusionary, particularly because many studies have excluded patients above age 75 and thus, sufficient outcome data are not available *(49)*. Because DBS is an investigational treatment for epilepsy, pain, and several neuropsychiatric conditions, there are no published, widely agreed upon neurobehavioral inclusion and exclusion criteria.

Further reasons for pre-operative evaluation include establishment of a baseline against which to evaluate potential postoperative changes, and differential diagnosis if a patient meets an exclusionary criterion. For example, if a patient has dementia, is this dementia related to depression or medications and, thus, potentially reversible? Neuropsychological evaluation in epilepsy surgery is also used to provide corroborating evidence about the laterality and location of epileptic foci, prediction of postoperative seizure control, and neuropsychological outcome *(75)*. Evaluation can also assist in identifying persons with non-epileptic seizures even though individual tests probably do not yield consistent differences between those with nonepileptic and epileptic seizures *(76)*.

The capacity to consent to treatment, including the ability to perceive a choice to seek and refuse a given treatment, to choose among possible treatments, and the ability to appreciate the possible consequences of each of these courses of action, can be addressed by presurgical evaluation. Evaluation of cognition, mood state and coping can facilitate decisions regarding a patient's ability to cooperate with the arduous presurgical evaluation process, operation and postoperative care.

All this information can be used by the treatment team to provide the patient and family with tools to make a sound decision regarding the likely outcomes and risks of surgical intervention, or lack thereof. Careful discussion of expectations is indicated, because marital conflict may arise in cases where PD patient and caregiver expectations of post-surgical improvement and increased functional independence are unmet *(77)*. It may be that patients with milder PD have greater expectations for restoration of function *(78)* and thus, might be at greater risk of having unmet expectations. Similarly, unmet seizure reduction and psychosocial improvement expectations are associated with lesser postoperative satisfaction and poorer psychosocial outcome after ablative epilepsy surgery *(79–81)*, and the issue of pre-operative expectations and satisfaction with DBS in MS has also been addressed *(82)*.

**Purposes of Postoperative Neuropsychological Evaluation**

Postoperative neuropsychological evaluation is advocated at a minimum in PD patients in whom this is clinically indicated *(83)*, though an argument may be made for more systematic and thorough cognitive evaluation given the insensitivity of screening instruments to cognitive changes after STN DBS *(84)*. Postoperative evaluation is also done fairly routinely after epilepsy surgery, and certainly, given the very limited available neuropsychological outcome data for DBS in epilepsy, pain, TS, dystonia, OCD, and depression, there is an onus on clinicians and researchers to objectively document the neuropsychological safety and outcomes of investigational DBS.

In the event that "delayed" complications emerge, it becomes possible to determine via neuropsychological evaluation whether cognitive, emotional and behavioral changes are related to surgical intervention or operative complications, DBS, medications or other alternative treatments, disease progression, seizure activity, or emotional and psychosocial factors. In the event of significant neurobehavioral changes after surgery, postoperative evaluation can clearly delineate the extent and nature of these changes, thereby facilitating rehabilitation planning. Such intervention is of importance given that neurobehavioral symptoms not only compromise the PD patient's QOL, but also that of the care partner *(85)*, and because treatment side effects impact intractable epilepsy patients' and care partners' QOL *(86)*.

**Methods of Neuropsychological Evaluation**

Comprehensive neuropsychological evaluation entails a review of medical records, interviews with patient and family, observation of behavior, and administration and scoring of psychometric test instruments. These sources of information are integrated to arrive at a description of the patient's neurobehavioral strengths and weaknesses, inferences about the etiology of cognitive and emotional dysfunction, and the suitability of DBS intervention for that person. It is important to emphasize that, given the current state of knowledge about the neuropsychological effects of DBS and risk factors for morbidity, prognostic statements are best phrased in terms of broad bands of probability, such as a person being at average, greater than average, or less than average risk of neurobehavioral morbidity.

Several papers recommend specific tests to be employed in the neuropsychological evaluation of surgical candidates with PD *(47, 51, 52, 87)* and TS *(50)*, but no papers propose specific tests for the evaluation of DBS candidates with other disorders. Specific neuropsychological tests proposed for evaluation of PD surgery candidates by various position and review papers overlap, but are not identical. Because there is probably less disagreement about which areas of cognition to evaluate than about which specific tests to utilize, recent consensus statements have suggested the domains of neurobehavioral functioning to be evaluated and potential test choices for these domains rather than prescribed test batteries *(49)*. In addition, several general considerations in neuropsychological evaluation for PD surgery *(49)* and epilepsy *(88)* might apply to a range of disorders to be treated by DBS. Tests to be used in clinical decision making rather than research should be standardized, have adequate normative data, reliability, validity, and preferably test–retest data specifically for the condition being evaluated. Except in unusual circumstances, such as unavailability of standardized tests in a given country or language, experimental tests, while of utility in research studies, should not be used in clinical decision making. In addition, test selection should consider local relevance of tests, ethnicity, and culture of the test-taker. Limitations of tests should be considered and probably mentioned explicitly in clinical reports when such limitations might compromise the validity of the assessment.

Contents of test batteries for evaluation of DBS candidates with disorders such as MS, ET, dystonia, epilepsy, and neuropsychiatric disorders may ultimately be different than for PD, depending upon the neurobehavioral patterns and pathophysiology observed in those conditions and test sensitivity. However, until adequate data are available, a similar subset or core of neuropsychological tests, supplemented with tests specifically designed for or sensitive to cognitive and behavioral changes in a given condition, might be used in DBS evaluations for different conditions. Such use of overlapping test batteries would permit comparison of neurobehavioral outcomes across disorders. Indeed, an examination of tests recommended for evaluations in epilepsy surgery *(55)*, MS *(89–91)*, and already used in studies of DBS in epilepsy *(56)*, OCD *(92, 93)*, and depression *(11)* reveals a pre-existing overlap with tests recommended for use in PD and TS.

**Areas of Functioning Assessed in Neuropsychological Evaluations**

The domains of functioning assessed in most evaluations include intelligence or overall level of cognitive functioning, attention and working memory, executive functions, language, visuoperceptual and spatial functions, motor function,

**Table 21.3** Examples of standardized tests used in neuropsychological evaluation for deep brain stimulation.

| Type of Test | Specific Tests |
|---|---|
| Estimate of pre-morbid function | North American Adult Reading Test, Barona Demographic Equations, Wechsler Test of Adult Reading |
| General cognitive functioning | Raven's Progressive Matrices, Wechsler Adult Intelligence Scale, Wechsler Abbreviated Scale of Intelligence (WASI), Kaufman Brief Intelligence Test, Mattis Dementia Rating Scale, Mini Mental Status Examination,[2] Cambridge Cognitive Examination[2] |
| Language | Controlled Oral Word Association Test,[3] Boston Diagnostic Aphasia Examination's Animal Naming and Boston Naming Tests, Multilingual Aphasia Examination's Sentence Repetition and Token Test |
| Attention and working memory | Paced Auditory Serial Attention Test (PASAT), Stroop Color and Word Interference Test, Brief Test of Attention, Digit and Visual Memory (Spatial) Span, WMS-III Letter-Number Sequencing, Digit Symbol/Symbol Digit, Trailmaking Test[3] |
| Executive function | Wisconsin Card Sorting Test (or WCST-64), Cognitive Estimation Test, Booklet Category Test, Delis-Kaplan Executive Function System, Matrix Reasoning, Tower tests |
| Memory | Benton Visual Retention Test, Wechsler Memory Scales (revisions) Logical Memory, Rey-Osterreith Complex Figure Test (not for patients with notable motor impairment), Rey Auditory Verbal Learning Test, Hopkins Verbal Learning Test,[3] California Verbal Learning Test-II, Wechsler Memory Scale III Family Pictures and Faces; Selective Reminding Test |
| Motor | Finger Tapping, Grooved Pegboard (for patients with mild movement disorder)[3] |
| Visuoperceptual-spatial | Benton Judgment of Line Orientation,[3] Benton Facial Recognition Test, Benton Visual Discrimination Test, Hooper Visual Organization Test, Block Design |
| Mood and personality | Profile of Mood States, Beck Depression Inventory,[1] State-Trait Anxiety Inventory, Zung Depression Index, Beck Anxiety Inventory, Minnesota Multiphasic Personality Inventory (MMPI), Frontal Systems Behavior Scale (FrSBe), Hospital Anxiety and Depression Scale, Neuropsychiatric Inventory, Montgomery-Åsberg Depression Scale,[1] Hamilton Depression Rating Scale or Inventory,[1] Hamilton Anxiety Rating Scale |
| Quality of life | Sickness Impact Profile (SIP), Parkinson's Disease Questionnaire (PDQ), Nottingham Health Profile, Quality of Life in Epilepsy Inventory (QOLIE), Quality of Life in Depression Scale |
| Stressors | Life Stressors and Social Resources Inventory |
| Coping | Coping Responses Inventory |
| Experimental tasks | Tower of London (or Hanoi or Toronto), Conditional Associative Learning Test, Emotional Stroop task |
| Computerized or Web-based tests | CANTAB |

[1]Recommended by the American Academy of Neurology Practice Parameter *(406)* for screening of depression in Parkinson's disease
[2]Recommended by the American Academy of Neurology Practice Parameter *(406)* for screening of dementia in Parkinson's disease
[3]Recommended for assessment for DBS for Tourette's syndrome *(50)*

memory, mood state, and QOL. We also recommend a formal assessment of coping responses and stressors. Examples of tests of each of these domains, many of which have been used in published studies of movement disorders surgery, epilepsy surgery, and MS are listed in Table 21.3.

### *Intelligence*

Except in cases of dementia, intelligence is preserved in PD, ET, dystonia, OCD, depression, and MS. Nonetheless, PD patients may perform poorly on some tests of the Wechsler scales (particularly some of the Performance scale subtests which are timed and have significant motor demands) due to bradyphrenia and bradykinesia. The pattern of lower Performance than Verbal IQs in MS, when observed, may be attributable to sensory and motor factors *(94)*. In epilepsy, lower intelligence has been associated with seizure onset before age 5, extent of cortical dysplasia, greater frequency of generalized seizures, repeated status epilepticus, type of seizure syndrome (e.g., Landau-Kleffner), seizure type (generalized tonic-clonic), and even medications (e.g., lamotrigine, Phenobarbital; ref. *95*). However, declines in intelligence can also be observed in focal epilepsies such as mesial temporal lobe epilepsy *(96)*.

In practice it is rare that a patient has previously undergone intelligence testing while healthy (i.e., premorbidly). Consequently, indirect methods (such as performance on oral word reading tests resistant to decline subsequent to cerebral dysfunction, or equations utilizing demographic information) are used to estimate premorbid intelligence and infer whether current performance represents a decline from once higher levels.

### Cognitive Screening

Brief screening measures, or measures of overall level of cognitive functioning, are convenient and inexpensive to use. However, such scales may lack sensitivity, meaning that impaired performance is revealing of disease, but intact performance does not imply absence of mild to moderate or selective cognitive deficits. Consequently, use of such a test early in the evaluation process is helpful in sparing the significantly impaired patient further arduous testing for surgical evaluation (although further testing may be indicated for differential diagnosis).

### Attention and Working Memory

Working memory is a limited-capacity, multi-component system involved in the temporary storage and manipulation of information. This system, and the allocation of attention resources, is often compromised by PD, some of the medications used to treat the disease, and by surgical treatments *(97–100)*. Working memory is usually preserved in mesial temporal lobe epilepsy *(96)*, but may be compromised in persons with focal frontal and generalized epilepsies *(101, 102)*. Antiepileptic drugs (AEDs) may also impair attention and working memory *(103)*. Attentional and working memory deficits are relatively common in MS *(104)*, are seen to variable extent in depression *(105)*, and have recently been observed in ET *(106)* and dystonia *(107)*.

### Executive Functions

Executive functions include conceptualization, abstraction, planning, insight, cognitive flexibility, the ability to monitor, regulate, and initiate and inhibit responses. These functions depend, among other factors, on frontal lobe and fronto-striatal integrity and are vulnerable to PD and its surgical treatment *(84, 108, 109)*. Executive function deficits are also among the most prominent of the cognitive alterations observed in OCD *(110, 111)* and depression *(105, 112)* and have been observed in as many as one third of persons with MS *(113)*. Although cognition is thought to be intact in ET and dystonia, subtle changes in executive functions have been reported in both ET *(106, 114–118)* and some but not all studies of dystonia *(107, 119–121)*. Executive deficits are also observed in TS *(122)* and poor performance on tasks of conceptualization and cognitive flexibility may be related to the obsessive characteristics often observed in TS *(123)*.

Assessment of executive functions is of particular relevance and importance in DBS candidates with PD, because executive deficit in PD is linked to diminution of capacity to consent to medical treatment *(124)*, ability to carry out instrumental activities of daily living *(125)*, and capacity to deploy a range of effective coping strategies *(126)*. Similarly, seemingly mild cognitive deficits in MS can compromise ability to engage in activities of daily living *(127)*, and in adults and children with epilepsy, neuropsychological, and especially executive function, is related to independent living and/or behavioral adaptation *(128, 129)*.

### Language

Performance on verbal fluency tasks, requiring oral generation within a time limit of words beginning with a given letter of the alphabet, or belonging to a given semantic category such as animals, is frequently disrupted by neurosurgical interventions for PD *(36, 130)*. Verbal fluency may or may not be disrupted in PD without dementia, but almost always is disrupted in dementia *(131)*. Verbal fluency impairments may be a harbinger of incipient dementia in PD *(73, 132, 133)*. In contrast to verbal fluency, other language functions such as repetition, comprehension, word knowledge, and visual confrontation naming are preserved in PD. When impairments are observed in such functions, the diagnostic possibility of a dementia, especially one not due to PD, needs to be considered.

Language functions are rarely disturbed in OCD and depression, although performance on timed fluency tasks may be *(134)*. Language functions are also rarely affected in MS and decrements in verbal fluency tasks may reflect information processing speed or word retrieval difficulties *(94)*. Patients with temporal lobe epilepsy (TLE), and especially left TLE, as a group show impairments in naming and verbal fluency *(135, 136)*, though such deficits may be observed in only a minority of patients *(137)*. In addition, despite precautionary measures such as language mapping by functional neuroimaging or electrical cortical stimulation, language may decline after temporal lobectomy *(135)*.

### Visuoperceptual Functions

Visuoperceptual deficits have been observed in numerous studies of PD, but not in others, and it is also a matter of debate whether these deficits are true visuoperceptual deficits or secondary to executive deficits *(138)*. Surgical treatment has only rarely been reported to impact these functions. Visuoperceptual disturbances have been among the more commonly reported cognitive changes in OCD, though they can be quite mild *(110)* and may be seen only in persons with OCD onset after age 21 *(134)*. Difficulties with facial processing and spatial judgment occur in about 10 to 20% of patients with MS *(104)*. Impoverished visuospatial task performance can also be observed in mesial TLE *(96)*. Visuomotor integration deficits are among the most common observed deficits in TS *(122)*. In contrast, visuospatial skills are usually preserved in ET, dystonia, and depression.

## Memory and Learning

Profound memory impairment is not a hallmark of PD. The ability to recall new information is generally compromised, but recognition is relatively intact. Such dissociation between recall and recognition has been interpreted as indicating a retrieval deficit in PD. While this interpretation is probably correct, there is evidence that PD patients also have encoding deficits (139). The exact extent to which encoding and retrieval deficits reflect executive deficits remains debated (140). Similarly, both encoding and retrieval deficits probably underlie the memory impairments commonly observed in MS (141, 142), and depression (143, 144). In contrast, TLE has been associated with memory impairments related to deficient encoding, storage, and retrieval (145). Though there are often assumed to be material-specific memory differences between left and right TLE, these differences have been difficult to elicit reliably, and verbal memory deficits are probably more readily appreciated in left TLE than are nonverbal memory deficits in right TLE (96). Frontal epilepsy surgery may impact memory indirectly (146). Although verbal memory impairment is rarely found in OCD, some patients have difficulty organizing memoranda for later retrieval (147) and nonverbal memory impairment is observed quite consistently (147). Remote memory (recollection of information from the distant past) is preserved in PD, and a retrograde amnesia is typically associated only with dementia (148).

Nonverbal memory tests with significant motor components are not recommended in surgical candidates with PD given their severe motor disability (bradykinesia, tremor, dyskinesia) and motor fluctuations. The Wechsler Memory Scale –III includes several visual tasks without motor components (Faces and Family Pictures) that are more appropriate.

## Mood State and Behavioral Symptoms

Anxiety and depression symptoms are common in PD: about 50% of persons with PD become depressed at some point during their illness (149, 150), and a similar lifetime risk of depression has been reported for MS (151). Depression is the most common psychiatric comorbidity in patients with epilepsy, and 40 to 60% of persons with TLE may have depression (152). Assessment of depression is of particular relevance in DBS candidates for at least three reasons: depression can exacerbate cognitive impairment in PD (153–155) and MS (156); depression has been associated with poorer surgical outcome in movement disorders (157); and pre-operative depression confers higher risk of continued depression after epilepsy surgery (81, 158). Depression also compromises the patient's cooperation during surgery while awake and reduces resources to cope with peri- and postoperative stressors. It is probably prudent to treat and re-evaluate the patient with marked depression before making a final decision about the appropriateness of surgical treatment (49).

Assessment of anxiety may also allow prognosis concerning patient ability to cooperate with an arduous evaluation and surgical procedure. In assessing anxiety by questionnaires, care should be taken to scrutinize items that are endorsed. Many questionnaires contain symptom items that might reflect symptoms of PD rather than anxiety (159). Patients who report phobic experiences and generalized anxiety may have difficulty tolerating an MRI procedure without sedation. In our experience, patients who have difficulty dealing with the stress of a neuropsychological evaluation prior to surgery are more apt to have difficulty tolerating protracted work-up and surgery. Patient education, including preparation for surgery, can be extremely helpful in this regard.

Because surgical intervention can lead to "frontal" personality changes or exaggeration of presurgical behavioral characteristics and psychopathology *(160)*, evaluation of personality structure by interview or formal assessment is indicated. Measures that have been used in PD include the Neuropsychiatric Inventory *(161)*, the Frontal Lobe Personality Scale *(162)* (now called the Frontal Systems Behavior Scale *[163]*) and the Minnesota Multiphasic Personality Inventory *(164)*, although the latter is long and difficult to complete for the patient who easily fatigues and has a movement disorder. Personality and mood assessment is also often used in epilepsy surgery *(165, 166)*, and is obviously required in DBS for neuropsychiatric disorders.

### Stressors and Coping

Informal assessment is frequently made of patients' stressors, resources, and coping mechanisms during the interview. However, self-report questionnaires, permitting a quantitative assessment, are also available. The importance of considering a person's response to stress in predicting movement disorder surgery outcome was already commented upon by Diller et al. in 1956 *(167)*. Stressors can contribute to anxiety and depression, and an assessment of current stressors permits judgments about the timing of surgery. In general, if a patient has numerous other ongoing stressors, one might consider delaying surgery until these stressors are resolved. The evaluation, surgical procedure, and recovery may be stressful and adding such significant stressors to an already stressful environment heightens risk for exacerbation of mood disturbance.

The impact that stressors have on a patient is mediated by social resources (such as financial reserves, social support networks) and coping mechanisms. The patient with significant stressors, limited social assets, and restricted coping abilities is likely to be a poorer surgical candidate than one who has significant stressors but a wide range of assets and is able to utilize a diversity of coping strategies. For example, greater social resources and fewer stressors have been associated with a better QOL after pallidotomy *(168)*.

### Quality of Life

Adequate definitions and conceptualizations of QOL are elusive. Pragmatically, health-related QOL is defined as the patient's perception and evaluation of the impact that an illness, its treatment, and its consequences have on their life. In general, most agree that physical, psychological, social, economic, vocational, and spiritual factors contribute to overall QOL. QOL is not only becoming an outcome measure of increasing significance in its own right *(169)*, but QOL measures form the basis of modern cost-effectiveness analyses, including of DBS *(170)*. Assessment of QOL is particularly important in movement disorders surgery because the treatment is not curative but designed primarily to improve function and QOL *(171, 172)*. Explicit evaluation of QOL in surgery for movement disorders *(173–175)* and in neurosurgery more generally *(176)* is of recent origin. Assessment of QOL in epilepsy surgery has a more robust history, particularly since such assessment was recommended by consensus in 1990 *(177)*.

Measures of QOL and functional status fall into two broad categories: generic and disease-specific. The advantage of generic measures is that they permit comparison of QOL across diseases and conditions. Disease-specific measures, in contrast, earn their utility from their sensitivity to issues specific and important to individuals with a given disease. In ideal circumstances, assessment should be achieved using both generic and disease-specific measures. Numerous disease-specific QOL measures are now available for PD and DBS *(178–180)*, epilepsy and epilepsy surgery *(181)*, MS *(182)*, ET *(183)*, and depression *(184)*.

## Interpretative and Practical Challenges for the Neuropsychologist

Several issues need be kept in mind while planning the evaluation of patients before and after DBS and in comparing and interpreting pre-and postoperative test results.

### *Medication Effects*

Dopaminergic drugs can impact cognitive functions, and in particular working memory and executive functions, although effects on different functions within a given domain of cognition can be heterogeneous *(99, 131, 185)*. Antiepileptic medications can adversely affect attention, reaction time, language, and memory *(186, 187)*. Antidepressants can have both negative and positive effects on cognition *(188)*. Patients should always be questioned about when they take their medication and asked to bring medications with them to appointments. Deviations from dosage regimens may result in unpredictable fluctuations in motor symptoms of patients with movement disorders or inadequate seizure control in patients with epilepsy, thus complicating neuropsychological testing. The complete (neurologic, neuropsychological, neurodiagnostic and neurosurgical) pre-surgical work-up is time consuming and extensive, sometimes necessitating evaluation over more than one day. It is preferable for the patient to be tested on their usual medications, and indeed this has been formally recommended in the case of PD *(49)*.

Medication effects also need to be considered in comparing pre- and postoperative test performance. Particularly after subthalamic DBS, medication dosage is often dramatically reduced. Although such effect is expected to be mild, medication reduction can both positively and negatively impact cognitive functions and mood state. Of greater complexity is the possibly interactive effect of surgery and medication: it has recently been shown that pallidotomy may alter the effect levodopa has on certain cognitive functions *(189)*. Alterations in medication regimens after surgery can similarly complicate interpretation of neuropsychological evaluation results in epilepsy and neuropsychiatric conditions.

### *Consideration of Motor Symptoms and Seizures*

Neuropsychological evaluation is extremely challenging when the parkinsonian patient is in the "off" state. Not only may the patient be bradykinetic, in a "frozen" state, and bradyphrenic, but also speech may become so hypophonic and dysarthric as to be unintelligible. Although comparison of cognitive functioning in the "on" and "off" states is of interest, such a comparison is rarely feasible from a practical standpoint. Consequently, it is recommended that patients be tested, so far as possible, within their self-described "on" state. Surgical candidates may have levodopa or dopamine agonist induced dyskinesias during portions of the "on" state. The best way to achieve a valid neuropsychological evaluation is to plan ahead: the patient and caregiver should be questioned about duration of "on" state, occurrence and duration of dyskinesias, and duration of "off" state. The rapidly fluctuating patient presents a particular challenge, and testing may have to be interrupted where feasible and spread over several relatively brief sessions. Consideration also needs to be given to the motor and vocal tics of patients with TS and the postural abnormalities and painful muscle contractions of persons with dystonia. Similarly, the extent and nature of motor deficits in patients with MS should be considered in planning the evaluation and potential accommodations in the test process.

The patient with epilepsy should be evaluated interictally. If a seizure occurs during testing, it is helpful to know from interview or history how long it typically takes a patient to return to a pre-ictal cognitive state and for possible confusion to clear. Evaluation should be carried out once the patient's sensorium and confusion have cleared, though brief, informal evaluation of memory and observation of language or speech arrest during a seizure can be informative.

### *Practice Effects*

When individuals undergo repeated evaluations using the same or similar test instruments, it is conceivable that scores may "improve" because the individual remembers and has experience with the test. Several strategies are available to minimize practice effects, such as utilizing alternate test forms (two versions of the test differing in specific content, but not difficulty), maximizing the test–retest interval, or utilizing statistical techniques *(190, 191)*. Even when alternate test forms are used, a familiarity effect may occur, meaning the individual performs better on tests due to becoming more test sophisticated or "test wise".

An important issue is whether comparable test–retest effects observed in normative samples are evident in clinical populations. There is some suggestion that such practice effects may not occur in PD on numerous tests *(192)*. If a practice effect does not occur in PD, then possible score gains after surgery represent improvements rather than practice effects. Conversely, if practice effects are seen in PD, than a lack of gain might actually represent a decline, and a score gain would have to exceed the practice effect before it is considered an "improvement." Of greater complexity in interpreting individual patient test score changes is the issue of a possible interaction between surgery, medication, stimulation and practice effects.

Similar considerations apply to repeated evaluations of persons with other disorders, and in some instances, normative data (such as reliable change indices) are available to facilitate determination of whether a test score change is significant or unusual in epilepsy *(193, 194)*, and statistical methods are available to calculate similar indices for other disorders *(195)*.

### *Length and Breadth of Test Battery and the Role of Screening*

Saint-Cyr and Trépanier *(52)*, York and colleagues *(191)*, and Green and Barnhart *(190)* have commented on the issue of how long a test battery for PD surgery candidates should be, and whether the battery should be broad or narrow in focus. Given the fatigability and motor fluctuations of most PD surgery candidates, the battery should be as short as possible, but still broad enough to answer the referral question and to develop clear and valid diagnostic and prognostic impressions. Similar considerations drive the selection of tests within a battery of tests for other conditions, such as epilepsy, MS, dystonia, depression, TS, and OCD.

In clinical endeavors we suggest that the test battery be selected on the basis of: a) referral question; b) known neurobehavioral effects of a given disease; c) known neurobehavioral risks of a given treatment; d) patient ability to cooperate with tests; and e) findings uncovered during evaluation. Choice of specific tests is also based on consideration of each test's assets and liabilities (normative data, test–retest data, validity and reliability, availability of alternate forms, sensitivity, and ability of the test to delineate mechanisms underlying deficient task performance).

While persons selected to undergo DBS should undergo full neuropsychological evaluation, it seems reasonable that persons suspected to have severe cognitive or psychiatric impairments that might contraindicate DBS undergo a shorter screening examination so as to reduce patient burden. Indeed, it has been recommended that, in the case of PD, patients failing screening be referred only for full neuropsychological evaluation if the failure is borderline or if the reason for failure is unclear and might be due to reversible, transient, or educational, cultural and linguistic factors *(49)*. Furthermore, decisions about a candidate's neuropsychological suitability for DBS should never be based on a single test or test score. It should also be noted that cognitive screening measures should be used as such; their lack of sensitivity suggests that they are probably inadequate as outcome measures.

## DBS and Neurobehavioral Outcomes in PD

### Thalamic Stimulation

*Cognition, Language, and Memory*
One study mentions in passing that no significant neuropsychological deficits were observed in 10 PD patients after thalamic DBS *(196)*. However, only three studies have reported detailed neuropsychological outcomes after thalamic DBS for PD. Neither Caparros-Lefebvre et al. *(197)* nor Tröster and co-workers *(198)* found changes in overall level of cognitive functioning in their small samples of nine patients after surgery. Similarly, in their heterogeneous sample of five PD, two ET, and two MS patients undergoing unilateral thalamic DBS, Loher and colleagues *(199)* failed to find global cognitive changes. In contrast to thalamotomy, thalamic stimulation, at least in PD, seems to be unassociated with declines in verbal fluency or memory, though Loher et al. did find, in a comparison of patients on and off stimulation, statistically significantly poorer verbal memory in those having left thalamic DBS. Studies have also reported some improvements (possibly practice effects) on certain tasks. Caparros–Lefebvre et al. observed better performance on a card sorting task 4 to 10 days after surgery, while Tröster et al. found that patients demonstrated improved delayed recall of prose and recognition of a word list, and somewhat better naming, about 4 months after surgery. In a 12-month follow-up of five patients reported upon by Tröster et al. *(198)*, Woods and colleagues *(200)* found that gains in verbal fluency and memory were maintained.

Interpretation of post-DBS changes in cognition is probably even more complex than interpretation of changes after ablation. In addition to medication and/or test practice effects, neurobehavioral changes may reflect a transient microthalamotomy effect. Furthermore, effects on cognition may depend on stimulation parameters (unipolar vs. bipolar; amplitude, frequency, pulse width). The importance of considering stimulation parameters is amplified by the findings of Hugdahl and colleagues *(201–203)*. These authors found that intra-operative high-frequency stimulation did not predict the effect on memory of thalamotomy; this is in contrast to the prediction of post-thalamotomy memory deficits afforded by low-frequency stimulation *(204)*.

Interpretative complexities of DBS effects on cognition are also illustrated by a case study. Tröster and colleagues *(205)* evaluated cognitive functioning in a PD patient before surgery, and in four conditions after surgery: with the stimulator turned on when the patient was either on or withdrawn from medication, and again with the stimulator turned off, while the patient was either on or off medication. A postoperative decrement in verbal fluency was observed, but stimulation in both medication conditions was associated with improved verbal fluency. In essence, based on this case, surgery and stimulation apparently may have opposite effects on this function.

### *Mood State, Behavioral Changes, and QOL*

Caparros-Lefebvre et al. *(197)* found an improvement in mood state (depressive symptoms) 4 to 10 days after surgery. QOL improvements did not attain statistical significance in the study by Straits-Tröster et al. *(206)*, but this may reflect the fact that a generic QOL measure, probably less sensitive to change than a disease-specific measure was used, and that the sample was small. Indeed, among five patients, QOL gains on the disease-specific PDQ were still observed 12 months after unilateral thalamic DBS *(200)*. Alternatively, the lack of significant QOL impact of thalamic DBS (which alleviates tremor), may reflect the observation that tremor may be a less important determinant of QOL in PD than other symptoms such as bradykinesia, postural instability, and gait difficulties *(207)*.

### **Pallidal Stimulation**

#### *Cognition, Language, and Memory*

Tröster and colleagues *(208)*, in nine patients undergoing unilateral pallidal DBS, found that none of the patients experienced significant changes in overall level of cognitive functioning 3 months after surgery. As a group, the patients demonstrated statistically significant declines in visuoconstructional ability and in verbal fluency, but the changes were rarely of clinical significance.

Subsequent studies have yielded similar findings. Vingerhoets et al. *(209)*, in 20 patients, found no statistically significant declines in cognitive functioning after unilateral pallidal DBS. These authors also calculated an impairment index (percentage of measures falling below impairment criterion) for each patient. Using an extremely liberal criterion of impairment (a score falling 1 SD below the mean of normative samples), they noted that only six of the 20 patients showed *any* decrement (i.e., any magnitude increase in percentage of tests in the impaired range). These patients tended to be older and were taking higher medication dosages prior to surgery than patients showing no change or improvement. Merello et al. *(210)*, among six unilateral GPi DBS cases, observed no significant changes in mean scores on neuropsychological tests, but this might reflect the lack of statistical power attributable to the small sample size.

Safety of bilateral GPi DBS has been addressed in only a few studies, but the majority of these suggest that the procedure is relatively safe from a cognitive standpoint. Ardouin et al. *(211)*, among 13 bilateral GPi DBS cases, found no significant changes in average test scores 3 months (Grenoble subjects, $n = 8$) or 6 months (Paris subjects, $n = 5$) after surgery. Pillon et al. *(212)* found no cognitive morbidity, using clinical tests, in a very similar group of patients at 12-month follow-up. Unlike STN patients, the performance on experimental tasks of five GPi patients at 6 months was no different on and off levodopa. Ghika et al. *(213)* found no significant changes in neuropsychological test scores 3 months after bilateral GPi DBS electrode implantation in six patients.

To determine whether the second surgery carries cognitive risks relative to the first surgery, Fields et al. *(214)* examined neuropsychological functioning in six patients undergoing staged bilateral GPi DBS electrode implantation. Patients were evaluated before surgery, 2 months after the first operation, and again 3 months after the second operation. No patient experienced significant declines in cognition and delayed recall was improved relative to baseline following the second operation. Rothlind and colleagues *(215)* recently reported on a randomized comparison of staged, bilateral GPi and STN DBS in 42 patients and found that minimal cognitive changes ensued from the second relative to the first operation. However, semantic verbal fluency declined after left DBS regardless of whether the left side was operated first or second. Though phonemic verbal fluency also declined only after left DBS, a significant effect of the second surgery was not demonstrated.

Only a single case study with MRI-confirmed electrode location has reported significant executive dysfunction after bilateral GPi DBS *(216)*. Importantly, this study indicates the role stimulation played in this impairment. When the stimulators were turned off, the impairment was partially reversed. Relatively isolated cognitive impairments were reported by the Toronto group *(217)*. Among four patients, there was a significant decrease only in backward digit span. Verbal fluency testing was administered to only one patient, who demonstrated a decline on this task. The decline sometimes seen in verbal fluency after GPi DBS *(208, 218)* may be related to word search or executive strategy changes: patients seem to shift less efficiently between word categories when searching for words *(219)*.

Whether unilateral GPi DBS is cognitively safer than pallidotomy has not been adequately addressed, but studies by Merello et al. *(210)* and Fields et al. *(220)* found the cognitive safety of the procedures to be comparable. Although, there is suggestion to date that bilateral GPi DBS may entail less cognitive morbidity than bilateral STN DBS *(221–223)*, the only randomized comparison of the cognitive effects of GPi and STN DBS has failed to show substantial differences between the two treatments *(215)*. Whereas Digit Symbol test performance (a measure of psychomotor speed and visual working memory) declined more after STN than GPi DBS, performance on an auditory working memory task (backward digit span) declined more after GPi than STN DBS.

### Mood State, Behavioral Changes, and QOL

Vingerhoets et al. *(224)* administered a generic QOL measure (Sickness Impact Profile; SIP) to 20 patients before and 3 months after unilateral GPi DBS. Significant improvements were evident in the Physical, Psychosocial, and Total scores. Among the 12 subscales, improvements were observed for ambulation, body care and movement, communication, sleep and rest, and eating. Straits-Tröster et al. *(206)*, in their sample of nine unilateral GPi DBS patients, also observed significant improvements in the Physical and Total scales of the SIP, but did not analyze scores on subscales.

Studies employing measures of mood state (Beck Depression Inventory) did not find improvements in depressive symptomatology *(206, 209, 211, 213, 224)* but Fields et al. *(214)* noted that patients experienced a reduction in anxiety. Higginson and colleagues *(225)* observed improvements in the autonomic, neurophysiologic, and subjective symptoms of anxiety in patients having undergone either unilateral GPi ablative surgery or DBS. As others *(226–228)* have noted, the clinical significance of these group (mean) changes on symptom inventories is unclear, and future studies would do well to deal with caseness, i.e., report on the number of cases meeting diagnostic criteria for a certain condition such as depression before and after surgery. One report detailed hypomania and manic episodes after unilateral or bilateral GPi DBS *(229)* in a single patient but this morbidity may have been related to an interaction between stimulation and medication. Similarly, it is unclear whether hypersexuality reported in isolated cases *(230, 231)* reflects a possible dopamine dysregulation syndrome, medication–stimulation interactions, or a phenomenon that is part of hypomania.

## Subthalamic Stimulation

### Cognition, Language, and Memory

Neurobehavioral outcomes after bilateral STN DBS for PD have been published more frequently than for any other form of DBS. Despite this relatively rich literature, notable controversy exists about the frequency, nature, and extent of cognitive changes and the factors accounting for such changes. The reported frequencies with which cognitive changes occur after STN DBS is quite variable and this probably reflects differences in ascertainment methods (informal review suggests that studies using formal neuropsychological evaluation are more likely to find changes than studies using undefined methods or screening instruments), patient selection criteria, operative technique, and pre- and postoperative patient management strategies. A recent review *(232)* estimated that cognitive problems are observed in 41% of patients after STN DBS, but the extent and nature of such problems was not elaborated upon.

Examination of clinical studies suggests that profound or wide ranging changes in cognition are probably fairly rare. Rodriguez-Oroz and colleagues *(222)*, who were careful to operationally define severity of impairment, found that severe impairments (meaning those that are incapacitating) occurred in 1 to 2% of cases. Moderate impairments (requiring treatment or having mild functional impact), and mild deficits (having no functional impact) were more common, occurring in about 20% of patients. This latter number is similar to that reported in another series *(233)*, but considerably higher than the approximately 4% incidence of cognitive impairment observed in a recently published, controlled multicenter trial (although it is not clear how this impairment was established or defined; ref. *234*).

Studies utilizing formal neuropsychological evaluation methods have generally observed small and confined cognitive changes *(87, 211, 212, 215, 235–252)*. Three groups of researchers have reported more wide-ranging adverse cognitive and behavioral effects *(217, 235, 248, 253–255)*. Saint-Cyr, Trépanier, and their colleagues found poorer performance on the Trailmaking Test (Part B), poorer delayed recall and recognition of a word list, diminished verbal fluency, and poorer visual memory 3 to 6 months after than before bilateral DBS surgery in 11 patients. These deficits were still evident in patients returning for 12-month follow-up (up to nine patients for some tests; ref. *255*). Declines in some other functions were observed at 12 but not 3 to 6 months, and these changes, thus, probably relate to disease progression, subject selection bias, and/or attrition. Alegret and co-workers similarly found significant declines in average verbal memory, verbal fluency, complex visual attention, and visuospatial task scores 3 months after surgery in a group of 15 patients tested off medications. In contrast to Saint-Cyr and colleagues, however, Alegret et al. *(253)* interpreted the observed cognitive changes *not* to be of clinical significance. Smeding and her colleagues *(248)*, in their controlled study (the largest sample to date having undergone formal, detailed neuropsychological evaluation) reported declines on a range of tasks the authors felt were reflective of executive deficits (this study is discussed further under the three studies that have evaluated neuropsychological changes relative to an unoperated PD control group).

Morrison et al. *(87)* were the first investigators to publish neuropsychological findings pertaining to unilateral STN DBS. In their group of three patients, few cognitive changes were observed. Two of three patients (one left and one right DBS) showed improved category fluency, while two (one left, one right DBS) showed decrements in letter verbal fluency. Two patients (both left DBS) also showed poorer performance on the Stroop task and on an alternating fluency task. Although the sample is too small to evaluate laterality effects of STN DBS, it appears changes can occur after both left and right STN DBS. A more recent study of staged GPI and STN DBS, which afforded the opportunity to observe neuropsychological changes after unilateral surgery, found declines in verbal fluency after left DBS *(215)*.

*Controlled Studies of Neuropsychological Outcome:* Given that many of the neuropsychological studies of bilateral STN DBS have small sample sizes, it is probably prudent to rely more on controlled than uncontrolled studies, meaning those studies that compare neuropsychological changes in operated and unoperated PD groups. Unfortunately, to date, there are only three such studies and each has significant methodological and/or conceptual limitations. The first published controlled neuropsychological study of STN DBS by Gironell and co-workers *(241)* compared the outcomes in eight patients with bilateral STN DBS, eight patients undergoing unilateral pallidotomy, and eight unoperated PD patients. Surgical patients were tested on their medication 1 month before and 6 months after surgery, while the control group was retested after 6 months. In that study, a selective decline in semantic verbal fluency was observed in the STN DBS group.

The second controlled study made similar observations, although the methodology differed. This study by Morrison and colleagues *(245)* evaluated 17 patients (two of whom had had a prior pallidotomy) before and 3 to 4 months after STN DBS, and 11 PD patients on medical therapy on two occasions, about 9 weeks apart. The impact of medical therapy in the STN DBS patients is difficult to evaluate because 5 of the 17 patients were tested off medication, while 12 were tested on medication. A desirable feature of the study is that a subset of 13 STN DBS patients were tested twice after surgery, once with the stimulators turned on, and once with the devices turned off. The surgery effect (operationally defined as the difference between baseline and post-surgical "stimulation off" scores relative to the change in the control group's scores) was limited to mild decrements in language and attention. The procedure as a whole (the effect of surgery plus stimulation) was associated with subtle declines in delayed verbal recall and language. However, the effect of stimulation per se (comparing test performance with stimulators turned on and off relative to change observed in the control group) revealed no significant changes.

The most recent, controlled study by Smeding and associates *(248)* evaluated 99 STN DBS patients on medication, within 3 months before surgery and 6 months after surgery. The change in neuropsychological test scores was compared to the change observed among 36 medically treated PD patients tested twice, 6 months apart. Relative to the control group, the STN DBS group was reported to have more marked decline in overall level of cognitive function (approaching statistical significance), verbal fluency, delayed recall, and visual attention. Although QOL was apparently improved and depression scores improved, the STN DBS group also showed diminished positive affect and increased emotional lability after surgery.

Although this study is probably among the best available, given the use of a control group and a fairly large sample, several important limitations, including several discussed by the study's authors, should be borne in mind when considering the potential significance of the findings. The study was not randomized. In addition, no comparison was made of neuropsychological functioning on and off stimulation so that it is not possible to determine whether stimulation per se exerted a negative effect on cognition. Accuracy of electrode placement is also unknown. Even though some of the comparisons are statistically significant, the effect sizes associated with them are small to moderate. Perhaps a more critical issue is the statistical treatment of the data. The study's authors argue that a liberal statistical approach (using nonparametric statistics, not correcting for chance findings associated with a multitude of statistical comparisons, and the use of one-tailed significance tests) is appropriate since safety of the procedure is a primary consideration and one would presumably rather err by incorrectly concluding that a difference exists (Type I error) than to miss a true difference (Type II error). This position has merit, but some may question whether a more conservative approach might still be adequately liberal. In particular, given that there usually is some heterogeneity among patients' test score changes (some show improvements, some declines, some no change on any given test), one might wonder whether a one-tailed significance testing approach can be justified. Such an approach assumes a priori that a uni-directional change (presumably a decline) will occur, an assumption not supported by findings by others that reveal variability among individuals' outcomes and the observation that some test scores improve in groups of patients *(211, 238)*. Unfortunately, the frequency of sizeable negative and positive changes was not reported. Also, as noted by the authors, some effects may have been medication-related: for example, the decline in memory was no longer significant from the change in the control group once anticholinergic medication intake was accounted for.

*Meta-analysis of Neuropsychological Outcomes*: A major issue in interpreting the somewhat discordant neuropsychological findings is that the vast majority of studies have relatively small sample sizes. Woods and colleagues *(256)* found that only two of 30 studies had adequate power (above 0.80, where maximal power is 1 and minimal power is 0) to detect large cognitive effects, and that none had sufficient power to detect cognitive changes associated with conventionally small or medium effect sizes. Given this limited power, and the general absence of effect sizes in statistical analyses our laboratory recently undertook a quantitative meta-analysis of findings to date *(84)*. That study was based on a literature search of peer-reviewed, English language studies from 1990 to April 2006 that reported interval or ratio data, provided pre- and postoperative data on at least one standardized neuropsychological test, and provided sufficient information to allow calculation of effect sizes. Given the large number of different tests used in the literature, tests were assigned to the functional domains they are commonly accepted to primarily measure (e.g., verbal memory, language, attention). Of 40 studies identified, 28 met inclusion criteria, and this yielded a maximum combined sample size of 612 for calculation of the effect size of changes in the various domains of cognition. Analyses revealed that STN DBS (considered as a whole treatment procedure) was associated with moderate declines in verbal fluency and mild declines in verbal memory and executive function. Mild improvements were observed in psychomotor/information processing speed. Overall, the uncontrolled, controlled, and meta-analytic findings are in general accord that STN DBS is relatively safe from a cognitive perspective. One might bear in mind, however, that meta-analysis does not, despite attaching greater weight to studies with larger samples, redress methodological shortcomings of the studies included in the analyses.

*Factors Underlying Cognitive Changes After STN DBS*: Studies to date do not convincingly identify the factors that underlie cognitive changes after STN DBS. One possibility is that suboptimal electrode placement or spread to nonmotor (that is, limbic and associative) circuits *(257–259)* accounts for these cognitive and behavioral changes. However, to date, a relationship has not been found between cognitive change and active electrode coordinates *(260)*. Similarly, although one might assume that less accurate electrode placement is associated with poorer motor outcome and that patients with poorer motor outcome would thus be expected to have more pronounced cognitive changes, a relationship has not been found between motor improvement (a proxy measure of electrode placement accuracy) and cognitive outcome *(248, 260)*. Of course, this lack of relationship might be explained away by arguing that there is, at least among experienced treatment centers, little range (and variability) in electrode location making it difficult to obtain a significant correlation between location and cognitive outcome. Similarly, one might argue that suboptimal electrode placement can be compensated for by adjusting stimulation parameters, such that even patients with cognitive and behavioral changes may still have good motor outcomes.

Unfortunately, attempts to clearly delineate a relationship between stimulation parameters and cognitive outcome have met with limited success, probably in large part because four stimulation parameters (polarity, frequency, amplitude, pulse width) can be varied, yielding an almost infinite set of possible combinations of parameter adjustments. Consequently, the relationships of stimulation parameters to neuropsychological outcome have been explored retrospectively within narrow ranges of motorically beneficial or therapeutic stimulation settings. Another issue is that while it is known that various PD motor signs have different time-response curves *(261)*, the time course of various cognitive responses to DBS is not known. Thus, it is not known how soon after turning stimulation on or off changes in cognition may become apparent. A report that various aspects of stimulation (such as higher frequency) are related to cognitive change *(262)* must be tempered by the observation that parameters other than the one being evaluated were not being held constant, making it difficult to identify clearly which parameters influence cognition and how they do so.

Another strategy to isolate effects of stimulation on cognition is to compare test performance with stimulators turned on and off. In general, such comparisons have yielded few replicable effects *(212, 242, 245, 246, 250, 263, 264)* and, even when statistically significant, clinical significance of such effects remains a matter of conjecture, as do their implications for brain–behavior relationships in the absence of precise electrode localization. Only one study appears to have examined different STN stimulation frequency effects on cognition and that study reported differential effects of low frequency, high frequency, and no stimulation on verbal fluency *(265)*, namely facilitation by low frequency stimulation and diminution by high frequency stimulation. A potential future avenue for exploring effects of STN stimulation on cognition is to do so intra-operatively, though the amount of testing that can be done with awake patients intra-operatively is very limited.

Examinations of other possible factors that might account for cognitive changes between pre-and postoperative evaluations have failed to disclose relationships between cognitive change and depression *(260)* and dopaminergic medication changes *(84, 248, 260)*. Although a relationship between cognitive impairment and apathy may emerge 6 months to several years after STN DBS *(240, 251)*, such a relationship was not evident 3 months after surgery *(251)*. Other potential risk factors for cognitive deterioration have not been established, but include more advanced age (>69 years; refs. *87, 217, 255*) and pre-existing cognitive deficits *(266–268)*. While age appears to predispose to postoperative confusional episodes *(269)* and poorer executive function outcome in the long term after STN DBS *(240)*, it does not necessarily confer risk for poorer cognitive short-term outcomes *(215)*.

The identification of reliable prognostic indicators is of urgency given the heterogeneity of cognitive outcomes among individual patients as exemplified by the findings of Dujardin and her colleagues *(238)*. Among 9 patients studied on medication 3 months after surgery, these researchers observed declines in average verbal recall and verbal fluency scores, but gains in reaction time and simple attention (forward digit span). However, when examining change in individual patients, one third of patients showed overall declines in cognitive functioning (defined by declines of at least one standard deviation on at least

20% of the tests). On the positive side, among the 6 patients followed to 12 months, none showed such declines, and importantly, the one patient among the six who had shown significant overall decline at 3 months, had recovered by 1-year follow-up.

*Mechanisms Underlying Verbal Fluency Declines*: That verbal fluency can be directly impacted by STN DBS (rather than the treatment procedure as a whole) was elegantly shown in a study utilizing randomized, double-blinded, high-frequency (130 Hz), low-frequency (10 Hz), and sham stimulation (presumably bilateral). Low-frequency stimulation improved performance on four 1-minute verbal fluency tasks, whereas high-frequency stimulation tended to produce a diminution. Regardless of the debate about whether electrodes properly placed in sensorimotor STN or misplaced electrodes account for cognitive changes, two potential mechanistic explanations for verbal fluency declines are probably the most credible: motor speech and cognitive. If one were to speculate that motor speech mechanisms underlie verbal fluency decrements, it would be sufficient to posit an effect of STN DBS on cortical-basal ganglionic motor circuits. In contrast, were one to propose cognitive, and more specifically semantic or executive mechanisms as fundamental to DBS-induced verbal fluency changes, it would be necessary to speculate that: stimulation spreads beyond the motor circuit, active electrode contacts are placed outside the putative motor area, different stimulation patterns affect different basal ganglia structures and cortical regions *(270, 271)*, or basal ganglia circuits are more open and inter-connected than held by accepted models (see Joel & Weiner *[272]*).

A motor speech explanation of declines in verbal fluency after STN DBS would appear to be paradoxical given motor improvements with DBS. However, one might argue that the range of effective stimulation for limb and speech motor programs is different *(273)*. The majority of studies find an improvement or no change in dysarthria after STN DBS *(273–277)* and these improvements are related to normalization of cerebral metabolic patterns associated with speech activation *(273)*, a finding paralleling the normalization of cortical metabolism in good responders but not non-responders to DBS. When negative effects on motor speech do occur *(278)*, they may be related to misplacement of electrodes or stimulation at suboptimal parameters, dyskinesias related to medication and stimulation interactions *(276, 279)*, or an imbalance between right and left stimulation *(277)*. Törnqvist et al. *(280)* have shown that using typical stimulation settings, there was no difference on and off stimulation in speech intelligibility, but that intelligibility declined with higher stimulation frequencies and amplitudes.

Empirical evidence, albeit largely indirect, probably favors a non-motor speech explanation for verbal fluency changes. Support for a cognitive rather than motor mechanism underlying verbal fluency changes comes from a study with seven patients undergoing PET while carrying out verbal fluency tasks with and without STN stimulation. Whereas motor function improved with stimulation, verbal fluency performance declined by 15%. In addition, verbal fluency differences between on and off stimulation were correlated with regional cerebral blood flow activation decrements during on vs off stimulation in the left inferior frontal and temporal gyri. Other evidence supporting cognitive and linguistic mechanisms underlying verbal fluency decrements are that: STN DBS affects semantic processing *(249)*, motor speech decrements would affect performance on a range of expressive language tasks, yet verbal fluency decrements may be specific in that they can be accompanied by improvements on other expressive language tasks, including visual confrontation naming *(281)*, and reductions in verbal fluency after pallidal surgery are associated with diminution of patients' efficiency in switching between lexical-semantic categories during word search and retrieval, thus implicating specific cognitive mechanisms in verbal fluency deterioration *(219, 282)*. Consistent with the latter findings, STN DBS is reported to be associated with diminished switching between categories, whereas clustering remains unchanged *(283)*.

*Changes in Attention and Working Memory*: Numerous clinical, experimental and animal studies reveal that the thalamus and basal ganglia are involved in multiple aspects of attention, especially visuo-spatial attention, divided attention, selective attention and working memory and response inhibition *(284–286)*. Furthermore, because attention and working memory are susceptible to disruption by PD and dopaminergic treatment *(287, 288)* the impact of STN DBS on these functions may merit special attention. Sizeable changes in attention and working memory have generally not been reported in clinical studies of STN DBS but clinical studies using tasks such as the Trail Making Test (or variants of the Stroop) task have observed both positive *(212, 242)* and negative *(238, 242, 244, 254)* effects of STN DBS on attention and working memory *(130)*. Thus, like pharmacotherapy *(185)*, STN DBS may exert heterogeneous effects on different tasks, and indeed, affect performance differently than GPi DBS *(242)*. Whether or not STN DBS affects attention and working memory may depend on the cognitive load imposed by the tasks, such that impairments are observed only on tasks placing high demands on cognitive control and memory load *(264)*.

The biological mechanisms underlying these subtle attentional changes are poorly understood. One study found that one physiological index of frontal activity related to response preparation improves with STN DBS (i.e., the contingent negative variation amplitude increases over the frontal and fronto-central regions with bilateral STN DBS; ref. *289*). Using PET, Schroeder and colleagues *(290)* identified impaired executive attention task performance to be related to decreased activation in right anterior cingulate cortex (ACC) and right ventral striatum during STN stimulation.

Only a few studies have examined the influence of DBS on isolated attentional functions so as to elucidate possible cognitive mechanisms underlying changes on more complex attention and working memory tasks. Witt et al. *(291)* identified an influence of STN stimulation on visuo-spatial orientation by showing that left-sided STN-DBS increased the reaction times of both hands to visual stimuli within the left visual hemispace. In contrast, Heber and colleagues *(292)* detected changes in visuo-spatial scanning patterns in both visual hemifields, dependent on stimulation amplitude differences between left and right STN. DBS induced a gain of speed in detecting targets ipsilateral to the site with the higher amplitude. Both studies indicate an imbalance in cortico-subcortical circuits monitoring visuo-spatial attention and oculomotor function, induced by unilateral or imbalanced stimulation respectively.

*Experimental Cognitive and Social Neuroscience Studies*: One criticism of early movement disorder surgery studies was that they failed to take into account the role of human basal ganglia in cognition and behavior *(293)*.

Efforts are underway to avoid such a conclusion in the current era of movement disorder surgery. Recent studies have, for example, revealed an improvement in time estimation with STN DBS *(294)* and impaired recognition of facial expressions with compared to without stimulation *(295)* and after as compared to before surgery *(296, 297)*. In addition to studies examining isolated aspects of attention and working memory outlined in the preceding section, recent studies have revealed a potentially positive impact of STN DBS on aspects of nondeclarative memory *(298)*.

*Mood State, Behavioral Changes, and QOL*
Recent meta-analysis of 22 studies carried out between 1993 and 2004 *(299)* yielded estimates that 6.8% of patients develop depression after STN DBS, that hypomania or a manic episode occurs in 1.9%, and that other psychiatric disorders such as hypersexuality, lability, psychosis, and hallucinations occur in 3.5% of patients. Similar figures were reported in a review by Temel and colleagues *(232)*: depression 8%, hypomania or mania 4%, anxiety disorders less than 2%, personality changes, hypersexuality, apathy, and aggressiveness less than 0.5%. These findings coincide with the overall rate of psychiatric issues requiring treatment of 9% reported in a controlled study of 99 patients *(248)*. However, the range in incidence of various behavioral alterations reported by different studies may be quite broad *(227)*: depression 1.5 to 25%, attempted and completed suicide 0.5 to 2.9%, and (hypo)mania 4 to 15%. Factors underlying this heterogeneity of outcomes may relate to patient selection/exclusion criteria, especially with regard to psychiatric illness, ascertainment and definition methods, surgical and postoperative management differences, and rigor of study methodology.

Informal inspection of published studies raises the hypothesis that historically earlier studies, studies with small samples, and studies with longer follow-up are apt to report a higher incidence of postoperative psychiatric morbidity. For example, one study of 11 patients over 5 years reported mania/hypersexuality in almost 20% and apathy in almost 10% *(237)*. Another study of 37 cases collected between 1996 and 1999, using 5-year follow-up, reported attempted suicide or suicide in 13.5%, apathy in 22%, disinhibition in 35%, psychosis and/or hallucinations in 27%, aggression in 8%, and dopamine dysregulation syndrome (levodopa addiction) in 8% *(300)*. By contrast, a recent, controlled study of 78 patients at 6 months follow-up reported depression in 5%, suicide in 1%, and psychosis in 5% *(234)*. It is premature, however, to draw conclusions about the mechanisms of such behavioral changes and about the similarities and differences in long-term outcomes between patients having DBS and those subjected to other treatments. Certainly, given the progressive nature of PD, one expects behavioral changes to emerge more frequently with longer disease duration. Potential mechanisms underlying psychiatric phenomena after DBS include pre-operative vulnerability *(301)*, effects of stimulation, effects of surgery, psychosocial stressors and adaptation, and alterations in medication after surgery. STN stimulation has been observed to lead to visual hallucinations *(302)*, pseudobulbar crying *(303)*, laughter and euphoria *(9, 304)* and depression *(305, 306)*. Acute mood changes tend to be provoked by stimulation dorsal or ventral to the target for optimal motor control *(307)*, whereas apathy is associated with ventral and medial STN DBS *(251)*, and delusions perhaps with medial stimulation *(308)*. Aggression occurs with stimulation in the region of the triangle of Sano *(309)*, though aggression has also been observed with presumably accurately placed STN electrodes *(310)*.

Of interest is the apparent disconnect between studies reporting postoperative depression and those using symptom rating scales and self-report inventories showing improvements in average scores of symptom severity. Several studies have reported improvement in depressive symptomatology *(211, 223, 255, 311)* when considering self-report mood state questionnaires. Similarly, studies disagree whether apathy does or does not increase after STN DBS *(251, 312)*. On one hand, studies reporting postoperative behavioral changes typically do not report change in caseness from pre-operative state, leaving it possible that incidence of psychiatric conditions actually improves from pre-operative levels. Indeed, it has been shown that the incidence of psychiatric illness may be greater among PD surgical candidates than among the PD population in general *(313)*. Alternatively, patients completing inventories or responding to questions on rating scales may underestimate or be relatively unaware of behavioral changes as indicated by discrepancies in the report of patients and their care partners *(255)*.

Another topic of increasing interest has been the phenomenon of pathological gambling, isolated examples of which have been reported after DBS *(248)*. A large, retrospective study *(314)* identified seven persons who had displayed pathological gambling prior to surgery among 598 patients who underwent STN DBS. In all patients gambling improved after surgery, resolving on average 18 months after surgery, but in two patients the condition worsened transiently. The improvement in gambling and other symptoms of dopamine dysregulation syndrome (e.g., off period dysphoria, non-motor fluctuations) paralleled the course of dopaminergic medication reduction after electrode implantation.

Several studies have convincingly shown that QOL improves after STN DBS *(315)*. Not only does QOL improve after DBS, but also it improves more than with medical treatment as revealed by a controlled study *(234)*. In addition to improving patients' QOL, STN DBS also translates into gains in QOL of care partners for at least 2 years *(316)*. However, not all domains of QOL improve comparably and gains may be limited to physical aspects of QOL such as bodily discomfort, activities of daily living, mobility, and perceived stigma *(317, 318)*, though several studies have also found improvement in satisfaction with social, psychological and emotional functioning, 1 to 3 years after surgery *(319, 320)*. There appear to be no strong presurgical predictors of QOL improvement *(319)*, but improvement in bradykinesia appears to be one of the strongest correlates of QOL improvement *(319, 321)*. How much of the effect of motor improvement on QOL is direct is still unclear, and some of the benefit may be indirect via improving depressive symptoms *(322)*. Whether verbal fluency decline, the most common cognitive morbidity after STN DBS, has a significant impact on QOL is unknown. Two studies have found significantly decreased satisfaction with communication *(239, 317)*, but the factors responsible for those specific QOL declines were not identified.

Few studies have attended to social adaptation after surgery, a complex issue that has been more adequately addressed in the epilepsy surgery literature. Recent studies consistently provide evidence that gains in motor function and QOL do not necessarily translate into improved social integration and adaptation *(323, 324)*. Familial relationships can be compromised after DBS

*(77, 324)*, presumably when expectations of outcomes and perceived levels of functioning diverge between patient and care partner. In addition, despite improvements in motor function and QOL, patients may not return to work. In one study, only 9/16 who worked before surgery had returned to work by 18 to 24 months after surgery *(324)*. Predictors of barriers to social adjustment remain to be identified.

## DBS and Neurobehavioral Outcomes in ET

Several studies have demonstrated the effectiveness of thalamic DBS in the reduction of postural and action tremor in patients with ET with some showing that improvements persist for 6 years *(325–328)*. Limited case studies also suggest that DBS of the white matter adjacent to the STN may also be effective for ET *(329–331)*.

### Cognition, Language, and Memory

Detailed neuropsychological data pertaining to unilateral thalamic DBS in ET were presented by Tröster and colleagues *(174)*. Another study *(196)* mentions in passing that one of four ET patients experienced transient slowing of information processing. Tröster et al. *(174)* found that among 40 patients with ET, the only decrement observed involved lexical verbal fluency (in contrast to the absence of such an effect in PD). Improvements, possibly impacted by test–retest effects, were observed in visuoconstructional skill and visuoperceptual gestalt formation, backward visual span, delayed prose recall and word list recognition (also seen in PD after thalamic DBS). In a follow-up study 12 months following surgery largely similar results were reported *(332)*. Improvements in delayed verbal memory, visual construction, visual perception, and dominant hand manual dexterity were maintained relative to baseline and patients demonstrated additional improvement from baseline on a measure of verbal learning, perhaps reflecting a practice effect. Significant increases in performance were found between the 3- and 12-month evaluations on measures of verbal learning and concept formation. Twelve months following surgery, no significant declines were noted on any measures in comparison to baseline. However, four patients with baseline deficits in verbal fluency showed substantial further decrements following surgery, suggesting that persons with poor verbal fluency prior to surgery may be more susceptible to exacerbation of this deficit by DBS.

Few studies have compared neuropsychological test performance with and without stimulation. One case report found that thalamic DBS may improve verbal fluency *(333)*. No differences were noted in other measures of attention, verbal memory, or visual perception. However, another study comparing performance on and off stimulation found that thalamic DBS may disrupt recall of a word list *(199)*. Because only two of the nine patients in this study had ET it is difficult to discern whether similar findings would obtain in a larger sample of ET patients.

Research has rarely examined the surgical and stimulation parameters that might predict cognitive or ADL changes after DBS in ET. One study compared the characteristics of 27 ET patients with mild cognitive declines following surgery with those of 22 patients without such declines *(334)*. There were no significant differences between the two groups in baseline neuropsychological performance, disease duration and onset, demographics, or postoperative motor functioning, but a larger proportion of patients with cognitive declines had undergone left rather than right thalamic DBS. A significantly higher pulse width (PW) was used in the group with cognitive declines and there was a significant association between cognitive decline and pulse width greater than 119 microseconds. It should be noted that not all stimulation parameters' relationship to verbal fluency could be evaluated simultaneously, and therefore the specific role of pulse width in verbal fluency declines remains unknown. Onset of ET after age 37 was another significant predictor of worse cognitive outcome.

**Mood State, Behavioral Changes, and QOL**

Several studies demonstrate effective reduction of disability and significant improvements in activities of daily living (ADL) such as writing and pouring, following DBS for ET *(335)*. Clinicians and patients have rated similar levels of improvement, ranging from 40 to 60%, on measures of ADLs such as the TADLS *(336, 337)*. Improvements of ADLs have been noted in comparisons of baseline and post surgical scores, in comparisons of stimulation turned on and off *(336, 338)*, and these improvements occur after both unilateral and bilateral DBS *(326)*. Such ADL improvements are associated with gains in QOL. Tröster and colleagues *(174)* found a reduction in anxiety symptoms 3 months after unilateral thalamic DBS surgery for ET. On the SIP (a generic QOL measure), improvements were found in Total and Psychosocial scores, and on the modified PDQ (a disease-specific measure), patients expressed significantly increased satisfaction with ADLs, communication, emotional functioning, and stigma. At 12-month follow-up, gains were maintained on the SIP Psychosocial scale and the modified PDQ Stigma, Activities of daily Living and Emotional Well-being scales *(339)*.

## DBS and Neurobehavioral Outcomes in Dystonia

Primary or idiopathic dystonias vary in the body parts they affect but all involve involuntary muscle contractions that lead to abnormal posture, twisting, and repetitive movements. The earliest attempts to treat torticollis and dystonia with stimulation targeted the thalamus *(340, 341)*. Findings of recent case reports that bilateral pallidal stimulation alleviates dystonia have been confirmed in larger series using blinded evaluation *(342)* and sham stimulation controls *(343)*, but relatively few studies have evaluated neuropsychological functioning, mood and behavioral changes, and QOL.

In an early case series Morrison et al. *(87)* reported minimal cognitive change in two patients with dystonia who underwent right GPi DBS. One patient experienced a decline in verbal fluency, but both patients experienced improvements on some tests of attention and memory. In the most detailed neuropsychological study to date evaluating overall level of cognition, attention, executive functions, verbal fluency, verbal learning, mood state and QOL in 15 patients, Hälbig et al. *(344)* reported improvement in motor function following bilateral GPi DBS ranging from 26 to 93%. As compared to baseline there was no deterioration in patients' cognitive scores 3 to 12 months following surgery as a group, although there was some variability in outcome such that some patients showed declines or improvements on one or more tests. Slight overall improvements were noted in Part A of the Trailmaking test, a test of psychomotor speed and visual attention. There were no marked changes on measures of depression, anxiety, psychosis and mania. Overall QOL, measured with the PDQ designed for PD, improved 37% after DBS.

The study by Vidailhet et al. *(342)* of 22 patients using a blinded evaluation protocol found that mean dystonia severity scores improved by an average of 51% 12 months after surgery. These authors found that, compared to pretreatment baseline testing, none of the patients experienced statistically significant declines in cognitive functioning 12 months after surgery, but evaluation was carried out only with the MMSE which may not be sensitive to the circumscribed cognitive dysfunction occasionally observed in dystonia. QOL evaluated with the Medical Outcomes Study (MOS) 36-item Short-Form General Health Survey (SF-36) revealed significant improvements in only two of the eight domains evaluated (General Health and Physical Functioning). Pillon et al. *(345)* conducted a more comprehensive neuropsychological evaluation of abstract reasoning, verbal intelligence, attention, executive function, verbal fluency, and verbal learning memory, and depressive symptomatology in this same patient population, and also observed no negative impacts on cognition at the 1-year study endpoint. Pillon and colleagues further noted that, as a group, patients showed mild but statistically significant improvements relative to baseline on measures of concept formation and reasoning, executive function, and memory. Whether these gains exceed expected practice or familiarity effects is unclear.

## DBS and Neurobehavioral Outcomes in Epilepsy

Surgery for medically intractable epilepsy has been carried out for a long time and there are a large variety of ablative procedures that have been used for different syndromes. Numerous neuroanatomical structures (see Table 21.1) have been utilized to treat small numbers of epileptic patients with stimulation *(346, 347)*, with the earliest work by Cooper targeting the anterior thalamus and cerebellum *(340, 348, 349)*. The relative dearth of empirically documented neuropsychological outcomes is somewhat surprising given the central role of neuropsychological evaluation in ablative epilepsy surgery.

Hodaie and colleagues *(350)* reported on anterior thalamic DBS in five patients with generalized tonic-clonic or secondarily generalized seizures. It was reported that the family witnessed no behavioral changes, and that the families of three patients reported improved cognition and activities of daily living. However, no objective data were provided. Similarly, a pilot study of 14 patients *(351)*, which did not provide detailed neuropsychological data, noted that two patients experienced depression and another two experienced increased irritability.

A placebo-controlled pilot study of centromedian nucleus stimulation in seven patients with either tonic-clonic, tonic, or complex partial seizures utilized a neuropsychological test battery including tests of intelligence, speech and language, visual and verbal memory, visuospatial functions, attention, executive functions, and motor speed *(352)*. Detailed neuropsychological findings were not presented but it was reported that no differences were observed between baseline scores and those on and off stimulation after DBS.

Hippocampal stimulation has been used in patients deemed at excessive risk of cognitive (memory) deficit after potential temporal lobe resection. One study has reported neuropsychological evaluation results in four patients with complex partial seizures with or without secondary generalization who underwent left hippocampal DBS *(353)*. Patients underwent a 3-month baseline evaluation period and were again evaluated after DBS after 3 months on and 3 months off stimulation. Except for one patient no detailed data were presented but it was reported that no changes were observed in neuropsychological function when comparing test performance on and off stimulation and to baseline. A recent study failed to observe any significant cognitive changes after mammillothalamic DBS in three patients, though detailed data were not provided *(354)*.

## DBS and Neurobehavioral Outcomes in MS

DBS does not represent a comprehensive treatment for MS, but, like other surgical interventions used in this condition *(355)*, has application in the amelioration of tremor. The target used is generally the thalamic ventral intermediate nucleus (VIM), although the ventralis oralis posterior and anterior (VOP and VOA) nuclei have been stimulated in conjunction with VIM *(356)*. A review of studies published from 1980 to 2002 makes clear that detailed neuropsychological outcome data remain unavailable *(357)*.

## DBS and Neurobehavioral Outcomes in Depression

Based on functional neuroimaging findings implicating the subgenual cingulate in negative mood states and antidepressant treatment effects, Mayberg and colleagues *(11)* undertook DBS of white matter tract adjacent to the subgenual cingulate gyrus in six patients with major depression (MDD) refractory to other therapies. Four of the six patients appeared to respond to the treatment (50% reduction of symptoms at 6 months) and the patients did not experience significant declines in cognitive functioning as a result of surgery. While, at the time of this writing, a detailed discussion of neuropsychological test results has not yet been published, Mayberg and colleagues reported that when compared to pretreatment baseline evaluation, intelligence, language, and basic visual-spatial functioning remained stable after 3 and 6 months of stimulation. Moreover, improvements were noted in visuo-motor function, and on tests said to be sensitive to dorsolateral frontal function (verbal fluency), ventral prefrontal function, and orbital frontal function.

Greenberg et al. *(358)*, in a 3-month study of five MDD patients undergoing bilateral DBS in the ventral portion of the anterior limb of the internal capsule and the adjacent dorsal ventral striatum (VC/VS), found that three patients experienced more than 50% improvement in depressive symptoms while two other patients showed 24% and 17% improvements, respectively. Detailed neuropsychological data were not reported. Similarly, single case studies of thalamic peduncle DBS for depression *(359)* and of GPi stimulation for dyskinesia in a depressed patient associated with amelioration of depression *(360)* did not report cognitive outcomes.

## DBS and Neurobehavioral Outcomes in OCD

Only a few studies discuss the effect on cognition of bilateral DBS in the anterior limb of the internal capsule for treatment-refractory OCD. Greenberg et al. *(361)* monitored treatment progress in eight of the original ten OCD patients in their study, and found that chronic DBS over a 3-year period induced a 25% or greater reduction in OCD symptom severity in six patients. Neuropsychological test results obtained after a mean of approximately 10 months after surgery revealed that, as a group, these patients experienced no significant declines in cognitive performance relative to baseline testing, and no individual patient demonstrated a clear pattern of decline. Significant overall improvements in passage recall were reported, even when correcting for practice effects.

Gabriëls and co-workers *(93)* found that two of three patients they studied with OCD also experienced a significant reduction in symptom severity subsequent to DBS surgery. Neuropsychological assessments, focusing especially on executive functions and attention, were performed prior to and 1 year after treatment. No significant deterioration in cognitive abilities was observed with DBS, but one patient tended to make more errors on a card-sorting task after 1 year and visual memory tended to improve.

More variable neuropsychological outcomes were reported in another study of four patients undergoing DBS of the anterior limb of the internal capsule for refractory OCD *(92)*. In those patients who underwent DBS in a randomized "on-off" stimulation sequence of four 3-week blocks, evaluation of attention, working memory, processing speed, verbal fluency, and cognitive flexibility revealed no consistent pattern of change across subjects comparing baseline and four post-surgical evaluations. A more extensive test battery done at baseline and after 6 months of continuous stimulation also revealed no consistent neuropsychological alterations. However, isolated patients did show improvements and declines in executive function tests.

Aouizerate and colleagues *(362)* found that an OCD patient undergoing DBS in the ventral caudate experienced a clinically significant reduction in symptom severity after 1 year of stimulation at 130 Hz. A comparison of pretreatment cognitive test scores to those obtained 1 and 6 months following chronic stimulation showed no impairment of cognition and revealed improvements in attentional and executive functions as well as in visual and verbal memory. Pool *(28)* had already used chronic caudate stimulation in a depressed patient in 1948, though cognitive outcome was not reported. A report of right nucleus accumbens stimulation did not provide neuropsychological data *(363)*. One case study of intra-operative stimulation during electrode placement for OCD in the anterior limb of the internal capsule in the vicinity of the nucleus accumbens showed that fear and panic could be induced with stimulation and reliably replicated by turning the stimulation on or off *(364)*. This finding parallels the observation of anxiety symptoms elicited by intra-operative rostral cingulate stimulation in the course of ablative surgery for various psychiatric conditions in the past *(365)*.

## DBS and Neurobehavioral Outcomes in TS

Few patients with TS have undergone DBS, and it currently remains unclear whether thalamic or pallidal targets are preferable. Both have been used *(366)*. To assess the impact of DBS for TS on cognition, Visser-Vandewalle et al. *(367)* studied three patients whose electrodes were implanted at the level of the centromedian nucleus, substantia periventricularis, and nucleus ventrooralis internus. After chronic stimulation for a period of 5 years in the first patient, 1 year for the second patient, and 8 months for the third patient, motor and vocal tics subsided completely. Neuropsychological test results were only reported for the first and third patient. No significant changes between pre- and postoperative cognitive test scores were noted in the first patient. Postoperative test scores for the third patient, however, demonstrated a decline in ability on timed tasks relative to baseline testing. Improvements were noted in both patients on verbal memory and facial recognition tests.

In a single TS patient, bilateral thalamic and/or GPi DBS at approximately 130 Hz resulted in a 70% improvement in the frequency of tics and self-injurious behavior *(368)*, and bilateral GPi DBS in another patient yielded a 73% reduction in vocal tics per minute after 14 months of treatment *(369)*. When compared to preoperative cognitive testing, the patient in the former study demonstrated improvements in attention, episodic and working memory, and cognitive flexibility. The latter study noted that when compared to the baseline evaluation, cognitive test results did not change significantly on or off stimulation at the 14-month study endpoint. Another case study found mild declines in memory 6 months after GPi DBS *(370)*. However, ratings of psychiatric co-morbidity improved, as did performance on some tests of executive function (verbal abstract reasoning, cognitive flexibility), psychomotor speed, and visual perception. Thus, to date, neurocognitive findings after DBS for TS have been quite variable.

## DBS and Neurobehavioral Outcomes in Other Conditions

Posterior hypothalamic DBS has recently been used to treat cluster headaches *(371)* and posterior-medial hypothalamic stimulation was reported to decrease aggressive and disruptive behavior in two persons with mental retardation *(372)*. These studies, and studies using DBS for neuropathic pain *(373)*, have not reported neuropsychological outcomes. Tarsy and co-workers *(374)* reported that STN DBS in a patient with multiple system atrophy (MSA) developed speech problems (dysarthria), but neuropsychological outcome was not detailed. In a case with Huntington's disease, a single case study of GPi stimulation noted no neuropsychological changes 12 months after DBS, but details were not provided *(375)*.

## Conclusions

The past decade has seen an explosion in the number of medically refractory conditions and neuroanatomical structures targeted for DBS treatment. The extension of DBS to use fully implantable systems to new conditions was slow to gain momentum in the 1980s, but has witnessed exponential growth since the 1990s, perhaps related to the success and relative safety of DBS demonstrated in movement disorders. While a review of the literature and meta-analyses indicates DBS for movement disorders to be quite safe from a neurobehavioral standpoint (while effective in treating motor symptoms and producing gains in the QOL of patient and care partner), it is also clear that a small subset of patients experienced moderate or severe neurobehavioral morbidity. If one combines the various cognitive and psychiatric morbidities reported across studies, it is probably reasonable to approximate that about 10% of patients with PD undergoing DBS will have one or another neurobehavioral adverse events. Furthermore, what remains unclear and is deserving of detailed empirical investigation, is the initial observation in a few small studies that improvements in motor symptoms and QOL may not necessarily translate into social (re)adjustment. That is, patients' occupational, interpersonal, familial, and marital functioning may not change dramatically. Perhaps, as in epilepsy surgery, treatment success does not ensure enhanced social functioning, but instead provides a new platform upon which to build or rebuild these social roles. Perhaps a much greater role of ancillary health services, such as speech therapy, occupational and physical therapy, neuropsychology, and psychotherapy needs to be contemplated if outcomes after DBS are to be optimized. Health care providers should not rely on subjective impression or spontaneous patient report to identify neurobehavioral and psychosocial issues. There is ample empirical evidence that even seasoned movement disorders clinicians may be inaccurate in identifying persons with, for example depression, and that non-motor symptoms are under treated *(376–378)*. The recent formulation of consensus statements on patient selection, treatment, and outcome evaluation *(49, 83, 379)* should facilitate greater uniformity in outcome reporting and identification of neurobehavioral risk.

What has proved elusive to this point, despite an increase in the volume of available literature, is the identification of reliable predictors and risk factors for such neurobehavioral changes. Ethical concerns and seemingly intractable methodological limitations hinder the initiation of more sophisticated, controlled, blinded, comparative trials with large numbers of subjects needed to isolate such predictors of neurobehavioral and QOL outcomes. Similarly, it is difficult to conclude at present that stimulation per se is associated with neurobehavioral morbidity, though in some cases, there is a replicable effect on mood and cognition when stimulation is turned on and off. In the case of PD, and likely many of the disorders for which DBS is beginning to be investigated, outcomes may be related to an interaction of the surgical procedure and stimulation as well as subsequent changes in medications, psychosocial factors and pre-operative vulnerability. Conclusions that DBS is neuropsychologically safe in conditions such as dystonia, depression, OCD, TS, epilepsy, MS and others must be considered highly preliminary until adequate controlled trials are completed.

The emergence of cognitive and social neuroscience studies of DBS *(291, 294, 295, 298, 380)*, particularly in the accompaniment of functional imaging (and the possibility of functional magnetic resonance imaging in DBS; refs. *381* and *382*) are encouraging signs that DBS might be used as a vehicle to better understand the cognitive and behavioral role of the basal ganglia. Such endeavors would prevent future critics from proclaiming that surgical studies have proved to be a failure in understanding the behavioral functions of the basal ganglia, as stated by Crown *(293)* three decades ago.

# References

1. Koller W, Hristova A (1996) Efficacy and safety of stereotaxic surgical treatment of tremor disorders. Eur J Neurol 3:507–514.
2. Laitinen LV (2000) Behavioral complications of early pallidotomy. Brain Cognit 42(3):313–323.
3. Hassler R, Riechert T, Mundinger F, Umbach W, Ganglberger JA (1960) Physiological observations in stereotaxic operations in extrapyramidal motor disturbances. Brain 83:337–350.
4. Siegfried J, Lippitz B (1994) Chronic electrical stimulation of the VL-VPL complex and of the pallidum in the treatment of movement disorders: personal experience since 1982. Stereotact Funct Neurosurg 62(1–4):71–75.
5. Benabid AL, Pollak P, Gross C, et al (1994) Acute and long-term effects of subthalamic nucleus stimulation in Parkinson's disease. Stereotact Funct Neurosurg 62(1–4):76–84.
6. Benabid AL, Pollak P, Louveau A, Henry S, de Rougemont J (1987) Combined (thalamotomy and stimulation) stereotactic surgery of the VIM thalamic nucleus for bilateral Parkinson disease. Appl Neurophysiol 50(1–6):344–346.
7. Siegfried J, Lippitz B (1994) Bilateral chronic electrostimulation of ventroposterolateral pallidum: a new therapeutic approach for alleviating all parkinsonian symptoms. Neurosurgery 35(6):1126–1129; discussion 1129–1130.
8. Velasco F, Velasco M, Velasco AL, Menez D, Rocha L (2001) Electrical stimulation for epilepsy: stimulation of hippocampal foci. Stereotact Funct Neurosurg 77(1–4):223–227.
9. Benabid AL, Koudsié A, Benazzouz A, et al (2001) Deep brain stimulation of the corpus luysi (subthalamic nucleus) and other targets in Parkinson's disease. Extension to new indications such as dystonia and epilepsy. J Neurol 248 (Suppl 3):37–47.
10. Benabid AL, Minotti L, Koudsie A, de Saint Martin A, Hirsch E (2002) Antiepileptic effect of high-frequency stimulation of the subthalamic nucleus (corpus luysi) in a case of medically intractable epilepsy caused by focal dysplasia: a 30-month follow-up: technical case report. Neurosurgery 50(6):1385–1391; discussion 1391–1382.
11. Mayberg HS, Lozano AM, Voon V, et al (2005) Deep brain stimulation for treatment-resistant depression. Neuron 45(5):651–660.
12. Nuttin B, Cosyns P, Demeulemeester H, Gybels J, Meyerson B (1999) Electrical stimulation in anterior limbs of internal capsules in patients with obsessive-compulsive disorder. Lancet 354(9189):1526.
13. Guridi J, Lozano AM (1997) A brief history of pallidotomy. Neurosurgery 41(5):1169–1180.
14. Ostertag CB, Lücking CH, Mehdorn HM, Deuschl G (1997) Stereotaktische Behandlung der Bewegungstörungen. Nervenarzt 68(6):477–484.
15. Siegfried J, Blond S (1997) The Neurosurgical Treatment of Parkinson's Disease and Other Movement Disorders. London: Williams & Wilkins Europe Ltd.
16. Gabriel EM, Nashold BS Jr (1998) Evolution of neuroablative surgery for involuntary movement disorders: an historical review. Neurosurgery 42(3):575–590.
17. Gildenberg PL (1998) The history of surgery for movement disorders. Neurosurg Clin N Am 9(2):283–294.
18. Speelman JD, Bosch DA (1998) Resurgence of functional neurosurgery for Parkinson's disease: a historical perspective. Mov Disord 13(3):582–588.
19. Gildenberg PL (2000) History of movement disorder surgery. In: Lozano AM, ed. Movement Disorder Surgery. Basel: Karger, pp. 1–20.

20. Iskandar BJ, Nashold BS Jr (1995) History of functional neurosurgery. Neurosurg Clin N Am 6(1):1–25.
21. Kopell BH, Greenberg B, Rezai AR (2004) Deep brain stimulation for psychiatric disorders. J Clin Neurophysiol 21(1):51–67.
22. Mashour GA, Walker EE, Martuza RL (2005) Psychosurgery: past, present, and future. Brain Res Brain Res Rev 48(3):409–419.
23. Gildenberg PL (2006) History of electrical neuromodulation for chronic pain. Pain Med 7(Suppl 1):S7–S13.
24. Wallace BA, Ashkan K, Benabid AL (2004) Deep brain stimulation for the treatment of chronic, intractable pain. Neurosurg Clin N Am 15(3): 343–357, vii.
25. Kellinghaus C, Loddenkemper T, Moddel G, et al (2003) Electric brain stimulation for epilepsy therapy. Nervenarzt 74(8):664–676.
26. Penfield W, Boldrey E (1937) Somatic motor and sensory representation in the cerebral cortex of man as studied by electrical stimulation. Brain 60:389–443.
27. Spiegel EA, Wycis HT, Marks M, Lee AJ (1947) Stereotaxix apparatus for operations on the human brain. Science 106:349–350.
28. Pool JL (1954) Psychosurgery in older people. J Am Geriatr Soc 2(7):456–466.
29. Delgado JM, Hamlin H, Chapman WP (1952) Technique of intracranial electrode implacement for recording and stimulation and its possible therapeutic value in psychotic patients. Confin Neurol 12(5–6):315–319.
30. Heath RG (1954) Studies in schizophrenia: a multidisciplinary approach to mind-brain relationships. Cambridge, MA: Harvard University Press.
31. Heath RG, Monroe RR, Mickle WA (1955) Stimulation of the amygdaloid nucleus in a schizophrenic patient. Am J Psychiatry 111(11):862–863.
32. Bechtereva NP, Bondartchuk AN, Smirnov VM, Meliutcheva LA, Shandurina AN (1975) Method of electrostimulation of the deep brain structures in treatment of some chronic diseases. Confinia Neurologica 37(1–3):136–140.
33. Sem-Jacobsen CW (1965) Depth electrographic stimulation and treatment of patients with Parkinson's disease including neurosurgical technique. Acta Neurol Scand Suppl 13 Pt 1:365–377.
34. Brice J, McLellan L (1980) Suppression of intention tremor by contingent deep-brain stimulation. Lancet 1(8180):1221–1222.
35. Gross CE, Boraud T, Guehl D, Bioulac B, Bezard E (1999) From experimentation to the surgical treatment of Parkinson's disease: prelude or suite in basal ganglia research? Progr Neurobiol 59(5):509–532.
36. Tröster AI, Fields JA (2003) The role of neuropsychological evaluation in the neurosurgical treatment of movement disorders. In: Tarsy D, Vitek JL, Lozano AM, eds. Surgical Treatment of Parkinson's Disease and Other Movement Disorders. Totowa, NJ: Humana Press, pp. 213–240.
37. Tröster AI, Wikinson SB (1998) Surgical interventions in neurodegenerative disease: impact on memory and cognition. In: Tröster AI, ed. Memory in neurodegenerative disease: biological, cognitive, and clinical perspectives. Cambridge: Cambridge University Press, pp. 362–376.
38. Riklan M, Levita E (1966) Psychological studies in parkinsonism: effects of subcortical surgery. J Gerontol 21(3):372–379.
39. Ford PJ, Kubu CS (2006) Stimulating debate: ethics in a multidisciplinary functional neurosurgery committee. J Med Ethics 32(2):106–109.
40. Greenberg BD (2004) Deep brain stimulation in psychiatry. In: Lisanby SH, ed. Brain stimulation in psychiatric treatment. Washington, D.C.: American Psychiatric Publishing, pp. 53–65.
41. Fins JJ (2003) From psychosurgery to neuromodulation and palliation: history's lessons for the ethical conduct and regulation of neuropsychiatric research. Neurosurg Clin N Am 14(2):303–319, ix–x.

42. Heller AC, Amar AP, Liu CY, Apuzzo ML (2006) Surgery of the mind and mood: a mosaic of issues in time and evolution. Neurosurgery 59(4):720–733; discussion 733–729.
43. Gao G, Wang X, He S, et al (2003) Clinical study for alleviating opiate drug psychological dependence by a method of ablating the nucleus accumbens with stereotactic surgery. Stereotact Funct Neurosurg 81(1–4):96–104.
44. Hall W (2006) Stereotactic neurosurgical treatment of addiction: minimizing the chances of another 'great and desperate cure'. Addiction 101(1):1–3.
45. Orellana C (2002) Controversy over brain surgery for heroin addiction in Russia. Lancet Neurol 1(6):333.
46. Bronstein JM, DeSalles A, DeLong MR (1999) Stereotactic pallidotomy in the treatment of Parkinson disease: an expert opinion. Arch Neurol 56(9):1064–1069.
47. Defer G-L, Widner H, Marié R-M, Rémy P, Levivier M (1999) Core assessment program for surgical interventional therapies in Parkinson's disease (CAPSIT-PD). Mov Disord 14(4):572–584.
48. Hallett M, Litvan I (1999) Evaluation of surgery for Parkinson's disease: a report of the Therapeutics and Technology Assessment Subcommittee of the American Academy of Neurology. Neurology 53(9):1910–1921.
49. Lang AE, Houeto JL, Krack P, et al (2006) Deep brain stimulation: preoperative issues. Mov Disord 21(Suppl 14):S171–S196.
50. Mink JW, Walkup J, Frey KA, et al (2006) Patient selection and assessment recommendations for deep brain stimulation in Tourette syndrome. Mov Disord 21(11):1831–1838.
51. Pillon B (2002) Neuropsychological assessment for management of patients with deep brain stimulation. Mov Disord 17(Suppl 3):S116–S122.
52. Saint-Cyr JA, Trépanier LL (2000) Neuropsychologic assessment of patients for movement disorder surgery. Mov Disord 15(5):771–783.
53. Cross JH, Jayakar P, Nordli D, et al (2006) Proposed criteria for referral and evaluation of children for epilepsy surgery: recommendations of the Subcommission for Pediatric Epilepsy Surgery. Epilepsia 47(6):952–959.
54. Siegel AM (2004) Presurgical evaluation and surgical treatment of medically refractory epilepsy. Neurosurg Rev 27(1):1–18; discussion 19–21.
55. Lassonde M, Sauerwein HC, Gallagher A, Theriault M, Lepore F (2006) Neuropsychology: traditional and new methods of investigation. Epilepsia 47(Suppl 2):9–13.
56. Tellez-Zenteno JF, Dhar R, Hernandez-Ronquillo L, Wiebe S (2006) Long-term outcomes in epilepsy surgery: antiepileptic drugs, mortality, cognitive and psychosocial aspects. Brain.
57. Dodrill CB, Morris GL (2001) Effects of vagal nerve stimulation on cognition and quality of life in epilepsy. Epilepsy and Behavior 2:46–53.
58. Hamberger MJ, Drake EB (2006) Cognitive functioning following epilepsy surgery. Curr Neurol Neurosci Rep 6(4):319–326.
59. Sackeim HA, Keilp JG, Rush AJ, et al (2001) The effects of vagus nerve stimulation on cognitive performance in patients with treatment-resistant depression. Neuropsychiatry Neuropsychol Behav Neurol 14(1):53–62.
60. Schachter SC (2004) Vagus nerve stimulation: mood and cognitive effects. Epilepsy Behav 5(Suppl 1):S56–S59.
61. Sjogren MJ, Hellstrom PT, Jonsson MA, Runnerstam M, Silander HC, Ben-Menachem E (2002) Cognition-enhancing effect of vagus nerve stimulation in patients with Alzheimer's disease: a pilot study. J Clin Psychiatry 63(11):972–980.
62. Mindus P, Nyman H, Rosenquist A, Rydin E, Meyerson BA (1988) Aspects of personality in patients with anxiety disorders undergoing capsulotomy. Acta Neurochir Suppl (Wien) 44:138–144.

63. Nyman H, Andreewitch S, Lundback E, Mindus P (2001) Executive and cognitive functions in patients with extreme obsessive-compulsive disorder treated by capsulotomy. Appl Neuropsychol 8(2):91–98.
64. Nyman H, Mindus P (1995) Neuropsychological correlates of intractable anxiety disorder before and after capsulotomy. Acta Psychiatr Scand 91(1):23–31.
65. Oliver B, Gascon J, Aparicio A, et al (2003) Bilateral anterior capsulotomy for refractory obsessive-compulsive disorders. Stereotact Funct Neurosurg 81(1–4):90–95.
66. Ruck C, Andreewitch S, Flyckt K, et al (2003) Capsulotomy for refractory anxiety disorders: long-term follow-up of 26 patients. Am J Psychiatry 160(3):513–521.
67. Ruck C, Svanborg P, Meyerson BA (2005) Lesion topography in capsulotomy for refractory anxiety—is the right side the right side? Stereotact Funct Neurosurg 83(4):172–179.
68. Calev A, Gaudino EA, Squires NK, Zervas IM, Fink M (1995) ECT and non-memory cognition: a review. Br J Clin Psychol 34(Pt 4):505–515.
69. Fujita A, Nakaaki S, Segawa K, et al (2006) Memory, attention, and executive functions before and after sine and pulse wave electroconvulsive therapies for treatment-resistant major depression. J Ect 22(2):107–112.
70. Martis B, Alam D, Dowd SM, et al (2003) Neurocognitive effects of repetitive transcranial magnetic stimulation in severe major depression. Clin Neurophysiol 114(6):1125–1132.
71. Sackeim HA, Prudic J, Fuller R, Keilp J, Lavori PW, Olfson M (2006) The Cognitive Effects of Electroconvulsive Therapy in Community Settings. Neuropsychopharmacology.
72. Levy G, Jacobs DM, Tang MX, et al (2002) Memory and executive function impairment predict dementia in Parkinson's disease. Mov Disord 17(6):1221–1226.
73. Woods SP, Troster AI (2003) Prodromal frontal/executive dysfunction predicts incident dementia in Parkinson's disease. J Int Neuropsychol Soc 9(1):17–24.
74. Pilitsis JG, Rezai AR, Boulis NM, Henderson JM, Busch RM, Kubu CS (2005) A preliminary study of transient confusional states following bilateral subthalamic stimulation for Parkinson's disease. Stereotact Funct Neurosurg 83(2–3):67–70.
75. Dodrill CB, Wilkus RJ, Ojemann LM (1992) Use of psychological and neuropsychological variables in selection of patients for epilepsy surgery. Epilepsy Res Suppl 5:71–75.
76. Bortz JJ, Prigatano GP, Blum D, Fisher RS (1995) Differential response characteristics in nonepileptic and epileptic seizure patients on a test of verbal learning and memory. Neurology 45(11):2029–2034.
77. Perozzo P, Rizzone M, Bergamasco B, et al (2001) Deep brain stimulation of subthalamic nucleus: behavioural modifications and familiar relations. Neurolog Sci 22(1):81–82.
78. Melnick ME, Dowling GA, Aminoff MJ, Barbaro NM (1999) Effect of pallidotomy on postural control and motor function in Parkinson disease. Arch Neurol 56(11):1361–1365.
79. Wheelock I, Peterson C, Buchtel HA (1998) Presurgery expectations, postsurgery satisfaction, and psychosocial adjustment after epilepsy surgery. Epilepsia 39(5):487–494.
80. Wilson SJ, Saling MM, Kincade P, Bladin PF (1998) Patient expectations of temporal lobe surgery. Epilepsia 39(2):167–174.
81. Rose KJ, Derry PA, McLachlan RS (1995) Patient expectations and postoperative depression, anxiety, and psychosocial adjustment after temporal lobectomy: a prospective study. Int J Behav Med 2(1):27–40.
82. Berk C, Carr J, Sinden M, Martzke J, Honey CR (2002) Thalamic deep brain stimulation for the treatment of tremor due to multiple sclerosis: a prospective study of tremor and quality of life. J Neurosurg 97(4):815–820.

83. Deuschl G, Herzog J, Kleiner-Fisman G, et al (2006) Deep brain stimulation: postoperative issues. Mov Disord 21(Suppl 14):S219–S237.
84. Parsons TD, Rogers SA, Braaten AJ, Woods SP, Tröster AI (2006) Cognitive sequelae of subthalamic nucleus deep brain stimulation in Parkinson's disease: a meta-analysis. Lancet Neurol 5(7):578–588.
85. Aarsland D, Larsen JP, Karlsen K, Lim NG, Tandberg E (1999) Mental symptoms in Parkinson's disease are important contributors to caregiver distress. International J Geriat Psychiatry 14(10):866–874.
86. Wheless JW (2006) Intractable epilepsy: A survey of patients and caregivers. Epilepsy Behav 8(4):756–764.
87. Morrison CE, Borod JC, Brin MF, et al (2000) A program for neuropsychological investigation of deep brain stimulation (PNIDBS) in movement disorder patients: development, feasibility, and preliminary data. Neuropsych Neuropsychol Behavior Neurol 13(3):204–219.
88. Baker GA, Goldstein LH (2004) The dos and don'ts of neuropsychological assessment in epilepsy. Epilepsy Behav 5(Suppl 1):S77–S80.
89. Benedict RH, Fischer JS, Archibald CJ, et al (2002) Minimal neuropsychological assessment of MS patients: a consensus approach. Clin Neuropsychol 16(3): 381–397.
90. Boringa JB, Lazeron RH, Reuling IE, et al (2001) The brief repeatable battery of neuropsychological tests: normative values allow application in multiple sclerosis clinical practice. Mult Scler 7(4):263–267.
91. Peyser JM, Rao SM, LaRocca NG, Kaplan E (1990) Guidelines for neuropsychological research in multiple sclerosis. Arch Neurol 47(1):94–97.
92. Abelson JL, Curtis GC, Sagher O, et al (2005) Deep brain stimulation for refractory obsessive-compulsive disorder. Biol Psychiatry 57(5):510–516.
93. Gabriels L, Cosyns P, Nuttin B, Demeulemeester H, Gybels J (2003) Deep brain stimulation for treatment-refractory obsessive-compulsive disorder: psychopathological and neuropsychological outcome in three cases. Acta Psychiatr Scand 107(4):275–282.
94. Tröster AI, Arnett PJ (2006) Assessment of movement and demyelinating disorders. In: Snyder PJ, Nussbaum PD, Robins DL, eds. Clinical Neuropsychology: A Pocket Handbook for Assessment, second ed. Washington, DC: American Psychological Association.
95. Aldenkamp AP, Bodde N (2005) Behaviour, cognition and epilepsy. Acta Neurol Scand Suppl 182:19–25.
96. Hermann BP, Seidenberg M, Schoenfeld J, Davies K (1997) Neuropsychological characteristics of the syndrome of mesial temporal lobe epilepsy. Arch Neurol 54(4):369–376.
97. Gabrieli JDE, Singh J, Stebbins G, Goetz CG (1996) Reduced working memory span in Parkinson's disease: evidence for the role of a frontostriatal system in working and strategic memory. Neuropsychology 10:322–332.
98. Owen AM, Iddon JL, Hodges JR, Summers BA, Robbins TW (1997) Spatial and non-spatial working memory at different stages of Parkinson's disease. Neuropsychologia 35(4):519–532.
99. Owen AM, Sahakian BJ, Hodges JR, Summers BA, Polkey CE, Robbins TW (1995) Dopamine-dependent fronto-striatal planning deficits in early Parkinson's disease. Neuropsychology 9:126–140.
100. Stebbins GT, Gabrieli JD, Shannon KM, Penn RD, Goetz CG (2000) Impaired frontostriatal cognitive functioning following posteroventral pallidotomy in advanced Parkinson's disease. Brain Cognit 42(3):348–363.
101. Swartz BE, Halgren E, Simpkins F, et al (1996) Primary or working memory in frontal lobe epilepsy: An 18FDG-PET study of dysfunctional zones. Neurology 46(3):737–747.

102. Swartz BE, Simpkins F, Halgren E, et al (1996) Visual working memory in primary generalized epilepsy: an 18FDG-PET study. Neurology 47(5):1203–1212.
103. Meador KJ (2006) Cognitive and memory effects of the new antiepileptic drugs. Epilepsy Res 68(1):63–67.
104. Rao SM, Leo GJ, Bernardin L, Unverzagt F (1991) Cognitive dysfunction in multiple sclerosis. I. Frequency, patterns, and prediction. Neurology 41(5):685–691.
105. Marvel CL, Paradiso S (2004) Cognitive and neurological impairment in mood disorders. Psychiatr Clin North Am 27(1):19–36, vii–viii.
106. Tröster AI, Tucker KA (2005) Impact of essential tremor and its medical and surgical treatment on neuropsychological functioning, activities of daily living, and quality of life. In: Lyons KE, Pahwa R, eds. Handbook of Essential Tremor and Other Tremor Disorders. Boca Raton, FL: Taylor and Francis, pp. 117–131.
107. Scott RB, Gregory R, Wilson J, et al (2003) Executive cognitive deficits in primary dystonia. Mov Disord 18(5):539–550.
108. Cools R, Barker RA, Sahakian BJ, Robbins TW (2001) Mechanisms of cognitive set flexibility in Parkinson's disease. Brain 124(Pt 12):2503–2512.
109. Pillon B, Boller F, Levy R, Dubois B (2001) Cognitive deficits and dementia in Parkinson's disease. In: Boller F, Cappa SF, eds. Handbook of Neuropsychology, second ed. Amsterdam: Elsevier, pp. 311–371.
110. Anderson KE, Savage CR (2004) Cognitive and neurobiological findings in obsessive-compulsive disorder. Psychiatr Clin North Am 27(1):37–47, viii.
111. Cavedini P, Gorini A, Bellodi L (2006) Understanding obsessive-compulsive disorder: focus on decision making. Neuropsychol Rev 16(1):3–15.
112. Tavares JV, Drevets WC, Sahakian BJ (2003) Cognition in mania and depression. Psychol Med 33(6):959–967.
113. Calabrese P (2006) Neuropsychology of multiple sclerosis—an overview. J Neurol 253(Suppl 1):I10–I15.
114. Lombardi WJ, Woolston DJ, Roberts JW, Gross RE (2001) Cognitive deficits in patients with essential tremor. Neurology 57(5):785–790.
115. Lacritz LH, Dewey R Jr, Giller C, Cullum CM (2002) Cognitive functioning in individuals with "benign" essential tremor. J Int Neuropsycholog Soc 8(1):125–129.
116. Tröster AI, Woods SP, Fields JA, et al (2002) Neuropsychological deficits in essential tremor: an expression of cerebello-thalamo-cortical pathophysiology? Eur J Neurol 9(2):143–151.
117. Duane DD, Vermilion KJ (2002) Cognitive deficits in patients with essential tremor. Neurology 58(11):1706.
118. Gasparini M, Bonifati V, Fabrizio E, et al (2001) Frontal lobe dysfunction in essential tremor: a preliminary study. J Neurol 248(5):399–402.
119. Duane DD, Vermilion KJ (2004) Cognition and affect in patients with cervical dystonia with and without tremor. Advance Neurol 94:179–189.
120. Jahanshahi M, Rowe J, Fuller R (2003) Cognitive executive function in dystonia. Mov Disord 18(12):1470–1481.
121. Balas M, Peretz C, Badarny S, Scott RB, Giladi N (2006) Neuropsychological profile of DYT1 dystonia. Mov Disord 21(12):2073–2077.
122. Como PG (2001) Neuropsychological function in Tourette syndrome. Adv Neurol 85:103–111.
123. Bornstein RA (1991) Neuropsychological correlates of obsessive characteristics in Tourette syndrome. J Neuropsychiatry Clin Neurosci 3(2):157–162.
124. Dymek MP, Atchison P, Harrell L, Marson DC (2001) Competency to consent to medical treatment in cognitively impaired patients with Parkinson's disease. Neurology 56(1):17–24.
125. Cahn DA, Sullivan EV, Shear PK, Pfefferbaum A, Heit G, Silverberg G (1998) Differential contributions of cognitive and motor component processes to

physical and instrumental activities of daily living in Parkinson's disease. Arch Clin Neuropsychol 13:575–583.
126. Tröster AI, Fields JA, Straits-Tröster KA, et al (2000) Executive function, coping, mood state, and quality of life in Parkinson's disease patients being evaluated for pallidotomy. J Int Neuropsycholog Soc 6(2):207.
127. Higginson CI, Arnett PA, Voss WD (2000) The ecological validity of clinical tests of memory and attention in multiple sclerosis. Arch Clin Neuropsychol 15(3):185–204.
128. Culhane-Shelburne K, Chapieski L, Hiscock M, Glaze D (2002) Executive functions in children with frontal and temporal lobe epilepsy. J Int Neuropsychol Soc 8(5):623–632.
129. Batzel LW, Dodrill CB (1984) Neuropsychological and emotional correlates of marital status and ability to live independently in individuals with epilepsy. Epilepsia 25(5):594–598.
130. Woods SP, Fields JA, Tröster AI (2002) Neuropsychological sequelae of subthalamic nucleus deep brain stimulation in Parkinson's disease: a critical review. Neuropsychol Rev 12(2):111–126.
131. Tröster AI, Woods SP (2003) Neuropsychological aspects of Parkinson's disease and parkinsonian syndromes. In: Pahwa R, Lyons KE, Koller WC, eds. Handbook of Parkinson's Disease, third ed. New York: Marcel Dekker, pp. 127–157.
132. Jacobs DM, Marder K, Cote LJ, Sano M, Stern Y, Mayeux R (1995) Neuropsychological characteristics of preclinical dementia in Parkinson's disease. Neurology 45(9):1691–1696.
133. Mahieux F, Fenelon G, Flahault A, Manifacier MJ, Michelet D, Boller F (1998) Neuropsychological prediction of dementia in Parkinson's disease. J Neurol Neurosurg Psychiatry 64(2):178–183.
134. Hwang SH, Kwon JS, Shin YW, Lee KJ, Kim YY, Kim MS (2007) Neuropsychological profiles of patients with obsessive-compulsive disorder: early onset versus late onset. J Int Neuropsychol Soc 13(1):30–37.
135. Saykin AJ, Stafiniak P, Robinson LJ, et al (1995) Language before and after temporal lobectomy: specificity of acute changes and relation to early risk factors. Epilepsia 36(11):1071–1077.
136. Tröster AI, Warmflash V, Osorio I, Paolo AM, Alexander LJ, Barr WB (1995) The roles of semantic networks and search efficiency in verbal fluency performance in intractable temporal lobe epilepsy. Epilepsy Res 21(1):19–26.
137. Bartha L, Benke T, Bauer G, Trinka E (2005) Interictal language functions in temporal lobe epilepsy. J Neurol Neurosurg Psychiatry 76(6):808–814.
138. Pahwa R, Paolo A, Tröster A, Koller W (1998) Cognitive impairment in Parkinson's disease. Eur J Neurol 5(5):431–441.
139. Buytenhuijs EL, Berger HJ, Van Spaendonck KP, Horstink MW, Borm GF, Cools AR (1994) Memory and learning strategies in patients with Parkinson's disease. Neuropsychologia 32(3):335–342.
140. Tröster AI, Fields JA (1995) Frontal cognitive function and memory in Parkinson's disease: toward a distinction between prospective and declarative memory impairments? Behavioural Neurology 8:59–74.
141. Griffiths SY, Yamamoto A, Boudreau VG, Ross LK, Kozora E, Thornton AE (2005) Memory interference in multiple sclerosis. J Int Neuropsychol Soc 11(6):737–746.
142. Thornton AE, Raz N, Tucke KA (2002) Memory in multiple sclerosis: contextual encoding deficits. J Int Neuropsychol Soc 8(3):395–409.
143. Backman L, Forsell Y (1994) Episodic memory functioning in a community-based sample of old adults with major depression: utilization of cognitive support. J Abnorm Psychol 103(2):361–370.
144. Bearden CE, Glahn DC, Monkul ES, et al (2006) Patterns of memory impairment in bipolar disorder and unipolar major depression. Psychiatry Res 142(2–3):139–150.

145. Leritz EC, Grande LJ, Bauer RM (2006) Temporal lobe epilepsy as a model to understand human memory: the distinction between explicit and implicit memory. Epilepsy Behav 9(1):1–13.
146. McDonald CR, Bauer RM, Grande L, Gilmore R, Roper S (2001) The role of the frontal lobes in memory: evidence from unilateral frontal resections for relief of intractable epilepsy. Arch Clin Neuropsychol 16(6):571–585.
147. Kuelz AK, Hohagen F, Voderholzer U (2004) Neuropsychological performance in obsessive-compulsive disorder: a critical review. Biol Psychol 65(3):185–236.
148. Huber SJ, Shuttleworth EC, Paulson GW (1986) Dementia in Parkinson's disease. Arch Neurol 43(10):987–990.
149. McDonald WM, Richard IH, DeLong MR (2003) Prevalence, etiology, and treatment of depression in Parkinson's disease. Biologic Psychiatry 54(3):363–375.
150. Tröster AI, Letsch EA (2004) Evaluation and treatment of anxiety and depression in Parkinson's disease. In: Pahwa R, Lyons KE, Koller WC, eds. Therapy of Parkinson's Disease, third ed. New York: Marcel Dekker, pp. 423–445.
151. Sadovnick AD, Remick RA, Allen J, et al (1996) Depression and multiple sclerosis. Neurology 46(3):628–632.
152. Grabowska-Grzyb A, Jedrzejczak J, Naganska E, Fiszer U (2006) Risk factors for depression in patients with epilepsy. Epilepsy Behav 8(2):411–417.
153. Boller F, Marcie P, Starkstein S, Traykov L (1998) Memory and depression in Parkinson's disease. Eur J Neurol 5(3):291–295.
154. Kuzis G, Sabe L, Tiberti C, Leiguarda R, Starkstein SE (1997) Cognitive functions in major depression and Parkinson disease. Arch Neurol 54(8): 982–986.
155. Tröster AI, Paolo AM, Lyons KE, Glatt SL, Hubble JP, Koller WC (1995) The influence of depression on cognition in Parkinson's disease: a pattern of impairment distinguishable from Alzheimer's disease. Neurology 45(4):672–676.
156. Arnett PA (2005) Longitudinal consistency of the relationship between depression symptoms and cognitive functioning in multiple sclerosis. CNS Spectr 10(5): 372–382.
157. Burchiel KJ, Taha JM, Favre J (1997) Posteroventral pallidotomy for Parkinson's disease patients. In: Rengachary SS, Wilkins RH, eds. Neurosurgical operative atlas. Park Ridge, IL: Am. Assoc. of Neurol. Surgeons, pp. 13–26.
158. Altshuler L, Rausch R, Delrahim S, Kay J, Crandall P (1999) Temporal lobe epilepsy, temporal lobectomy, and major depression. J Neuropsychiatry Clin Neurosci 11(4):436–443.
159. Higginson CI, Fields JA, Koller WC, Tröster AI (2001) Questionnaire assessment potentially overestimates anxiety in Parkinson's disease. J Clin Psychol Med Settings 8(2):95–99.
160. Saint-Cyr JA, Trépanier LL (2000) Neuropsychological considerations in movement disorder surgery. In: Lozano AM, ed. Movement Disorder Surgery. Basel: Karger, pp. 266–271.
161. Cummings JL, Mega M, Gray K, Rosenberg-Thompson S, Carusi DA, Gornbein J (1994) The Neuropsychiatric Inventory: comprehensive assessment of psychopathology in dementia. Neurology 44(12):2308–2314.
162. Grace J, Stout JC, Malloy PF (1999) Assessing frontal lobe behavioral syndromes with the frontal lobe personality scale. Assessment 6(3):269–284.
163. Grace J, Malloy PF (2001) Frontal Systems Behavior Scale: Professional Manual. Lutz, FL: Psychological Assessment Resources, Inc.
164. Narabayashi H, Miyashita N, Hattori Y, Saito K, Endo K (1997) Posteroventral pallidotomy: its effect on motor symptoms and scores of MMPI test in patients with Parkinson's disease. Parkinsonism Relate Disord 3(1):7–20.
165. Derry PA, Harnadek MC, McLachlan RS, Sontrop J, Blume WT, Girvin JP (2002) A longitudinal study of the effects of seizure symptoms on the Minnesota

Multiphasic Personality Inventory-2 (MMPI-2) clinical interpretation. J Clin Psychol 58(7):817–826.
166. Dodrill CB, Wilkus RJ, Ojemann GA, et al (1986) Multidisciplinary prediction of seizure relief from cortical resection surgery. Ann Neurol 20(1):2–12.
167. Diller L, Riklan M, Cooper IS (1956) Preoperative response to stress as a criterion of the response to neurosurgery in Parkinson's disease. J Am Geriat Soc 4:1301–1308.
168. Tröster AI, Fields JA, Straits-Tröster KA, et al (1998) Motoric and psychosocial correlates of quality of life in Parkinson's disease four months after unilateral pallidotomy. Neurology 50(Suppl 4):A299.
169. Tröster AI (2000) Clinical neuropsychology, functional neurosurgery, and restorative neurology in the next millennium: beyond secondary outcome measures. Brain Cogn 42(1):117–119.
170. Tomaszewski KJ, Holloway RG (2001) Deep brain stimulation in the treatment of Parkinson's disease: a cost- effectiveness analysis. Neurology 57(4):663–671.
171. Hailey D, Harstall C (1998) Posteroventral pallidotomy for Parkinson's disease: assessment and policy on a technology in transition. Health Policy 43(1):55–64.
172. Thompson PD (2001) Deep brain stimulation is superior to ablative surgery for Parkinson's disease: the case against. J Clin Neurosci 8(3):291–292; discussion 293–294.
173. López-Lozano JJ, Mata M (1999) Surgical treatment for Parkinson's disease: impact on the patient's quality of life. In: Martínez-Martín P, Koller WC, eds. Quality of life in Parkinson's disease. Barcelona: Masson, pp. 107–136.
174. Tröster AI, Fields JA, Pahwa R, et al (1999) Neuropsychological and quality of life outcome after thalamic stimulation for essential tremor. Neurology 53(8):1774–1780.
175. Tröster AI, Lyons KE, Straits-Tröster KA (1999) Determinants of health-related quality of life changes in Parkinson's disease. In: Martínez-Martín P, Koller WC, eds. Quality of Life in Parkinson's Disease. Barcelona: Masson, pp. 55–77.
176. Laing RJ (2000) Measuring outcome in neurosurgery. Br J Neurosurg 14(3): 181–184.
177. Vickrey BG (1993) A procedure for developing a quality-of-life measure for epilepsy surgery patients. Epilepsia 34(Suppl 4):S22–S27.
178. Kuehler A, Henrich G, Schroeder U, Conrad B, Herschbach P, Ceballos-Baumann A (2003) A novel quality of life instrument for deep brain stimulation in movement disorders. J Neurol Neurosurg Psychiatry 74(8):1023–1030.
179. Peto V, Jenkinson C, Fitzpatrick R (1998) PDQ-39: a review of the development, validation and application of a Parkinson's disease quality of life questionnaire and its associated measures. J Neurol 245(Suppl 1):S10–S14.
180. Marinus J, Ramaker C, van Hilten JJ, Stiggelbout AM (2002) Health related quality of life in Parkinson's disease: a systematic review of disease specific instruments. J Neurol Neurosurg Psychiatry 72(2):241–248.
181. Hermann BP (1995) The evolution of health-related quality of life assessment in epilepsy. Qual Life Res 4(2):87–100.
182. Vickrey BG, Hays RD, Harooni R, Myers LW, Ellison GW (1995) A health-related quality of life measure for multiple sclerosis. Qual Life Res 4(3):187–206.
183. Tröster AI, Pahwa R, Fields JA, Tanner CM, Lyons KE (2005) Quality of Life in Essential Tremor Questionnaire (QUEST): development and initial validation. Parkinsonism Relat Disord 11(6):367–373.
184. Hunt SM, McKenna SP (1992) The QLDS: a scale for the measurement of quality of life in depression. Health Policy 22(3):307–319.
185. Lange KW, Robbins TW, Marsden CD, James M, Owen AM, Paul GM (1992) L-dopa withdrawal in Parkinson's disease selectively impairs cognitive performance in tests sensitive to frontal lobe dysfunction. Psychopharmacology 107(2–3):394–404.

186. Aldenkamp AP, De Krom M, Reijs R (2003) Newer antiepileptic drugs and cognitive issues. Epilepsia 44(Suppl 4):21–29.
187. Ortinski P, Meador KJ (2004) Cognitive side effects of antiepileptic drugs. Epilepsy Behav 5(Suppl 1):S60–S65.
188. Kennedy SH (2006) A review of antidepressant treatments today. Eur Neuropsychopharmacol 16(Suppl 5):S619–S623.
189. Alegret M, Vendrell P, Junqué C, et al (2000) Effects of unilateral posteroventral pallidotomy on 'on-off' cognitive fluctuations in Parkinson's disease. Neuropsychologia 38(5):628–633.
190. Green J, Barnhart H (2000) The impact of lesion laterality on neuropsychological change following posterior pallidotomy: a review of current findings. Brain Cognit 42(3):379–398.
191. York MK, Levin HS, Grossman RG, Hamilton WJ (1999) Neuropsychological outcome following unilateral pallidotomy. Brain 122(Pt 12):2209–2220.
192. Schmand B, de Bie RM, Koning-Haanstra M, de Smet JS, Speelman JD, van Zomeren AH (2000) Unilateral pallidotomy in PD: a controlled study of cognitive and behavioral effects. The Netherlands Pallidotomy Study (NEPAS) group. Neurology 54(5):1058–1064.
193. Martin R, Sawrie S, Gilliam F, et al (2002) Determining reliable cognitive change after epilepsy surgery: development of reliable change indices and standardized regression-based change norms for the WMS-III and WAIS-III. Epilepsia 43(12):1551–1558.
194. Sawrie SM, Chelune GJ, Naugle RI, Luders HO (1996) Empirical methods for assessing meaningful neuropsychological change following epilepsy surgery. J Int Neuropsychol Soc 2(6):556–564.
195. Temkin NR, Heaton RK, Grant I, Dikmen SS (1999) Detecting significant change in neuropsychological test performance: a comparison of four models. J Int Neuropsycholog Soc 5(4):357–369.
196. Blond S, Caparros-Lefebvre D, Parker F, et al (1992) Control of tremor and involuntary movement disorders by chronic stereotactic stimulation of the ventral intermediate thalamic nucleus. J Neurosurg 77(1):62–68.
197. Caparros-Lefebvre D, Blond S, Pécheux N, Pasquier F, Petit H (1992) Evaluation neuropsychologique avant et après stimulation thalamique chez 9 parkinsoniens. Revue Neurologique 148(2):117–122.
198. Tröster AI, Fields JA, Wilkinson SB, et al (1997) Neuropsychological functioning before and after unilateral thalamic stimulating electrode implantation in Parkinson's disease [electronic manuscript]. Neurosurg Focus 2(3):Article 9, pp. 1–6.
199. Loher TJ, Gutbrod K, Fravi NL, Pohle T, Burgunder JM, Krauss JK (2003) Thalamic stimulation for tremor. Subtle changes in episodic memory are related to stimulation per se and not to a microthalamotomy effect. J Neurol 250(6): 707–713.
200. Woods SP, Fields JA, Lyons KE, et al (2001) Neuropsychological and quality of life changes following unilateral thalamic deep brain stimulation in Parkinson's disease: a 12-month follow-up. Acta Neurochir 143:1273–1278.
201. Hugdahl K, Wester K (1997) Lateralized thalamic stimulation: effects on verbal memory. Neuropsych Neuropsychol Behav Neurol 10(3):155–161.
202. Wester K, Hugdahl K (1997) Thalamotomy and thalamic stimulation: effects on cognition. Stereotact Funct Neurosurg 69(1–4):80–85.
203. Hugdahl K, Wester K (2000) Neurocognitive correlates of stereotactic thalamotomy and thalamic stimulation in Parkinsonian patients. Brain Cogn 42(2):231–252.
204. Ojemann GA, Hoyenga KB, Ward AA Jr (1971) Prediction of short-term verbal memory disturbance after ventrolateral thalamotomy. J Neurosurg 35(2): 203–210.

205. Tröster AI, Wilkinson SB, Fields JA, Miyawaki K, Koller WC (1998) Chronic electrical stimulation of the left ventrointermediate (VIM) thalamic nucleus for the treatment of pharmacotherapy-resistant Parkinson's disease: a differential impact on access to semantic and episodic memory? Brain Cogn 38(2):125–149.
206. Straits-Tröster K, Fields JA, Wilkinson SB, et al (2000) Health-related quality of life in Parkinson's disease after pallidotomy and deep brain stimulation. Brain Cogn 42(3):399–416.
207. Lyons KE, Pahwa R, Tröster AI, Koller WC (1997) A comparison of Parkinson's disease symptoms and self-reported functioning and well-being. Parkinsonism Relat Disord 3:207–209.
208. Tröster AI, Fields JA, Wilkinson SB, et al (1997) Unilateral pallidal stimulation for Parkinson's disease: neurobehavioral functioning before and 3 months after electrode implantation. Neurology 49(4):1078–1083.
209. Vingerhoets G, van der Linden C, Lannoo E, et al (1999) Cognitive outcome after unilateral pallidal stimulation in Parkinson's disease. J Neurol Neurosurg Psychiatry 66(3):297–304.
210. Merello M, Nouzeilles MI, Kuzis G, et al (1999) Unilateral radiofrequency lesion versus electrostimulation of posteroventral pallidum: a prospective randomized comparison. Mov Disord 14(1):50–56.
211. Ardouin C, Pillon B, Peiffer E, et al (1999) Bilateral subthalamic or pallidal stimulation for Parkinson's disease affects neither memory nor executive functions: a consecutive series of 62 patients. Ann Neurol 46(2):217–223.
212. Pillon B, Ardouin C, Damier P, et al (2000) Neuropsychological changes between "off" and "on" STN or GPi stimulation in Parkinson's disease. Neurology 55(3):411–418.
213. Ghika J, Villemure JG, Fankhauser H, Favre J, Assal G, Ghika-Schmid F (1998) Efficiency and safety of bilateral contemporaneous pallidal stimulation (deep brain stimulation) in levodopa-responsive patients with Parkinson's disease with severe motor fluctuations: a 2-year follow-up review. J Neurosurg 89(5):713–718.
214. Fields JA, Tröster AI, Wilkinson SB, Pahwa R, Koller WC (1999) Cognitive outcome following staged bilateral pallidal stimulation for the treatment of Parkinson's disease. Clin Neurol Neurosurg 101(3):182–188.
215. Rothlind JC, Cockshott RW, Starr PA, Marks WJ (2007) Neuropsychological performance following staged bilateral pallidal or subthalamic nucleus deep brain stimulation for Parkinson's disease. J Int Neuropsychol Soc 13(1):68–79.
216. Dujardin K, Krystkowiak P, Defebvre L, Blond S, Destee A (2000) A case of severe dysexecutive syndrome consecutive to chronic bilateral pallidal stimulation. Neuropsychologia 38(9):1305–1315.
217. Trépanier LL, Kumar R, Lozano AM, Lang AE, Saint-Cyr JA (2000) Neuropsychological outcome of GPi pallidotomy and GPi or STN deep brain stimulation in Parkinson's disease. Brain Cognit 42(3):324–347.
218. Volkmann J, Allert N, Voges J, Sturm V, Schnitzler A, Freund HJ (2004) Long-term results of bilateral pallidal stimulation in Parkinson's disease. Ann Neurol 55(6):871–875.
219. Tröster AI, Woods SP, Fields JA, Hanisch C, Beatty WW (2002) Declines in switching underlie verbal fluency changes after unilateral pallidal surgery in Parkinson's disease. Brain Cognit 50(2):207–217.
220. Fields JA, Tröster AI, Wilkinson SB, et al (1998) Comparison of the cognitive safety of unilateral pallidal stimulation and pallidotomy. Neurology 50(Suppl 4):A389.
221. Anderson VC, Burchiel KJ, Hogarth P, Favre J, Hammerstad JP (2005) Pallidal vs subthalamic nucleus deep brain stimulation in Parkinson disease. Arch Neurol 62(4):554–560.

222. Rodriguez-Oroz MC, Obeso JA, Lang AE, et al (2005) Bilateral deep brain stimulation in Parkinson's disease: a multicentre study with 4 years follow-up. Brain.
223. Volkmann J, Allert N, Voges J, Weiss PH, Freund H-J, Sturm V (2001) Safety and efficacy of pallidal or subthalamic nucleus stimulation in advanced PD. Neurology 56(4):548–551.
224. Vingerhoets G, Lannoo E, van der Linden C, et al (1999) Changes in quality of life following unilateral pallidal stimulation in Parkinson's disease. J Psychosomat Res 46(3):247–255.
225. Higginson CI, Fields JA, Tröster AI (2001) Which symptoms of anxiety diminish after surgical interventions for Parkinson's disease. Neuropsych Neuropsychol Behav Neurol 14(2):117–121.
226. Burn DJ, Tröster AI (2004) Neuropsychiatric complications of medical and surgical therapies for Parkinson's disease. J Geriatr Psychiatry Neurol 17(3):172–180.
227. Voon V, Kubu C, Krack P, Houeto JL, Tröster AI (2006) Deep brain stimulation: neuropsychological and neuropsychiatric issues. Mov Disord 21(Suppl 14):S305–S327.
228. Voon V, Moro E, Saint-Cyr JA, Lozano AM, Lang AE (2005) Psychiatric symptoms following surgery for Parkinson's disease with an emphasis on subthalamic stimulation. In: Anderson KE, Weiner WJ, Lang AE, eds. Behavioral Neurology of Movement Disorders, second ed. Philadelphia: Lippincott, Williams & Wilkins, pp. 130–147.
229. Miyawaki E, Perlmutter JS, Tröster AI, Videen TO, Koller WC (2000) The behavioral complications of pallidal stimulation: a case report. Brain Cognit 42(3):417–434.
230. Krause M, Fogel W, Heck A, et al (2001) Deep brain stimulation for the treatment of Parkinson's disease: subthalamic nucleus versus globus pallidus internus. J Neurol Neurosurg Psychiatry 70(4):464–470.
231. Roane DM, Yu M, Feinberg TE, Rogers JD (2002) Hypersexuality after pallidal surgery in Parkinson disease. Neuropsych Neuropsychol Behav Neurol 15(4):247–251.
232. Temel Y, Kessels A, Tan S, Topdag A, Boon P, Visser-Vandewalle V (2006) Behavioural changes after bilateral subthalamic stimulation in advanced Parkinson disease: a systematic review. Parkinsonism Relat Disord 12(5):265–272.
233. Kleiner-Fisman G, Fisman DN, Sime E, Saint-Cyr JA, Lozano AM, Lang AE (2003) Long-term follow up of bilateral deep brain stimulation of the subthalamic nucleus in patients with advanced Parkinson disease. J Neurosurg 99(3):489–495.
234. Deuschl G, Schade-Brittinger C, Krack P, et al (2006) A randomized trial of deep-brain stimulation for Parkinson's disease. N Engl J Med 355(9):896–908.
235. Castelli L, Perozzo P, Zibetti M, et al (2006) Chronic deep brain stimulation of the subthalamic nucleus for Parkinson's disease: effects on cognition, mood, anxiety and personality traits. Eur Neurol 55(3):136–144.
236. Brusa L, Pierantozzi M, Peppe A, et al (2001) Deep brain stimulation (DBS) attentional effects parallel those of l- dopa treatment. J Neural Trans 108(8–9):1021–1027.
237. Contarino MF, Daniele A, Sibilia AH, et al (in press) Cognitive outcome five years after bilateral chronic stimulation of subthalamic nucleus in patients with Parkinson's disease. J Neurol Neurosurg Psychiatry.
238. Dujardin K, Defebvre L, Krystkowiak P, Blond S, Destée A (2001) Influence of chronic bilateral stimulation of the subthalamic nucleus on cognitive function in Parkinson's disease. J Neurol 248:603–611.
239. Erola T, Karinen P, Heikkinen E, et al (2005) Bilateral subthalamic nucleus stimulation improves health-related quality of life in Parkinsonian patients. Parkinsonism Relat Disord 11(2):89–94.

240. Funkiewiez A, Ardouin C, Caputo E, et al (2004) Long term effects of bilateral subthalamic nucleus stimulation on cognitive function, mood, and behaviour in Parkinson's disease. J Neurol Neurosurg Psychiatry 75(6):834–839.
241. Gironell A, Kulisevsky J, Rami L, Fortuny N, Garcia-Sanchez C, Pascual-Sedano B (2003) Effects of pallidotomy and bilateral subthalamic stimulation on cognitive function in Parkinson disease. A controlled comparative study. J Neurol 250(8):917–923.
242. Jahanshahi M, Ardouin CM, Brown RG, et al (2000) The impact of deep brain stimulation on executive function in Parkinson's disease. Brain 123(Pt 6): 1142–1154.
243. Moretti R, Torre P, Antonello RM, et al (2001) Effects on cognitive abilities following subthalamic nucleus stimulation in Parkinson's disease. Eur J Neurol 8(6):726–727.
244. Moretti R, Torre P, Antonello RM, et al (2003) Neuropsychological changes after subthalamic nucleus stimulation: a 12 month follow-up in nine patients with Parkinson's disease. Parkinsonism Relat Disord 10(2):73–79.
245. Morrison CE, Borod JC, Perrine K, et al (2004) Neuropsychological functioning following bilateral subthalamic nucleus stimulation in Parkinson's disease. Arch Clin Neuropsychol 19(2):165–181.
246. Perozzo P, Rizzone M, Bergamasco B, et al (2001) Deep brain stimulation of the subthalamic nucleus in Parkinson's disease: comparison of pre- and postoperative neuropsychological evaluation. J Neurolog Sci 192(1–2):9–15.
247. Smeding HM, Esselink RA, Schmand B, et al (2005) Unilateral pallidotomy versus bilateral subthalamic nucleus stimulation in PD—a comparison of neuropsychological effects. J Neurol 252(2):176–182.
248. Smeding HM, Speelman JD, Koning-Haanstra M, et al (2006) Neuropsychological effects of bilateral STN stimulation in Parkinson disease: a controlled study. Neurology 66(12):1830–1836.
249. Whelan BM, Murdoch BE, Theodoros DG, Hall B, Silburn P (2003) Defining a role for the subthalamic nucleus within operative theoretical models of subcortical participation in language. J Neurol Neurosurg Psychiatry 74(11): 1543–1550.
250. Witt K, Pulkowski U, Herzog J, et al (2004) Deep brain stimulation of the subthalamic nucleus improves cognitive flexibility but impairs response inhibition in Parkinson disease. Arch Neurol 61(5):697–700.
251. Drapier D, Drapier S, Sauleau P, et al (2006) Does subthalamic nucleus stimulation induce apathy in Parkinson's disease? J Neurol 253(8):1083–1091.
252. De Gaspari D, Siri C, Landi A, et al (2006) Clinical and neuropsychological follow up at 12 months in patients with complicated Parkinson's disease treated with subcutaneous apomorphine infusion or deep brain stimulation of the subthalamic nucleus. J Neurol Neurosurg Psychiatry 77(4):450–453.
253. Alegret M, Junqué C, Valldeoriola F, et al (2001) Effects of bilateral subthalamic stimulation on cognitive function in Parkinson disease. Arch Neurol 58(8): 1223–1227.
254. Alegret M, Valldeoriola F, Marti M, et al (2004) Comparative cognitive effects of bilateral subthalamic stimulation and subcutaneous continuous infusion of apomorphine in Parkinson's disease. Mov Disord 19(12):1463–1469.
255. Saint-Cyr JA, Trépanier LL, Kumar R, Lozano AM, Lang AE (2000) Neuropsychological consequences of chronic bilateral stimulation of the subthalamic nucleus in Parkinson's disease. Brain 123(Pt 10):2091–2108.
256. Woods SP, Rippeth JD, Conover E, Carey CL, Parsons TD, Tröster AI (2006) Statistical power of studies examining the cognitive effects of subthalamic nucleus deep brain stimulation in Parkinson's disease. Clin Neuropsychol 20:27–38.

257. Temel Y, Blokland A, Steinbusch HW, Visser-Vandewalle V (2005) The functional role of the subthalamic nucleus in cognitive and limbic circuits. Prog Neurobiol 76(6):393–413.
258. Perlmutter JS, Mink JW (2006) Deep brain stimulation. Annu Rev Neurosci 29:229–257.
259. Wichmann T, Delong MR (2006) Deep brain stimulation for neurologic and neuropsychiatric disorders. Neuron 52(1):197–204.
260. Perriol MP, Krystkowiak P, Defebvre L, Blond S, Destee A, Dujardin K (2006) Stimulation of the subthalamic nucleus in Parkinson's disease: cognitive and affective changes are not linked to the motor outcome. Parkinsonism Relat Disord 12(4):205–210.
261. Hristova A, Lyons K, Tröster AI, Pahwa R, Wilkinson SB, Koller WC (2000) Effect and time course of deep brain stimulation of the globus pallidus and subthalamus on motor features of Parkinson's disease. Clin Neuropharmacol 23(4):208–211.
262. Francel P, Ryder K, Wetmore J, et al (2004) Deep brain stimulation for Parkinson's disease: association between stimulation parameters and cognitive performance. Stereotact Funct Neurosurg 82(4):191–193.
263. Jahanshahi M, Brown RG, Rothwell JC, Pollak P, Limousin P (1997) Subthalamic nucleus (STN) and globus pallidus (GPi) stimulation in Parkinson's disease (PD): II. effects on executive function and working memory. Mov Disord 12(Suppl 1):130.
264. Hershey T, Revilla FJ, Wernle A, Gibson PS, Dowling JL, Perlmutter JS (2004) Stimulation of STN impairs aspects of cognitive control in PD. Neurol 62(7):1110–1114.
265. Wojtecki L, Timmermann L, Jorgens S, et al (2006) Frequency-dependent reciprocal modulation of verbal fluency and motor functions in subthalamic deep brain stimulation. Arch Neurol 63(9):1273–1276.
266. Hariz MI, Johansson F, Shamsgovara P, Johansson E, Hariz GM, Fagerlund M (2000) Bilateral subthalamic nucleus stimulation in a parkinsonian patient with preoperative deficits in speech and cognition: persistent improvement in mobility but increased dependency: a case study. Mov Disord 15(1):136–139.
267. Valldeoriola F, Tolosa E, Alegret M, et al (2006) Cognitive changes in Parkinson's disease during subthalamic stimulation: a clinicopathologic study. J Neurol Neurosurg Psychiatry 77(4):565–566.
268. Jarraya B, Bonnet AM, Duyckaerts C, et al (2003) Parkinson's disease, subthalamic stimulation, and selection of candidates: a pathological study. Mov Disord 18(12):1517–1520.
269. Benabid AI, Koudsié A, Benazzouz A, et al., eds (1999) Neurosurgical therapy in Parkinson's disease. Utrecht, The Netherlands: Academic Pharmaceutical Productions.
270. Montgomery EB Jr (2005) Effect of subthalamic nucleus stimulation patterns on motor performance in Parkinson's disease. Parkinsonism Relat Disord 11(3):167–171.
271. Schulz GM, Grant MK (2000) Effects of speech therapy and pharmacologic and surgical treatments on voice and speech in Parkinson's disease: a review of the literature. J Commun Disord 33(1):59–88.
272. Joel D, Weiner I (1997) The connections of the primate subthalamic nucleus: indirect pathways and the open-interconnected scheme of basal ganglia-thalamocortical circuitry. Brain Res Rev 23(1–2):62–78.
273. Pinto S, Thobois S, Costes N, et al (2004) Subthalamic nucleus stimulation and dysarthria in Parkinson's disease: a PET study. Brain.

274. Gentil M, Garcia-Ruiz P, Pollak P, Benabid AL (1999) Effect of stimulation of the subthalamic nucleus on oral control of patients with parkinsonism. J Neurol Neurosurg Psychiatry 67(3):329–333.
275. Gentil M, Pinto S, Pollak P, Benabid A-L (2003) Effect of bilateral stimulation of the subthalamic nucleus on parkinsonian dysarthria. Brain Lang 85(2): 190–196.
276. Rousseaux M, Krystkowiak P, Kozlowski O, Ozsancak C, Blond S, Destee A (2004) Effects of subthalamic nucleus stimulation on parkinsonian dysarthria and speech intelligibility. J Neurol 251(3):327–334.
277. Santens P, De Letter M, Van Borsel J, De Reuck J, Caemaert J (2003) Lateralized effects of subthalamic nucleus stimulation on different aspects of speech in Parkinson's disease. Brain Lang 87(2):253–258.
278. Moretti R, Torre P, Antonello RM, et al (2003) 'Speech initiation hesitation' following subthalamic nucleus stimulation in a patient with Parkinson's disease. Eur Neurol 49(4):251–253.
279. Pinto S, Gentil M, Krack P, et al (2005) Changes induced by levodopa and subthalamic nucleus stimulation on parkinsonian speech. Mov Disord 20(11): 1507–1515.
280. Tornqvist AL, Schalen L, Rehncrona S (2005) Effects of different electrical parameter settings on the intelligibility of speech in patients with Parkinson's disease treated with subthalamic deep brain stimulation. Mov Disord 20(4): 416–423.
281. Zanini S, Melatini A, Capus L, Gioulis M, Vassallo A, Bava A (2003) Language recovery following subthalamic nucleus stimulation in Parkinson's disease. Neuroreport 14(3):511–516.
282. York MK, Levin HS, Grossman RG, Lai EC, Krauss JK (2003) Clustering and switching in phonemic fluency following pallidotomy for the treatment of Parkinson's disease. J Clin Exp Neuropsychol 25(1):110–121.
283. De Gaspari D, Siri C, Di Gioia M, et al (2006) Clinical correlates and cognitive underpinnings of verbal fluency impairment after chronic subthalamic stimulation in Parkinson's disease. Parkinsonism Relat Disord 12(5):289–295.
284. Fimm B, Zahn R, Mull M, et al (2001) Asymmetries of visual attention after circumscribed subcortical vascular lesions. J Neurol Neurosurg Psychiatry 71(5):652–657.
285. Gitelman DR, Nobre AC, Parrish TB, et al (1999) A large-scale distributed network for covert spatial attention: further anatomical delineation based on stringent behavioural and cognitive controls. Brain 122(Pt 6):1093–1106.
286. Uslaner JM, Robinson TE (2006) Subthalamic nucleus lesions increase impulsive action and decrease impulsive choice—mediation by enhanced incentive motivation? Eur J Neurosci 24(8):2345–2354.
287. Kensinger EA, Shearer DK, Locascio JJ, Growdon JH (2003) Working memory in mild Alzheimer's disease and early Parkinson's disease. Neuropsychology 17(2):230–239.
288. Kulisevsky J, García-Sánchez C, Berthier ML, et al (2000) Chronic effects of dopaminergic replacement on cognitive function in Parkinson's disease: a two-year follow-up study of previously untreated patients. Mov Disord 15(4): 613–626.
289. Gerschlager W, Alesch F, Cunnington R, et al (1999) Bilateral subthalamic nucleus stimulation improves frontal cortex function in Parkinson's disease. An electrophysiological study of the contingent negative variation. Brain 122(Pt 12):2365–2373.
290. Schroeder U, Kuehler A, Haslinger B, et al (2002) Subthalamic nucleus stimulation affects striato-anterior cingulate cortex circuit in a response conflict task: a PET study. Brain 125(Pt 9):1995–2004.

291. Witt K, Kopper F, Deuschl G, Krack P (2006) Subthalamic nucleus influences spatial orientation in extra-personal space. Mov Disord 21(3):354–361.
292. Heber IA, Kronenbuerger M, Fromm C, Coenen VA, Block F, Fimm B (2006) Attentional functions in Parkinson's disease patients treated with deep brain stimulation. Eur J Neurol 13(Suppl 2):76.
293. Crown S (1971) Psychosomatic aspects of Parkinsonism. J Psychosomat Res 15(4):451–459.
294. Koch G, Brusa L, Caltagirone C, et al (2004) Subthalamic deep brain stimulation improves time perception in Parkinson's disease. Neuroreport 15(6):1071–1073.
295. Schroeder U, Kuehler A, Hennenlotter A, et al (2004) Facial expression recognition and subthalamic nucleus stimulation. J Neurol Neurosurg Psychiatry 75(4):648–650.
296. Biseul I, Sauleau P, Haegelen C, et al (2005) Fear recognition is impaired by subthalamic nucleus stimulation in Parkinson's disease. Neuropsychologia 43(7):1054–1059.
297. Dujardin K, Blairy S, Defebvre L, et al (2004) Deficits in decoding emotional facial expressions in Parkinson's disease. Neuropsychologia 42(2):239–250.
298. Hälbig TD, Gruber D, Kopp UA, et al (2004) Subthalamic stimulation differentially modulates declarative and nondeclarative memory. Neuroreport 15(3):539–543.
299. Kleiner-Fisman G, Herzog J, Fisman DN, et al (2006) Subthalamic nucleus deep brain stimulation: summary and meta-analysis of outcomes. Mov Disord 21(Suppl 14):S290–S304.
300. Schüpbach WM, Chastan N, Welter ML, et al (2005) Stimulation of the subthalamic nucleus in Parkinson's disease: a 5 year follow up. J Neurol Neurosurg Psychiatry 76(12):1640–1644.
301. Houeto JL, Mesnage V, Mallet L, et al (2002) Behavioural disorders, Parkinson's disease and subthalamic stimulation. J Neurol Neurosurg Psychiatry 72(6):701–707.
302. Diederich NJ, Alesch F, Goetz CG (2000) Visual hallucinations induced by deep brain stimulation in Parkinson's disease. Clin Neuropharmacol 23(5):287–289.
303. Okun MS, Raju DV, Walter BL, et al (2004) Pseudobulbar crying induced by stimulation in the region of the subthalamic nucleus. J Neurol Neurosurg Psychiatry 75(6):921–923.
304. Kumar R, Lozano AM, Sime E, Halket E, Lang AE (1999) Comparative effects of unilateral and bilateral subthalamic nucleus deep brain stimulation. Neurology 53(3):561–566.
305. Bejjani BP, Damier P, Arnulf I, et al (1999) Transient acute depression induced by high-frequency deep-brain stimulation. N Engl J Med 340(19):1476–1480.
306. Houeto JL, Damier P, Bejjani PB, et al (2000) Subthalamic stimulation in Parkinson disease: a multidisciplinary approach. Arch Neurol 57(4):461–465.
307. Okun MS, Green J, Saben R, Gross R, Foote KD, Vitek JL (2003) Mood changes with deep brain stimulation of STN and GPi: results of a pilot study. J Neurol Neurosurg Psychiatry 74(11):1584–1586.
308. Chen SY, Lin SZ, Lee TW (2004) Subthalamic nucleus stimulation and the development of delusion. J Psychiatr Res 38(6):637–638.
309. Bejjani BP, Houeto JL, Hariz M, et al (2002) Aggressive behavior induced by intraoperative stimulation in the triangle of Sano. Neurology 59(9):1425–1427.
310. Sensi M, Eleopra R, Cavallo MA, et al (2004) Explosive-aggressive behavior related to bilateral subthalamic stimulation. Parkinsonism Relat Disord 10(4):247–251.
311. Kalteis K, Standhardt H, Kryspin-Exner I, Brucke T, Volc D, Alesch F (2006) Influence of bilateral Stn-stimulation on psychiatric symptoms and psychosocial

functioning in patients with Parkinson's disease. J Neural Transm 113(9): 1191–1206.
312. Czernecki V, Pillon B, Houeto JL, et al (2005) Does bilateral stimulation of the subthalamic nucleus aggravate apathy in Parkinson's disease? J Neurol Neurosurg Psychiatry 76(6):775–779.
313. Voon V, Saint-Cyr J, Lozano AM, Moro E, Poon YY, Lang AE (2005) Psychiatric symptoms in patients with Parkinson disease presenting for deep brain stimulation surgery. J Neurosurg 103(2):246–251.
314. Ardouin C, Voon V, Worbe Y, et al (2006) Pathological gambling in Parkinson's disease improves on chronic subthalamic nucleus stimulation. Mov Disord 21(11):1941–1946.
315. Diamond A, Jankovic J (2005) The effect of deep brain stimulation on quality of life in movement disorders. J Neurol Neurosurg Psychiatry 76(9):1188–1193.
316. Lezcano E, Gomez-Esteban JC, Zarranz JJ, et al (2004) Improvement in quality of life in patients with advanced Parkinson's disease following bilateral deep-brain stimulation in subthalamic nucleus. Eur J Neurol 11(7):451–454.
317. Drapier S, Raoul S, Drapier D, et al (2005) Only physical aspects of quality of life are significantly improved by bilateral subthalamic stimulation in Parkinson's disease. J Neurol 252(5):583–588.
318. Martínez-Martín P, Valldeoriola F, Tolosa E, et al (2002) Bilateral subthalamic nucleus stimulation and quality of life in advanced Parkinson's disease. Mov Disord 17(2):372–377.
319. Siderowf A, Jaggi JL, Xie SX, et al (2006) Long-term effects of bilateral subthalamic nucleus stimulation on health-related quality of life in advanced Parkinson's disease. Mov Disord 21(6):746–753.
320. Lagrange E, Krack P, Moro E, et al (2002) Bilateral subthalamic nucleus stimulation improves health-related quality of life in PD. Neurology 59(12):1976–1978.
321. Lyons KE, Pahwa R (2005) Long-term benefits in quality of life provided by bilateral subthalamic stimulation in patients with Parkinson disease. J Neurosurg 103(2):252–255.
322. Tröster AI, Fields JA, Wilkinson S, Pahwa R, Koller WC, Lyons KE (2003) Effect of motor improvement on quality of life following subthalamic stimulation is mediated by changes in depressive symptomatology. Stereotact Funct Neurosurg 80(1–4):43–47.
323. Houeto JL, Mallet L, Mesnage V, et al (2006) Subthalamic stimulation in Parkinson disease: behavior and social adaptation. Arch Neurol 63(8):1090–1095.
324. Schüpbach M, Gargiulo M, Welter ML, et al (2006) Neurosurgery in Parkinson disease: a distressed mind in a repaired body? Neurology 66(12):1811–1816.
325. Kumar R, Lozano AM, Sime E, Lang AE (2003) Long-term follow-up of thalamic deep brain stimulation for essential and parkinsonian tremor. Neurology 61(11):1601–1604.
326. Limousin P, Speelman JD, Gielen F, Janssens M (1999) Multicentre European study of thalamic stimulation in parkinsonian and essential tremor. J Neurol Neurosurg Psychiatry 66(3):289–296.
327. Pahwa R, Lyons KL, Wilkinson SB, et al (1999) Bilateral thalamic stimulation for the treatment of essential tremor. Neurology 53(7):1447–1450.
328. Rehncrona S, Johnels B, Widner H, Tornqvist AL, Hariz M, Sydow O (2003) Long-term efficacy of thalamic deep brain stimulation for tremor: double-blind assessments. Mov Disord 18(2):163–170.
329. Plaha P, Patel NK, Gill SS (2004) Stimulation of the subthalamic region for essential tremor. J Neurosurg 101(1):48–54.
330. Kitagawa M, Murata J, Kikuchi S, et al (2000) Deep brain stimulation of subthalamic area for severe proximal tremor. Neurology 55(1):114–116.

331. Murata J, Kitagawa M, Uesugi H, et al (2003) Electrical stimulation of the posterior subthalamic area for the treatment of intractable proximal tremor. J Neurosurg 99(4):708–715.
332. Fields JA, Tröster AI, Woods SP, et al (2003) Neuropsychological and quality of life outcomes 12 months after unilateral thalamic stimulation for essential tremor. J Neurol Neurosurg Psychiatry 74(3):305–311.
333. Lucas JA, Rippeth J, Uitti R, Obwegeser A, Wharen R (2000) Cognitive, motor, and mood-related effects of left thalamic stimulation in the treatment of parkinsonian and essential tremor. J Int Neuropsycholog Soc 6(4):392.
334. Woods SP, Fields JA, Lyons KE, Pahwa R, Tröster AI (2003) Pulse width is associated with cognitive decline after thalamic stimulation for essential tremor. Parkinsonism Relate Disord 9:295–300.
335. Ondo W, Jankovic J, Schwartz K, Almaguer M, Simpson RK (1998) Unilateral thalamic deep brain stimulation for refractory essential tremor and Parkinson's disease tremor. Neurology 51(4):1063–1069.
336. Bryant JA, De Salles A, Cabatan C, Frysinger R, Behnke E, Bronstein J (2003) The impact of thalamic stimulation on activities of daily living for essential tremor. Surg Neurol 59(6):479–484; discussion 484–475.
337. Lyons KE, Pahwa R, Busenbark KL, Tröster AI, Wilkinson S, Koller WC (1998) Improvements in daily functioning after deep brain stimulation of the thalamus for intractable tremor. Mov Disord 13(4):690–692.
338. Sydow O, Thobois S, Alesch F, Speelman JD (2003) Multicentre European study of thalamic stimulation in essential tremor: a six year follow up. J Neurol Neurosurg Psychiatry 2003;74(10):1387–1391.
339. Fields JA, Tröster AI, Woods SP, et al (2003) Neuropsychological and quality of life outcomes 12 months after unilateral thalamic stimulation for essential tremor. J Neurol Neurosurg Psychiatry 74(3):305–311.
340. Cooper IS, Upton AR, Amin I (1980) Reversibility of chronic neurologic deficits. Some effects of electrical stimulation of the thalamus and internal capsule in man. Appl Neurophysiol 43(3–5):244–258.
341. Andy OJ (1983) Thalamic stimulation for control of movement disorders. Appl Neurophysiol 46(1–4):107–111.
342. Vidailhet M, Vercueil L, Houeto JL, et al (2005) Bilateral deep-brain stimulation of the globus pallidus in primary generalized dystonia. N Engl J Med 352(5):459–467.
343. Kupsch A, Benecke R, Muller J, et al (2006) Pallidal deep-brain stimulation in primary generalized or segmental dystonia. N Engl J Med 355(19):1978–1990.
344. Hälbig TD, Gruber D, Kopp UA, Schneider GH, Trottenberg T, Kupsch A (2005) Pallidal stimulation in dystonia: effects on cognition, mood, and quality of life. J Neurol Neurosurg Psychiatry 76(12):1713–1716.
345. Pillon B, Ardouin C, Dujardin K, et al (2006) Preservation of cognitive function in dystonia treated by pallidal stimulation. Neurology 66(10):1556–1558.
346. Polkey CE (2004) Brain stimulation in the treatment of epilepsy. Expert Rev Neurother 4(6):965–972.
347. Theodore WH, Fisher RS (2004) Brain stimulation for epilepsy. Lancet Neurol 3(2):111–118.
348. Cooper IS, Amin I, Upton A, Riklan M, Watkins S, McLellan L (1977) Safety and efficacy of chronic stimulation. Neurosurgery 1(2):203–205.
349. Cooper IS, Upton AR (1978) Effects of cerebellar stimulation on epilepsy, the EEG and cerebral palsy in man. Electroencephalogr Clin Neurophysiol Suppl 34:349–354.
350. Hodaie M, Wennberg RA, Dostrovsky JO, Lozano AM (2002) Chronic anterior thalamus stimulation for intractable epilepsy. Epilepsia 43(6):603–608.

351. Graves NM, Fisher RS (2005) Neurostimulation for epilepsy, including a pilot study of anterior nucleus stimulation. Clin Neurosurg 52:127–134.
352. Fisher RS, Uematsu S, Krauss GL, et al (1992) Placebo-controlled pilot study of centromedian thalamic stimulation in treatment of intractable seizures. Epilepsia 33(5):841–851.
353. Tellez-Zenteno JF, McLachlan RS, Parrent A, Kubu CS, Wiebe S (2006) Hippocampal electrical stimulation in mesial temporal lobe epilepsy. Neurology 66(10):1490–1494.
354. Duprez TP, Serieh BA, Raftopoulos C (2005) Absence of memory dysfunction after bilateral mammillary body and mammillothalamic tract electrode implantation: preliminary experience in three patients. AJNR Am J Neuroradiol 26(1):195–197; author reply 197–198.
355. Patwardhan RV, Minagar A, Kelley RE, Nanda A (2006) Neurosurgical treatment of multiple sclerosis. Neurol Res 28(3):320–325.
356. Foote KD, Seignourel P, Fernandez HH, et al (2006) Dual electrode thalamic deep brain stimulation for the treatment of posttraumatic and multiple sclerosis tremor. Neurosurgery 58(4 Suppl 2):ONS-280–285; discussion ONS-285–286.
357. Wishart HA, Roberts DW, Roth RM, et al (2003) Chronic deep brain stimulation for the treatment of tremor in multiple sclerosis: review and case reports. J Neurol Neurosurg Psychiatry 74(10):1392–1397.
358. Greenberg B, Friehs G, Carpenter L, Tyrka A, Malone D, Rezai A, Shapira N, Foote K, Okun M, Goodman W, Rasmussen S, Price L (2005) Deep brain stimulation: clinical findings in intractable depression and OCD. Neuropsychopharmacology 29:S32.
359. Jimenez F, Velasco F, Salin-Pascual R, et al (2005) A patient with a resistant major depression disorder treated with deep brain stimulation in the inferior thalamic peduncle. Neurosurgery 57(3):585–593; discussion 585–593.
360. Kosel M, Sturm V, Frick C, et al (2006) Mood improvement after deep brain stimulation of the internal globus pallidus for tardive dyskinesia in a patient suffering from major depression. J Psychiatr Res.
361. Greenberg BD, Malone DA, Friehs GM, et al (2006) Three-year outcomes in deep brain stimulation for highly resistant obsessive-compulsive disorder. Neuropsychopharmacology 31(11):2384–2393.
362. Aouizerate B, Cuny E, Martin-Guehl C, et al (2004) Deep brain stimulation of the ventral caudate nucleus in the treatment of obsessive-compulsive disorder and major depression. Case report. J Neurosurg 101(4):682–686.
363. Sturm V, Lenartz D, Koulousakis A, et al (2003) The nucleus accumbens: a target for deep brain stimulation in obsessive-compulsive- and anxiety-disorders. J Chem Neuroanat 26(4):293–299.
364. Shapira NA, Okun MS, Wint D, et al (2006) Panic and fear induced by deep brain stimulation. J Neurol Neurosurg Psychiatry 77(3):410–412.
365. Laitinen LV (1979) Emotional responses to subcortical electrical stimulation in psychiatric patients. Clin Neurol Neurosurg 81(3):148–157.
366. Ackermans L, Temel Y, Cath D, et al (2006) Deep brain stimulation in Tourette's syndrome: two targets? Mov Disord 21(5):709–713.
367. Visser-Vandewalle V, Temel Y, Boon P, et al (2003) Chronic bilateral thalamic stimulation: a new therapeutic approach in intractable Tourette syndrome. Report of three cases. J Neurosurg 99(6):1094–1100.
368. Houeto JL, Karachi C, Mallet L, et al (2005) Tourette's syndrome and deep brain stimulation. J Neurol Neurosurg Psychiatry 76(7):992–995.
369. Diederich NJ, Kalteis K, Stamenkovic M, Pieri V, Alesch F (2005) Efficient internal pallidal stimulation in Gilles de la Tourette syndrome: a case report. Mov Disord 20(11):1496–1499.

370. Shahed J, Poysky J, Kenney C, Simpson R, Jankovic J (2007) GPi deep brain stimulation for Tourette syndrome improves tics and psychiatric comorbidities. Neurology 68(2):159–160.
371. Leone M (2004) Chronic cluster headache: new and emerging treatment options. Curr Pain Headache Rep 8(5):347–352.
372. Franzini A, Marras C, Ferroli P, Bugiani O, Broggi G (2005) Stimulation of the posterior hypothalamus for medically intractable impulsive and violent behavior. Stereotact Funct Neurosurg 83(2–3):63–66.
373. Bittar RG, Kar-Purkayastha I, Owen SL, et al (2005) Deep brain stimulation for pain relief: a meta-analysis. J Clin Neurosci 12(5):515–519.
374. Tarsy D, Apetauerova D, Ryan P, Norregaard T (2003) Adverse effects of subthalamic nucleus DBS in a patient with multiple system atrophy. Neurology 61(2):247–249.
375. Hebb MO, Garcia R, Gaudet P, Mendez IM (2006) Bilateral stimulation of the globus pallidus internus to treat choreathetosis in Huntington's disease: technical case report. Neurosurgery 58(2):E383; discussion E383.
376. Shulman LM, Taback RL, Rabinstein AA, Weiner WJ (2002) Non-recognition of depression and other non-motor symptoms in Parkinson's disease. Parkinsonism Relate Disord 8:193–197.
377. Weintraub D, Moberg PJ, Duda JE, Katz IR, Stern MB (2003) Recognition and treatment of depression in Parkinson's disease. J Geriat Psychiatry Neurol 16(3):178–183.
378. Weintraub D, Morales KH, Moberg PJ, et al (2005) Antidepressant studies in Parkinson's disease: a review and meta-analysis. Mov Disord 20(9):1161–1169.
379. Rezai AR, Kopell BH, Gross RE, et al (2006) Deep brain stimulation for Parkinson's disease: surgical issues. Mov Disord 21(Suppl 14):S197–S218.
380. Schroeder U, Kuehler A, Lange KW, et al (2003) Subthalamic nucleus stimulation affects a frontotemporal network: a PET study. Ann Neurol 54(4):445–450.
381. Stefurak T, Mikulis D, Mayberg H, et al (2003) Deep brain stimulation for Parkinson's disease dissociates mood and motor circuits: a functional MRI case study. Mov Disord 18(12):1508–1516.
382. Phillips MD, Baker KB, Lowe MJ, et al (2006) Parkinson disease: pattern of functional MR imaging activation during deep brain stimulation of subthalamic nucleus–initial experience. Radiology 239(1):209–216.
383. Gross C, Rougier A, Guehl D, Boraud T, Julien J, Bioulac B (1997) High-frequency stimulation of the globus pallidus internalis in Parkinson's disease: a study of seven cases. J Neurosurg 87(4):491–498.
384. Plaha P, Gill SS (2005) Bilateral deep brain stimulation of the pedunculopontine nucleus for Parkinson's disease. Neuroreport 16(17):1883–1887.
385. Pagni CA, Altibrandi MG, Bentivoglio A, et al (2005) Extradural motor cortex stimulation (EMCS) for Parkinson's disease. History and first results by the study group of the Italian neurosurgical society. Acta Neurochir Suppl 93:113–119.
386. Plaha P, Ben-Shlomo Y, Patel NK, Gill SS (2006) Stimulation of the caudal zona incerta is superior to stimulation of the subthalamic nucleus in improving contralateral parkinsonism. Brain 129(Pt 7):1732–1747.
387. Siegfried J (1993) Therapeutic stereotactic procedures on the thalamus for motor movement disorders. Acta Neurochir (Wien) 124(1):14–18.
388. Schulder M, Sernas T, Mahalick D, Adler R, Cook S (1999) Thalamic stimulation in patients with multiple sclerosis. Stereotact Funct Neurosurg 72(2–4):196–201.
389. Nandi D, Chir M, Liu X, et al (2002) Electrophysiological confirmation of the zona incerta as a target for surgical treatment of disabling involuntary arm movements in multiple sclerosis: use of local field potentials. J Clin Neurosci 9(1):64–68.

390. Bereznai B, Steude U, Seelos K, Bötzel K (2002) Chronic high-frequency globus pallidus internus stimulation in different types of dystonia: a clinical, video, and MRI report of six patients presenting with segmental, cervical, and generalized dystonia. Mov Disord 17(1):138–144.
391. Chang JW, Choi JY, Lee BW, Kang UJ, Chung SS (2002) Unilateral globus pallidus internus stimulation improves delayed onset post-traumatic cervical dystonia with an ipsilateral focal basal ganglia lesion. J Neurol Neurosurg Psychiatry 73(5):588–590.
392. Sellal F, Hirsch E, Barth P, Blond S, Marescaux C (1993) A case of symptomatic hemidystonia improved by ventroposterolateral thalamic electrostimulation. Mov Disord 8(4):515–518.
393. Chou KL, Hurtig HI, Jaggi JL, Baltuch GH (2005) Bilateral subthalamic nucleus deep brain stimulation in a patient with cervical dystonia and essential tremor. Mov Disord 20(3):377–380.
394. Eltahawy HA, Feinstein A, Khan F, Saint-Cyr J, Lang AE, Lozano AM (2004) Bilateral globus pallidus internus deep brain stimulation in tardive dyskinesia: a case report. Mov Disord 19(8):969–972.
395. Trottenberg T, Volkmann J, Deuschl G, et al (2005) Treatment of severe tardive dystonia with pallidal deep brain stimulation. Neurology 64(2):344–346.
396. Moro E, Lang AE, Strafella AP, et al (2004) Bilateral globus pallidus stimulation for Huntington's disease. Ann Neurol 56(2):290–294.
397. Huang Y, Garrick R, Cook R, O'Sullivan D, Morris J, Halliday GM (2005) Pallidal stimulation reduces treatment-induced dyskinesias in "minimal-change" multiple system atrophy. Mov Disord 20(8):1042–1047.
398. Burbaud P, Vital A, Rougier A, et al (2002) Minimal tissue damage after stimulation of the motor thalamus in a case of chorea-acanthocytosis. Neurology 59(12):1982–1984.
399. Guehl D, Cuny E, Tison F, et al (2007) Deep brain pallidal stimulation for movement disorders in neuroacanthocytosis. Neurology 68(2):160–161.
400. Chkhenkeli SA, Sramka M, Lortkipanidze GS, et al (2004) Electrophysiological effects and clinical results of direct brain stimulation for intractable epilepsy. Clin Neurol Neurosurg 106(4):318–329.
401. Velasco F, Carrillo-Ruiz JD, Brito F, et al (2005) Double-blind, randomized controlled pilot study of bilateral cerebellar stimulation for treatment of intractable motor seizures. Epilepsia 46(7):1071–1081.
402. Kumar K, Toth C, Nath RK (1997) Deep brain stimulation for intractable pain: a 15-year experience. Neurosurgery 40(4):736–746; discussion 746–737.
403. Green AL, Owen SL, Davies P, Moir L, Aziz TZ (2006) Deep brain stimulation for neuropathic cephalalgia. Cephalalgia 26(5):561–567.
404. Vandewalle V, van der Linden C, Groenewegen HJ, Caemaert J (1999) Stereotactic treatment of Gilles de la Tourette syndrome by high frequency stimulation of thalamus. Lancet 353(9154):724.
405. Flaherty AW, Williams ZM, Amirnovin R, et al (2005) Deep brain stimulation of the anterior internal capsule for the treatment of Tourette syndrome: technical case report. Neurosurgery 57(4 Suppl):E403; discussion E403.
406. Miyasaki JM, Shannon K, Voon V, et al (2006) Practice Parameter: evaluation and treatment of depression, psychosis, and dementia in Parkinson disease (an evidence-based review): report of the Quality Standards Subcommittee of the American Academy of Neurology. Neurology 66(7):996–1002.

# 22
# Deep Brain Stimulation Safety: MRI and Other Electromagnetic Interactions

Kenneth B. Baker and Michael D. Phillips

## Abstract

The potential for interaction between medical implants and electromagnetic (EM) energy generated by devices in the patient's environment has long been a safety concern for health care professionals. The magnitude and subsequent effect of such an interaction will depend on the strength of the EM field as well as the susceptibility and location of the device. For most implants, particularly those that are passive in nature (e.g., aneurysm clips, stents), newer materials and manufacturing techniques have led to dramatic improvements in the susceptibility of implants. The situation is more complex, however, for active implants like those used in cardiac or neurostimulation therapy, where the electronic, conductive, and typically elongated nature of the implant increases its overall susceptibility to EM fields. To date, reported interactions for patients with implanted deep brain stimulation (DBS) systems have ranged from inadvertent switching of the pulse generators between the on and off state to the induction of permanent, neurological deficit. While the total number of documented adverse events over the past decade is relatively small in comparison to the 30,000 plus patient implants performed to date, patients and physicians need to be aware of the potential sources and effects of EM interactions. This chapter presents an overview of those sources and their potential impact on the DBS hardware and subsequently the patient, with particular emphasis on the MRI environment and recent data on MRI-related heating.

**Keywords:** deep brain stimulation, magnetic resonance imaging, safety, magnetic resonance imaging, bioeffects, neurostimulation

## Introduction

EM energy is an increasingly pervasive aspect of our world, whether in the medical or non-medical environment. When such energy disrupts or otherwise interferes with the functionality of a secondary device it is considered EM interference (EMI). The unwelcome energy may arrive at the implanted device through radiation, conduction, or induction. While the most obvious example of radiation is broadcast radio or television signals, EM radiation is a byproduct of essentially any active electronic circuit. The potential for EMI arises as a result of the radiated emission coupling with the metallic components of the receiving device and generating unwanted electrical currents. Examples of radiated EM interference are common in society and include the interference caused by overhead power lines when listening to AM radio or television interference caused by vacuum cleaners. EMI is also what airlines and the Federal Aeronautics Administration seek to avoid when passengers are asked to stow electronic devices, in particular cell phones and other devices that actively radiate EM energy for the purpose of data transmission. Interference can also arise from energy that is transferred via induction, a situation that occurs when there is magnetic or capacitive coupling between two devices (e.g., pulsed gradients during MRI). As with a radiated EM field, induction does not require direct contact between the transmitting and receiving devices. Finally, as its name implies, conduction involves the transfer of EM energy across a physical connection, as in the use of electrocautery *(1–3)* or cardiac defibrillation *(4)*.

Concern over the threat of EMI to an implantable pulse generator (IPG) and lead system was not newly founded with chronic neurostimulation applications like DBS, but rather became well appreciated in the mid-1960s *(1–3, 5–8)*, shortly after the introduction of the cardiac pacemaker. Conductive transfer was reported as a consequence of electrocautery *(1–3, 5)* or as a result of equipment malfunction (e.g., improper grounding *[7]*) and radiated transfer was observed with proximity to large power sources *(6–8)*. In 1968, Furman et al. *(7)* described a patient who developed an irregular heart rate with perceived fluttering when in proximity to an open television set. Reports in the early 1970s included symptomatic interactions (e.g., syncope) resulting from radiation arising from proximity to microwave ovens *(9–11)* as well as medical devices that included induction casting machines *(12)* and diathermy *(13)*. Although advances have been made in the past few decades in both the susceptibility of implants (i.e., shielded leads) as well as the allowed EM leakage levels of electronic appliances and equipment, the potential for EM interactions with implantable devices continues to be cause for concern for both cardiac and neurostimulation systems.

Regardless of the method of transfer, the degree of EMI produced during an interaction depends on the magnitude of the ingress, which is in turn related to the strength of the signal as it reaches the receiving device (a product of source strength and distance) and the susceptibility of the receiving device. In the case of DBS systems, reported interactions to date have ranged from inadvertent switching of the DBS pulse generator between on and off states *(14)* to several cases of permanent, neurological deficit *(4, 15, 20, 21)*. While simple malfunction of the device, in the form of a failure to function or unintended deactivation, is unlikely to be life threatening for patients with movement disorders; abrupt, unanticipated, and undetected cessation of therapeutic stimulation may have a greater impact on newer applications of DBS, including psychiatric conditions where the rate of occurrence and magnitude of such rebound effects have yet to be determined. Beyond malfunction, the generation of anomalous currents within the lead/extension system of the DBS lead can lead to functional stimulation of neural tissue or to tissue heating. The following sections review the components that comprise the DBS therapy system, the potential sources and effects of EMI, and summarize the reported cases of known or suspected EMI with an implanted DBS system. Special emphasis will be given to addressing the potential hazards associated with MRI, as this otherwise safe and noninvasive diagnostic technique holds perhaps the greatest potential for significant EMI-related interactions with DBS implants.

## Components and Materials Used in DBS

Three separate components comprise the current, commercially available DBS system: (1) a pacemaker-like IPG, (2) the DBS lead with four cylindrical contacts at one end, and (3) an extension cable connecting those two components. The three are pressure coupled together intra-operatively during a single procedure or a series of two procedures. During normal operation, pulsed electrical current is passed from the IPG through the extension lead to the neural tissue, with the return (i.e., anode) portion of the circuit being one or more additional contacts at the distal tip of the lead or the metal case of the IPG.

Three generations of IPGs have been marketed to date by Medtronic for use in DBS therapy: the Itrel II™, the Soletra™, and the Kinetra™. Each essentially consists of a battery cell and electronic circuitry hermetically sealed within a titanium shell. While the Itrel II™ will be encountered with increasing rarity, as that the model line was replaced by the Soletra™ in 2000, there is very little distinction between the two from a patient or programming perspective. Both are single chamber systems with only slight differences in the range of possible stimulation parameters and features. With the recent addition of the Kinetra™ model IPG, a second chamber was added, enabling the unit to deliver stimulation through two separate extension/lead combinations. As might be expected, this addition came with an increase in the overall volume (82%) and weight (98%) of the device *(16, 17)*. Of interest from an EMI perspective, however, an additional feature of the Kinetra™ IPG is the availability of the Therapy Controller (Model 7436). This device provides the patients with the option to activate or deactivate the IPG without the use of the small, handheld magnet that has been standard for the Itrel II™ and Soletra™. Although the option to use the handheld magnet to activate and deactivate the Kinetra™ still exists, that magnet function can be disabled using a physician programmer. One possible benefit of this feature may be to reduce inadvertent switching of the device state (on/off) that can result from EMI, as discussed later *(14)*.

The current generation of extensions and implantable leads contains no active, electronic components. The leads have four cylindrical, platinum/iridium contacts at the distal end that are interconnected by four non-interlacing, spiral wound, fluropolymer-insulated platinum/iridium wires to a set of four cylindrical, nickel alloy contacts at the other end. The remainder of the lead is comprised of polyurethane tubing *(18)*. The contacts at the proximal end of the lead serve as the connection point between the lead and the distal aspect of the extension cable, while those at the distal tip interface with neural tissue. The cylindrical contacts are 1.27 mm in diameter, with the specific length and spacing variable based on lead model and application. For patients with movement disorders, two lead models are currently available. Both have contacts that are 1.5 mm in length, but are distinguished by having either 1.5-mm (Model 3387) or 0.5-mm (Model 3389) inter-contact spacing. For psychiatric applications, a lead is available whose four contacts are each 3 mm in length and separated by a 4-mm span of insulation (Model 3387-IES). The wires within the extension cable are largely composed of a non-magnetic, nickel-cobalt based alloy (MP35), with the newer, low-impedance model adding a silver core *(18)*. Various lengths of extensions (25–95 cm) and leads (28–40 cm) are available to accommodate different size patients as well as alternate placements of the IPGs (e.g., abdomen vs chest). However some differences in lead availability may exist between different global markets.

In all, the relatively complex nature of the DBS system affords several opportunities for EMI to cause problems. The system is comprised of metal components and thus subject to magnetic interactions, both static and pulsed. Moreover, the system is elongated and conductive, thereby increasing its susceptibility to induction and radiated EM transfer. As mentioned previously, those currents can lead to unwanted stimulation of neural tissue with potential for perceived neurologic effects or may lead to heat generation through ohmic or resistive heating as the energy passes from electrode to tissue. Finally, the IPG contains electronic circuitry and switches that may be damaged or modified either by magnetic or electrical forces. The following sections review reported interactions to date.

## Potential Interactions

In the United States, the Center for Devices and Radiological Health, a division of the Food and Drug Administration (FDA), regulates issues related to device EM compatibility. Changes in labeling, including advisories concerning possible EMI sources and interactions are submitted by device manufacturers to the FDA for approval. The various patient manuals provided with the Activa® Therapy System from Medtronic provide a relatively comprehensive overview of the possible sources and consequences of EMI *(16–19)*. The major potential sources of EMI to be encountered in the non-medical environment provided are listed in Table 22.1. These sources are classified by their likelihood of generating interference, reflecting the overall power of the EM field radiated by the source *(16, 17, 19)*. As the potential for EMI is directly related to the strength of the EM field at a given distance and inversely proportional to the distance between the two devices, items listed under "possible" interference are essentially those that generate relatively weak EM fields or are unlikely to come in close proximity to the DBS hardware under normal use. For example, stereo speakers can be found listed under this category as they may contain magnets that are sufficiently strong to switch the IPG between on and off states. However, the risk is small given that such an interaction is only likely to occur if the magnet is in extremely close proximity to the IPG, such as if the patient were to hold the speaker close to his body at a level corresponding to the IPG location. Otherwise, under normal use, such an event is extremely unlikely. The manual also covers a number of sources that, while historically associated with producing EMI (e.g., microwave ovens *[9–11]*), are no longer considered to pose a significant threat so long as those devices are operating normally. To that end, patient education is perhaps the most important component for avoiding interactions from objects in the non-medical environment, and certainly some consideration should be given to younger patients where potential occupational hazards may be of concern (e.g., welder, mechanic).

**Table 22.1** Non-medical Sources of Potential EMI.

**Interference likely**

    Theft detectors/security gates
    Citizen band or ham radio antenna
    Electric arc or resistance welding
    Electric induction heaters
    Industrial electric steel furnaces
    Power lines
    TV and radio transmit towers
    Electric substations and power generators
    Therapeutic magnets

**Interference possible**[*]

    Refrigerator/freezer magnetic strip
    Telephone (standard, cordless or cellular)
    Stereo speakers
    Sewing machine (motor)
    Salon hair dryer (motor)
    Induction range
    Power tools

**Safe from interference**[**]

    Microwave ovens
    Electric blankets and heating pads
    Major appliances
    Hand held hair dryers, shavers
    Home security systems
    Personal computers, electric typewriters
    Photocopiers and fax machines
    Televisions, AM/FM radios and stereos
    Vacuum cleaners and electric brooms

[*]Very close proximity typically required for interaction
[**]Assumes units in good operating condition

Significant interactions between a medical implant or device and environmental EMI can be difficult to track. Generally, the probability of a patient reporting an adverse event to his or her physician is likely to be directly related to the severity of the event, such that while inadvertent switching of the IPG from the "on" to the "off" state with no change in the therapeutic benefit once the patient re-activates his or her unit may go unreported, the same state change associated with a perceived electrical "jolt" or "shock" is likely to be reported. Certainly an instance in which the event is associated with persistent morbidity is highly likely to make its way to the physician, assuming that an association, assumed or otherwise, is made between the device and the event. Even at that level, however, the dissemination or reporting of that information to the device manufacturer or regulatory agencies is not known. The Manufacturers and User Facility Device Experience (MAUDE) database, operated by the Center for Devices and Radiological Health of the FDA, attempts to track such events through voluntary reports made by health care providers, manufacturers, and distributors. Given its voluntary nature however, the listed events are likely to underestimate the actual incidence of such events.

In September 2006, we searched the MAUDE database using each of the following brand name keywords "DBS," "Activa," "Itrel," "Soletra," and "Kinetra" individually for reports received over the past 10 years (available date range: June 30, 1996–June 29, 2006). When the brand name "Itrel" was searched, the record was thoroughly reviewed for evidence that it referred to a DBS application and not spinal cord stimulation. In the event that the distinction could not be made based on the details provided in the record, the entire record was excluded. A secondary search was also performed using only the product code "MHY" and "GZB," codes associated with neurostimulation devices in the database, to identify any remaining records that were not already retrieved. For all searches, the manufacturer search field was left blank, as were the product problem, product class, and event type. Although this type of search resulted in a large number of extraneous hits, it was determined through initial search attempts that reporting errors in the database would limit the number of true "hits" obtained if the search criteria were construed in a narrow fashion. It should be noted that the details provided on the MAUDE database are brief and there is little consistency in the language used across reports.

The majority of hits generated by the search were related to device removal or replacement secondary to infection, followed next by physical damage (e.g., lead breakage). A total of 38 reports were identified where the cause of the adverse event was suspected or known to be related to EMI. Of those, the majority ($n = 26$) were attributed to the patient passing in proximity to an electronic article surveillance (EAS) system (i.e., theft detector or metal detector). The magnitude of the event, as reported, ranged from simple switching of the device off to reports of patients feeling "zapped" or "jolted." The range of effects reported from these increasingly common systems is not unusual considering the variety of different technologies in use. The systems are common in shopping centers and libraries and consist of one or more pylons located at the entrance or exit of the building. In general, all of these systems sense a "tag" or marker placed on a product by emitting an EM field that "interrogates" a region of space some distance from it. The nature of the EM field can be quite different, however, with respect to the frequency range used or the use of pulsed EM energy. There has been at least one report of older, Itrel II model IPGs being replaced with Kinetra IPGs for the purpose of eliminating frequent EMI-related issues *(14)*. Illustrations that depict ways to minimize the potential for significant EMI with EAS systems are included in the manuals provided by the manufacturer *(16, 17)*. Events of similar magnitude have also been reported, albeit less frequently, in relation to telephones ($n = 2$), home security systems ($n = 1$), medical X-ray ($n = 1$), and unspecified devices ($n = 1$).

While patients should be made aware of potential interactions in the non-medical environment, the most severe adverse events have been associated with EM energy sources in the medical environment. Indeed, the two primary contraindications for DBS therapy *(16, 17)* relate to the use of radiofrequency (RF) sources for medical treatment or diagnosis: diathermy and MRI. From the MAUDE database, these sources included cardioversion ($n = 1$), therapeutic ultrasound or diathermy ($n = 3$), electrocautery ($n = 2$), and MRI ($n = 1$). In the published literature, which overlaps somewhat with those events reported in MAUDE, there have been at least four case reports involving adverse events associated with medical treatment *(4, 15, 20, 21)*. The earliest report came from Yamamoto et al. *(4)* concerning a 56-year-old man with a lead (Model 3380) placed in the thalamus for the treatment of uncontrolled action tremor involving the left hand. Importantly, the system was unlike those currently in use, as the implanted lead was connected to a RF receiver placed at the level of the chest. This relatively passive antenna-like device then required continuous input from an external power source and transmitting antenna placed over the anterior chest wall in order to achieve therapeutic benefit. After 3 years of good benefit, the patient underwent cardioversion (100–200 Joules) for paroxysmal atrial fibrillation, which was followed by cessation of the patient's tremor in the absence of stimulation. Although no evidence of a thalamic lesion could be appreciated in the area of the implanted lead using CT imaging, the effect persisted throughout an additional 4-year follow-up period. For current DBS systems, the safety of cardioversion has still not been established. If considered necessary for patient survival, however, the manufacturer recommends using the lowest clinically appropriate energy output with the paddles positioned perpendicular to the implanted system and as far from the neurostimulators as possible (for details, see refs. *16* and *17*).

Ultrasonic diathermy is used to generate therapeutic deep heating of tissues and is contraindicated for patients with DBS implants. The MAUDE database includes three adverse events associated with diathermy *(22–24)*, of which at least one has appeared as a published case report *(21)*. The published case was a 70-year-old man with bilateral STN leads who underwent diathermy following extraction of his maxillary teeth *(21)*. At the end of the diathermy treatment, the patient was nonresponsive with pinpoint pupils and shortly thereafter developed decerebrate posturing with occasional myoclonic jerks and a positive Babinski sign. Subsequent MRI revealed symmetrical lesions throughout the pons, midbrain, cerebral peduncles, and posterior limbs of the internal capsule. The second report was of a patient with bilateral pallidal leads who underwent bipolar, high-frequency ultrashortwave therapy of the thoracolumbar region as part of his physical therapy treatment *(24)*. During treatment, the patient's presented with deficits marked by impaired mental status, aphasia, hemiplegia, eye deviation, and positive Babinski sign. At 2 days post, MRI revealed signal abnormalities around the tips of the leads bilaterally. As of the report date, the patient was able to follow commands, but remained emaciated and somnolent with inability to voluntarily open the eyes. Finally, a 2003 report describes a patient with a thalamic lead for treatment of tremor who experienced persistent numbness and tingling in association with diathermy for the treatment of pain *(22)*.

Additional sources of potential EMI in the medical environment are reviewed in the current manufacturer labeling for DBS *(16, 17)*, with a listing of potential sources provided in Table 22.2. Despite the absence of reported incidents to date, caution is warranted and if their use is deemed necessary, any and all guidelines provided by the implant manufacturer should be followed. The following section reviews the risks to patients with DBS implants presented by the MRI environment.

Table 22.2 Medical Sources of Potential EMI.

**Interference Likely**

Diathermy (Therapeutic Ultrasound)
Magnetic Resonance Imaging (MRI)
Electrocautery
Lithotripsy
External Defibrillators
Radiation Therapy (e.g., gamma radiation)
Electroshock
Transcranial Magnetic Stimulation

**Interference Possible**

Electrolysis
Dental Drills and Ultrasonic Probes
Mammography
Implantable Cardiac Sensing Devices
- (e.g., implantable defibrillator, pacemaker)

**Safe from Interference**

Computerized Axial Tomography (CT)
Diagnostic Ultrasound
Diagnostic X-rays

## The MRI Environment

MRI involves the application of a static, homogenous magnetic field for the purpose of hydrogen nuclei polarization, a combination of time-varying magnetic fields to change the frequency of the hydrogen nuclei by spatial location, and an RF field that is used to excite the hydrogen nuclei from low to high energy levels (the RF is then recorded as the nuclei fall back to the lower energy level for image generation purposes). In presenting this rather distinct combination of static and time-varying magnetic fields as well as pulsed electrical fields, the MRI environment is fairly unique in its hostility towards medical implants and devices. More than 1,400 objects are listed in the 2006 "Reference Manual for Magnetic Resonance Safety, Implants, and Devices," a 520-page guidebook that provides the MR-safety status of various medical and non-medical objects in the MR environment (25). While the list is dominated by passive implants such as aneurysm clips, coils, stents, and heart valve prostheses; active devices including cardiac stimulators, infusion pumps, and neurostimulators also are included. In the past, patients with such electronically activated implants have generally been strictly prohibited from undergoing MRI procedures (26–28), as adverse events including serious injuries and deaths had been reported (15, 26, 27, 29). However, the guidebook, as well as all related literature (30–44), serve to underscore the importance of using MRI for the continued care and management of patients with certain electronically activated implants. Indeed, it is somewhat ironic that the patient with an implanted neurostimulation system and, thus, somewhat complicated medical condition, is more likely to be considered for MRI than the general population. There are several scenarios that require MRI procedures in patients with implanted DBS electrodes. These include verification of lead position; poor or worsening clinical outcome of DBS and/or significant side effects or lack of effect where precise localization of the electrode with respect to the target needs to be confirmed; the need to replace DBS electrodes or place contralateral or additional DBS electrodes; and the need to evaluate other intracranial pathologies related or unrelated to the DBS electrodes, such as strokes, hemorrhages, and other mass lesions.

Our group has conducted a series of experiments over the past 5 years in an effort to better understand the types and magnitude of potential interactions between the MRI environment and implanted DBS systems and to determine if, and under what conditions, MRI can be safely performed in patients with neurostimulation systems. Hazards and problems that may occur with implanted devices are related to magnetic field-induced movement or dislodgment, excessive heating, the induction of electrical currents, disruption of functional aspects, and the misinterpretation of an imaging artifact as an abnormality *(27, 45–49)*.

## MRI: Potential Interactions

### Static Field Interactions

The potential interactions between the static, magnetic field of the MRI environment, and an implanted medical device involve the development of displacement and torsion forces. The displacement force, a translational force caused by exposure of ferromagnetic material to the spatial gradient of the magnetic field is perhaps most readily associated with the concept of "projectile hazard," evoking images of oxygen cylinders stuck in the bore of the magnet or metal fragments lodged in the eye. Meanwhile, torsion forces are involved in the tendency of the implanted device to rotate or align itself relative to the magnetic field, which can translate into shifting of the device within the patient. The magnitude of these interactions will be proportional to the field strength and spatial gradient of the MR system *(50)*, as well as to the characteristics of the object itself, including its mass and shape as well as the magnetic susceptibility of the material from which it is made. Considerable discomfort or injury can occur in a patient that has a metallic implant that exhibits substantial force or torque in association with exposure to the MR environment *(25, 32, 49)*.

Standard procedures for assessing displacement force and torque effects on implants are provided and continue to be refined by the American Society for Testing and Materials (ASTM; refs. *51* and *52*). The test methods are relatively straightforward, with displacement force measured using the deflection angle test. Here, the test item is suspended from a lightweight string at specific areas relative to the MRI system and the angle of deflection recorded. Torque testing involves assessing the amount of force required to rotate the test item, positioned along each of its three orthogonal axes, at a defined location within the bore of the magnet. We have recently shown that, for DBS implants, the magnitude of static field interactions, both force and torque measured at a field strength of 1.5-Tesla, have steadily diminished with successive models of IPGs *(53)*. The latest generation of IPGs for DBS show interactions with the 1.5-Tesla field that are up to twice that which would be expected based on gravity alone, compared to values of 25x or more for older RF receiver models. Our pilot experiments (unpublished observations), as well as the work of others *(54)*, failed to demonstrate any effect of the static field on either the leads or extensions used for DBS.

In interpreting any such data however, it is important to consider the intended *in vivo* application *(55, 56)*. Once implanted, substantial "retentive" forces are provided by sutures or other means of fixation, including tissue in-growth, scarring, and granulation. The latter features are obviously impacted by the length of time that the device has been implanted.

### *Gradient-Induced Currents*

Unlike the static magnetic field that is always active even when imaging is not being performed, the gradient magnetic field, manifested as the audible ticking or knocking sound made by the system, is active only during imaging. This low-frequency, spatial variation in the magnetic field is known to induce neural activation, including peripheral nerve stimulation in patients without implanted devices. The probability of such activation depends on the type of sequence applied, as those with fast switching gradients (i.e., higher dB/dt) are associated with a greater effect. The DBS lead system, or any metallic implant for that matter, will tend to concentrate this effect, and Nyenhuis et al. *(57)* have shown that the magnitude of the induced current may on the order of 5 Volts/meter. Thus, over an approximately 60-cm length DBS system, a voltage of as much as 3 Volts may be induced. However, the overall impedance of the lead system will tend to limit the magnitude of the gradient-induced currents *(58)*, and attempts to measure these currents using an *ex vivo* model have thus far failed to reveal appreciable current levels *(54)*. Moreover, there have been no reported incidents (e.g., "tingling," contractions) attributable to neural stimulation in association with MRI.

### *The RF Field*

The pulsed RF field, which is also only present during an imaging sequence, is used to induce precession in the hydrogen nuclei. Similar to the peripheral nerve stimulation induced by the pulsed gradient field, concern regarding RF-induced heating is not limited to patients with implants. Rather, tissue heating is a universal concern in MRI, with specific absorption rate (SAR) developed as an index of the amount of RF power absorbed per unit of mass of an objected in units of Watts/kg *(59)*. The International Electrotechnical Commission (IEC) and the FDA regulate allowable SAR limits during imaging to avoid overheating of tissue. Again similar to the issue of pulsed gradients, concerns over RF-related heating are compounded by the presence of conductive implants in the body, particularly those that are electronically activated or have an elongated configuration. The presence of such implants can locally increase these currents and, under certain MR operational conditions, generate excessive heating of biomedical devices *(59)*.

Empirical data supporting the development of substantial RF-related temperature elevations during MRI have been reported for cardiac pacemakers, indwelling catheters with metallic components (e.g., thermodilution catheters), and guide wires resulting in first-, second-, and third-degree burns *(27, 29, 49, 60–64)*. In 1997, Achenbach et al. *(60)* reported a temperature increase at the tip of a cardiac pacing electrode of up to 63.1 °C during 90 seconds of scanning. Interestingly, however, two of the earliest reports for a DBS system yielded negative results with respect to MRI-related heating. Tronnier et al. *(65)* studied unilateral Itrel II and Itrel III neurostimulation systems (Medtronic, Minneapolis, MN) in 0.2-, 0.25-, and 1.5-T MR systems during MR imaging using standard spin-echo pulse sequences. An infrared camera was used to measure heating of the neurostimulation systems applied to the surface of a water phantom. Because an infrared camera was used, all metallic surfaces of the neurostimulation systems were covered with black paint to prevent reflection of heat radiation from other objects in the RF area. Experiments were performed using the head and body RF coils, with the tips of the leads placed in air, saline or connected to a resistor. Tronnier et al. *(65)* reported that "no heat induction was observed in any part of the hardware." However, the methods used in this study have several major limitations, including the fact that an infrared camera was used to evaluate heating. It is not possible to measure the temperature at the tip of the lead while it is immersed in saline using an infrared camera and neurostimulation system was not surrounded by conductive media to simulate human tissue. Moreover, it is unknown whether painting the metal parts impacted the results of MRI-related heating and the levels of RF power that were used in the experiments were not reported.

Schueler et al. *(35)* examined MRI-related heating in a phantom simulating unilateral Itrel II and Itrel III system placement in a 1.5-T MR system operating at SARs that did not exceed a whole body averaged SAR of 0.4 W/kg (i.e., 10 times less than the highest level currently recommended by the FDA). In this case, experiments were performed with the neurostimulation systems outside (i.e., in air) and inside of a saline bath. The authors reported that "no heating of any devices, catheters, extensions, or leads was detected in several experiments in which the location and orientation of objects within the magnet bore were varied" *(35)*. However, the authors did not measure the temperature of the electrodes and the components that they did study were not expected to exhibit any heating. Also, the work by Schueler et al. is problematic because of the use of a saline-filled phantom. A phantom filled with gel that simulates the conductive qualities of human tissue is preferred over a saline-filled phantom for evaluation of MRI-related heating of devices because the use of a saline-filled phantom greatly underestimates temperature changes for electrically conductive devices, such as neurostimulation systems *(31, 66)*.

Since that time, a number of phantom-based experiments carried out by our group have demonstrated rather clearly the potential for excessive heating of DBS devices *(37, 41, 67–69)*, in particular the electrical contacts at the distal tip of the DBS lead. Findings from our early investigations demonstrated that MR procedures conducted at whole body averaged SAR of 3.9 W/kg yielded 25.3 °C after 15 minutes when a transmit/receive body coil configuration was used *(37)*. When the transmit/receive head coil was used, with a whole-body average SAR of 0.24 W/kg, a maximum temperature of 7.1 °C was observed after 15 minutes of scanning *(37)*. These data indicate that substantial heating occurs for certain conditions, while others produce relatively minor, physiologically inconsequential temperature increases. Of perhaps greater concern was the exponential rate at which the temperature increased, with the majority of the heating occurring within the first minute of scanning and reaching a "steady-state" within 15 minutes.

Since these early reports, our group has been actively investigating factors that influence the amount of heat generated in a neurostimulation system used for DBS during MRI. Such factors include the electrical characteristics of the particular neurostimulation system; the field strength of the MR system (and consequent change in the frequency of the transmitted RF energy); the orientation or routing of the IPG, extension lead (the extension is the cable that connects the IPG to the implanted lead), and stimulating lead relative to the source of RF energy *(67)*; the lengths and routing of the extension and lead, the type of RF coil used (e.g., transmit/receive body coil, transmit body coil with receive-only head coil, transmit/receive head coil); the anatomy imaged (e.g., the landmark position *[67]* or the anatomic site undergoing MR imaging that is associated with heating depends on the geometry of the RF coil and the amount of the DBS lead contained within this coil); the amount of RF energy delivered (i.e., the SAR); and how the SAR is calculated by a given MR system *(68, 69)*.

A key finding over the past several years, having even contributed to recent changes in the upper limit of SAR in the DBS manufacturer's guidelines, has concerned the use of SAR as an index of RF-related heating of DBS leads. Originally, Finelli et al. *(41)* demonstrated that the relationship between console-reported values of SAR was linearly related to the observed temperature change on the MR system used for evaluation. The original labeling provided by the DBS hardware manufacturer cited three MR systems from which empirical data had been acquired and on which MRI safety guidelines were based *(70)*. As early as 1984, in reviewing the effects of MRI on implantable pulse generators, Fetter et al. *(71)* noted that devices from different manufacturers and even for different applications behave differently and data derived for one device will not necessarily apply to all others. Indeed, since the initial work by Finelli et al. *(41)*, we have demonstrated that SAR-based indices of implant heating do not generalize across MR systems, even those from the same manufacturer *(68)*. In 2004, we compared the amount of heat generated per unit of whole body averaged SAR ($\Delta T/SAR-W$) across two different MR systems from the same manufacturer, using the transmit/receive body coil configuration, and found more than a 80-fold difference *(68)* depending on the landmark location and the lead contact monitored. More recently, these experiments were repeated using the transmit/receive head coil configuration in accordance with the DBS manufacturer guidelines *(69)*. The difference across the two systems was smaller, but remained significant, ranging from three- to fivefold depending on the site from which temperature was measured. These findings have been further substantiated by additional heating experiments conducted in cardiac pacemakers evaluated in three different 1.5-Tesla MR systems *(34)*. Consequently, console-reported values of SAR currently should not be considered an appropriate metric for the development of safety criterion. This topic has attracted the attention of the FDA and intercomparison protocols are being developed.

Even within a given MR system, the magnitude of the $\Delta T/SAR$ has been shown to be sensitive to changes in lead routing or configuration as well as the overall length of the leads. In their preliminary work, Rezai et al. *(37)* found that the 25.3 °C temperature rise they measured dropped to 6.1 °C when two small loops (approximately 2.5 cm in diameter) were placed in an axial orientation at the top of the head portion of the phantom. This effect was demonstrated more directly in 2005 using a custom burrhole cap that allowed the lead to be reproducibly configured in concentric loops as it exited the burrhole *(67)*. A linear relationship was observed between the number of loops (range: 0–2.75) and the measured temperature change, with an overall reduction of up to 74% seen when all excess lead was configured around the burrhole device. The mechanism(s) behind this effect is not clear; however, it is probable that the loops may have added a reactive inductance that yielded a source or impedance near the end of the electrode, thereby reducing the induced RF current in the wire.

Changing the overall length of the lead and extension system also will impact how it interacts, or the degree of coupling with the transmitted RF field. For any lead or wire placed in a uniform electric field, there will be a length at which RF coupling, and consequently the potential for heating, is greatest. Although some characteristics of the lead, including its material and the presence and nature of any insulating materials, will influence this resonant length, coupling will typically be maximal when the lead length is approximately half a wavelength. Thus, this effect will be a combined effect of the DBS hardware as well as the field strength of the MR system, insofar as the field strength determines the frequency at which the RF energy is transmitted in order to produce precession of the magnetic moments of the hydrogen nuclei (optimal frequency for protons is 42.58 MHz/Tesla). Nyenhuis et al. *(72)* examined the effect of lead length on RF-induced temperature rise by successively cutting a capped lead and measuring the maximum temperature change after 6 minutes of RF application in a 1.5-T system. Under these conditions, maximal heating was observed at an overall length of approximately 40 cm.

Finally, the magnitude of the measured $\Delta T/SAR$ has also been shown to change as a function of landmark (i.e., the portion of the body placed at the isocenter of the MR system) when the transmit/receive body coil configuration is used *(67)*. In phantom experiments, the greatest $\Delta T/SAR$ was observed when the landmark of the MR system was placed over the distal tip of the leads, while caudal movements, including placing the landmark over the IPGs, resulted in relatively less heating. However, those data were derived from a single MR system and the degree to which the behavior observed on that system generalizes to others is unclear. It is clear however, from the case report discussed below, that even placing the landmark relatively low on the body (i.e., lumbar spine) can result in excessive heating at the distal tip of the DBS leads some distance away.

Overall, the interaction between neurostimulation systems and the MR environment is extremely complex. If nothing else, the number of potential permutations of implanted systems across patients is extensive and there is a need for mathematical modeling to bridge the gap between sets of empirical data. Moreover, much of the data reported to date has been derived from normal-functioning, intact systems, and changes in the system, including short circuiting or lead breakage would be expected to drastically alter the heating effect.

## *Artifacts*

Although not strictly a safety issue, MRI artifacts associated with the presence of neurostimulation components may prevent the proper diagnostic use of MRI *(36, 73–76)*. Susceptibility artifact in MRI arises when a material distorts the linear magnetic field gradients generated by the MR system, thereby interfering with the signal derived from the area surrounding the implant. Although this effect will be greatest for ferromagnetic materials like iron and nickel, it occurs in the presence of paramagnetic (e.g., aluminum, magnesium) as well as diamagnetic materials (e.g., gold, bismuth, plastic). Platinum and iridium, which comprise the metal contacts and wiring of the DBS leads *(18)*, are paramagnetic material; and while they may have relatively low magnetic susceptibility levels, under certain MR conditions observed artifacts can be substantial and limit the interpretability of diagnostic scans.

The net effect for patients is the presence of voids on the developed images in proximity to the implanted material. Within the brain, these voids can, under certain conditions, extend to well over 5 mm despite the 1.27-mm diameter of the lead itself *(77)*. Moreover, the distortion of the image is not limited to the void area, but extends beyond to interfere with image accuracy in a fringe region surrounding the void. Another area that can be greatly impacted by susceptibility artifact is at the level of the cortex, particularly in regions where the excess, subcutaneously routed lead has been coiled. The magnitude of this effect will be related to the field strength of the MR system as well as the type of sequence applied. Overall, the amount of artifact can be reduced by using sequences with high bandwidth and short echo times, and gradient echo sequences tend to be more sensitive to susceptibility artifact than spin echo or fast spin echo sequences *(78)*.

**DBS Manufacturer Labeling**

The most recent guidelines provided by the current manufacturer of DBS hardware are extensive and precise and will not be reproduced here. The reader interested in performing MRI on patients with DBS implants is encouraged to refer to those guidelines in their entirety *(16–18)*. In general, however, those guidelines restrict imaging to 1.5-Tesla MR systems, and then only those outfitted with a transmit/receive head coil. This latter requirement may become increasingly difficult to deal with as most MR system manufacturers seem to be moving towards doing away with the transmit/receive head coil in favor of a transmit body/receive head configuration. Moreover, the guidelines practically eliminate imaging any part of the body other than the head.

The current upper limit of SAR averaged over the head is set at 0.1 W/kg, down from the 0.4 W/kg that was the upper limit just over a year ago. As mentioned before, this change was instigated in part by the finding of inconsistencies in the console-reported values of SAR across MR systems as well as the general complexity of the overall issue. Unfortunately, this upper limit is extremely low and restricts the range of sequences that can be applied almost to the point of impracticality. Still, it is important to consider that there have been no reported adverse events to date when the guidelines have been followed. While there is evidence in the literature of patients having been scanned with sequences that are typically associated with much higher SAR values *(79–81)* without any reported overt adverse effects, this cannot be taken as proof principle of safety in light of the complexity of the interaction.

**Published and Reported Adverse Events**

Unfortunately, two case reports underscore the potentially serious consequences of heating at the DBS tip in an MRI. Spiegel et al. *(20)* reported the case of a 73-year-old patient who underwent MRI in the transmit/receive head coil configuration of a 1.0-Tesla system (not the recommended 1.5-Tesla). The patient, who had bilateral DBS leads implanted for Parkinson's disease, exhibited dystonic and partially ballistic movements of the left leg immediately after imaging. The second case, reported by Henderson et al. *(15)*, had a much more severe outcome. The patient was a 56-year-old male who had undergone bilateral implantation of DBS leads. As the patient enjoyed hunting, the IPG for the left DBS lead was placed in the abdomen away from the shoulder the patient used to brace his rifle. Several months after implantation, the patient underwent MRI of the lumbar spine at 1.0-Tesla using a transmit/receive body coil. Upon completion of the MRI procedure, the patient was noted to have sustained a neurological deficit marked in part by the development of a right hemiparesis *(15)*. Subsequent neurological examination was significant for aphasia, right hemiplegia, bilateral extensor plantar responses, and eye deviation. Follow-up T2-weighted MRI performed 2 days after the event revealed the presence of a large (several centimeter diameter) hyperintense signal at the level of the left DBS lead. At last report, the patient had persistent deficits marked by dysarthria, right hemiparesis, and mild dysconjugate gaze. Both incidents occurred with scanning that was performed outside of the guidelines provided by the device manufacturer and further emphasize the danger of generalizing or trivializing the safety recommendations.

## Conclusions

Electromagnetic interference is a reality of modern times. Patients with implanted medical devices, including DBS hardware, are constantly exposed to varying degrees of EM energy, particularly via EM radiation. In most cases, such fields are weak and pose little or no risk to the patient. However, as reviewed previously, there are particular situations that physicians and patients need to be aware of in order to avoid potential adverse events. As is often the case, minimizing patient risk from these potential EM interactions depends largely on increasing education and awareness. As threats come from both non-medical and medical environments and considering that the potential for injury is probably great, both the patient and members of the medical community need to be made aware of the potential sources of EMI. The impact of any restrictions on the care and management of the patient's primary or secondary medical conditions imposed by the presence of the implanted DBS system should be considered and discussed with the patient prior to surgery. This is particularly true with respect to the exclusion of whole body MRI from subsequent clinical management.

In the MRI environment, future progress in ensuring patient safety will depend greatly on the identification of a universal metric of RF power delivery as well as a greater understanding of the impact of device routing and configuration. Some of these concerns may be ameliorated through advancements in the DBS hardware itself, including, for example, the inclusion of capacitive filtering systems that are tuned to the frequency bands associated with MRI or the inclusion of fiber-optic components *(82)*. Other modifications that have been proposed include changing the coiling technique of the wires within the lead *(83)* or external shielding techniques involving the placement of some type of material over the device to limit infiltration of RF. The latter is by no means a novel idea, as it is similar to a report by Butrous et al. *(84)* of two patients with cardiac pacemakers who were able to return to work at an electrical substation only with specially designed suits to shield their bodies from the high intensity electric fields. However, for DBS systems, which tend to involve more elongated and elaborate routing techniques than those used for cardiac applications, such shielding techniques may not be feasible. In any case, until additional data become available or until any secondary technique for reducing MRI-related heating is developed, current manufacturer guidelines for MRI should be followed explicitly. Finally, at least within the realm of DBS, the current situation is made relatively simple by the existence of only a single device manufacturer with a limited offering of IPGs, leads, and extensions. This situation will evolve further as new device manufacturers enter the marketplace, bringing with them DBS hardware systems composed of different designs and materials.

## References

1. Fein RL (1967) Transurethral electrocautery procedures in patients with cardiac pacemakers. JAMA 202(1):101–103.
2. Wajszczuk WJ, Mowry FM, Dugan NL (1969) Deactivation of a demand pacemaker by transurethral electrocautery. N Engl J Med 280(1):34–35.
3. Smith RB, Wise WS (1971) Pacemaker malfunction from urethral electrocautery. JAMA 218(2):256.
4. Yamamoto T, Katayama Y, Fukaya C, Kurihara J, Oshima H, Kasai M (2000) Thalamotomy caused by cardioversion in a patient treated with deep brain stimulation. Stereotact Funct Neurosurg 74(2):73–82.
5. Titel JH, el-Etr AA (1968) Fibrillation resulting from pacemaker electrodes and electrocautery during surgery. Anesthesiology 29(4):845–846.
6. Lichter I, Borrie J, Miller WM (1965) Radio-frequency hazards with cardiac pacemakers. Br Med J 1965;1(5449):1513–1518.
7. Furman S, Parker B, Krauthamer M, Escher DJ (1968) The influence of electromagnetic environment on the performance of artificial cardiac pacemakers. Ann Thorac Surg 6(1):90–95.
8. Carleton RA, Sessions RW, Graettinger JS (1964) Environmental Influence on Implantable Cardiac Pacemakers. JAMA 190:938–940.
9. Bonney CH, Rustan PL Jr, Ford GE (1973) Evaluation of effects of the microwave oven (915 and 2450 MHz) and radar (2810 and 3050 MHz) electromagnetic radiation on noncompetitive cardiac pacemakers. IEEE Trans Biomed Eng 20(5):357–364.
10. Rustan PL, Hurt WD, Mitchell JC (1973) Microwave oven interference with cardiac pacemakers. Med Instrum 7(3):185–188.
11. King GR, Hamburger AC, Parsa F, Heller SJ, Carleton RA (1970) Effect of microwave oven on implanted cardiac pacemaker. JAMA 212(7):1213.
12. (1973) Possible electromagnetic interference with cardiac pacemakers from dental induction casting machines and electrosurgical devices. Council on Dental Materials and Devices. J Am Dent Assoc 86(2):426.
13. Orland HJ, Jones D (1975) Cardiac pacemaker induced ventricular fibrillation during surgical diathermy. Anaesth Intensive Care 3(4):321–326.
14. Blomstedt P, Hariz MI (2005) Hardware-related complications of deep brain stimulation: a ten year experience. Acta Neurochir (Wien) 147(10):1061–1064; discussion 1064.
15. Henderson JM, Tkach J, Phillips M, Baker K, Shellock FG, Rezai AR (2005) Permanent neurological deficit related to magnetic resonance imaging in a patient with implanted deep brain stimulation electrodes for Parkinson's disease: case report. Neurosurgery 57(5):E1063; discussion E.
16. Medtronic (2006) Kinetra: Dual Program Neurostimulator for Deep Brain Stimulation— Technical Manual. Minneapolis: Medtronic, Inc.
17. Medtronic (2006) Soletra: Neurostimulator for Deep Brain Stimulation—Physician and Hospital Staff Manual. Minneapolis: Medtronic, Inc.
18. Medtronic (2006) DBS: Lead Kid for Deep Brain Stimulation—Implant Manual. Minneapolis: Medtronic, Inc.

19. Medtronic (2005) MRI and Activa Therapy Manual. Minneapolis: Medtronic, Inc.
20. Spiegel J, Fuss G, Backens M, et al (2003) Transient dystonia following magnetic resonance imaging in a patient with deep brain stimulation electrodes for the treatment of Parkinson disease. Case report. J Neurosurg 99(4):772–774.
21. Nutt JG, Anderson VC, Peacock JH, Hammerstad JP, Burchiel KJ (2001) DBS and diathermy interaction induces severe CNS damage. Neurology 56(10):1384–1386.
22. MAUDE Database (2003) ID# 460649. U.S. Food and Drug Administration. Accessed Sept. 30, 2006, at www.accessdata.fda.gov/scripts/cdrh/cfdocs/cfMAUDE/Detail.cfm?MDRFOI__ID=460649.
23. MAUDE Database (2001) ID# 315109. U.S. Food and Drug Administration. Accessed Sept. 30, 2006, at www.accessdata.fda.gov/scripts/cdrh/cfdocs/cfMAUDE/Detail.CFM?MDRFOI__ID=315109.
24. MAUDE Database (2006) ID# 330144. U.S. Food and Drug Administration. Accessed Sept. 30, 2006, at www.accessdata.fda.gov/scripts/cdrh/cfdocs/cfMAUDE/Detail.CFM?MDRFOI__ID=330144.
25. Shellock FG (2006) Reference Manual for Magnetic Resonance Safety, Implants, and Devices. Los Angeles: Biomedical Research Publishing Group.
26. Zaremba L (2001) FDA guidance for MR system safety and patient exposures: current status and future considerations. In: Shellock FG, ed. Magnetic Resonance Procedures: Health Effects and Safety. Boca Raton: CRC Press, pp. 183–196.
27. Shellock FG (2001) Magnetic Resonance: Health Effects and Safety. Boca Raton: CRC Press.
28. Hayes DL, Holmes DR Jr, Gray JE (1987) Effect of 1.5 tesla nuclear magnetic resonance imaging scanner on implanted permanent pacemakers. J Am Coll Cardiol 10(4):782–786.
29. Gangarosa RE, Minnis JE, Nobbe J, Praschan D, Genberg RW (1987) Operational safety issues in MRI. Magn Reson Imaging 5(4):287–292.
30. Sommer T, Vahlhaus C, Lauck G, et al (2000) MR imaging and cardiac pacemakers: in-vitro evaluation and in-vivo studies in 51 patients at 0.5 T. Radiology 215(3):869–879.
31. Smith CD (2001) Health effects of induced electrical currents: Implications for implants. In: Shellock FG, ed. Magnetic Resonance: Health Effects and Safety. Boca Raton: CRC Press, pp. 393–413.
32. Shellock FG, Shellock VJ (1999) Metallic stents: evaluation of MR imaging safety. AJR 173(3):543–547.
33. Shellock FG, Hatfield M, Simon BJ, et al (2000) Implantable spinal fusion stimulator: assessment of MR safety and artifacts. J Magn Reson Imaging 12(2):214–223.
34. Shellock FG, Fieno DS, Thomson LJ, Talavage TM, Berman DS (2006) Cardiac pacemaker: in vitro assessment at 1.5 T. Am Heart J 151(2):436–443.
35. Schueler BA, Parrish TB, Lin JC, et al (1999) MRI compatibility and visibility assessment of implantable medical devices. J Magn Reson Imaging 9(4):596–603.
36. Rezai AR, Lozano AM, Crawley AP, et al (1999) Thalamic stimulation and functional magnetic resonance imaging: localization of cortical and subcortical activation with implanted electrodes. Technical note. J Neurosurg 90(3):583–590.
37. Rezai AR, Finelli D, Rugieri P, Tkach J, Nyenhuis JA, Shellock FG (2001) Neurostimulators: potential for excessive heating of deep brain stimulation electrodes during magnetic resonance imaging. J Magn Reson Imaging 14(4):488–489.
38. Liem LA, van Dongen VC (1997) Magnetic resonance imaging and spinal cord stimulation systems. Pain 70(1):95–97.
39. Heller JW, Brackmann DE, Tucci DL, Nyenhuis JA, Chou CK (1996) Evaluation of MRI compatibility of the modified nucleus multichannel auditory brainstem and cochlear implants. Am J Otol 17(5):724–729.
40. Gleason CA, Kaula NF, Hricak H, Schmidt RA, Tanagho EA (1992) The effect of magnetic resonance imagers on implanted neurostimulators. Pacing Clin Electrophysiol 15(1):81–94.

41. Finelli DA, Rezai AR, Ruggieri PM, et al (2002) MR imaging-related heating of deep brain stimulation electrodes: in vitro study. AJNR Am J Neuroradiol 23(10):1795–1802.
42. Chou CK, McDougall JA, Chan KW (1997) RF heating of implanted spinal fusion stimulator during magnetic resonance imaging. IEEE Trans Biomed Eng 44(5):367–373.
43. Chou CK, McDougall JA, Can KW (1995) Absence of radiofrequency heating from auditory implants during magnetic resonance imaging. Bioelectromagnetics 16(5):307–316.
44. Schaefer DJ, Bourland JD, Nyenhuis JA (2000) Review of patient safety in time-varying gradient fields. J Magn Reson Imaging 12(1):20–29.
45. Shellock FG (2001) MR imaging and electronically activated devices. Radiology 219(1):294–295.
46. Sawyer-Glover AM, Shellock FG (2000) Pre-MRI procedure screening: recommendations and safety considerations for biomedical implants and devices. J Magn Reson Imaging 12(3):510.
47. Nyenhuis JA, Kildishev AV, Foster KS, Graber G, Athey W (1999) Heating near implanted medical devices by the MRI RF-magnetic field. IEEE Trans Magn 35:4133–4135.
48. New PF, Rosen BR, Brady TJ, et al (1983) Potential hazards and artifacts of ferromagnetic and nonferromagnetic surgical and dental materials and devices in nuclear magnetic resonance imaging. Radiology 147(1):139–148.
49. Shellock FG (2001) Pocket guide to metallic implants and MR procedures: update 2001. New York: Lippincott-Raven Healthcare.
50. Shellock FG, Tkach JA, Ruggieri PM, Masaryk TJ (2003) Cardiac pacemakers, ICDs, and loop recorder: evaluation of translational attraction using conventional ("long-bore") and "short-bore" 1.5- and 3.0-Tesla MR systems. J Cardiovasc Magn Reson 5(2):387–397.
51. ASTM (2002) Standard test method for measurement of magnetically induced torque on passive implants in the magnetic resonance environment, standard F2213-02. In: ASfTaM, ed. Annual Book of ASTM Standards. West Conshohocken: ASTM, pp. 19,428–19,959.
52. ASTM (2002) Standard test method for measurement of magnetically induced displacement force on passive implants in the magnetic resonance environment. Designation: F 2052. In: ASfTaM, ed. Annual Book of ASTM Standards, Section 13, Medical Devices and Services, Volume 1301 Medical Devices; Emergency Medical Services. West Conshohocken: ASTM, pp. 1576–1580.
53. Baker KB, Nyenhuis JA, Hrdlicka G, Rezai AR, Tkach JA, Shellock FG (2005) Neurostimulation systems: assessment of magnetic field interactions associated with 1.5- and 3-Tesla MR systems. J Magn Reson Imaging 21(1):72–77.
54. Georgi JC, Stippich C, Tronnier VM, Heiland S (2004) Active deep brain stimulation during MRI: a feasibility study. Magn Reson Med 51(2):380–388.
55. Shellock FG (2005) In: Shellock FG, ed. Reference Manual for Magnetic Resonance Safety, Implants, and Devices, 2005 edition. Los Angeles: Biomedical Research Publishing Group, pp. 122–134.
56. Schenk J (2001) Health effects and safety of static magnetic fields. In: Shellock FG, ed. Magnetic Resonance Procedures: Health Effects and Safety. Boca Raton: CRC Press, pp. 1–29.
57. Nyenhuis JA (2001) Health effects and safety of intense MRI gradient fields. In: Shellock FG, ed. Magnetic Resonance Procedures: Health Effects and Safety. Boca Raton: CRC Press, pp. 31–54.
58. Geddes LA, Baker LE (1989) Principles of Applied Biomedical Instrumentation, third edition. Wiley and Sons.
59. IEC (2002) Medical electrical equipment, particular requirements for the safety of magnetic resonance equipment for medical diagnosis. International Standard IEC 60601-2-33.

60. Achenbach S, Moshage W, Diem B, Bieberle T, Schibgilla V, Bachmann K (1997) Effects of magnetic resonance imaging on cardiac pacemakers and electrodes. Am Heart J 134(3):467–473.
61. Brown TR, Goldstein B, Little J (1993) Severe burns resulting from magnetic resonance imaging with cardiopulmonary monitoring. Risks and relevant safety precautions. Am J Phys Med Rehab/Assoc Acad Physiatrists 72(3):166–167.
62. Konings MK, Bartels LW, Smits HF, Bakker CJ (200) Heating around intravascular guidewires by resonating RF waves. J Magn Reson Imaging 12(1):79–85.
63. Ladd ME, Quick HH (2000) Reduction of resonant RF heating in intravascular catheters using coaxial chokes. Magn Reson Med 43(4):615–619.
64. Nitz WR, Oppelt A, Renz W, Manke C, Lenhart M, Link J (2001) On the heating of linear conductive structures as guide wires and catheters in interventional MRI. J Magn Reson Imaging 13(1):105–114.
65. Tronnier VM, Staubert A, Hahnel S, Sarem-Aslani A (1999) Magnetic resonance imaging with implanted neurostimulators: an in vitro and in vivo study. Neurosurgery 44(1):118–125; discussion 25–26.
66. Park SM, Nyenhuis JA, Smith CD, et al (2003) Gelled versus nongelled phantom material for measurement of MRI-induced temperature increases with bioimplants. IEEE Trans Magnet 39(5):3367–3371.
67. Baker KB, Tkach J, Hall JD, Nyenhuis JA, Shellock FG, Rezai AR (2005) Reduction of magnetic resonance imaging-related heating in deep brain stimulation leads using a lead management device. Neurosurgery 57(4 Suppl):392–397; discussion 397.
68. Baker KB, Tkach JA, Nyenhuis JA, et al (2004) Evaluation of specific absorption rate as a dosimeter of MRI-related implant heating. J Magn Reson Imaging 20(2):315–320.
69. Baker KB, Tkach JA, Phillips MD, Rezai AR (2006) Variability in RF-induced heating of a deep brain stimulation implant across MR systems. J Magn Reson Imaging.
70. Medtronic (2001) Soletra neurostimulator for dep brain stimulation—model 7246 physician and hospital staff manual. Minneapolis: Medtronic, Inc.
71. Fetter J, Aram G, Holmes DR, Jr., Gray JE, Hayes DL (1984) The effects of nuclear magnetic resonance imagers on external and implantable pulse generators. Pacing Clin Electrophysiol 7(4):720–727.
72. Nyenhuis JA, Park SM, Kamondetdacha R, Amjad A, Shellock FG, Rezai A (2005) MRI and Implanted Medical Devices: Basic Interactions with an Emphasis on Heating. IEEE Trans Dev Mat Reliab 5(3):467–480.
73. Alterman RL, Reiter GT, Shils J, et al (1999) Targeting for thalamic deep brain stimulator implantation without computer guidance: assessment of targeting accuracy. Stereotact Funct Neurosurg 72(2–4):150–153.
74. Lemaire JJ, Durif F, Boire JY, Debilly B, Irthum B, Chazal J (1999) Direct stereotactic MRI location in the globus pallidus for chronic stimulation in Parkinson's disease. Acta Neurochir (Wien) 141(7):759–765; discussion 766.
75. Mobin F, De Salles AA, Behnke EJ, Frysinger R (1999) Correlation between MRI-based stereotactic thalamic deep brain stimulation electrode placement, macroelectrode stimulation and clinical response to tremor control. Stereotact Funct Neurosurg 72(2–4):225–232.
76. Suh JS, Jeong EK, Shin KH, et al (1998) Minimizing artifacts caused by metallic implants at MR imaging: experimental and clinical studies. Ajr 171(5):1207–1213.
77. Pollo C, Villemure JG, Vingerhoets F, Ghika J, Maeder P, Meuli R (2004) Magnetic resonance artifact induced by the electrode Activa 3389: an in vitro and in vivo study. Acta Neurochir (Wien) 146(2):161–164.
78. Petersilge CA, Lewin JS, Duerk JL, Yoo JU, Ghaneyem AJ (1996) Optimizing imaging parameters for MR evaluation of the spine with titanium pedicle screws. Ajr 166(5):1213–1218.

79. Schrader B, Hamel W, Weinert D, Mehdorn HM (2002) Documentation of electrode localization. Mov Disord 17(Suppl 3):S167–S174.
80. Ryu SI, Romanelli P, Heit G (2004) Asymptomatic transient MRI signal changes after unilateral deep brain stimulation electrode implantation for movement disorder. Stereotact Funct Neurosurg 82(2–3):65–69.
81. Hariz MI, Krack P, Melvill R, et al (2003) A quick and universal method for stereotactic visualization of the subthalamic nucleus before and after implantation of deep brain stimulation electrodes. Stereotact Funct Neurosurg 80(1–4):96–101.
82. Greatbatch W, Miller V, Shellock FG (2002) Magnetic resonance safety testing of a newly-developed fiber-optic cardiac pacing lead. J Magn Reson Imaging 16(1):97–103.
83. Gray RW, Bibens WT, Shellock FG (2005) Simple design changes to wires to substantially reduce MRI-induced heating at 1.5T: implications for implanted leads. Magn Reson Imaging 23(8):887–891.
84. Butrous GS, Bexton RS, Barton DG, Male JC, Camm AJ (1983) Interference with the pacemakers of two workers at electricity substations. Brit J Ind Med 40(4):462–465.

# 23

# Deep Brain Stimulation Fault Testing

Jay L. Shils, Ron L. Alterman, and Jeffrey E. Arle

## Abstract

As deep brain stimulation (DBS) has become a treatment standard for medically refractory Parkinson's disease (PD), essential tremor, and dystonia, more is being learned about the longevity and function of the implantable stimulator and its components. Early reports have related a 15 to 30% failure and infection rate associated with this device *(1–7)*. As the number of medical conditions treated with DBS increases, the total number of device failures will also rise. Therefore, a systematic method for troubleshooting device failures is required in order to minimize both DBS "downtime" and the number of surgeries required to identify and replace failed components.

**Keywords:** deep brain stimulation, DBS, troubleshooting, testing, noninvasive, invasive, open circuit, closed circuit

## Introduction

The present standard of care for medically refractory Parkinson's disease, essential tremor, and dystonia is the surgical placement of a deep brain stimulating (DBS) system. The degree of hardware related failures in any implantable system varies, but for the DBS system reports describe a 15 to 30% failure and infection rate (1-7). Thus as more patients are implanted, both for present indications and as future indications are developed, it seems clear that the total number of hardware related failures will rise. With this in mind, our groups have devised a methodology for troubleshooting device related failures in order to both minimize DBS "downtime" and to reduce the number of surgical incisions and hardware replacements required for repair.

Surgery to isolate and fix device malfunctions takes time, is expensive, and exposes the patient to additional risk. Therefore, it is important to evaluate completely the patient who is responding poorly to DBS before manipulating his/her device surgically. The potential causes of a poor response to DBS include inaccurately placed leads, an incorrect initial diagnosis, inadequate stimulator

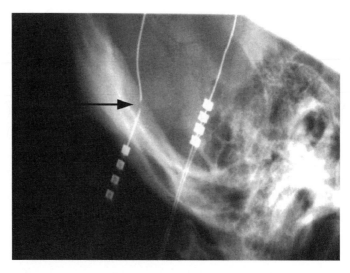

**Figure 23.1** A sagittal X-ray showing a break in one of the leads (black arrow). This break is across all four of the electrode wires

programming, and a worsening disease state *(8)*. If specific symptoms or electrophysiological data derived through device interrogation do not suggest a device failure (see later), these clinical issues must be ruled out before assuming that a device malfunction exists. However, even when it is clear that a malfunction is present, it is essential to make every possible attempt to localize the fault noninvasively before embarking on surgical interventions.

Unless a lead fracture is visible on X-ray (Figure 23.1), locating short or "open" circuits in system components is very difficult with current manufacturer-supplied hardware and software. Intermittent system problems are especially difficult to locate, and the differentiation of an intermittent problem from a *pseudo* problem can be nearly impossible. In this chapter, we describe a noninvasive means to localize system failures, which we have used successfully to guide the surgical repair of malfunctioning DBS systems. Illustrative cases are also provided.

## The DBS System

The DBS system consists of: a four-contact stimulating lead *(9)*, a combination implantable pulse control system and self-contained power supply *(10)*, and an extension cable *(11)* that connects the two (Figure 23.2). At this time there are two Food and Drug Administration (FDA)-approved leads: Medtronic models 3387 and 3389. Each of these leads has four contacts that are 1.5mm long by 1.27mm diameter that are composed of platinum/iridium. Each contact is connected via a coiled platinum/iridium wire to a nickel alloy (MP35N) cylinder on the opposite end of the lead, which exits the skull and is connected to an extension cable. Individual wires are insulated with a fluoropolymer to prevent contact shorting. The four lead wires are contained in a type 80A urethane jacket. The coils and the insulation allow for limited lead motion to accommodate patient movement[1]. The maximum impedance of the lead is less than 100Ω.

---

[1] At the time of this writing, the only FDA-approved device is made by Medtronic, Inc. All techniques discussed in this chapter were developed on these systems. These techniques should be acceptable for other systems when approved for use.

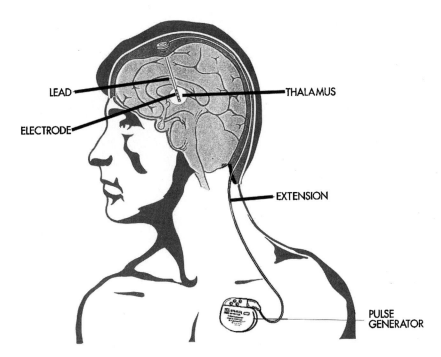

**Figure 23.2** A graphical representation of the implanted DBS system. This is the only FDA-approved system at the time of this writing

The lead is secured where it exits the skull by one of several acceptable means. The excess length of lead wire is neatly coiled beneath the scalp and connected to the extension (11), which is thicker and more durable than the lead. The conductors in the extension are made from silver core MP35N. Each conductor is coiled and set in an individual cylindrical opening which reduces the chance of shorting. The extension is passed through a subcutaneous tract that traverses the retrosigmoid region and neck to an ipsilateral subcutaneous pocket in the subclavicular area of the upper chest where the extension lead is connected to the implantable pulse generator (IPG). For a dual-stimulation device, each lead is connected to a single extension wire via a 'Y'-adapter ('Y' in shape only – all contacts are still individual). A silastic cover (boot) is placed over the lead/extension connection and two ties are placed on each end creating a water tight seal for the connection (Figure 3). The connector screws are made from titanium and the connector blocks from stainless steel. The extension insulation is silicone rubber and polyurethane while the connector block is sealed in silicone rubber and siloxane coated silicone rubber. The maximum resistance of the complete extension wire is 7 $\Omega$.

## The DBS Circuit

For current to flow through an electrical circuit, the circuit needs to be configured in a closed loop. The electrical circuit that contains the DBS system is depicted in Figure 23.2. The power source provides a constant voltage pulse of

**Figure 23.3** A photograph of the lead–extension connection. The silastic boot is covering the connection and there are two black ties on each end of the boot to seal the connection. This is supposed to keep a water-tight seal around the connection in order to protect the connection and reduce the chance for shorting

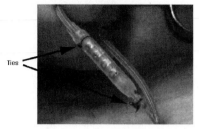

potential V that, when activated, sends a current around the circuit. The current (I) is determined by the potential (V) and the impedance (Z) that the potential needs to overcome.

$$I = \frac{V}{Z} \qquad (1)$$

For DBS, the impedance includes both the circuit resistance and the effects of capacitance and inductance at the biomechanical interface of the electrode and tissue. Therefore, the total circuit impedance is composed of three elements: (1) the connections between the system components; (2) the impedances of the conductors (wires) used in both the extension cable (< 7 Ω *[11]*) and the lead (<100 Ω *[9]*); and (3) the brain–body–electrode interface, which contributes the largest impedance. It is also important to note that the impedance of brain tissue varies with the stimulation frequency, therefore, comparing impedances over time is only useful if the same test frequency and pulse width were used. Presently, the only FDA-approved device uses a 30-Hz test frequency, which differs considerably from the frequencies most commonly used for DBS therapy (typically 130–185 Hz). In general, as the frequency increases the measured impedance of the biologic material decreases *(12–14)*. For an intact system, normal impedance values for a test pulse of 210 μsec at 30 Hz, when referenced to the IPG case (i.e., monopolar configuration), should range between 600 and 2000 ohms with a current between 9 and 25 μA using 2.0 volts. This is true for electrodes located within the STN, GPi, and VIM when using the Medtronic model 8840 programmer in the electrode impedance test mode, but not during therapy measurement testing. Future systems may use different test parameters and will yield different normal impedance values. Also, normal impedance values in other brain regions may differ from those observed in these three areas.

The literature describes very little anatomical change at the electrode/brain interface as a consequence of chronic DBS *(15–17)*. Therefore, one may conclude that a major change in the measured electrical properties of impedance and current over time will most likely occur at the other two primary circuit impedance points (the conductors and connection points). It should be noted, however, that within 3 months of implantation there may be large changes in impedance, likely due to surgical healing. Three types of electrical failure modes have been identified in DBS systems: (1) foreign body accumulation at the connection points; (2) an open circuit (i.e., a break in the circuit path); and (3) a "short," which is a new unexpected and unwanted circuit pathway between what should be independent circuit elements. An internal failure of the IPG is exceedingly rare, but possible; however, locating a problem in the IPG is more complex and is arrived at through a process of elimination, when all other testing, to be described later, fails to localize the failure.

Under the open circuit condition, current is unable to flow due to a break in the pathway (Figure 23.4). If the circuit is completely open, the measured current will be zero and the impedance will be infinite. If the circuit contains an intermittent open and closed condition, current will flow some of the time (transient mode failure), during which current flow through the circuit may appear normal. Intermittent open circuits are very difficult to troubleshoot, and may only be found during the actual open period. An intermittent open circuit could be seen when a break in the conductor allows the two ends to remain close proximity. When the ends are in contact the circuit will function normally, however, if the extension or the lead are moved (for example, while turning the head) the ends separate and the open circuit condition occurs.

In patients with tremor, which varies quickly in relation to the state of stimulation, the ability to diagnose an intermittent open circuit is easier than in patients whose symptoms change more slowly. If the intermittent condition is very brief no abnormality may be detected. Patients with brief intermittent open circuits may derive benefit from stimulation, but the results will be suboptimal. Therefore, if a patient presents with an unexplained reduction in therapeutic efficacy, but the system appears to be functioning properly, one must consider a transient mode failure.

In a short circuit situation, current is shunted away from the electrode contacts in the brain. This is because the new circuit pathway, created by the short, is of lower impedance and draws current away from the lead tip. For the DBS system there may be multiple short-circuit types. The first type involves a break (open-circuit) in the extension or lead insulation. The wires on the IPG side of the break may touch each other causing the current to flow only in the

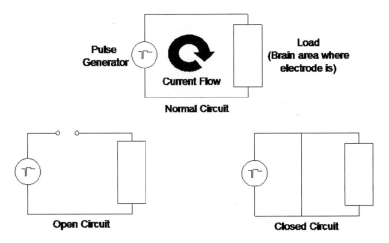

**Figure 23.4** A schematic representation of current flow in an electrical circuit. The top image shows a normal circuit. The lower left image shows an open circuit where no current can flow into the load. The lower right image shows a short circuit where current will be shunted away from the load via the short

electrical circuit and not in the body. Under this condition, one will measure very low impedance and very high current during the therapeutic test (see later). The term "high" and "low" are used because the normal values depend on the therapeutic settings being employed. For stimulation with pulse widths of 60 to 90 μsec, one or two active contacts, and voltages under 3.7 volts, the stimulation current should be less than 150 μA. However, for a pulse width of 210 μsec or higher, and/or a voltage of >3.6 volts, and/or more than two activated contacts, the current can exceed 200 μA and still be considered normal. Thus, it is critical to look at the therapeutic parameters at each visit so that a reference exists for each particular patient.

A second type of short occurs if the insulation between the conductors in the extension breaks down and the conductors begin to short due to contact with biological tissue. Because there is no open circuit, some of the current flows back to the IPG via the shorted wire while the rest flows to the conductors in the brain. Consequently, some inactive contacts may transmit current, stimulating unintended areas of the brain. Short circuits can cause excessive current flow because when the impedance trends toward zero, the current will exceed the maximum desired, rapidly draining the power source. One dangerous problem with short circuits, and the high current that results, is that this high current may break down the insulation, causing additional unwanted current paths. Also, higher current can generate heat at the site of the short, which will in turn heat adjacent tissue, generating potential burns. In Figure 23.5, burns can be seen on both the left and right extensions wires removed from this patient.

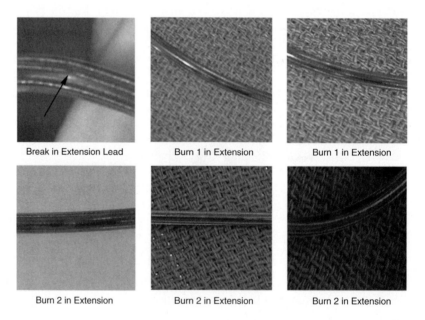

**Figure 23.5** This is a series of photographs from a damaged lead taken from a patient who had a DBS system implanted in the thalamus for chronic pain. There was a break in the extension that in turn allowed fluid to contact the leads causing a short. As the blood started to dry in the extension the short energy was high enough to generate burns internal to the insulation. The patient described some sharp electrical shocks for about 6 hours and then nothing. This was probably during the time the battery was draining

A third type of short circuit condition can arise when fluid enters the connection between the extension and the lead or the extension and the IPG. The fluid can act as a conductor, shunting the current away from the DBS electrode surfaces to other unintended contacts. In monopolar configuration, the shunted current may activate an alternate conductor, again sending current to an inactive electrode, stimulating an area of brain inadvertently.

Monopolar and bipolar stimulation behave somewhat differently in failure modes due to the differing return pathways for the current. During monopolar stimulation, the return is the casing of the IPG, which is usually placed in the chest area. If the lead and extension wire insulations are intact (i.e., the break is inside an intact insulation), the insulation will create a very high resistance thus still allowing the current to flow to the lead in the brain and not from the break point. However, if the insulation has a break, current will escape from the opening back to the IPG and the patient may feel a shock at the break point. For the short circuit situation in monopolar configuration, the current will be split between the two shorting leads if only one lead is active. No changes will be seen if both of the leads are active, assuming the insulation is not broken. If the short is between the connector and the IPG the patient may feel intense pain at the IPG site. A note of caution: under normal circumstances thin patients may feel a sensation at the chest area during monopolar stimulation, which may be mistaken for a short circuit. However, interrogation of the system will reveal normal impedance. If the insulation is broken, a shock may be felt at the break point. If the impedance at the break point is lower than that of the electrode contacts in the brain, current will pass from the break point to the case, taking the path of least resistance.

During bipolar stimulation multiple types of open circuit situations can occur. If the insulation is intact, no current will flow in the circuit. If, however, the insulation surrounding one of the conductors is broken, current will flow along two pathways. The first pathway is from the insulation break to the reference electrode in the brain. The second is the intended pathway between the active and reference electrodes.[2] The amount of current flowing at the break will depend on the relative impedance in each pathway. In fact, no problem may be noticed by the patient in the case where the impedance at the break point is very large. If both conductors are broken, current will most likely flow at the break point.

Short circuits also present in multiple ways depending on the state of the insulation and the state of the conductors at the location of the short. If the insulation and the conductors are fully intact, minimal current will get to the brain because the impedance at the short is very low. If the insulation is intact and multiple electrodes are being employed for therapy, two conditions could arise. First, if the short is between the active contact and another (an electrode not used for the patients particular therapy program), or the reference and another, the current will be split between the normal circuit and the new path, stimulating an unintended region of the brain. Second, if the short is

---

[2] At first, one may think that if there is a break in the wire and conductor then no current will get to the brain. Yet if there is fluid in the conductor between the breaks, a current pathway may exist for energy to reach the brain.

between two active contacts or between two reference contacts, no difference will be seen. If the insulation is broken, the current has multiple pathways it can travel and the current to the brain electrodes will most likely be reduced due to the low power supply resistance.

Note that in contrast to constant voltage devices, the internal resistance of constant-current stimulators must be very high to ensure that the power supply and not the load controls the current delivered. In every day life load typically controls current. For example, when we turn on a brighter light at home, the lamp draws more current from the power supply. In a patient, the electronics need to operate in reverse, so that when there is a short, the power supply will automatically limit the current to a safe level. In the home, there are fuses and circuit breakers for protection.

## Noninvasive Testing

When evaluating a patient with a reduction in DBS efficacy, signs of a potential device failure include: (1) a sudden change in the therapeutic benefit of stimulation; (2) strange electrical shocks along the circuit pathway; (3) a sudden onset of muscle contractions; (4) a sudden onset of continuous or intermittent paresthesias; (5) a sudden change in vision; and (6) battery depletion long before expected. The techniques and methods for troubleshooting a malfunctioning DBS device fall into two categories: noninvasive testing performed in the clinic and invasive testing performed in the operating room.

Initial testing is performed with the clinical patient programmer. Observe and record the following:

(1) device state (on/off)
(2) number of activations since the previous visit
(3) percentage of on time since the previous visit
(4) battery voltage
(5) therapeutic impedance
(6) therapeutic current
(7) monopolar impedances
(8) monopolar currents
(9) bipolar impedances
(10) bipolar currents

All 10 of these details are discernable with the programmer. It is critical that at the end of each visit the internal counters in the implanted IPG are reset so items 2 and 3 in the list are accurate. If the device is off, the clinician must attempt to determine why and when it turned off. One way to estimate the length of time the device was shut off, if a singular event, is to determine the amount of time the device has been off. This can be estimated by observing the date of the last reset and subtracting the total hours used from the total hours since the last reset and calculating the intervening hours by:

$$\sim DaysSinceOff = \frac{(NumberOfDaysSince\,Reset \times 24) - HoursUsed}{24} \quad (2)$$

The patient should be questioned about specific events within a few days of this estimated time. Ask the patient about recent travel, shopping, or other excursions. Ask if he or she was near large power lines or electrical substations or close to large neon signs. Ask whether power tools or welders were used. Finally, ask about any impacts they may have taken to the chest area. Newer DBS systems (i.e., post-2003) are less susceptible to external magnetic interference, but the patient's recent history to such exposure should be recorded. If the patient cannot recall any specific event (the most common case), turn the device back on and run both the electrode specific impedance and current checks as well as the therapeutic parameter check. If all parameters are within the normal range, no other changes are necessary. Recommend that the patient keep a diary of potential causative external events (as cited earlier) to have a record if the same situation arises in the future.

If the measured parameters are outside of the normal range then more investigation is necessary. The battery voltage gives an indication of how much battery energy is left. Our experience has shown that when battery voltages for Medtronic devices drop below 3.65 volts, the IPG should be replaced. The Medtronic product manuals recommend a lower voltage before device change, but in the authors' experience, when the voltage drops below 3.65 volts, the therapeutic voltage must be raised to achieve a similar, though not quite as beneficial result, as compared to a fresh battery that is delivering its full output potential. After IPG replacement, the therapeutic values are typically the same as those prior to battery voltage reduction. (For other manufacturers devices these guidelines will need to be determined.)

If the battery voltages test at a reasonable level (i.e. above 3.65 volts), the next step is to examine the circuit integrity. To accomplish this, both the electrode circuit test (each electrode and each electrode combination is checked) and the therapeutic test (current and impedance at the therapeutic settings) need to be performed. Both are needed since an acceptable therapeutic test will not always identify a short circuit involving an "inactive" electrode, which could be the cause of paresthesia, contractions, visual problems, or poor therapeutic results due to the stimulus being shunted from desirable to undesirable brain areas. When performing the therapeutic parameters test, major impedance and current changes (i.e., >200 ohms and >20 mA, respectively) since the last visit will indicate a problem. However, remember that during the first 3 to 6 months after implantation, changes of this order may be observed as a result of the normal brain healing process.

The results of the bipolar component of the electrode testing program help one to make sense of abnormalities or changes found during the therapeutic test. During bipolar testing it is critical to look at all of the electrode combinations, not just those involving active contacts. A low impedance value and a high current value between any electrode pair that includes an active electrode indicates that a nonplanned current is being delivered. For the case where the active electrode is paired with an inactive electrode, current is being delivered to an area of the brain that should not be receiving any current. For the case where the active electrode is paired with another active electrode of opposite polarity, an inappropriate amount of current is being delivered. Either of these cases will require replacement of some system component. If the short is between two inactive electrodes, no changes may be required. If no abnormal values are noted then more investigation is necessary.

Monopolar impedances and currents should also be investigated using the electrode test program as the problem may not involve a specific electrode pair but could reside within a single conductor or within the IPG switching matrix. An open circuit (very large impedances and very low currents) in electrodes that are inactive could indicate a future problem in an active electrode or an intermittent fault. Intermittent faults are generally the most difficult to localize. This is because they may not show as faults during normal testing with the clinical programmer. A break in an inactive electrode is good evidence that there may be a transient fault in an active lead in the event of a sudden change in therapeutic benefit. Another way to identify intermittent faults is to manipulate the lead connector lightly under the skin while asking the patient if they feel any changes. If the intermittent fault is causing motor or sensory phenomena this technique has a good chance of exposing it. When manipulating near or at the break point, the patient may experience sharp paresthesias or contractions. If no paresthesias or contractions are found when manipulating the lead or extension wire, but a transient fault is still suspected, a lateral and A-P X-ray of the chest, head, and neck may be useful in locating a troubled area in the lead or extension. A potential troubled area is one where there is a sharp bend in the lead or extension, or one where the wires appear to be broken. It has been the author's experience that near the connector, the wires may appear broken even when they are intact. Utilizing information from the X-ray, push on the wire at the point where the X-ray indicates a problem and then retest the system using the electrode test program. Manipulating the lead and extension at the break point may cause a change that can be detected. It is especially important to do this testing at the connections (i.e., the lead to extension connection and the IPG to extension connection). X-rays may also be used to determine if there are large breaks in the lead or extension wire (Figure 23.1).

## Noninvasive Active Testing

To identify more complex failures such as transient failures or better localize a failure, we developed a technique that utilizes either an oscilloscope or an intra-operative neurophysiological monitoring system with electromyography (EMG) software to visualize the electrical pulse traveling through the circuit. By analyzing the shape and amplitude of the recorded wave one may determine: whether or not a fault exists; the type of fault; and potentially the exact location of the fault. Figure 23.6 shows the placement of the recording electrodes along the DBS system. Figure 23.7 shows the theoretical shape of the IPG wave, and a normal IPG wave recorded at the surface of the skin via the set up shown in Figure 23.6. The testing is performed in both monopolar and bipolar modes. This technique is based on the principles underlying surface EMG and far field evoked potentials. The electrical potential generated in the muscle or nerve synapse forms an electric field (Figure 23.8) that can be recorded on the skin. The primary measured impedance is that from the electrode contact in the brain and the case and is represented by the grey rectangles in Figure 23.9. This impedance consists of all the energy that is dissipated in all the tissue along the pathway, including the skin. Thus, by placing recording leads on the skin the voltage gradient between the two leads can be recorded. If all the wired connections are intact then signal that is recorded on the surface of the skin will be similar for all leads and

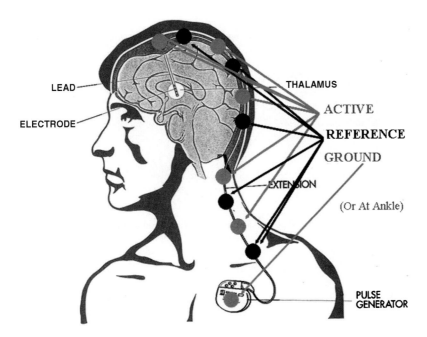

**Figure 23.6** These are the locations of the test points on the surface of the skin. The ground is placed over the IPG while the active and reference leads are moved over the wires

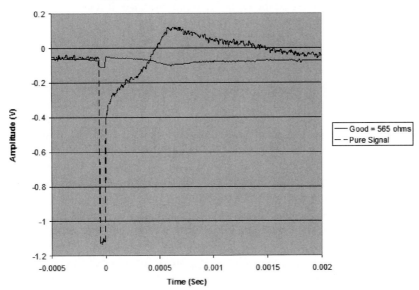

**Figure 23.7** Examples of the DBS signal recorded from a system in a simulated body load and from a surface recoding where the impedance was 560 ohms. The initial negative peak is the cathodal stimulation amplitude that is represented by the voltage value that is set on the programmer. The positivity represents the charge balanced component of the wave form

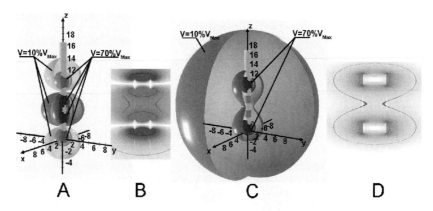

**Figure 23.8** Graphical representations of an analytic solution to the voltage (A and C) and electric (B and D) fields generated by the Medtronic DBS lead. The hot colors (yellow and red) represent the anodal field while the cool colors (blue and green) represent the cathodal field. (To view this figure in color, see insert)

skin locations measured[3]. If there is a break in one of the wired elements, then the potential that is generated on the skin during stimulation with that lead will be different as compared to the other leads. Depending upon the relationship of the open circuit to the recording electrodes (i.e., distance from the open circuit, space between the active and reference electrode, and whether or not the open circuit is located between the recording electrodes or not) the signal will either be larger or smaller than when it is between the other leads. In the normal intact DBS system, the primary signal is a far field signal that is generated at the electrode brain interface. If there is a break in the lead or a short between wires then a new *synaptic* point is created. This new point will divert some, or all, of the signal from the electrode tip–brain interface. If the signal diversion is kept completely inside of the insulation and the diversion is an open circuit, the far field amplitude at the electrode brain interface will have a smaller amplitude than the normally operating system. If the signal diversion is kept completely inside of the insulation and the diversion is a short circuit bringing an inactive electrode into play, the far field amplitude at the electrode brain interface may be larger in either the positive or negative direction during bipolar stimulation or in both directions during monopolar stimulation. This is due to the larger spread of energy in the brain. If the signal diversion is kept completely inside of the insulation and the diversion is a break with a short to another contact the far field amplitude at the electrode brain interface may show either an increase in amplitude or a decrease in amplitude, but a change will be noted. If the diversion is at a point where the insulation is broken there will likely be an increase in the signal at the point of the break for an open circuit, or the amplitude will decrease as the recording electrodes are moved away from the short in the case of a short circuit.

---

[3] There will actually be a slight amplitude variation due to impedance differences in the leads. This difference will be well below any change that is detected from a fault.

During monopolar stimulation the circuit pathway includes the IPG, extension, lead, and body back to the IPG (Figure 23.9). Monopolar testing is performed in two different steps (note that by monopolar we mean the IPG stimulation configuration). The first step is to place the reference electrode over the skull where the lead enters the brain and then move the active recording electrode along skin overlying the system pathway. Large changes in the recorded voltage indicate that the active recording electrode is near the area of a failure. The second step is to separate the active and reference electrodes by about 3 cm and move the pair along the system. While moving the electrodes, carefully palpate the wire between the leads. If the wires are intact the recorded amplitude should change only 5 to 10% owing to geometry and normal body impedances. Larger changes indicate the site of a break. This procedure should be done while activating each of the DBS contacts in monopolar configuration.

One problem with this technique occurs when the break is very close to the IPG or is within the IPG-extension connector. This is because the IPG generates the signal and therefore it is difficult to determine if an increase in the recorded amplitude is resulting from a break or simply reflects proximity to the stimulus source. Figure 23.10 shows an example of an open circuit test when the active and reference electrodes are placed on either side of a transient break in the extension. When the wire was manipulated the open circuit occurred. Patient 1 in the case reports section is an example of such a situation. A variation of this testing method is performed by keeping the reference electrode at one end of

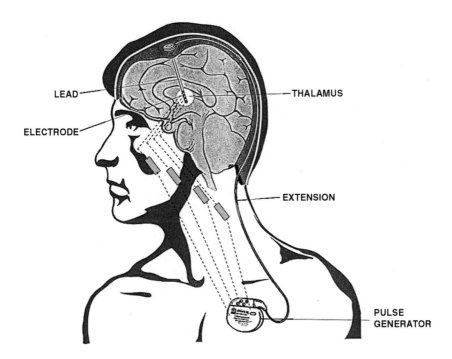

**Figure 23.9** A representation of the impedance pathways in the body when recording on the skin. In an intact system the pathway is from the lead tips to the case. If there is a short or open circuit these pathways change

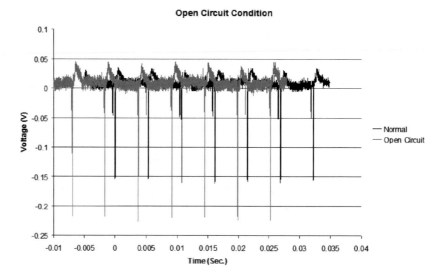

**Figure 23.10** A test that demonstrates a transient open circuit in the system. The active lead is placed 3 cm from the area with the break. As the broken lead is moved the current changes from flowing in the lead to flowing through multiple conductors in the lead. The reduced impedance causes an increase in current and thus a jump in the potential. This is recorded from the patient in example 1

the circuit and moving the active lead along the extension wire and lead external to the skull. When the active lead and the reference point are on the same side as the break the potential will be very small. When the active lead comes close to the break point the potential will start to increase rapidly. This situation is represented by patient 2 described in the case reports section.

Testing for faults when the system is in a bipolar configuration allows for better localization of short circuits. When a short exists, two, three, or all four wires may be implicated. If all four leads are shorted the signal passing through the wire will encounter a nearly zero impedance and thus the field generated in the surrounding tissue will be too small to be detected if it exists at all. If the short exists at a point where there is a break in the insulation or at a connection point, due to the introduction of some biological tissue or fluid, the signal may be large enough to be detected up at the surface of the skin. If there is a question as to whether a short exists, all bipolar combinations need to be checked. If it is already known that a short exists then the shorted wires should be checked relative to a good wire (shorted wires as cathode, good wire as anode). By placing the active and reference surface electrodes furthest from the IPG, recording a signal, and then manipulating the wire through the skin while moving along the wire, one may see a change in the signal at the break area. The purpose of the manipulation is to break and make the short, which will change the impedance and thus the signal picture.

## Invasive Testing

Despite our best efforts there are still instances where noninvasive testing cannot indicate the defective element to replace. Replacing the brain lead obviously poses the greatest risk and inconvenience to the patient. Therefore, it is imperative that every effort be made to rule out faults in the other system components before proceeding with lead replacement. When necessary, we perform invasive testing under general anesthesia with endotracheal intubation. Unless the IPG is known to be defective, or the battery needs replacement, the first incision is made at the extension–lead connection so that the lead may be tested independent of the other system components. The incision is made directly over the connector and is of sufficient length (typically 3 cm), to provide enough room to remove and replace the boot. The incision should avoid crossing or "T"-ing into a prior incision made during the original placement. Care must be taken at every step not to damage the lead (even cleaning and drying it with a gauze pad can inadvertently catch and pull a contact free of its connector). It is best to avoid monopolar cautery, use of which may cause heating of the implanted electrodes and injury to the surrounding brain. It is essential to note every detail of the tissue and the state of the hardware when it is initially encountered. In particular, fluid type, amount, and location, as well as the exact configuration of the wires, boot, and sutures may be important and should be appreciated before disturbing the hardware for evaluation. Avoidance of local anesthetic injections is recommended as inadvertent needle damage to a wire or the introduction of fluid within the boot can confound the intra-operative evaluation.

The extension–lead connection is examined first. We have sometimes found that fluid becomes trapped within the plastic boot that is placed over the lead–extension connection, causing a short between the connections. The exterior of the boot can be gently patted dry. Do not press too firmly when drying the boot as fluid can be forced out thereby erasing the evidence. The two sutures on each end of the boot should be removed and the boot slid off of the connector. The connection should be opened using the small hexdriver supplied by the manufacturer. Both the lead and extension connection should be dried. Using a small suction tip, the inside of the female end of the connector can also be dried. The boot should be checked for cracks, holes or other defects, and replaced if any defect is found. In rare cases, each tiny set screw should be removed and cleaned and its connector threading cleaned and dried as well.

If the boot is intact and no fluid is observed in the connection, the extension should be the next component tested. It is tested by using the implanted IPG as the power generator and recording signal on the exposed end. We use small sterile alligator clips to attach to the small connections on the exposed end of the extension. The wires attached to the clips are passed from the sterile field and connected to an oscilloscope across a 1 K$\Omega$ resistor. The IPG programming head is placed in a sterile bag and positioned over the IPG. All electrode combinations are tested. For these tests the IPG parameters are set to 2.0 volts, 60 Hz, and 210 μsec. During each test the surgeon manipulates the extension through the skin. Both shorts and open circuits will cause a reduction in the signal observed on the scope and will show a flat or much reduced trace. If this occurs while testing any electrode combination, the extension wire should be replaced. In our experience, the two locations at which we most commonly identify open circuits are the retromastoid region and the extension–lead connection.

The next step is to test the brain lead itself. This is somewhat more difficult because we do not have access to the full lead, specifically the end that is in the brain. In the authors' experience, we have encountered only one case

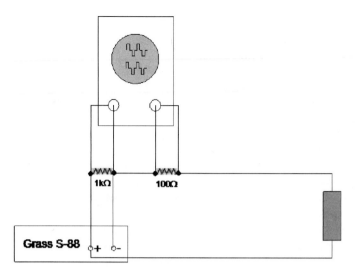

**Figure 23.11** A circuit to test the impedance of the lead wire in the implanted patient

where the lead was defective *inside* the skull. That was determined using the following technique. Using a grass S-88 stimulator, a circuit (Figure 23.11) was built to determine the impedance of the leads (similar to the circuit depicted in Figure 1 of ref. *13*). The test stimulus was as follows: frequency, 30 Hz; pulse width, 210 µSec; voltage, 2.0 volts. By measuring the current and voltage across scalp regions R1 and R2 the impedance of the lead/brain system can be calculated. An impedance that is either infinite or less than 50 Ω demonstrates a definite fault in the system. Because the brain tissue acts as the primary component of the impedance in the intact system, the measured values should be between 500 Ω and 5000 Ω. Impedance values that fall between 50 Ω and 500 Ω represent a gray area. A general rule of thumb used by the authors is that impedances below 300 Ω should be investigated as a potential short circuit. Two areas that should be checked when investigating the lead are the area near the extension–lead connection and the area near the cranial locking mechanism.

If the lead and the extension are intact, and the boot had no fluid in it, the IPG must be exposed to test its integrity. The continuity of the IPG-extension connection is tested in a similar fashion to the lead–extension connection, using small alligator clips attached to the battery end connector of the extension wire. During the test the extension connector should be manipulated to elicit any transient fault. The IPG should be inspected for fluid and cleaned. If the circuit is intact the sole remaining possibility is that the IPG has an intermittent fault and needs to be replaced.

### Testing Methodology

Initial interrogations of devices with suspected malfunctions are performed with either the Medtronic model 8840 N-vision clinician programmer or model 7432 Physician programmer (Medtronic Inc, Minneapolis, MN). All contacts are tested in both monopolar and bipolar stimulation modes. For VIM patients, the stimulator test parameters are: 1.5 volts, 30 Hz, 210 μsec. For STN and GPi patients, the parameters are: 2.0 volts, 30 Hz, 210 μsec. A higher test voltage is used at the STN and GPi because impedances in these areas are greater than 2000 Ω at the lower test voltage. A measured impedance more than 2000 Ω with a current less than 7 μA indicates a potential open circuit. An impedance less than 500 Ω with a current more than 200 μA, indicates a potential short circuit. In addition, when testing in monopolar configuration, the presence of identical impedances and currents (to within ± 5 Ω and ± 1 μA) in any two leads suggests a short circuit, which should be further investigated with bipolar testing. With the newer FDA-approved programmers (Medtronic model 8840) this step is automatically performed. However, with the older stimulator programmer (Medtronic model 7432, Medtronic, Inc., Minneapolis, MN) this bipolar testing must be done manually. During bipolar testing (same test parameters as described earlier) impedances less than 200 Ω and currents more than 200 μA indicate a short between the tested leads.

When a fault is identified or if an intermittent fault is suspected, we proceed to our noninvasive detection technique. Nicolet skin recording electrodes (model 019-420800, Viasys Healtcare, Madison, WI) are preferred. The reference and ground electrodes (for the EMG/IOM machine [Nicolet Viking IV, Madison, WI]) are placed over the IPG and then over the lead–extension connector (Figure 23.6). Prior to placing the leads, the skin is prepped with alcohol and dried. Skin prep is not used in order to minimize the risk of skin breakdown over the length of the system. Thus far, all measured skin electrode impedances were below 1 kΩ when using the EMG/IOM machine. The oscilloscope (Tektronix model TDS 3032, Beaverton, OH) impedances measured with an impedance meter (Grass Model F-EZM5, Grass Telefactor, Warwick, RI) were similar to the values given earlier. The instrumentation is set up as follows: the time base of the oscilloscope is set to 100 μsec/div and 2 msec/div. The time base of the Nicolet Viking IV is adjusted to 10 msec/screen. The output of the IPG is adjusted to 2.0 volts. The pulse width and frequency are unchanged from the values of the clinically effective settings. For some EMG machines it may be easier to see the wave when using a larger pulse width. It is important to note that in this configuration the anodal component of the charge balanced pulse will have a larger amplitude and shorter pulse length and will therefore look a little different than the waves depicted in Figure 23.7.

The contacts are tested in sequential order starting at the most ventral contact (contact 0). The scale of the recording device is adjusted so the full wave is visible on the screen. A short segment of each contact is recorded, noting both the amplitude and phase of the signal. After each contact is tested, the amplitudes are compared. If no major amplitude changes (greater or less than approximately 25% of most of the leads) are observed, each contact is tested again. During the second test the extension and connector are all tapped with a finger. In later tests, both of these techniques were combined. The skin over each element is also gently manipulated. Any system amplitude and phase perturbations are investigated further. Figure 10 shows an example of such a signal change. In many cases the location of the failure can be found by gentle manipulation of the system.

For an open circuit with two faulty conductors, moving the active test electrode over the implanted extension and lead will record a large reduction in amplitude at the site of the break during manipulation. This due to the two open leads shorting during the manipulation. For a single DBS wire open circuit, one may or may not observe a large amplitude decrease. For the single lead open case (where the lead has penetrated through the insulation only) the test needs to be performed in a bipolar mode and the stimulation voltage may need to be increased to 3 or 4 volts. Care must be taken when doing this to avoid causing the patient any discomfort.

## Case Histories

### Patient 1

The patient is a 44-year-old male with an 8-year history of PD. The patient underwent implantation of bilateral STN DBS systems in January 2001 at another treatment facility. In February 2002, the patient came to our hospital complaining of reduced stimulation efficacy and intermittent shocks. The patient had recently been in an automobile accident. The patient was observed in the hospital for 3 days. Noninvasive interrogation of the IPGs revealed that the left IPG had inexplicably turned on and off multiple times. Both IPGs were replaced. Later, in September 2002, the patient noted intense electrical shocks while combing his hair and returned for evaluation. Standard impedance and electrical tests were performed using the Medtronic patient programmer (Model 8840). Impedance, current, and voltage were normal for each contact.

Upon palpating the skin near the lead/extension connector, the patient experienced shocks in his scalp overlying the connector. An oscilloscope was used to evaluate the intact IPG system in real-time. Electrodes were placed as follows: ground placed on the skin overlying the chest; reference placed over the extension wire at the clavicle; and the active lead placed on the skin over the IPG burr hole cap (Medtronic model 3350, Minneapolis, MN).

Because the general location of the failure was known to be near the lead–extension junction, location testing was not necessary. With the oscilloscope set at a time base of 5 to 100 msec per screen, we observed 1 to 20 pulses from the IPG. Each of the contacts was tested in monopolar and bipolar configurations with no manipulation of the lead and no abnormalities were seen. The IPG was then programmed to the patient's treatment settings and the patient was asked to comb his hair. The scope displayed a 47% (0.15–0.22 relative volts) increase in amplitude as the patient pulled the comb back through his hair (see Figure 23.10).

Because the comb covered a relatively large area of the head, minute finger manipulation of the lead was performed to determine if the transient fault was in the lead, the connector between the lead and extension, or in the extension wire. Neither manipulation on the lead side of the connector nor manipulation of the connector itself elicited a change in amplitude; however, manipulation of the extension about 2 to 3 cm from the connector, elicited the signal shown in Figure 23.10. It was apparent that the extension wire was faulty and needed replacement. The patient was taken to the operating room where the area over the lead/extension connector was opened and the extension wire disconnected. To demonstrate that the lead was still intact a low current impedance meter (BAK model IMP-1, Germantown, MD) was used. Note that we were not interested in exact impedance measures, only the detection of open and short circuits. Testing was done in bipolar configuration. Each of the conductors exhibited impedances of approximately 1 KΩ[4]. No open or short circuits were identified. The extension wire was replaced and the patient returned to his previous satisfactory performance level.

**Patient 2**

The patient is a 37-year-old male with primary generalized DYT-1 dystonia for which the patient underwent implantation of bilateral globus pallidus DBS systems. The patient's primary complaint was pronounced torticollis. The postoperative course was uneventful. During the first month of therapy, the voltage and pulse width were slowly raised to 3.3 volts and 400 μsec, respectively, at which point the patient began to improve. However, after 4 months of therapy, the patient's symptoms returned. Device interrogation with the Medtronic programmer demonstrated an open circuit in leads 1 and 2 with impedances more than 2000 Ω and currents less than 7 μA.

Gentle palpation over the lead and extension demonstrated no adverse sensations. The other two contacts were normal. We thought there might be fluid within the connector. An oscilloscope was used but manipulation of the connector did not change the results. When we placed the active lead near the connector and the reference over the connector, no signal was recorded for contacts 1 and 2. When testing contact 1, the active electrode was moved towards the IPG. As the electrode passed the mastoid area and moved onto the neck, a signal was located. The same result occurred for contact 2. The break was determined to be in the extension wire in the area of the mastoid. The extension wire was replaced and the patient has enjoyed an excellent result.

**Patient 3**

Patient 3 is a 57-year-old male with essential tremor who had enjoyed 3 years of excellent tremor control following left Vim thalamic DBS surgery. For 6 months prior to presentation, the patient had noted a progressive worsening of his speech and some return of his right hand tremor. Interrogation of his device with the Medtronic programmer showed no clear short or open circuits. Contacts 0 and 3 demonstrated similar currents and impedances, but only one-third of the time.

Palpation over the lead and extension elicited no adverse sensations. However, the intermittent impedance and current similarities noted for contacts 0 and 3 indicated a potential problem. In many cases the impedance and current will vary slightly over short periods of time. Typically these variations are small, on the order of ± 10 Ω and ± 1 μA, respectively. In this case, two contacts were being affected in the same way, some of the time.

---

[4] The accuracy of that meter at that range is poor but adequate for the purpose.

A reference lead was placed over the IPG and the active lead was placed over the lead–extension connector. When the IPG was set to monopolar mode, each conductor exhibited acceptable electrical specifications, but when the system was placed in bipolar mode and the recording was taken during stimulation with contact 0 set negative and contact 3 positive, the amplitude dropped by about 40% as compared to the other bipolar settings. Palpation over the extension wire was normal except for a single brief amplitude increase during this test. We concluded that the failure was within the extension wire, even though the noninvasive demonstration was not as definitive as the previous two cases. The extension wire was replaced and the patient improved.

**Patient 4**

Patient 4 is a 75-year-old male with PD. The patient underwent staged bilateral STN DBS implants in the fall of 2000. Two and a half years later the patient presented with electrical shock sensations down the anterior and posterior aspects of his leg and arm. He stated that these sensations were sometimes associated with movement of his neck, but not one specific movement. Manipulation of the battery and extension wires failed to reproduce the symptoms. No abnormalities were found with the programmer. We hypothesized that a transient short was present due to the paresthesias in the leg and arm. Because the sensations were on the left side it was felt that the problem was with the right IPG.

Figure 23.12 shows the results of the EMG signal tests. A reference lead was placed over the IPG and the active lead was placed over the lead–extension connector. When the IPG was set to monopolar mode (Figures 23.12A–D), contacts 0 and 3 showed a full signal while contacts 1 and 2 exhibited an amplitude reduction of more than 50%. Bipolar testing was then performed. Figure 23.12E shows the results of the bipolar test with no pressure on the extension. Figure 23.12F shows the results of the test when pressure was applied over the right mastoid region, the only place where pressure elicited this change. Figures 23.12G and 23.12H show the same type of testing on the left IPG with no changes in the signal. Based on these results, the right extension was replaced with a resolution of the difficulties.

## Conclusion

The testing paradigms described in this chapter have been developed through more than 10 years of experience with DBS systems. Our current testing algorithm is exhibited in Figure 23.13. Clinic testing times range from 30 minutes to 2 hours depending on how complex the fault mode is. Unfortunately, even after working through all of the testing described herein there will be a small number of cases where the failure may not be localized noninvasively. Often, in such cases, simply opening the system and cleaning the connections has restored proper device function. We have assumed that in these cases, failure was due to fluid in the connector, but were not able to prove this. Nevertheless, we are typically able to localize system faults accurately while minimizing the number of surgeries and the number of surgical incisions needed to fix the problem.

# 23 Deep Brain Stimulation Fault Testing

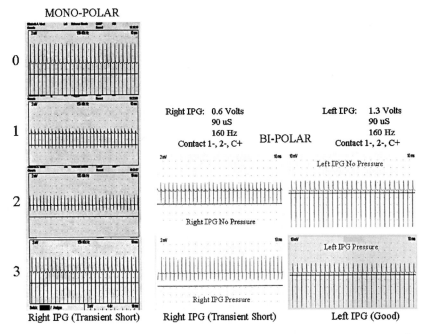

**Figure 23.12** This series of tests shows how a transient short is seen on the output of a EMG machine as compared to the good side. It was thought that reduction in amplitude was due to a partial short where there was still some continuity between the IPG and the lead, but the wires were touching in the insulation also

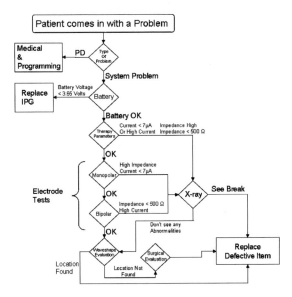

**Figure 23.13** This flow chart is designed to offer a general pathway through trouble shooting staring from the simplest noninvasive tests to the most complex invasive tests. Even though the most complex tests may offer instantaneous results, we feel that the invasiveness to the patients is not warranted until all other options have been met

## References

1. Beric A, Kelly PJ, Rezai A, Sterio D, Mogilner A, Zonenshayn M, Kopell B (2001) Complications of deep brain stimulation surgery. Stereotact Funct Neurosurg 77(1–4):73–78.
2. Oh MY, Abosch A, Kim SH, Lang AE, Lozano AM (2002) Long-term hardware related complications of deep brain stimulation. Neurosurgery 50:1268–1276.
3. Umemura A, Jaggi JL, Hurtig HI, Siderowf AD, Colcher A, Stern MB, Baltuch GH (2003) Deep brain stimulation for movement disorders: morbidity and mortality in 109 patients. J Neurosurg 98:779–784.
4. Joint C, Nandi D, Parkin S, Gregory R, Aziz T (2002) Hardware-related problems of deep brain stimulation. Mov Disord 17(Suppl 3):S175–S180.
5. Lyons KE, Wilkinson SB, Overman J, Pahwa R (2004) Surgical and hardware complications of subthalamic stimulation. A series of 160 procedures. Neurology 63:612–616.
6. Constantoyannis C, Berk C, Honey CR, Mendez I, Brownstone RM (2005) Reducing hardware-related complications of deep brain stimulation. Can J Neurol Sci 32(2):194–200.
7. Goodman RR, Kim B, McClelland, III S, Senatus PB, Winfield LM, Pullman SL, Yu Q, Ford B, McKhann II GM (2006) Operative techniques and morbidity with subthalamic nucleus deep brain stimulation in 100 consecutive patients with advanced Parkinson's disease J Neurol Neurosurg Psychiatry 77:12–17.
8. Okun MS, Tagliati M, Pourfar M, Fernandez HH, Rodriguez RL, Alterman RL, Foote KD (2005) Management of refereed deep brain stimulation failures: a retrospective analysis from 2 movement disorders centers. Arch Neurol 62(8):1250–1255.
9. (2006) Medtronic model 3387 and 3389 DBS lead kit for deep brain stimulation implant manual.
10. (2006) Medtronic model 7426 DBS neurostimulator kit for deep brain stimulation physician and hospital staff manual.
11. (2006) Medtronic model 7482 DBS Extension kit for deep brain stimulation implant manual.
12. Webster JG (1995) Medical Instrumentation: Application and Design. New York: John Wiley and Sons.
13. Shils JL, Patterson T, Stecker MM (2000) Electrical properties of metal microelectrodes. Am J Electroneurodiagnos Tech 40:143–153.
14. Geddes LA Electrodes and the Measurement of Bioelectric Events. New York: John Wiley and Sons, p. 1072.
15. Burbaud P, Vital A, Rougier A, Bouillot S, Guehl D, Cuny E, Ferrer X, Lagueny A, Bioulac B (2002) Minimal tissue damage after stimulation of the motor thalamus in a case of chorea-acanthocytosis. Neurology 59:1982–1984.
16. Haberler C, Alesch F, Mazal P, Pilz P, Jellinger K, Pinter M, Hainfellner J, Budka H (2000) No tissue damage by chronic deep brain stimulation in Parkinson's disease. Ann Neurol 48(3).
17. Caparros-Lefebvre D, Ruchoux MM, Blond S, Petit H, Percheron G (1994) Long-term thalamic stimulation in Parkinson's disease: postmortem anatomoclinical study. Neurology 44:1856–1860.

# 24
# Quality of Life and Cost Effectiveness of Deep Brain Stimulation in Movement Disorders

Alan Diamond and Joseph Jankovic

## Abstract

Health-related quality of life (HRQOL) refers to an individual's feelings, daily functioning, and coping strategies in response to his or her disease. Instruments that measure HRQOL may be utilized to quantify burden of disease. HRQOL is particularly impaired in patients with medication refractory Parkinson's disease (PD), essential tremor (ET), dystonia, and cerebellar outflow tremor. For these patients, deep brain stimulation (DBS) is a viable alternative that may favorably impact their HRQOL.

**Keywords:** quality of life, deep brain stimulation, Parkinson's disease, essential tremor, cerebellar tremor, dystonia

## Introduction

The World Health Organization defines the individual's health related quality of life (HRQOL) as "perception of their position in life in the context of the culture and value systems in which they live and in relation to their goals, expectations, standards and concerns" *(1)*. Instruments used to measure HRQOL capture variables related to the subject's feelings, daily functioning, and their coping strategies in response to their disease *(2)*. They can be used to ascertain therapeutic benefit in clinical trials and quantify burden of disease *(3, 4)*. There are two types of HRQOL instruments, generic and disease specific. Generic instruments are multidimensional questionnaires that cover a wide variety of areas and can be applied to many diseases and allow comparisons between diseases *(2, 5)*. A limitation of generic instruments is that they may lack the sensitivity to detect change in longitudinal studies specific to a particular disease. Disease-specific HRQOL questionnaires are tailored to what may be important in a particular patient population. They allow more accurate information regarding the impact of a specific disease on the overall health burden.

## PD

In PD, there is a strong association with advancing stages of disease, motor complications, and prolonged *off* states as well as poorer perceptions of health and a deterioration in HRQOL *(6)*. Dyskinesias may interfere with activities of daily living (ADLs), further impairing HRQOL, and increase healthcare costs *(7, 8)*. Diphasic dyskinesias have been reported to be associated with worse HRQOL than peak-dose dyskinesias *(9)*. Furthermore, young-onset PD patients have worse HRQOL, stigma of disease, loss of marital satisfaction, and worse depression *(10)*. In addition to the cardinal motor features of PD and motor complications related to levodopa, nonmotor manifestations of PD, including fatigue, drooling, sleep dysfunction, sexual dysfunction, confusion, autonomic disturbances, and sensory disturbances all adversely affect HRQOL *(11–13)*. Moreover, fatigue has also been associated with worsening depression and disability *(14)*. As PD progresses, family members may become the primary caregivers, resulting in increased caregiver burden *(15)*. The most troublesome symptoms experienced by the patients from a caregiver perspective are motor dysfunction and cognitive decline *(15)*.

High-frequency DBS of the subthalamic nucleus (STN) is associated with marked improvements in motor symptoms of PD *(16–19)* and reduction in daily levodopa equivalents *(19, 20)*. This therapy may lead to reduced levodopa-induced motor complications *(17–19, 21)*. DBS may therefore reduce the burden of disease and therefore have the potential to improve HRQOL.

Disease-specific HRQOL questionnaires for PD that have been used in various clinical trials have included the Parkinson's Disease Questionnaire (PDQ-39; refs. *2, 5, 22,* and *23*), Parkinson's Disease Quality of Life questionnaire (PDQL; ref. *24*), Parkinson's Disease Quality of Life Scale (PDQUALIF; ref. *25*), and Parkinson's Impact Scale (PIMS; ref. *26*). A drawback of these questionnaires is that they are not designed to address specific issues important to DBS, such as device conspicuousness, cumbersome control, lack of qualified medical care, and potential complications *(12)*. To address these issues, the Quality of Life Satisfaction Movement Disorder (QLS$^m$-MD) and Deep Brain Stimulation Modules (QLS$^m$-DBS) were developed *(12)*.

### STN DBS Effects on HRQOL in PD (Table 24.1)

The most commonly utilized HRQOL instrument used in assessing the treatment effects of STN DBS is the PDQ-39 *(27–34)*. In a randomized-pairs trial, 156 patients with advanced PD were assigned to bilateral STN DBS or best medical therapy *(33)*. At 6 months, there were significant improvements in the PDQ-39 summary index (SI) and Unified Parkinson's Disease Rating Scale (UPDRS) part III in the surgical group. STN DBS resulted in improvements of up to 38% in the PDQ-39 subscales for mobility, ADLs, emotional well-being, stigma, and bodily discomfort *(33)*. In other studies, compared with pre-operative scores, as much as 62% improvement has been reported in the PDQ-39SI at up to 24 months of follow up *(27–35)*. Dimensions assessing mobility, ADL, stigma, emotional well-being, and bodily discomfort showed consistently greater improvement. Social support, communication, and cognition were less consistently improved.

Utilizing another disease-specific HRQOL instrument, 34 patients were randomized to unilateral pallidotomy ($n = 14$) or to bilateral STN DBS ($n = 20$;

**Table 24.1** STN DBS effects on HRQOL in Parkinson's disease.

| Reference | Target | N | HRQOL Tool | Follow-up (Months) | HRQOL Improvements | |
|---|---|---|---|---|---|---|
| (36) | STN | S = 20 P = 14 | PDQL | 6 | Mean total PDQL improvement of 13 and 18 in P and S groups, respectively | |
| (37) | STN | 60 | PDQL | 12 | Total PDQL improved 43%* | Systemic symptoms improved 34%* |
| | | | | | Social function improved 63%* | Emotional function improved 29%* |
| | | | | | PD related symptoms improved 48%* | |
| (38) | STN | 95 | PDQL | 3, 12 | Mean PDQL total score improved from 95.1 ± 17.2 to 120.9 ± 23.8 | |
| | | | | | All subscores significantly improved. | |
| (33) | STN | M = 78 S = 78 | PDQ-39 SF-36 | 6 | **PDQ-39 SI:** S = 9.5 ± 15.3 *; M = 0.2 ± 11.2 | Bodily discomfort S = 11.3 ± 26.4*; M= −3.1 ± 18.1 |
| | | | | | Mobility S = 14.8 ± 27.7*; M = −0.8 ± 19.6 | |
| | | | | | ADL S = 20.7 ± 26.1*; M = −2.0 ± 17.9 | **SF-36** Physical S = −6.4 ± 8.0*; M = −0.5 ± 7.5 |
| | | | | | EWB S =11.5 ± 23.7*; M = −0.8 ± 16.8 | Mental S = −2.4 ± 12.3*; M = −0.3 ± 9.4 |
| | | | | | Stigma S =11.1 ± 22.4*; M = −0.1 ± 17.6 | |
| (31) | STN | 20 | PDQ-39 | 24 | PDQ-39 SI | 43.1 ± 13.1 to 30.9 ± 13.0* |
| | | | | | Mobility | 65.8 ± 17.4 to 48.5 ± 20.7* |
| | | | | | ADL | 48.8 ± 23.4 to 26.5 ± 18.0* |
| | | | | | Stigma | 48.8 ± 28.9 to 23.7 ± 23.0* |
| | | | | | Bodily discomfort | 57.5 ± 25.9 to 39.9 ± 25.7* |
| (35) | STN | 59 | PDQ-39 | >24 | PDQ-39 SI | 41.7 ± 11.8 to 32.7 ± 14.6 * |
| | | | | | Mobility | 56.3 ± 22.0 to 45.1 ± 23.1* |
| | | | | | ADL | 49.4 ± 20.4 to 33.4 ± 21.1* |
| | | | | | Stigma | 34.1 ± 21.8 to 22.2 ± 21.7* |
| | | | | | Bodily discomfort | 50.6 ± 23.3 to 32.6 ± 19.1* |
| (29) | STN | 17 | PDQ-39 | 6 | PDQ-39 SI 49%* | Bodily discomfort 40.64%* |
| | | | | | Mobility 60.5%* | Stigma 29.52%* |
| | | | | | EWB 21.99%* | ADL 69.21%* |
| (30) | STN | 16 | PDQ-39 | 12 | PDQ-39 SI 14%* | |
| | | | | | ADL 30%* | |
| | | | | | Stigma 21%* | |

(continued)

Table 24.1 (continued)

| Reference | Target | N | HRQOL Tool | Follow-up (Months) | HRQOL Improvements |
|---|---|---|---|---|---|
| (28) | STN | S = 11 | PDQ-39 | 3, 6 | PDQ-39 SI: mean improvement of 16.1* in surgically and −0.4 in medically treated groups. |
|  |  | M = 13 |  |  | Surgically treated showed significant improvements in mobility, cognition, bodily discomfort, ADLs, EWB, stigma. There were no significant improvements in subscales in the medically treated group. |
| (34) | STN | 14 | PDQ-39 | 12, 24 | PDQ-39 SI improved 62%* <br> PDQ-39 subscales: <br> Mobility 53%*  ADL 81%* <br> EWB 58%*  Stigma 38%* <br> Bodily discomfort 63%*  Com 60%* |
| (27) | STN | 26 | PDQ-39 | 3 | PDQ-39 SI improved from 42.8 to 29.4* |
| (39) | STN | 16 | SIP | 6 | Total SIP improvement of 58%* |

N, number; STN, subthalamic nucleus; HRQOL, health-related quality of life; PDQL, Parkinson's Disease Quality of Life questionnaire; P, pallidotomy; S, surgical group; M, medical group; PD, Parkinson's disease; SF-36, Medical Outcome Short Form-36; ADLs, activities of daily living; EWB, emotional well being; Com, communication; SIP, Sickness Impact Profile; *, $P < 0.05$; PDQ-39, Parkinson's Disease Questionnaire.

ref. 36). Both treatment groups showed similar improvements in mean PDQL total scores at 3 months, although there was a trend towards improvement in favor of the STN DBS group. This lack of significance was thought to be due to the lack of statistical power as the PDQL score was a secondary measure. In addition, the STN DBS treatment group was superior in improvement in dyskinesias and *off* UPDRS Part III scores. In a study of 60 consecutive patients treated with bilateral STN DBS, there was a statistically significant improvement of 43% in total PDQL score at 12 months *(37)*. Furthermore, all dimensions of the PDQL improved: social function (63%), PD-related symptoms (48%), systemic symptoms (34%), and emotional function (29%). Furthermore, there was significant improvement in depression. In another study, 95 PD patients who were treated with bilateral STN DBS were assessed with the PDQL. At the 3-month follow up, the blinded off-medication UPDRS part III was improved by 51% and the non-blinded evaluation at the 12-month follow up was improved by 57%. At 12 months, there was significant improvement in PDQL total score (28%) and all subscores. There were only minor changes in cognition or mood after STN DBS; however, in seven patients there were declines in cognitive function. In those patients there was no worsening in HRQOL measures *(38)*.

In addition to disease-specific HRQOL instruments, generic tools have been utilized. Spottke et al.evaluated 16 consecutive patients who were treated with bilateral STN DBS with the Sickness Impact Profile (SIP). There were significant postoperative improvements of 58% in the SIP summary index and 67% in physical dimensions at 6 months (39). Psychosocial dimensions failed to reach significance. Items most improved after surgery, as measured by generic

HRQOL instruments, included effects on body care and movement, ambulation, social interaction, sleep and rest, and recreation/pastimes.

### Pallidal-DBS effects on HRQOL in PD (Table 24.2)

Thirty-nine patients with PD were treated with unilateral pallidotomy ($n = 23$), unilateral globus pallidus internus (GPi) DBS ($n = 9$), or unilateral ventral intermediate nucleus (VIM) DBS ($n = 7$; see later; ref. *40*). The surgical option was selected based on the patient's symptoms. In the unilateral GPi DBS treated group, there were significant improvements in mean SIP total score and SIP physical impairment score. There was only a trend toward improvement in SIP psychosocial impairment. In addition, depression and anxiety also improved. There was no correlation between changes in neuropsychiatric measures or motor impairment and HRQOL.

### Thalamic-DBS effects on HRQOL in PD (Table 24.2)

At 12 months, six of 11 patients with unilateral VIM DBS were assessed with the PDQ-39 *(41)*. At follow up, only mean ADL and emotional well-being dimensions were significantly improved. The other dimensions and PDQ-39SI did not reach significance. In another study, seven patients were treated with unilateral VIM DBS (see earlier) and at 3 months there were non-significant improvements in mean SIP total score, physical dysfunction, and psychosocial dysfunction *(40)*. This was in contrast to the pallidotomy and GPi DBS-treated groups where there were improvements in the physical dysfunction and total SIP score. The lack of improvement in generic HRQOL questionnaires was possibly due to the fact that tremor does not affect HRQOL in PD patients as much as motor complications or the other cardinal features of PD. Alternatively, the SIP was not sensitive enough to detect longitudinal changes in tremor-dominant PD patients.

### Predictive Indicators for QOL in PD

Several studies have examined predictive factors of both motor and nonmotor manifestations on HRQOL instruments. Tröster et al. found that improvements in depression significantly correlated with improvements in HRQOL, whereas

Table 24.2 GPI and VIM DBS effects on HRQOL in Parkinson's disease.

| Reference | Target | N | HRQOL Tool | Follow-up (Months) | HRQOL Improvements |
|-----------|--------|---|------------|--------------------|--------------------|
| (41) | VIM | 6 | PDQ-39 | 12 | No significant improvement in HRQOL measures. |
| (40) | VIM | 7 | SIP | 3 | No significant improvement in HRQOL measures. |
| (40) | GPi | 9 | SIP | 3 | Total SIP score improved. |

N, number; HRQOL, health-related quality of life; SIP, Sickness Impact Profile; PDQ-39, Parkinson's Disease Questionnaire; GPi, internal globus pallidus; VIM, ventral intermediate nucleus.

changes in motor function did not *(27)*. This was in contrast to other groups who have found that improvements in levodopa-induced motor complications and UPDRS scores correlated with improvements in HRQOL *(29, 34)*. We found that more severe tremor, dyskinesias, akinesia, and postural instability at baseline strongly predicted HRQOL in PD patients after STN DBS *(42)*. Another study found that only bradykinesia and tremor were significantly correlated with HRQOL outcomes *(35)*. In addition, pooled analysis of the GPi DBS, pallidotomy, and VIM DBS treatment groups revealed that the level of motor dysfunction at baseline correlated with pre-operative anxiety and pre-operative depression correlated with SIP psychosocial function at follow-up *(40)*. STN DBS was associated with subtle declines in measures of verbal fluency and memory, color naming, and attention and an increase in emotional liability and cognitive complaints; however, other studies have failed to show a negative impact of these features on HRQOL *(43)*. This suggests that features other than mild cognitive difficulties may play a more important role in determining HRQOL after DBS in PD patients.

## ET

ET is the most common movement disorder encountered in practice, occurring in 0.4 to 3.9% of the population *(44)*. ET is characterized by postural and action tremor, but axial tremors may also be present *(45)*. Up to 50% of patients with ET have disabling tremors even with optimal medical therapy *(45)*. Severe tremor can lead to significant physical limitations and social embarrassment *(46)*. Compared to controls, patients with ET have worse HRQOL with domains measuring neuropsychiatric complications being significantly more affected over the age of 40 years *(47)*. Tremor severity correlated with HRQOL outcomes *(47)*.

In ET, VIM DBS is associated with a 50 to 100% improvement in extremity tremor *(48–50)* with resting and postural tremor being more improved than action tremor *(48)*. Axial tremor is less commonly improved *(48, 49, 51, 52)*. As would be expected, by improving extremity tremor, VIM DBS is associated with improved HRQOL, disability, and patient satisfaction. Utilizing a self reported questionnaire, the Tremor Activities of Daily Living Scale (TADLS), in patients with ET undergoing VIM DBS, there has been up to 58% improvement in functional measures *(53)*. In addition, there was a 54% improvement in clinician rated section of the TADLS *(53)*.

**Thalamic DBS Effects on HRQOL in ET (Table 24.3)**

Most studies have utilized generic or modified PD HRQOL questionnaires. Recently, a disease-specific HRQOL instrument was validated for ET *(54)*. Hariz et al. assessed 27 patients with ET and VIM DBS with the ADL taxonomy scale, Nottingham health profile (NHP), and a visual analog scale (55). At follow-up, there were significant improvements in ADL and the NHP dimensions measuring emotional reaction, social life, hobbies, and home maintenance and the visual analog scale. Although there were improvements in disability and HRQOL, 7.4% of patients felt surgery did not meet their expectations. Another study evaluated 40 patients with unilateral VIM DBS and found that at 12 months there was significant improvement in

SIP psychosocial subscore, whereas SIP overall score showed no improvement and the SIP physical subscore worsened *(56)*. The worsening physical subscore occurred in the setting of improved tremor scores. This discrepancy was possibly due to the lack of sensitivity of the SIP for changes in tremor. In addition, the modified PDQ-39 showed significant improvements in ADL, emotional well-being and stigma; however, there were subtle non-significant declines in emotional well being, stigma and ADL between 3 and 12 months.

## Dystonia

GPi DBS is effective in alleviating signs and symptoms in patients with segmental dystonia *(57, 58)*, cervical dystonia *(59, 60)*, tardive dystonia *(61)*, and generalized dystonia *(58, 62, 63)*. Because of impaired movement and disability, patients with dystonia have higher unemployment and lower self esteem *(64–66)*. Depression, anxiety, and worsening disease severity are associated with worse HRQOL in dystonia *(67)*. Longer disease duration and higher educational status likely result in better coping strategies and better HRQoL *(64)*.

### Pallidal DBS Effects on HRQOL in Dystonia (Table 24.3)

There are no disease-specific HRQOL questionnaires for dystonia and most studies have adapted modified PD or generic HRQOL questionnaires. Utilizing the SF-36 and Burke-Fahn-Marsden dystonia (BFMD) scale as outcomes, 22 consecutive patients with primary generalized dystonia who had bilateral GPi DBS showed significant improvement in motor and disability scores at 1 year *(63)*. These motor improvements were associated with improved overall HRQOL and measures of general health (16%), physical function (21%), and vitality (10%). There were no changes in mood or cognition. A series of 15 consecutive patients with mixed dystonia underwent bilateral GPi DBS. Follow-up was 3 to 12 months and included measures of cognition, mood, HRQOL, and motor scores. GPi DBS significantly improved dystonic symptoms and functional abilities. This correlated with improved HRQOL as measured by modified PDQ-39SI. There was no significant deterioration in cognitive or neuropsychiatric functions in patients with dystonia *(68)*. Smaller series have shown improvements in generic and modified PD specific HRQOL questionnaires and motor outcomes in segmental dystonia *(69)* and cervical dystonia *(70)*. There was no correlation between depression, anxiety, or degree of motor improvement on HRQOL measures.

## Multiple Sclerosis (MS)

MS is associated with action tremor in up to 75% of patients *(71–73)*. Even best medical treatment usually does not provide sufficient long-term tremor suppression *(74)*. For medication refractory tremor, VIM DBS has been associated with tremor suppression *(75)* and improvement in ADL *(76)*. Although VIM DBS is associated with tremor suppression, less social embarrassment, and improved ADL, this is not necessarily correlated with improved overall disability *(77–79)*. In MS most clinicians are concerned with physical problems whereas patients are most concerned with mental health, emotional

Table 24.3 Quality of life in essential tremor and dystonia.

| Reference | Dx | N | HRQOL Tool | Follow-up (Months) | HRQOL Improvements | |
|---|---|---|---|---|---|---|
| (56) | ET | 40 | mPDQ-39 SIP | 12 | Nonsignificant improvement in HRQOL measures | |
| (55) | ET | 27 | NHP VAS | 12 | NHP: Emotional reaction | 12.3 ± 3.4 to 7.1 ± 2.9* |
| | | | | | VAS | |
| | | | | | Improvement in "life as a whole" | 31.3* |
| | | | | | Improvement in "social life" | 36.3* |
| (63) | DYT | 22 | SF-36 | 12 | General health 16%*  Vitality 10%*  Physical function 21%* | |
| (69) | DYT | 5 | mPDQ-39  EuroQol 1  EuroQol 2 | 3–12 | mPDQ-39 SI 65%*  EuroQol 1 56%*  EuroQol 2 400%* | |
| (68) | DYT | 15 | mPDQ-39 | 3–12 | mPDQ-39 SI improved 66.3 ± 27.1 to 41.6 ± 26.7* | |

N, number; HRQOL, health-related quality of life; SIP, Sickness Impact Profile; mPDQ-39, modified Parkinson's Disease Questionnaire; Dx, diagnosis; ET, essential tremor; DYT, dystonia; NHP, Nottingham Health Profile.

problems, and vitality (80–84). In addition to tremor, other causes of disability, which adversely affect HRQOL in MS patients are gait abnormalities, pain, depression, loss of ability to work, incontinence, and disease stigma. Tremor can further decrease HRQOL by interfering with ADL, resulting in disability (85). Furthermore, depression, cognitive impairment, fatigue, and anxiety are independent predictors of HRQOL in MS (86, 87), although their effects on HRQOL outcomes in DBS have not been studied.

**Thalamic DBS Effects on HRQOL in MS**

A study of 12 patients with MS treated with VIM DBS and followed for 12 months showed significant improvements in resting (58%), postural (57%), and action tremors (70%), and overall tremor severity (63%). At 2 months, there were improvements in ability to feed oneself and a trend for improvement in dressing, but at 1 year the improvement in feeding was no longer significant. At 12 months, there were non-significant improvements in the SF-36 summary index or subscales. Although tremor was improved at 1 year, this did not correlate with improved HRQOL or ADL. These findings are consistent with previous reports of lack of efficacy in measures of disability in the setting of improved tremor with VIM DBS (77, 78). This is likely due to progression of MS, lack of appropriate tremor sensitive outcome measures, uncovering ataxia, unrealistic patient expectations, or because MS tremor does not make an important independent contribution to disability.

## Cost Effectiveness of DBS

Advancing PD is associated with early retirement, premature death, higher drug costs, and increased economic and societal burden *(88)*. The chronic and progressive nature of the disease has a detrimental impact and places an economic burden on society *(89)*. DBS is effective in alleviating the cardinal motor symptoms of PD and improving QOL; however, in today's medical climate decisions are partially based on cost effectiveness of treatment. The cost associated with STN DBS has been estimated to be $60,000 per patient over 5 years *(90)*. Almost 70% of these costs are attributable to the initial cost of the equipment and the follow-up, and likely replacement cost for the impulse generator (pacemaker; ref. *90*). The direct nonsurgical costs associated with PD care include hospitalizations, outpatient visits, auxiliary care, and medications. In a large study of 95 subjects, there was a cost reduction at 6 months after STN DBS *(38)*. The authors concluded that STN DBS would allow a return on investment in 2.2 years. A limitation in their estimates was the omission of the cost of replacing the neurostimulator battery *(38)*. Another study found an initial increase in cost in the first year after surgery, which was offset by a greater than 50% reduction by the end of the second year together with improved motor function *(91)*. In addition, patients with higher pre-operative medication costs had higher postoperative expenses. Pre-operative hospital admissions, disease severity, age, and duration of disease had no correlation with postoperative costs *(91)*.

One method to judge the therapeutic benefit of an expensive treatment is the use of cost utility analysis (CUA). CUA is a form of economic appraisal that focuses on the quality of health outcomes obtained by a specific treatment where health improvement is measured in quality adjusted life years (QALY) and results are expressed as cost per QALY gained *(92)*. The expression of health outcomes as QALY gained allows CUA to incorporate both an increase in quantity of life and increase in quality of life *(92)*. Consequently, CUA is relevant for evaluation of therapies where there is considerable impact on HRQOL through changes in disease severity *(92,93)*. A semi-Markov decision model estimated a QALY of 0.72 with STN DBS compared to best medical treatment for patients treated at age 55, assuming benefits lasted 4 years and gradually waned over 5 years *(94)*. The additional costs of surgery were estimated to be $35,000. The authors concluded that DBS is cost effective when it results in an improvement in HRQOL by at least 18%.

Preliminary studies suggest that in appropriately selected PD patients, DBS may be cost effective when compared to best medical treatment. Prospective, randomized, controlled DBS trials are needed to further elucidate the true economic gain.

## References

1. World Health Organization (2004) Introducing the WHOQOL instruments. Available at: www.who.int/evidence/assessment-instruments/qol/ql1.htm.
2. Jenkinson C, Fitzpatrick R, Peto V (1999) Health-related quality-of-life measurement in patients with Parkinson's disease. Pharmacoeconomics 15:157–165.
3. Deyo RA (1991) The quality of life, research, and care. Ann Intern Med 114:695–697.
4. Gage H, Hendricks A, Zhang S, Kazis L (2003) The relative health related quality of life of veterans with Parkinson's disease. J Neurol Neurosurg Psychiatry 74:163–169.

5. Jenkinson C, Peto V, Fitzpatrick R, Greenhall R, Hyman N (1995) Self-reported functioning and well-being in patients with Parkinson's disease: comparison of the short-form health survey (SF-36) and the Parkinson's Disease Questionnaire (PDQ-39). Age Ageing 24:505–509.
6. Chrischilles EA, Rubenstein LM, Voelker MD, Wallace RB, Rodnitzky RL (1998) The health burdens of Parkinson's disease. Mov Disord 13:406–413.
7. Damiano AM, McGrath MM, Willian MK, et al (2000) Evaluation of a measurement strategy for Parkinson's disease: assessing patient health-related quality of life. Qual Life Res 9:87–100.
8. Pechevis M, Clarke CE, Vieregge P, et al (2005) Effects of dyskinesias in Parkinson's disease on quality of life and health-related costs: a prospective European study. Eur J Neurol 12:956–963.
9. Chapuis S, Ouchchane L, Metz O, Gerbaud L, Durif F (2005) Impact of the motor complications of Parkinson's disease on the quality of life. Mov Disord 20:224–230.
10. Schrag A, Hovris A, Morley D, Quinn N, Jahanshahi M (2003) Young- versus older-onset Parkinson's disease: impact of disease and psychosocial consequences. Mov Disord 18:1250–1256.
11. Wilkinson, L., Rahman, S., Griffin, H., Quinn, N., Jahanshahi, M (2006) Quality of life in Parkinson's disease: the relative importance of the symptoms. Mov Disord 21:789.
12. Kuehler A, Henrich G, Schroeder U, et al (2003) A novel quality of life instrument for deep brain stimulation in movement disorders. J Neurol Neurosurg Psychiatry 74:1023–1030.
13. Martinez-Martin P (1998) An introduction to the concept of "quality of life in Parkinson's disease." J Neurol 245(Suppl 1):S2–S6.
14. Martinez-Martin P, Catalan MJ, Benito-Leon J, et al (2006) Impact of fatigue in Parkinson's disease: the Fatigue Impact Scale for Daily Use (D-FIS). Qual Life Res 15:597–606.
15. Lökk L (2006) Caregiver burden of patients with Parkinson's disease and the impact of disease duration. Mov Disord 21:569.
16. Limousin P, Pollak P, Benazzouz A, et al (1995) Effect of parkinsonian signs and symptoms of bilateral subthalamic nucleus stimulation. Lancet 345:91–95.
17. The Deep-Brain Stimulation for Parkinson's Disease Study Group (2001) Deep-brain stimulation of the subthalamic nucleus or the pars interna of the globus pallidus in Parkinson's disease. N Engl J Med 345:956–963.
18. Volkmann J, Allert N, Voges J, et al (2001) Safety and efficacy of pallidal or subthalamic nucleus stimulation in advanced PD. Neurology 56:548–551.
19. Kleiner-Fisman G, Herzog J, Fisman DN, et al (2006) Subthalamic nucleus deep brain stimulation: summary and meta-analysis of outcomes. Mov Disord 21(Suppl 14): S290–S304.
20. Houeto JL, Damier P, Bejjani PB, et al (2000) Subthalamic stimulation in Parkinson disease: a multidisciplinary approach. Arch Neurol 57:461–465.
21. Kleiner-Fisman G, Fisman DN, Sime E, et al (2003) Long-term follow up of bilateral deep brain stimulation of the subthalamic nucleus in patients with advanced Parkinson disease. J Neurosurg 99:489–495.
22. Jenkinson C, Fitzpatrick R, Peto V (1998) The Parkinson's disease questionnaire. User manual for the PDQ-39, PDQ-8, and PDQ summary index. Oxford: Joshua Horgan Print Partnership.
23. Peto V, Jenkinson C, Fitzpatrick R, Greenhall R (1995) The development and validation of a short measure of functioning and well being for individuals with Parkinson's disease. Qual Life Res 4:241–248.
24. de Boer AG, Wijker W, Speelman JD, de Haes JC (1996) Quality of life in patients with Parkinson's disease: development of a questionnaire. J Neurol Neurosurg Psychiatry 61:70–74.

25. Welsh M, McDermott MP, Holloway RG, et al (2003) Development and testing of the Parkinson's disease quality of life scale. Mov Disord 18:637–645.
26. Schulzer M, Mak E, Calne SM (2003) The psychometric properties of the Parkinson's Impact Scale (PIMS) as a measure of quality of life in Parkinson's disease. Parkinsonism Relat Disord 9:291–294.
27. Tröster AI, Fields JA, Wilkinson S, et al (2003) Effect of motor improvement on quality of life following subthalamic stimulation is mediated by changes in depressive symptomatology. Stereotact Funct Neurosurg 80:43–47.
28. Just H, OStergaard K (2002) Health-related quality of life in patients with advanced Parkinson's disease treated with deep brain stimulation of the subthalamic nuclei. Mov Disord 17:539–545.
29. Martinez-Martin P, Valldeoriola F, Tolosa E, et al (2002) Bilateral subthalamic nucleus stimulation and quality of life in advanced Parkinson's disease. Mov Disord 17:372–377.
30. Patel NK, Plaha P, O'Sullivan K, et al (2003) MRI directed bilateral stimulation of the subthalamic nucleus in patients with Parkinson's disease. J Neurol Neurosurg Psychiatry 74:1631–1637.
31. Houeto JL, Mallet L, Mesnage V, et al (2006) Subthalamic stimulation in Parkinson disease: behavior and social adaptation. Arch Neurol 63:1090–1095.
32. Erola T, Karinen P, Heikkinen E, et al (2005) Bilateral subthalamic nucleus stimulation improves health-related quality of life in Parkinsonian patients. Parkinsonism Relat Disord 11:89–94.
33. Deuschl G, Schade-Brittinger C, Krack P, et al (2006) A randomized trial of deep-brain stimulation for Parkinson's disease. N Engl J Med 355:896–908.
34. Lezcano E, Gomez-Esteban JC, Zarranz JJ, et al (2004) Improvement in quality of life in patients with advanced Parkinson's disease following bilateral deep-brain stimulation in subthalamic nucleus. Eur J Neurol 11:451–454.
35. Lyons KE, Pahwa R (2005) Long-term benefits in quality of life provided by bilateral subthalamic stimulation in patients with Parkinson disease. J Neurosurg 103:252–255.
36. Esselink RA, de Bie RM, de Haan RJ, et al (2004) Unilateral pallidotomy versus bilateral subthalamic nucleus stimulation in PD: a randomized trial. Neurology 62:201–207.
37. Lagrange E, Krack P, Moro E, et al (2002) Bilateral subthalamic nucleus stimulation improves health-related quality of life in PD. Neurology 59:1976–1978.
38. Fraix V, Houeto JL, Lagrange C, et al (2006) Clinical and economic results of bilateral subthalamic nucleus stimulation in Parkinson's disease. J Neurol Neurosurg Psychiatry 77:443–449.
39. Spottke EA, Volkmann J, Lorenz D, et al (2002) Evaluation of healthcare utilization and health status of patients with Parkinson's disease treated with deep brain stimulation of the subthalamic nucleus. J Neurol 249:759–766.
40. Straits-Troster K, Fields JA, Wilkinson SB, et al (2000) Health-related quality of life in Parkinson's disease after pallidotomy and deep brain stimulation. Brain Cogn 42:399–416.
41. Woods SP, Fields JA, Lyons KE, et al (2001) Neuropsychological and quality of life changes following unilateral thalamic deep brain stimulation in Parkinson's disease: a one-year follow-up. Acta Neurochir (Wien) 143:1273–1277.
42. Diamond A, Dat Vuong K, Jankovic J (2006) Deep brain stimulation of the subthalamic nucleus on Parkinson's disease: effects on quality of life. Mov Disord 21:1234.
43. Smeding HM, Speelman JD, Koning-Haanstra M, et al (2006) Neuropsychological effects of bilateral STN stimulation in Parkinson disease: a controlled study. Neurology 66:1830–1836.
44. Louis ED, Ottman R, Hauser WA (1998) How common is the most common adult movement disorder? Estimates of the prevalence of essential tremor throughout the world. Mov Disord 13:5–10.

45. Koller WC, Busenbark K, Miner K (1994) The relationship of essential tremor to other movement disorders: report on 678 patients. Essential Tremor Study Group. Ann Neurol 35:717–723.
46. Busenbark KL, Nash J, Nash S, Hubble JP, Koller WC (1991) Is essential tremor benign? Neurology 41:1982–1983.
47. Lorenz D, Schwieger D, Moises H, Deuschl G (2006) Quality of life and personality in essential tremor patients. Mov Disord 21:1114–1118.
48. Benabid AL, Pollak P, Gao D, et al (1996) Chronic electrical stimulation of the ventralis intermedius nucleus of the thalamus as a treatment of movement disorders. J Neurosurg 84:203–214.
49. Pahwa R, Lyons K, Wilkinson S, Koller W (1998) Bilateral thalamic stimulation for essential tremor. Neurology 51:A19.
50. Pahwa R, Lyons KE, Wilkinson SB, et al (2006) Long-term evaluation of deep brain stimulation of the thalamus. J Neurosurg 104:506–512.
51. Ondo W, Dat VK, Almaguer M, Jankovic J, Simpson RK (2001) Thalamic deep brain stimulation: effects on the nontarget limbs. Mov Disord 16:1137–1142.
52. Ondo W, Almaguer M, Jankovic J, Simpson RK (2001) Thalamic deep brain stimulation: comparison between unilateral and bilateral placement. Arch Neurol 58:218–222.
53. Lyons KE, Pahwa R, Busenbark KL, et al (1998) Improvements in daily functioning after deep brain stimulation of the thalamus for intractable tremor. Mov Disord 13:690–692.
54. Tröster AI, Pahwa R, Tanner C, Lyons K (2004) Validation of the Quality of Life in Essential Tremor Questionnaire (QUEST). Mov Disord 19:S405.
55. Hariz GM, Lindberg M, Bergenheim AT (2002) Impact of thalamic deep brain stimulation on disability and health-related quality of life in patients with essential tremor. J Neurol Neurosurg Psychiatry 72:47–52.
56. Fields JA, Troster AI, Woods SP, et al (2003) Neuropsychological and quality of life outcomes 12 months after unilateral thalamic stimulation for essential tremor. J Neurol Neurosurg Psychiatry 74:305–311.
57. Wohrle JC, Weigel R, Grips E, et al (2003) Risperidone-responsive segmental dystonia and pallidal deep brain stimulation. Neurology 61:546–548.
58. Kupsch A, Benecke R, Muller J, et al (2006) Pallidal deep-brain stimulation in primary generalized or segmental dystonia. N Engl J Med 355:1978–1990.
59. Bereznai B, Steude U, Seelos K, Botzel K (2002) Chronic high-frequency globus pallidus internus stimulation in different types of dystonia: a clinical, video, and MRI report of six patients presenting with segmental, cervical, and generalized dystonia. Mov Disord 17:138–144.
60. Krauss JK (2002) Deep brain stimulation for dystonia in adults. Overview and developments. Stereotact Funct Neurosurg 78:168–182.
61. Trottenberg T, Paul G, Meissner W, et al (2001) Pallidal and thalamic neurostimulation in severe tardive dystonia. J Neurol Neurosurg Psychiatry 70:557–559.
62. Coubes P, Cif L, El Fertit H, et al (2004) Electrical stimulation of the globus pallidus internus in patients with primary generalized dystonia: long-term results. J Neurosurg 101:189–194.
63. Vidailhet M, Vercueil L, Houeto JL, et al (2005) Bilateral deep-brain stimulation of the globus pallidus in primary generalized dystonia. N Engl J Med 352:459–467.
64. Ben Shlomo Y, Camfield L, Warner T (2002) What are the determinants of quality of life in people with cervical dystonia? J Neurol Neurosurg Psychiatry 72:608–614.
65. Gudex CM, Hawthorne MR, Butler AG, Duffey P (1998) Effect of dystonia and botulinum toxin treatment on health-related quality of life. Mov Disord 13:941–946.
66. Hilker R, Schischniaschvili M, Ghaemi M, Jacobs A, Rudolf J (2001) Health related quality of life is improved by botulinum neurotoxin type A in long term treated patients with focal dystonia. J Neurol Neurosurg Psychiatry 71:193–199.

67. Diamond A, Jankovic J (2005) The effect of deep brain stimulation on quality of life in movement disorders. J Neurol Neurosurg Psychiatry 76:1188–1193.
68. Halbig TD, Gruber D, Kopp UA, et al (2005) Pallidal stimulation in dystonia: effects on cognition, mood, and quality of life. J Neurol Neurosurg Psychiatry 76:1713–1716.
69. Kupsch A, Klaffke S, Kuhn AA, et al (2003) The effects of frequency in pallidal deep brain stimulation for primary dystonia. J Neurol 250:1201–1205.
70. Beyaert K, Suchowersky O, Eliasziw M, Tsui J, Kiss ZH (2006) Canadian multi-centre trial of bilateral pallidal deep brain stimulation for cervical dystonia. Mov Disord 21:1305.
71. Alusi SH, Glickman S, Aziz TZ, Bain PG (1999) Tremor in multiple sclerosis. J Neurol Neurosurg Psychiatry 66:131–134.
72. Alusi SH, Worthington J, Glickman S, Bain PG (2001) A study of tremor in multiple sclerosis. Brain 124:720–730.
73. Alusi SH, Aziz TZ, Glickman S, et al (2001) Stereotactic lesional surgery for the treatment of tremor in multiple sclerosis: a prospective case-controlled study. Brain 124:1576–1589.
74. Smith PF, Darlington CL (1999) Recent developments in drug therapy for multiple sclerosis. Mult Scler 5:110–120.
75. Brice J, McLellan L (1980) Suppression of intention tremor by contingent deep-brain stimulation. Lancet 1:1221–1222.
76. Wishart HA, Roberts DW, Roth RM, et al (2003) Chronic deep brain stimulation for the treatment of tremor in multiple sclerosis: review and case reports. J Neurol Neurosurg Psychiatry 74:1392–1397.
77. Hooper J, Whittle IR (2003) Costs of thalamic deep brain stimulation for movement disorders in patients with multiple sclerosis. Br J Neurosurg 17:40–45.
78. Schulder M, Sernas TJ, Karimi R (2003) Thalamic stimulation in patients with multiple sclerosis: long-term follow-up. Stereotact Funct Neurosurg 80:48–55.
79. Schuurman PR, Bosch DA, Bossuyt PM, et al (2000) A comparison of continuous thalamic stimulation and thalamotomy for suppression of severe tremor. N Engl J Med 342:461–468.
80. Riazi A, Hobart JC, Lamping DL, Fitzpatrick R, Thompson AJ (2002) Multiple Sclerosis Impact Scale (MSIS-29): reliability and validity in hospital based samples. J Neurol Neurosurg Psychiatry 73:701–704.
81. Riazi A, Hobart JC, Fitzpatrick R, Freeman JA, Thompson AJ (2003) Socio-demographic variables are limited predictors of health status in multiple sclerosis. J Neurol 250:1088–1093.
82. Riazi A, Hobart JC, Lamping DL, et al (2003) Using the SF-36 measure to compare the health impact of multiple sclerosis and Parkinson's disease with normal population health profiles. J Neurol Neurosurg Psychiatry 74:710–714.
83. Riazi A, Hobart JC, Lamping DL, Fitzpatrick R, Thompson AJ (2003) Evidence-based measurement in multiple sclerosis: the psychometric properties of the physical and psychological dimensions of three quality of life rating scales. Mult Scler 9:411–419.
84. Rothwell PM, McDowell Z, Wong CK, Dorman PJ (1997) Doctors and patients don't agree: cross sectional study of patients' and doctors' perceptions and assessments of disability in multiple sclerosis. BMJ 314:1580–1583.
85. Stolp-Smith KA, Carter JL, Rohe DE, Knowland DP III (1997) Management of impairment, disability, and handicap due to multiple sclerosis. Mayo Clin Proc 72:1184–1196.
86. Amato MP, Ponziani G, Rossi F, et al (2001) Quality of life in multiple sclerosis: the impact of depression, fatigue and disability. Mult Scler 7:340–344.
87. Benito-Leon J, Morales JM, Rivera-Navarro J (2002) Health-related quality of life and its relationship to cognitive and emotional functioning in multiple sclerosis patients. Eur J Neurol 9:497–502.

88. Keranen T, Kaakkola S, Sotaniemi K, et al (2003) Economic burden and quality of life impairment increase with severity of PD. Parkinsonism Relat Disord 9:163–168.
89. Scheife RT, Schumock GT, Burstein A, Gottwald MD, Luer MS (2000) Impact of Parkinson's disease and its pharmacologic treatment on quality of life and economic outcomes. Am J Health Syst Pharm 57:953–962.
90. McIntosh E, Gray A, Aziz T (2003) Estimating the costs of surgical innovations: the case for subthalamic nucleus stimulation in the treatment of advanced Parkinson's disease. Mov Disord 18:993–999.
91. Meissner W, Schreiter D, Volkmann J, et al (2005) Deep brain stimulation in late stage Parkinson's disease: a retrospective cost analysis in Germany. J Neurol 252:218–223.
92. Drummond MF, Stoddart GL, Torrance GW (1987) Cost utility analysis. Methods for the economic evaluation of health care programmes. Oxford: Oxford Medical Publications 112–139.
93. Torrance GW, Feeny D (1989) Utilities and quality-adjusted life years. Int J Technol Assess Health Care 5:559–575.
94. Tomaszewski KJ, Holloway RG (2001) Deep brain stimulation in the treatment of Parkinson's disease: a cost-effectiveness analysis. Neurology 57:663–671.

# Part IV

# Deep Brain Stimulation in Other Indications

# 25
# Deep Brain Stimulation in Depression: Background, Progress, and Key Issues

Benjamin D. Greenberg

## Abstract

Deep brain stimulation (DBS) is an approved adjunct therapy for severe, medication-refractory movement disorders, though it is currently investigational in neuropsychiatry and other neurological conditions. In movement disorders, DBS targets are based mainly on rationales derived from earlier lesion procedures and on knowledge of anatomical networks thought to be involved in pathophysiology of illness. In contrast to lesions DBS is nonablative and has the advantages of reversibility and adjustability. Thus, therapeutic effectiveness can be enhanced and stimulation-related side effects can be minimized during long-term patient management. Preclinical and clinical studies have shown effects of DBS on brain regions that are functionally connected to the stimulation target. Understanding the mechanism of action of DBS constitutes the current focus of a number of clinical and preclinical laboratories. Experience to date, which remains very limited, has suggested that DBS may offer hope to patients with severe and treatment-resistant neuropsychiatric illness. Thus far, work in obsessive–compulsive disorder (OCD), the first neuropsychiatric condition studied using modern DBS devices, has shown consistently positive results across multiple small-scale studies. Work in treatment-resistant depression, where there also may be therapeutic potential, is at an earlier stage. Early positive results have generated cautious optimism in this group of patients. Further development of DBS for these and other illnesses with primarily behavioral symptoms will require thoughtful collaboration among multiple disciplines. Psychiatrists and neurosurgeons, in particular, have only recently begun working together in a limited way. These and other disciplines will need to enhance their interactions as part of dedicated teams for best outcomes in research and ultimately in clinical practice.

## Introduction

### Background

The term depression connotes a group of conditions that impose a serious public health burden *(1)*. For unipolar major depressive disorder (MDD), conservative estimates reveal a population prevalence of 2.6 to 5.5% in men and 6.0 to 11.8% in women *(2)*. Most (50–85%) patients have recurrent illness *(3)*. In addition to marked distress, depression can cause profound disability with pervasive impairment in marital, parental, social, vocational, and academic functioning *(4)*. The Global Burden of Disease Study ranked depression as the leading cause of disability in adults in developed countries *(5)*. For comparison, disability due to unipolar major depression is almost three times greater than that due to chronic obstructive pulmonary disease *(6)*. Death from suicide is a major complication *(7)*. Moreover, depression is associated with increased mortality from co-occuring illnesses, such as cardiovascular disorders or cancer *(8, 9)*.

Conventional anti-depressants were largely developed after serendipitous observations that agents such as iproniazid and imipramine (originally developed for tuberculosis and psychosis, respectively) improved depression in patients treated for other illnesses. The insight that agents with effects on monoamine neurotransmitter systems improved depression led to successful attempts to "improve on serendipity" and ultimately resulted in discovery of drugs with fewer side effects. These drugs included selective serotonin transport inhibitors. Currently, more than 20 anti-depressants are commonly used in practice *(10)*. Their efficacy in general depressed populations is well established. The drugs are usually grouped by their chemical classes or pharmacological actions, such as: tricyclics and tetracyclics, selective serotonin reuptake inhibitors (SSRIs), monoamine oxidase inhibitors (MAOIs), and other drugs affecting biogenic amine systems. In practice, medications from different classes are frequently combined, particularly in refractory cases *(11)*.

**Treatment Resistance**

Conventional treatments, while they are effective, may have limitations. Medications, often used in conjunction with certain psychotherapies, alleviate symptoms in most but not all patients. Up to one-fifth of individuals with major depression have a poor outcome after 2 years, and about one-tenth do poorly even after 5 years of treatment *(12)*. Severe depression that resists medication and psychotherapy is often treated with electroconvulsive therapy (ECT), which is still a therapeutic gold standard after 70 years. ECT, however, is associated with significant adverse effects, particularly a variable memory loss *(13, 14)*, which can limit its acceptance. Moreover, ECT's therapeutic effects are transient in a large proportion of patients, and so continuation or "maintenance" treatment may be needed *(15)*. Although different definitions and levels of "treatment resistance" have been developed *(16)*, it is clear that individuals with the most resistant illnesses, and those who have an inadequate response to medications, psychotherapies, and ECT currently have little prospect of lasting recovery.

**Phenomenology**

In both the clinic and in research, depression is usually treated as a categorical construct, albeit one that comes in several varieties. However, depressive states can also be described by placing affected individuals along different symptom dimensions, a method that is finding favor in research on other psychiatric disorders (including OCD). This general approach is increasingly recognized as having potentially important implications for the genetics, pathophysiology, and treatment of depressive disorders. Factor analyses of depression rating instruments have resulted in different factor structures. This is not surprising, since the analyses can be influenced in part by differences in the scales themselves, and also in part by heterogeneity within studied patient groups. A full discussion of this emerging work is beyond the scope of this chapter but it is useful to note some of the symptom dimensions that have emerged from factor analyses of depression scales. They include various combinations of anhedonia (loss of pleasurable experiences), amotivation (impaired goal-directed behavior), depressed mood (a bias toward negative emotion), depressive cognitions (pessimistic thoughts, feelings of guilt, low self-esteem, and suicidal ideation), anxiety, diminished energy, other somatic symptoms (sleep and psychomotor disturbances, food-intake and body-weight dysregulation), and cognitive impairments. Different symptom dimensions may be differentially associated with activity in certain brain regions and networks *(17–19)*. Focal brain stimulation, which may prove effective for otherwise treatment-resistant patients, also may lend itself to modulation of networks that may underlie separable symptom dimensions.

**Pathophysiology**

Although the pathogenesis of depressive syndromes remains to be determined, evidence increasingly suggests that they result from interactions of genetic susceptibilities and environmental factors *(20–25)*. The task of integrating emerging etiological insights with the study of brain circuitry that mediates neuropsychiatric symptoms is at an early stage of development, but is now firmly placed on the research agenda.

Work on neuroanatomical networks and their possible associations with psychopathology has a relatively long history. It was proposed two decades ago that pathological changes in activity within cortical–limbic–thalamic–striatal networks might disrupt normal reinforcement contingencies, and contribute to the affective components of both psychiatric and neurologic disease states *(26)*. Cortico-basal circuits implicated in modulation of mood and reward signals have also figured prominently in neuroanatomical models of the pathophysiology of depressive illness, which have been developed more recently, based largely on functional neuroimaging *(27, 28)*. A recent review *(29)* described how this circuitry may relate to symptom improvement following lesion procedures that, while empirically derived *(30)*, target different nodes within these networks.

# DBS

**Background**

Several techniques to directly or indirectly alter the electrical activity of the brain are in current clinical use or in development for depression. In electroconvulsive therapy, current is delivered to the brain across the large electrical resistance of the scalp and skull. Transcranial magnetic stimulation and magnetic seizure therapy magnetically induce electrical currents in brain tissue using an electromagnetic coil placed on the scalp. Vagus nerve stimulation,vin contrast, utilizes electrodes wrapped around the vagus nerve in the neck to activate its afferent projections to target nuclei and related neural circuits.

Development of DBS for psychiatric illness, and specifically for depression, is not a new idea, although the devices are new and the theoretical models of depression-based neurocircuitry have advanced. For example, in 1948, Pool used implantation of a silver electrode in the caudate nucleus in an attempt to treat a woman with depression and anorexia *(31)*. The introduction of significant technical refinements, over the past 15 years, particularly in DBS for the treatment of movement disorders has resulted in a renaissance in functional neurosurgery. DBS has FDA-approved uses for the treatment of tremor *(32–34)* and Parkinson's disease *(35)* and, under a Humanitarian Device Exemption, for dystonia *(36, 37)*. This has spurred renewed interest in the use of such procedures for the treatment of other refractory neurologic conditions. Investigational uses in neurologic illness include epilepsy *(38, 39)*, pain *(40)*, cluster headache *(41)*, tardive dyskinesia *(42)*, Tourette's syndrome *(43)*, brain injury, and persistent vegetative states *(44, 45)*.

DBS for movement disorders is also associated with benefit in several dimensions of health-related quality of life *(46–48)*. There are numerous reports demonstrating the safety and efficacy of DBS surgery for intractable movement disorders. For example, studies of the outcome of DBS of the subthlamic nucleus and globus pallidus internus (GPi) for Parkinson's disease have shown improvements of 41 to 67% in standardized ratings of motor symptoms *(49–54)*.

In current practice, patients with tremor and Parkinson's disease who are potential candidates for this treatment have severe illness that has proven refractory to the best conventional medication therapies. Advancing understanding of anatomical networks underlying the pathophysiology of movement disorders has fueled research in DBS as an investigational treatment. Coming full circle, the therapeutic effectiveness of DBS in movement disorders has opened a new window on these brain circuits and their potential roles in pathophysiology.

Similarly, neurosurgical intervention has remained a therapeutic option for patients with otherwise untreatable and severe psychiatric illness. Ablative procedures like cingulotomy and capsulotomy are best known in the United States *(30)*. As in movement disorders, development of DBS for psychiatric illness, particularly the development of specific structural targets for stimulation, has derived, in part, from the clinical outcomes of ablative procedures.

**Technical Aspects**

Modern stereotactic surgery combines multiple imaging modalities, computerized surgical navigation, and physiological mapping to allow for targeting of intracranial structures *(55)*. As opposed to epidural and subdural surface electrodes, DBS involves the placement of multi-contact brain leads in subcortical nuclei or in specific white matter tracts *(56)*. Intra-operative physiological mapping is routine clinical practice for movement disorders, where targets are cell nuclei with characteristic physiological signatures (i.e., the GPi, subthalamic nucleus [STN], or thalamic nuclei). Several methods of intra-operative physiologic verification of the anatomical target exist: microelectrode recording (MER), semimicroelectrode recording, and macrostimulation. Both microelectrode and semimicroelectrode recording attempt to define the boundaries of a given structure based on the known spontaneous and/or evoked electrical activity of the target and surrounding structures. In some movement disorders, responses to intra-operative stimulation may help guide the final positioning of the electrodes. In DBS for essential tremor, initial electrode placement is guided via stereotactic coordinates and microelectrode recording. Changes in neuronal firing patterns are monitored as recording probes are advanced, which provide a guide to lead placement. With this approach, evidence that the electrodes have reached the desired target may be generated by concurrent activation of the electrodes and cessation of the patient's tremor. In a second surgical phase, the surgeon places the implantable neurostimulator or pulse generator subdermally in the upper chest wall and connects it via extension wires tunneled under the skin to the electrodes in the brain.

**Stimulation Technique**

The electrode used for DBS is a "lead" with multiple electrode contacts that are the sites of stimulation. A commonly used lead is 1.27 mm in diameter (Medtronic 3387), and is implanted stereotactically with millimeter accuracy into specific brain targets. There are typically four or more electrode contacts on each lead. Usually one lead is implanted on each side in a symmetrical fashion, for bilateral stimulation. The devices, sometimes called "brain pacemakers," are undergoing rapid refinements by several companies (Medtronic, Inc. [Minneapolis, MN], Advanced Neuromodulation Systems Inc. [Plano, TX] or NeuroPace, Inc. [Mountain View, CA]). Currently, only the Medtronic devices are approved for brain stimulation while the others are investigational. Since the leads have independently programmable electrode contact sites, the anatomical extent of stimulation is adjustable. By configuring a positive, negative or no charge at each of the contact sites, the shape and size of the stimulation field can be varied. Chronic stimulation can be unipolar, bipolar or multipolar, as each of the electrode contacts may be used as an anode or cathode. The frequency, intensity, and pulse width are also programmable for each lead, within safety limits that restrict the maximum density of the electrical charge induced. The stimulators are programmed via a portable device that communicates with the implanted generator via telemetry. Stimulation can be delivered continuously or intermittently, cycling on and off during fixed time intervals. Patient self-programming devices are also available. These allow patients to activate and deactivate the stimulator via handheld controllers and to modify a subset of the stimulation parameters within given limits set by the programming clinician.

**Mechanisms of DBS Action**

Most likely, DBS exerts its effects via a number of differing but interrelated mechanisms that come in to play depending on the site of stimulation, the illness being treated, and the stimulation parameters used. There is evidence supporting a number of potential mechanisms. High-frequency DBS (100 Hz or greater) has been proposed to modify transmission, for example, via synaptic fatigue or "neural jamming." Either of these phenomena would in effect produce a "functional lesion," mimicking the effect of a therapeutic ablative lesion. The parallel is inexact, however, since, in movement disorders, the clinical effects of lesions and of DBS do not always correspond. The limited available data from psychiatric uses of DBS suggest a disparity in time course of effects in that the therapeutic effects of stimulation may appear more rapidly than those of lesions. There are other possible mechanisms of action, including that stimulation does not inhibit information flow within key neural pathways but enhances it, reducing chaotic information processing via a phenomenon known as stochastic resonance *(60)*.

Importantly, the net effect of DBS on the functional state of a structure or pathway may change as distance from the electrode increases. The clinical effects seen with brain stimulation reflect a complex combination of inhibition and activation of cell bodies and axons. They also depend on the orientation of the electrode, the cytoarchitecture of the structure being stimulated and the frequency, pulse width, and duration of stimulation. Active research in clinical and preclinical laboratories *(61, 62)* is expected to help identify which of the proposed physiological mechanisms are most relevant to the clinical effects of DBS. Additional avenues for research concerning the functional effects of DBS include PET in humans. For example, preliminary studies have been carried out concerning acute *(63)* and longer-term effects of DBS in OCD patients *(57)* and in depression *(58)*. Work has also been done to examine potential predictors of response to DBS in OCD *(64)*. Recent findings that DBS devices are compatible with certain MRI systems *(65, 66)* have opened the avenue of functional MRI (fMRI) research on neuroanatomical networks affected by DBS.

**Adverse Effects**

Complications of DBS can be separated into those related to the surgical procedure, device-related problems and the stimulation itself. Adverse effects, including clinical deterioration, which are observed in clinical trials, may also be related to the underlying illness. The major risks of device implantation include intracerebral hemorrhage and infection *(67)*. Experience with DBS for movement disorders indicates these adverse effects range from about 2 to 3% for hemorrhage to 4 to 9% for infection *(68)*. Device-related complications include lead fracture, disconnection, lead movement, and lead malfunction. These have become less common with increasing surgical expertise and evolution of device technology.

Adverse effects due to stimulation are more common but reversible with changes in stimulation technique. The nature of these depends on the stimulation target and surrounding structures. Many of these effects are transient. Stimulation-induced sensorimotor effects may include parasthesias, muscle contraction, dysarthria, and diplopia. Subthalamic DBS has produced marked affective changes in movement disorder patients *(69, 70)*. Disturbances in memory, impulsivity or cognition have also been reported *(71)*. Patients with primary neuropsychiatric illness who undergo DBS may therefore also potentially experience untoward psychiatric effects. Distinguishing adverse effects of stimulation from symptomatology of the illness that is being treated may represent a challenge at times during a patient's course.

## Modern DBS in Psychiatry: OCD

As described elsewhere in this volume, the first contemporary reports of DBS for psychiatric illness focused on OCD. The rationale for development of DBS for OCD paralleled that for tremor, Parkinson's disease, and dystonia, whereby DBS was applied to the same structures where lesions had produced therapeutic effects.

While the pathogenesis of any psychiatric disorder remains unknown, there is a consistent body of functional neuroimaging evidence that implicates frontal-basal brain networks in OCD. The most common findings in untreated OCD patients are increased glucose metabolism or blood flow in the medial and orbitofrontal cortex (OFC) and anterior cingulate gyrus, the caudate nucleus, and, to a lesser extent, the thalamus. This implies a dysregulation in the basal ganglia and limbic striatal circuits that modulate neuronal activity in and between the OFC and the dorsomedial thalamus *(72, 73)*. To varying degrees the localized elevations in brain activity are, accentuated during symptom activation. Effective treatment with medications or behavior therapy tends to normalize activity in these regions. Modulation of these circuits by DBS could exert therapeutic effects by reducing drives to engage in repetitive, stereotyped behaviors and by alleviating the negative emotional charge associated with induction of such behaviors *(29)*.

Small-scale case studies of severely ill, treatment-resistant OCD patients treated with DBS of the anterior limb of the internal capsule and/or the adjacent striatum have been published. *(57, 59, 74–77)*. These reports have supported the therapeutic potential of DBS in this population, and have suggested that DBS is generally well-tolerated *(78)*.

For any surgical intervention for psychiatric illness, a key issue is long-term outcome. Therapeutic treatment decisions need to be made based on the probability that therapeutic effects will be durable while taking into account the burdens imposed by potential adverse effects. Based on our own experience and that of others with ablative lesion procedures for OCD *(30)*, it is very likely that beneficial changes in symptom severity, functioning, and quality of life may develop gradually in individuals who have had chronic and severely impairing illnesses that have disrupted not only the patients' functional capacities but also their family and social relationships.

To be judged adequately, the extent of benefits in multiple domains will require long-term follow-up. Our group *(79)* very recently reported on a series of OCD patients meeting stringent criteria for severity and treatment resistance who underwent DBS in a ventral internal capsule/ventral striatal (VC/VS) target. These patients had quadripolar stimulating leads implanted bilaterally in the VC/VS. DBS was activated in open fashion three weeks later. Eight patients were followed for at least 36 months. Group Yale-Brown Obsessive Compulsive Scale (YBOCS) scores decreased from 34.6 (mean) at baseline (severe range) to 22.3 (moderate range) at 36 months ($p < 0.001$). Four of eight patients had at least a 35% decrease in YBOCS severity (a stringent response criterion) at 36 months. In two other patients scores declined between 25 and 35% (a 25% response threshold is commonly used in recent medication trials for OCD). Depression and anxiety also improved. Global Assessment of Functioning scores improved from 36.6 at baseline to 53.8 at 36 months ($p < 0.001$). This corresponded to improvements in self-care, independent living, and work, school, and social functioning. Surgical adverse effects included an asymptomatic hemorrhage, a single intra-operative seizure, and a superficial infection. Psychiatric adverse effects included transient mood elevation that met the criteria for a hypomanic episode in one case. Notably, when DBS was interrupted by stimulator battery depletion, worsened depression was typically noted first, followed by a more gradual exacerbation of OCD symptoms. These observations were in accord with hypotheses that neurocircuitry mediating at least some components of depression and OCD may have important areas of overlap or convergence (29). Some patients gradually became able to successfully engage in cognitive behavioral therapy for OCD during DBS, which was not possible prior to stimulation. Moreover, two of the patients experienced persistent OCD improvement during periods of several months without stimulation, most likely representing lasting benefit from behavior therapy that was facilitated by DBS. On a mechanistic level, treatments that may modulate different primary neurocircuits might be expected to augment each other, since the cortico-basal-limbic networks most likely to be affected have reciprocal functional connections (80).

## Affective Effects of Depth Electrode Stimulation in the Mid-20th Century

Recent observations of affective effects of DBS used for movement disorders are potentially important in pointing to brain regions or networks that might represent potential therapeutic targets for psychiatric indications. Those observations, together with early attempts to both map effects of focal brain stimulation and use stimulation therapeutically highlight the multiple targets that may be clinically useful in this regard. A fuller understanding of target relationships and potential points at which brain stimulation effects may converge at the systems level has relatively recently become a tractable problem, due mainly to technical developments. It is useful to consider efforts made during an earlier era with a view towards eventually integrating these with our evolving anatomical models and the effects of successful treatments. Starting in the early 1950s, Sem-Jacobsen (81) studied effects of acute and chronic (several days) stimulation in 220 patients over more than two decades. Most patients subsequently underwent lesion procedures for Parkinson's disease but underwent ablation for primary psychopathology. Across patient types, stimulation of sites throughout the frontal lobes induced affective changes with apparent selectivity for ventromedial areas. Positive effects ranging from mild relaxation and feelings of tranquility to mild to marked euphoria were observed twice as often as negative effects, which ranged from mild tension or sadness to marked sadness with overt sobbing. Very similar responses were elicited by unilateral stimulation on the right or left sides of the brain (81). These observations suggest that stimulation of many different brain loci can induce positive and negative affective effects. Effects of opposite affective valence (e.g., mild tension and sadness vs mild euphoria) were sometimes seen with stimulation at sites 5 to 10 mm apart in the same individual.

DBS has been conceived of as a treatment for psychopathology since at least 1948 when caudate nucleus stimulation was attempted for treatment of depression and anorexia (31). In work that began soon afterwards, Heath et al. (82) stimulated the "septal region" in psychiatric patients, an area including the ventral anterior capsule and ventral striatum. Heath chose this region, in part, because tumors in this region had been related to psychiatric symptoms (82). Stimulation was limited to 1 to 3 days after electrode implantation in 20 patients with a formal diagnosis of schizophrenia with heterogenous symptoms including delusions, hallucinations, poverty of speech, mutism, depression, and compulsions. Stimulation amplitude was 2 to 15 mA. Three of the 20 patients had "no objective signs," and two more "could not be evaluated" during stimulation. The others reportedly had the following acute effects: 13 of 15 patients became more alert; there was increased motor activity and spontaneous speech production; previously inaudible or expressionless speech became louder with clearer enunciation. One of these, "who had been almost mute, became talkative and later almost hypomanic" *(83)*.

Accompanying and subsequent behavioral changes after stimulation was turned off included improved social interaction and enhanced emotional expression: There was improved "ability to relate to other people, increased responsiveness to pleasure, gradual appearance of sense of humor, and more overt expression of anxiety and ambivalence," There was also improved functioning with "less negativism as everyday problems were approached more realistically and more interest was shown in ward activities." Eleven patients described as generally "idle, seclusive, and withdrawn before operation, afterward participated actively in some or all of the ward activities." Improved emotional responsiveness in social settings was "even more dramatic." Twelve patients showed "significant improvement in their ability to relate to other people," one outstanding aspect was the "emergence of pleasurable feelings." Nine patients showed the "development of humor." Monroe and Heath believed that "… patients who respond particularly well … [were those] whose main abnormalities seem to consist of flattened affect or disturbed motor behavior" *(83)*. The time course and persistence of therapeutic benefit after stimulation ceased is not fully clear in this work although effects apparently could be transient. Some lasting or emerging benefit might have been due to concerted multidisciplinary therapies that were also used in these patients.

This work, carried out in the 1950s, did not use modern standardized diagnostic or severity measures or masked observer ratings thereby severely limiting interpretation. However, the observations of acute and subacute effects made by Monroe and Heath included behaviors that appear to have high face validity as manifestations of affective states, including enhanced production, volume, and prosody of speech; greater affective range, social relatedness, sense of humor; and more marked activation or hypomania.

## Affective Changes After DBS for Movement Disorders

### Background

Modern therapeutic uses of DBS for movement disorder patients have also sometimes produced dramatic effects on affective states. In one case report, a patient without a prior history of depression illustrated modulation of a mood-regulating network by DBS in the region of the STN *(84)*. When the stimulating electrodes, which were implanted slightly below the STN, were activated the subject experienced severe dysphoria that remitted when stimulation was interrupted. Other marked affective effects of DBS in STN, Fields of Forel, and zona incerta in patients with PD have been described *(35, 85)*, including hypomania *(86)*, merriment and involuntary laughter *(51)* and depressive dysphoria, anhedonia, apathy, and blunted affect *(87)*. These findings are extremely intriguing, although their relevance for development of therapeutic DBS for neurologically intact patients with primary depressive illness obviously remains to be determined.

## DBS for Primary Depressive Illness

The terms primary and secondary illness tend to be used somewhat differently in psychiatry and neurology. Descriptive psychopathology in psychiatry often designates a diagnosis as "primary" when its symptoms are what a patient is most distressed by and that result in their seeking treatment. In this tradition, which understandably arose in a field where the pathogenesis of illnesses are so often unknown, symptoms that appear later in the clinical course or are judged to be less pressing clinical issues are viewed as "secondary" or co-morbid.

Advances in clinical neuroscience are gradually moving psychiatry toward a position more familiar to neurologists in which specific mechanisms are invoked to explain the pathogenesis and pathophysiology associated with key features of psychiatric disorders. Recently, researchers armed with a body of functional neuroimaging research have targeted neuronal networks implicated in both the normal experience of sadness, in symptoms of depressive illness, and in responses to treatment. Using PET, Mayberg et al. *(58)* observed a link between changes in metabolism in subgenual cingulate cortex (Brodmann area 25) and the response to antidepressant medications. They used DBS to target these networks in refractory depression. Six patients were selected for notable but not extreme levels of treatment resistance and for a relative lack of psychiatric comorbidity. Stimulation of white matter tracts adjacent to the subgenual cingulate was associated with rapid improvement with substantial mean benefit one week after initiation of stimulation. Chronic DBS for up to 6 months was associated with sustained remission of depression in 4 of the 6 patients *(58)*. Three patients showed decreased metabolism in area 25 compared with pre-operative baseline PET scans, which was consistent with responses observed after other therapeutic modalities for depression. Interestingly, the subgenual white matter tracts that were targeted appear to overlap with those targeted with ablative procedures to treat mixed depressive and anxiety pathology in the 1970s *(88)*.

Other candidate target regions have recently been proposed *(89)* and are under investigation that follow in part empirical evidence gained from psychiatric neurosurgery. A group of ablative procedures with overlapping targets within cortico-basal-thalamic circuits (anterior capsulotomy, subcaudate tractotomy, and limbic leucotomy) have appeared to be effective in severe and resistant depression in multiple open studies, including large series of more than 1,000 patients for subcaudate tractotomy; refs. *30* and *90*). The extent to which these different targets may possibly affect similar neuronal networks via relationships at the systems level is a key research question.

Added to those prior data are findings from our collaborative work of consistent improvement in co-morbid depressive symptoms in OCD patients undergoing DBS in the ventral anterior limb of the internal capsule. Improvement in affect and mood appeared to precede improvement in OCD. We therefore began long-term studies of DBS in this target in patients with severe and disabling depression who were refractory to multiple trials of medications, medication combinations, psychotherapy, and bilateral electroconvulsive therapy. Data are currently being analyzed but preliminary results indicate benefit in most of the patients who have been stimulated to date (Malone et al., in preparation). Induction of transient, reversible mood elevation, which has occasionally reached the diagnostic threshold for DSM-IV hypomania, has been the most significant adverse effect of active stimulation. This effect is intensity-dependent, and has become less frequent with changes in stimulation technique.

A recent case report described the effects of bilateral DBS in the inferior thalamic peduncle (ITP) in a woman with refractory depression (Jimenez et al., World Stereotactic and Functional Neurosurgery Society Meeting, Rome, 2005). Such stimulation, due to effects propagated via ITP fibers that continue rostrally in the ventral portion of the anterior limb of the internal capsule, would be expected to modulate projections of the dorsolateral prefrontal cortex, the orbitofrontal cortex, and the ventromedial striatum to the dorsomedial and intralaminar thalamus. A substantial period of benefit followed insertion without stimulation suggesting some combination of a "microlesion" effect, placebo response, and possibly the course of illness itself since, unlike OCD, depression is typically episodic. Subsequently, however, the patient appeared to have long-term improvement associated with chronic DBS in this region, at relatively low stimulation intensities. This is of interest given that fibers coursing from rostral structures become more compact as they enter the ITP.

The effects of DBS of the STN in two patients with severe Parkinson's disease who also had moderately severe OCD have been reported *(91)*. Improvement in OCD symptoms was substantial within two weeks following the start of DBS *(91)*. In one of these patients, OCD improvement was seen despite little change in parkinsonism. Similar effects were seen more recently in one additional case *(92)*. A controlled trial of STN DBS is underway by a collaborative group of investigators in France. It will be interesting to see whether effects on co-morbid depression and anxiety symptoms in this trial will be similar to those observed after ventral capsule/ventral striatum DBS in prior OCD studies. There, rapid onset of anti-depressant or anti-anxiety effects with onset of DBS and rapid worsening in these domains after offset of DBS were observed, which seemed to precede changes in core OCD symptoms. Similar findings after stimulation of the "limbic" STN region would suggest convergence of circuits influenced at each target.

The effects experienced by patients treated with DBS for severe and resistant depression appear to be grounds for cautious optimism. However, relatively few patients have been studied. Moreover, the brain regions involved in dysregulation of mood and other symptom dimensions of depressive illness are inadequately understood. Sadness and depressive illness are both associated with decreased activity in dorsal neocortical regions and relative increased activity in ventral limbic and paralimbic areas *(93)*. In fact, increases in regional cerebral blood flow and metabolism have sometimes been shown in the amygdala, orbitofrontal cortex and medial thalamus and decreases in the dorsomedial and dorsal anterolateral prefrontal cortex, subgenual anterior cingulate cortex (ACC) and dorsal ACC relative to control subjects *(94)*. Dysregulation within functional networks including these areas has been hypothesized to explain the combination of clinical symptoms seen in depressed patients (i.e., mood, motor, cognitive, and vegetative symptoms; ref. *18*). These regions may be differentially affected in subtypes of depression *(95)*. Other important regions include the hippocampus *(96)*, insula *(97)*, and midbrain monoamine nuclei. Underlying structural abnormalities may also contribute to these dysfunctions *(98–100)*. Other factors to be considered in interpreting responses to DBS include the state of the disease, the inherited traits of the individual and genetic susceptibility *(101)*, and the type of response to treatment (i.e., how dimensions of depressive illness change). Mood, for example, is a continuous adaptive process. This implies that although certain localized activity changes may be identified, it is important to address the dynamic interplay within the system. The deactivations of subgenual cingulate with DBS reported in depression may be analogous to other anti-depressant treatments but they are also suggestive of a process of adaptation over time. Much work is still needed to understand the complex relationships between activity in different nodes of cortico-basal-thalamic-limbic networks.

## Future Developments: Issues and Recommendations

DBS is now a conventional therapeutic option for intractable movement disorders. The efficacy of the procedure is well-established, although questions remain about mechanisms of action, optimal stimulation targets, and methodologic techniques. While serious adverse events are possible, the overall side effect burden is favorable. The fact that interest in DBS is growing rapidly as a potential treatment for patients with severe neuropsychiatric illness is not surprising. Such patients experience extreme distress and inability to participate in social and occupational life. There are strong parallels with the application of DBS for intractable neurologic illness and its potential use in neuropsychiatry but there are also differences. The most salient of these arises from historical experience. The special concern over the use of neurosurgery for psychiatric illnesses is the legacy of the widespread use of destructive procedures, particularly frontal lobotomy, in the mid-20th century. Many patients underwent such surgery before adequate long-term safety data were obtained and without careful characterization of their primary disorder. Tragic consequences were frequent. These remain a vivid reminder of the need for caution in this area *(102)*. Currently, the practice of psychiatric neurosurgery is much more refined, restricted and regulated. Candidates must meet stringent criteria for severity and for resistance to conventional multimodal therapies. DBS is an invasive procedure and, although it is non-ablative in nature and theoretically reversible when stimulation is interrupted, the evidence that it may be useful in psychiatric disorders is limited to approximately 50 patients worldwide for OCD and to fewer cases of major depression.

It is important to remember that, unlike the model for Parkinson's disease, the development of animal models of human psychopathology has been very limited. There are, however, some potentially promising leads. Some recent work in model development has paralleled an interest in focusing on behavioral symptoms that are components of syndromes *(103)* and of predisposing and associated factors *(104)*. Such models, which represent major advances in conceptual sophistication and complexity, may enhance cross-species translational research.

Future work in this area may eventually yield advances in animal models. It is also notable that to date there have been few neuroimaging studies in patients with marked symptom severity and treatment resistance, in order to identify patients who might be considered potential candidates for neurosurgical interventions. It is possible that there may be subgroups of patients who differ meaningfully from the larger groups of patients with more common presentations, which have usually been studied.

Beyond that, the neurophysiological correlates of abnormal activity in patients with neuropsychiatric disorders as revealed by functional neuroimaging are not yet well established. There are some proposals that may have heuristic value in hypothesis generation in this regard. An example is the concept of thalamocortical dysrhythmia (TCD), which proposes that an increase in power of thalamocortical oscillatory activity in the theta range may underlie symptomatology of a number of neuropsychiatric conditions *(105)*. Understanding the role of synchrony and oscillatory activity may have important implications to the future applications of DBS in PD, movement disorders, and other neurological disorders. Studies using translational approaches, including integration of anatomical and physiological methods across species, are most likely to advance our understanding of how DBS might alter pathophysiology and thus exert therapeutic effects.

The clinical characteristics of patients with severe, chronic, and highly resistant psychiatric illness, which typically require multiple treatment modalities, will require close and long-term follow-up. A study of DBS in four OCD patients, using a more anterior capsular target than that of Nuttin et al. *(106)*, and a different stimulating electrode, reported significant benefit in three of the four patients with more than 35% reduction in YBOCS severity. Unfortunately, one patient in this series died by suicide during the trial. As noted earlier, co-morbid depression and demoralization, which can be severe, is the rule rather that the exception in such patients. In this patient, depression had been chronic before surgery and had shown some improvement during shorter-term stimulation *(57)*. While the relationship between DBS and suicidality in this patient is unclear, it serves as a stark reminder that individuals with the degree of illness severity with profound demoralization due to illness-related degradation in quality of life, are at potential risk of suicide after as well as before surgical intervention as there have been suicides of patients on waiting lists for psychiatric neurosurgery. Adverse behavioral outcomes, including some cases of suicide, have also been seen in patients treated with DBS for movement disorders *(107)*. Thus, close and expert monitoring and a long-term commitment to follow-up are essential for all DBS patients but the risks of adverse behavioral outcomes would seem greater *a priori* in patients treated for underlying psychiatric illness.

An interdisciplinary group of collaborators, which begun to systematically study the effectiveness and safety of DBS in psychiatric illness in the late 1990s, has recommended that certain minimum requirements be met, for psychiatrists and neurosurgeons contemplating using DBS for psychiatric indications *(108)*. This group recommended that, until FDA approval is provided, this work should be done only as part of an investigational protocol. This requires initial and ongoing review by an institutional review board or ethics committee. In the United States, there is additional review by the FDA via the Investigational Device Exemption (IDE) mechanism. As noted above, careful psychiatric assessment is an extremely important requirement. Psychiatrists must make certain that patient selection is appropriate. Patients must meet operational criteria for the neuropsychiatric disorder under study and for the severity of that illness. Proven medication and psychosocial/behavioral treatments must have already been given in adequate therapeutic trials. We propose that potential candidates for psychiatric DBS also undergo a second level of consideration by an interdisciplinary review committee with appropriate expertise, which should include bioethics, independent from the investigative team. Such research should be carried out at specialized academic centers with extensive experience in the treatment of patients with the neuropsychiatric condition in question. The neurosurgical team should also have substantial experience with DBS as currently practiced. Very recently, our recommendations in this realm have been updated *(108)*. Anticipating gradual expansion of research and clinical uses of DBS in psychiatry and stimulated by the emergence of vagus nerve stimulation, we have also sought to begin a discussion of issues concerning training and interdisciplinary collaborations raised by encouraging developments and future prospects of this field *(109)*.

## Conclusions

DBS is an investigational treatment in neuropsychiatry that has generated considerable interest. Although its mechanisms of action are incompletely understood, DBS can target precision regions and circuits within the brain proposed to be involved in the pathophysiology of some neuropsychiatric illnesses. It offers the advantages of reversibility and adjustability, which might permit the effectiveness of therapy to be enhanced or side effects to be minimized. Thus, DBS may offer a degree of hope for patients with severe and treatment-resistant neuropsychiatric illness. Most of the DBS work to date has focused on OCD where data from small-scale studies are encouraging. Early data from a few patients with major depression may also indicate some promise. Research to realize this potential will require a considerable commitment of resources, energy, and time across disciplines including psychiatry, neurosurgery, neurology, neuropsychology, bioengineering, and bioethics. Indications at the time of this writing suggest that, with appropriate multidisciplinary work, cautious optimism concerning the role of DBS in psychiatric treatment is justified.

## References

1. Kessler RC, McGonagle KA, Zhao S, et al (1994) Lifetime and 12-month prevalence of DSM-III-R psychiatric disorders in the United States. Results from the National Comorbidity Survey. Arch Gen Psychiatry 51(1):8–19.
2. Lehtinen V, Joukamaa M (1994) Epidemiology of depression: prevalence, risk factors and treatment situation. Acta Psychiatr Scand Suppl 1377:7–10.
3. Mueller TI, Leon AC, Keller MB, et al (1999) Recurrence after recovery from major depressive disorder during 15 years of observational follow-up. Am J Psychiatry 156(7):1000–1006.
4. Klerman GL, Weissman MM (1992) The course, morbidity, and costs of depression. Arch Gen Psychiatry 49(10):831–834.
5. Murray CJ, Lopez AD (1997) Global mortality, disability, and the contribution of risk factors: Global Burden of Disease Study. Lancet 349(9063):1436–1442.

6. Lopez AD, Murray CC (1998) The global burden of disease, 1990–2020. Nat Med 4(11):1241–1243.
7. Joukamaa M, Heliovaara M, Knekt P, Aromaa A, Raitasalo R, Lehtinen V (2001) Mental disorders and cause-specific mortality. Br J Psychiatry 179:498–502.
8. Glassman AH, Shapiro PA (1998) Depression and the course of coronary artery disease. Am J Psychiatry 155(1):4–11.
9. Wulsin LR, Vaillant GE, Wells VE (1999) A systematic review of the mortality of depression. Psychosom Med 61(1):6–17.
10. Agency for Healthcare Policy Research (1999) Evidence Report on Treatment for Depression- Newer Pharmacotherapies. San Antonio, TX: Evidence-Based Practice Centers.
11. Price LH, Lemmond K, Carpenter LC (1999) Refractory depression: Assessment and treatment. Direct in Psych 19:1–20.
12. Winokur G, Coryell W, Keller M, Endicott J, Akiskal H (1993) A prospective follow-up of patients with bipolar and primary unipolar affective disorder. Arch Gen Psychiatry 50(6):457–465.
13. Sobin C, Sackeim HA, Prudic J, Devanand DP, Moody BJ, McElhiney MC (1995) Predictors of retrograde amnesia following ECT. Am J Psychiatry 152(7):995–1001.
14. Lisanby SH, Maddox JH, Prudic J, Devanand DP, Sackeim HA (2000) The effects of electroconvulsive therapy on memory of autobiographical and public events. Arch Gen Psychiatry 57(6):581–590.
15. Gagne GG Jr, Furman MJ, Carpenter LL, Price LH (2000) Efficacy of continuation ECT and anti-depressant drugs compared to long-term anti-depressants alone in depressed patients. Am J Psychiatry 157(12):1960–1965.
16. Rush AJ, Thase ME, Dube S (2003) Research issues in the study of difficult-to-treat depression. Biol Psychiatry 53(8):743–753.
17. Dunn RT, Kimbrell TA, Ketter TA, et al (2002) Principal components of the Beck Depression Inventory and regional cerebral metabolism in unipolar and bipolar depression. Biol Psychiatry 51(5):387–399.
18. Milak MS, Parsey RV, Keilp J, Oquendo MA, Malone KM, Mann JJ (2005) Neuroanatomic correlates of psychopathologic components of major depressive disorder. Arch Gen Psychiatry 62(4):397–408.
19. Perico CA, Skaf CR, Yamada A, et al (2005) Relationship between regional cerebral blood flow and separate symptom clusters of major depression: a single photon emission computed tomography study using statistical parametric mapping. Neurosci Lett 384(3):265–270.
20. Wong ML, Licinio J (2001) Research and treatment approaches to depression. Nat Rev Neurosci 2(5):343–351.
21. Nestler EJ, Barrot M, DiLeone RJ, Eisch AJ, Gold SJ, Monteggia LM (2002) Neurobiology of depression. Neuron 34(1):13–25.
22. Caspi A, Sugden K, Moffitt TE, et al (2003) Influence of life stress on depression: moderation by a polymorphism in the 5-HTT gene. Science 301(5631):386–389.
23. Berton O, McClung CA, Dileone RJ, et al (2006) Essential role of BDNF in the mesolimbic dopamine pathway in social defeat stress. Science 311(5762):864–868.
24. Berton O, Nestler EJ (2006) New approaches to anti-depressant drug discovery: beyond monoamines. Nat Rev Neurosci 7(2):137–151.
25. Svenningsson P, Chergui K, Rachleff I, et al (2006) Alterations in 5-HT1B receptor function by p11 in depression-like states. Science 311(5757):77–80.
26. Swerdlow NR, Koob GF (1987) Dopamine, schizophrenia, mania and depression: toward a unified hypothesis of cortico-striatal-pallido-thalamic function. Behav Brain Sci 10:197–245.
27. Mayberg HS (2002) Modulating limbic-cortical circuits in depression: targets of anti-depressant treatments. Semin Clin Neuropsychiatry 7(4):255–268.

28. Phillips ML, Drevets WC, Rauch SL, Lane R (2003) Neurobiology of emotion perception II: Implications for major psychiatric disorders. Biol Psychiatry 54(5):515–528.
29. Rauch SL (2003) Neuroimaging and neurocircuitry models pertaining to the neurosurgical treatment of psychiatric disorders. Neurosurg Clin N Am. Apr 14(2): 213–223.
30. Greenberg BD, Price LH, Rauch SL, et al (2003) Neurosurgery for Intractable Obsessive-Compulsive Disorder and Depression: Critical Issues. Neurosurg Clin North Am 14(2):199–212.
31. Pool JL (1954) Psychosugery of older people. J Geriatr Assoc 2:456–465.
32. Tasker RR (1998) Deep brain stimulation is preferable to thalamotomy for tremor suppression. Surg Neurol 49(2):145–153; discussion 153–144.
33. Schuurman PR, Bosch DA, Bossuyt PM, et al (2000) A comparison of continuous thalamic stimulation and thalamotomy for suppression of severe tremor. N Engl J Med 342(7):461–468.
34. Deuschl G, Bain P (2002) Deep brain stimulation for tremor [correction of trauma]: patient selection and evaluation. Mov Disord 17(Suppl 3):S102–S111.
35. Pollak P, Fraix V, Krack P, et al (2002) Treatment results: Parkinson's disease. Mov Disord 17(Suppl 3):S75–S83.
36. Vercueil L, Krack P, Pollak P (2002) Results of deep brain stimulation for dystonia: a critical reappraisal. Mov Disord 17(Suppl 3):S89–S93.
37. Volkmann J, Benecke R (2002) Deep brain stimulation for dystonia: patient selection and evaluation. Mov Disord 17(Suppl 3):S112–S115.
38. Loddenkemper T, Pan A, Neme S, et al (2001) Deep brain stimulation in epilepsy. J Clin Neurophysiol 18(6):514–532.
39. Hodaie M, Wennberg RA, Dostrovsky JO, Lozano AM (2002) Chronic anterior thalamus stimulation for intractable epilepsy. Epilepsia 43(6):603–608.
40. Kumar K, Toth C, Nath RK (1997) Deep brain stimulation for intractable pain: a 15-year experience. Neurosurgery 40(4):736–746; discussion 746–737.
41. Leone M, Franzini A, Felisati G, et al (2005) Deep brain stimulation and cluster headache. Neurol Sci 26 Suppl 2:s138–139.
42. Schrader C, Peschel T, Petermeyer M, Dengler R, Hellwig D (2004) Unilateral deep brain stimulation of the internal globus pallidus alleviates tardive dyskinesia. Mov Disord 19(5):583–585.
43. Diederich NJ, Kalteis K, Stamenkovic M, Pieri V, Alesch F (2005) Efficient internal pallidal stimulation in Gilles de la Tourette syndrome: A case report. Mov Disord.
44. Schiff ND, Plum F, Rezai AR (2002) Developing prosthetics to treat cognitive disabilities resulting from acquired brain injuries. Neurol Res 24(2):116–124.
45. Yamamoto T, Kobayashi K, Kasai M, Oshima H, Fukaya C, Katayama Y (2005) DBS therapy for the vegetative state and minimally conscious state. Acta Neurochir Suppl 93:101–104.
46. Just H, Ostergaard K (2002) Health-related quality of life in patients with advanced Parkinson's disease treated with deep brain stimulation of the subthalamic nuclei. Mov Disord 17(3):539–545.
47. Erola T, Karinen P, Heikkinen E, et al (2005) Bilateral subthalamic nucleus stimulation improves health-related quality of life in Parkinsonian patients. Parkinsonism Relat Disord 11(2):89–94.
48. Tuite PJ, Maxwell RE, Ikramuddin S, et al (2005) Weight and body mass index in Parkinson's disease patients after deep brain stimulation surgery. Parkinsonism Relat Disord 11(4):247–252.
49. Voges J, Volkmann J, Allert N, et al (2002) Bilateral high-frequency stimulation in the subthalamic nucleus for the treatment of Parkinson disease: correlation of therapeutic effect with anatomical electrode position. J Neurosurg 96(2):269–279.

50. Volkmann J, Allert N, Voges J, Weiss PH, Freund HJ, Sturm V (2001) Safety and efficacy of pallidal or subthalamic nucleus stimulation in advanced PD. Neurology 56(4):548–551.
51. Limousin P, Krack P, Pollak P, et al (1998) Electrical stimulation of the subthalamic nucleus in advanced Parkinson's disease. N Engl J Med 339(16):1105–1111.
52. DBS for Parkinson's Disease Study Group (2001) Deep-brain stimulation of the subthalamic nucleus or the pars interna of the globus pallidus in Parkinson's disease. N Engl J Med 345(13):956–963.
53. Vingerhoets FJ, Villemure JG, Temperli P, Pollo C, Pralong E, Ghika J (2002) Subthalamic DBS replaces levodopa in Parkinson's disease: two-year follow-up. Neurology 58(3):396–401.
54. Peppe A, Pierantozzi M, Bassi A, et al (2004) Stimulation of the subthalamic nucleus compared with the globus pallidus internus in patients with Parkinson disease. J Neurosurg 101(2):195–200.
55. Rezai AR, Mogilner AY, Cappell J, Hund M, Llinas RR, Kelly PJ (1997) Integration of functional brain mapping in image-guided neurosurgery. Acta Neurochir Suppl 68:85–89.
56. Rezai AR, Hutchinson W, Lozano AM (1999) Chronic subthalamic nucleus stimulation for Parkinson's disease. In: Rezai AR, Hutchinson W, Lozano AM, eds. The Operative Neurosurgical Atlas, vol. 8. Rollings, IL: American Association of Neurosurgeons.
57. Abelson JL, Curtis GC, Sagher O, et al (2005) Deep brain stimulation for refractory obsessive-compulsive disorder. Biol Psychiatry 57(5):510–516.
58. Mayberg HS, Lozano AM, Voon V, et al (2005) Deep brain stimulation for treatment-resistant depression. Neuron 45(5):651–660.
59. Nuttin B, Cosyns P, Demeulemeester H, Gybels J, Meyerson B (1999) Electrical stimulation in anterior limbs of internal capsules in patients with obsessive-compulsive disorder. Lancet 354:1526.
60. Montgomery EB Jr, Baker KB (2000) Mechanisms of deep brain stimulation and future technical developments. Neurol Res 22(3):259–266.
61. Benabid AL, Benazzous A, Pollak P (2002) Mechanisms of deep brain stimulation. Mov Disord 17(Suppl 3):S73–S74.
62. McIntyre CC, Savasta M, Walter BL, Vitek JL (2004) How does deep brain stimulation work? Present understanding and future questions. J Clin Neurophysiol 21(1):40–50.
63. Rauch SL, Dougherty DD, Malone D, et al (2006) A functional neuroimaging investigation of deep brain stimulation in patients with obsessive-compulsive disorder. J Neurosurg 104(4):558–565.
64. Van Laere K, Nuttin B, Gabriels L, et al (2006) Metabolic imaging of anterior capsular stimulation in refractory obsessive compulsive disorder: a key role for the subgenual anterior cingulate and ventral striatum. J Nuc Med 47:740–747.
65. Rezai AR, Finelli D, Nyenhuis JA, et al (2002) Neurostimulation systems for deep brain stimulation: in vitro evaluation of magnetic resonance imaging-related heating at 1.5 tesla. J Magn Reson Imaging 15(3):241–250.
66. Li X, Walker J, Koola J, George MS, Bohning DE (2005) Using phase mapping to evaluate MRI-related DBS implant heating: initial report. Biol Psychiatry 57:113s.
67. Lyons KE, Wilkinson SB, Overman J, Pahwa R (2004) Surgical and hardware complications of subthalamic stimulation: a series of 160 procedures. Neurology 63(4):612–616.
68. Hariz MI (2002) Complications of deep brain stimulation surgery. Mov Disord 17(Suppl 3):S162–S166.
69. Landau WM, Perlmutter JS (1999) Transient acute depression induced by high-frequency deep-brain stimulation. N Engl J Med 341(13):1004.

70. Takeshita S, Kurisu K, Trop L, Arita K, Akimitsu T, Verhoeff NP (2005) Effect of subthalamic stimulation on mood state in Parkinson's disease: evaluation of previous facts and problems. Neurosurg Rev 28(3):179–186; discussion 187.
71. Witt K, Pulkowski U, Herzog J, et al (2004) Deep brain stimulation of the subthalamic nucleus improves cognitive flexibility but impairs response inhibition in Parkinson disease. Arch Neurol 61(5):697–700.
72. Insel TR (1992) Toward a neuroanatomy of obsessive-compulsive disorder. Arch Gen Psychiatry 49(9):739–744.
73. Baxter LR Jr, Saxena S, Brody AL, et al (1996) Brain mediation of obsessive-compulsive disorder symptoms: evidence from functional brain imaging studies in the human and nonhuman primate. Semin Clin Neuropsychiatry. 1(1):32–47.
74. Nuttin BJ, Gabriels LA, Cosyns PR, et al (2003) Long-term electrical capsular stimulation in patients with obsessive-compulsive disorder. Neurosurgery 52(6):1263–1272; discussion 1272–1264.
75. Anderson D, Ahmed A (2003) Treatment of patients with intractable obsessive-compulsive disorder with anterior capsular stimulation. Case report. J Neurosurg 98(5):1104–1108.
76. Sturm V, Lenartz D, Koulousakis A, et al (2003) The nucleus accumbens: a target for deep brain stimulation in obsessive-compulsive- and anxiety-disorders. J Chem Neuroanat 26(4):293–299.
77. Aouizerate B, Cuny E, Martin-Guehl C, et al (2004) Deep brain stimulation of the ventral caudate nucleus in the treatment of obsessive-compulsive disorder and major depression. Case report. J Neurosurg 101(4):682–686.
78. Gabriels L, Cosyns P, Nuttin B, Demeulemeester H, Gybels J (2003) Deep brain stimulation for treatment-refractory obsessive-compulsive disorder: psychopathological and neuropsychological outcome in three cases. Acta Psychiatr Scand 107(4):275–282.
79. Greenberg BD, Malone DA, Friehs GM, et al (2006) Three-year outcomes in deep brain stimulation for highly resistant obsessive-compulsive disorder. Neuropsychopharmacology 31:2384–2393.
80. Mayberg HS, Liotti M, Brannan SK, et al (1999) Reciprocal limbic-cortical function and negative mood: converging PET findings in depression and normal sadness. Am J Psychiatry 156(5):675–682.
81. Sem-Jacobsen CW (1968) Depth-electrographic stimulation of the human brain and behavior; from fourteen years of studies and treatment of Parkinson's disease and mental disorders with implanted electrodes. Charles C. Thomas: Springfield, IL, pp. 27–208.
82. Heath RG (1963) Electrical Self-stimulation of the Brain in Man. Am J Psychiatry 120:571–577.
83. Monroe RR, Heath RG (1954) Psychiatric observations. In: Heath RG, ed. Studies in Schizophrenia: A Multidisciplinary Approach to Mind-Brain Relationships. Cambridge, MA: Harvard University Press; pp. 345–389.
84. Bejjani B-P, Damier P, Arnulf I, et al. (1999) Transient acute depression induced by high-frequency deep brain stimulation. N Engl J Med 340:1476–1480.
85. Berney A, Vingerhoets F, Perrin A, et al (2002) Effect on mood of subthalamic DBS for Parkinson's disease: a consecutive series of 24 patients. Neurology 59(9):1427–1429.
86. Kulisevsky J, Berthier ML, Gironell A, Pascual-Sedano B, Molet J, Pares P (2002) Mania following deep brain stimulation for Parkinson's disease. Neurology 59(9):1421–1424.
87. Stefurak T, Mikulis D, Mayberg HS, et al (2003) Deep brain stimulation for parkinson's disease dissociates mood and motor circuits: a functional MRI case study. Mov Disord 18(12):1508–1541.
88. Vilkki J. (1977) Late psychological and clinical effects of subrostral cingulotomy and anterior mesoloviotomy in psychiatric illness. In: Sweet WH, Obrador S,

Martin-Rodriguez JG, eds. Neurosurgical Treatment in Psychiatry, Pain, and Epilepsy. Balitimore: University Park Press, pp. 253–259.
89. Kopell BH, Greenberg B, Rezai AR (2004) Deep brain stimulation for psychiatric disorders. J Clin Neurophysiol 21(1):51–67.
90. Cosgrove GR, Rauch SL (1995) Psychosurgery. Neurosurg Clin N Am 6:167–176.
91. Mallet L, Mesnage V, Houeto JL, et al (2002) Compulsions, Parkinson's disease, and stimulation. Lancet 360(9342):1302–1304.
92. Fontaine D, Mattei V, Borg M, et al (2004) Effect of subthalamic nucleus stimulation on obsessive-compulsive disorder in a patient with Parkinson disease. Case report. J Neurosurg 100(6):1084–1086.
93. Drevets WC, Bogers W, Raichle ME (2002) Functional anatomical correlates of anti-depressant drug treatment assessed using PET measures of regional glucose metabolism. Eur Neuropsychopharmacol 12(6):527–544.
94. Abercrombie HC, Schaefer SM, Larson CL, et al (1998) Metabolic rate in the right amygdala predicts negative affect in depressed patients. Neuroreport 9(14):3301–3307.
95. Sackeim HA, Prohovnik I (1993) Brain imaging studies of depressive disorders. In: Kupfer DJ, ed. The Biology of Depressive Disorders. New York: Plenum.
96. Sheline YI (2000) 3D MRI studies of neuroanatomic changes in unipolar major depression: the role of stress and medical comorbidity. Biol Psychiatry 48(8):791–800.
97. Elliott R, Rubinsztein JS, Sahakian BJ, Dolan RJ (2002) The neural basis of mood-congruent processing biases in depression. Arch Gen Psychiatry 59(7):597–604.
98. Ongur D, Drevets WC, Price JL (1998) Glial reduction in the subgenual prefrontal cortex in mood disorders. Proc Natl Acad Sci USA 95(22):13,290–13,295.
99. Drevets WC, Ongur D, Price JL (1998) Reduced glucose metabolism in the subgenual prefrontal cortex in unipolar depression. Mol Psychiatry 3(3):190–191.
100. Steingard RJ, Renshaw PF, Hennen J, et al (2002) Smaller frontal lobe white matter volumes in depressed adolescents. Biol Psychiatry 52(5):413–417.
101. Graff-Guerrero A, De la Fuente-Sandoval C, Camarena B, et al (2005) Frontal and limbic metabolic differences in subjects selected according to genetic variation of the SLC6A4 gene polymorphism. Neuroimage 25(4):1197–1204.
102. Fins JJ (2003) From psychosurgery to neuromodulation and palliation: history's lessons for the ethical conduct and regulation of neuropsychiatric research. Neurosurg Clin N Am 14(2):303–319, ix–x.
103. Joel D, Doljansky J, Schiller D (2005) 'Compulsive' lever pressing in rats is enhanced following lesions to the orbital cortex, but not to the basolateral nucleus of the amygdala or to the dorsal medial prefrontal cortex. Eur J Neurosci 21(8):2252–2262.
104. Coplan JD, Smith EL, Altemus M, et al (2006) Maternal-infant response to variable foraging demand in nonhuman primates: effects of timing of stressor on cerebrospinal fluid corticotropin-releasing factor and circulating glucocorticoid concentrations. Ann NY Acad Sci 1071:525–533.
105. Llinas RR, Ribary U, Jeanmonod D, Kronberg E, Mitra PP (1999) Thalamocortical dysrhythmia: A neurological and neuropsychiatric syndrome characterized by magnetoencephalography. Proc Natl Acad Sci USA 929(26):15,222–15,227.
106. Nuttin B, Gybels J, Cosyns P, et al (2003) Deep brain stimulation for psychiatric disorders. Neurosurg Clin N Am 14(2):xv–xvi.
107. Burkhard PR, Vingerhoets FJ, Berney A, Bogousslavsky J, Villemure JG, Ghika J (2004) Suicide after successful deep brain stimulation for movement disorders. Neurology 63(11):2170–2172.
108. Fins JJ, Rezai AR, Greenberg BD (2006) Psychosurgery: avoiding an ethical redux while advancing a therapeutic future. Neurosurgery 59(4):713–716.
109. Greenberg BD, Nuttin B, Rezai AR (2006) Education and neuromodulation for psychiatric disorders: a perspective for practitioners. Neurosurgery 59(4):717–719.

# 26
# Deep Brain Stimulation in Obsessive–Compulsive Disorder

Loes Gabriëls, Kris van Kuyck, Marleen Welkenhuyzen, Paul Cosyns, and Bart Nuttin

## Abstract

Obsessive–compulsive disorder (OCD) is a psychiatric disorder that often runs a chronic, fluctuating course. A minority of patients do not improve by any available psychopharmacological and/or psychotherapeutic treatment. Treatment-refractory OCD patients considered for stereotactic neurosurgery have a longstanding history of persistent and extremely incapacitating intrusive obsessions and repetitive compulsions. This disorder creates tremendous suffering and a deep sense of shame, resulting in social isolation and often depression. Although a specific brain abnormality has not been identified, a growing number of brain imaging studies have accumulated evidence for a neurobiological basis for OCD.

Eleven patients with severe, treatment refractory OCD were included in a double blind randomised crossover protocol. Electrical stimulation in the anterior limbs of the internal capsules and striatal gray matter inferiorly induced clinically significant therapeutic benefit in this patient group, not only in severity of OCD symptoms but also on the patient's mood scores. Technical aspects currently limit the use of capsular stimulation as a therapeutic option. This treatment option remains investigational for OCD patients and is not considered standard therapy.

**Keywords:** obsessive–compulsive disorder, neuromodulation, deep brain stimulation, psychosurgery, anterior capsulotomy

## Introduction

OCD is believed to be one of the most debilitating of the anxiety disorders. It affects approximately 2% of the general population (1). The cardinal symptoms of OCD are intrusive, persistent thoughts (obsessions) and/or repetitive behaviors (compulsions). Common themes are checking, washing and cleaning, excessive need for order and symmetry, unwanted aggressive thoughts, and counting. Symptoms may occupy many hours daily and lead to serious impairment in occupational, scholastic and/or social functioning. Most patients recognize the senselessness of their obsessions and compulsions but cannot dismiss the obsessional thoughts and continue to feel compelled to engage in rituals.

Co-morbid disorders such as major depression, personality disorders and anxiety disorders are frequently present and complicate and aggravate the clinical picture in OCD (2). Longitudinal research suggests that when OCD symptoms improve with effective treatment, depressive symptoms also disappear (3).

## Treatment Options

Both pharmacotherapy and cognitive behavioral therapy (CBT) can be effective in the treatment of OCD, either alone or in combination (4). As a rule, treatment adherence is necessary for lasting symptom relief but, even when effective, side effects of pharmacotherapy substantially hamper compliance (5–7). The cognitive behavioral approach of exposure and response prevention (ERP) yields significant and lasting therapeutic benefits for those OCD patients motivated to engage in the exercises (8).

Up to 7.1% of patients remain treatment refractory and run a chronic deteriorating course of OCD despite all available treatment (3). Spontaneous remission in severe, intractable and longstanding OCD is rare (2, 9).

## Capsulotomy for OCD

Clinical evidence suggests an improvement rate of about 50% of otherwise intractable cases of OCD produced by neurosurgical lesioning in the anterior limb of the internal capsule, a technique called capsulotomy (10–14). Irreversible destruction of brain tissue remains an obvious drawback but is counterbalanced by the potentially beneficial therapeutic effect for the despairing patient who is disabled by severe, chronic, treatment-refractory OCD (15, 16).

Although the target symptoms of obsessions, compulsions and anxiety are successfully reduced, side effects remain a major concern. These include weight gain, memory problems, attentional slowing, lower performance intelligence quotient, loss of initiative, disinhibition, elevated mood occasionally with an overshoot toward carelessness, emotional shallowness and, in rare cases, aggressive tendencies, poor impulse control and sexual assaults (11, 17–22).

## Capsular DBS for OCD

Development of electrical brain stimulation in the anterior limbs of the internal capsules (capsular stimulation) as a reversible treatment alternative for capsulotomy has opened a new avenue for research and treatment in OCD. The implantation of electrodes in the brain does not significantly damage brain tissue and stimulation can be modified or discontinued in the event of side effects. With informed consent from the patient, electrical current can be switched on or off in an experimental setting, or can be applied using different stimulation parameters (contact selection, amplitude, pulse width, frequency) without the patient's knowledge, in order to perform scientifically rigorous tests of efficacy.

The rationale for the choice of the anterior limb of the internal capsule as the target for electrical stimulation in OCD is similar to that for its current use in other indications as a treatment in tremor and Parkinson's disease, where the experience that ablative lesions produced therapeutic benefits was followed by high frequency deep brain stimulation (DBS) applied to the same structures.

**Experimental design**

Our protocol employs a two-branched, double blind, randomized crossover design. An episode with stimulation either switched on or off is followed by an episode of the opposite condition, with patient and evaluators blinded for the stimulation condition. Each patient serves as his own control. Behavioral measures were systematically assessed pre-operatively and during each phase of the randomization.

**Patient Selection**

All participating patients suffered from long-standing, severe, highly disabling OCD (300.30 according to the Diagnostic and Statistical Manual of Psychiatric Disorders, fourth edition; ref. *23*). Patients were screened and evaluated in the department of psychiatry of the University Hospital of Antwerp for complete psychiatric and neuropsychological assessment and underwent stereotactic neurosurgery in the University Hospital Gasthuisberg of Leuven. Both hospital Ethical Review Boards approved the study protocol.

Family history, present and past medical history and treatment surveys were documented. After scrutiny of the patient's case, a multidisciplinary advisory board for neurosurgical treatment for psychiatric disorders decided on the suitability of surgical treatment according to strict criteria *(24, 25)*, taking into account the written record, clinical examination, and formal referral from the patient's treating psychiatrist. Inclusion criteria required a primary diagnosis of OCD, by Structured Clinical Interview for DSM-IV (SCID-IV), judged to be of disabling severity, with a Yale-Brown Obsessive-Compulsive Scale (Y-BOCS; refs. *26* and *27*) score of at least 30/40 and a Global Assessment of Functioning (GAF) score of 45 or less. Reports of failure to respond to former OCD treatment were required: ineffectiveness or intolerance to adequate trials of at least three serotonin reuptake inhibitors and clomipramine, augmentation strategies with an antipsychotic drug, and an adequate trial of CBT. Age range was 18 to 60. Exclusion criteria were a current or past psychotic disorder, any clinically significant disorder or medical illness affecting brain function or structure (other than motor tics or Tourette's syndrome), prominent cluster B personality disorder or current or unstably remitted substance abuse. Personality disorders were assessed with the Structured Clinical Interview DSM-IV axis II (SCID-II; ref. *28*). Patients were to be able to understand and comply with instructions and provide their own written informed consent. The patient and a close family member were repeatedly and fully informed on both procedures (capsulotomy and capsular stimulation) and standard risks of both procedures were explained. If the patient did not improve after 1 year of capsular stimulation the option of anterior capsulotomy was to be considered.

Medication was tapered to an attainable minimum at least 6 weeks before surgical intervention and kept at a constant level for the first year after electrode

**Table 26.1** Patient characteristics at time of surgery.

| | M/F | Age onset OCD | Age surgery | Most severe OCD symptoms | Psychopharmacologic treatment |
|---|---|---|---|---|---|
| C1 | M | 12 | 35 | Obsession with the "sound of silence," fear of hair growth | Lormetazepam (0.5 mg) |
| C2 | F | 24 | 52 | Contamination, poisonous plants, checking, asking questions | Sertraline (150 mg/d) |
| | | | | | Prazepam (60 mg/d) |
| | | | | | Diazepam (10 mg/d) |
| | | | | | Trazodone (100 mg/d) |
| C3 | F | 16 | 38 | Obsession with "existence," touching things, counting, washing rituals | Fluoxetine (20 mg/d) |
| | | | | | Clomipramine (50 mg/d) |
| | | | | | Lorazepam (3.75 mg/d) |
| C4 | M | 12 | 35 | Extreme fear of poisoning others, obsessed with failing to assist people in need, checking, hand washing, cleaning rituals | Clomipramine (150 mg/d) Risperidone (6 mg/d) |
| | | | | | Alprazolam (4 mg/d) |
| | | | | | Lormetazepam (2 mg/d) |
| C5 | F | 14 | 40 | Contamination (urine, feces, sperm), washing rituals, toilet routine, repeating sentences and questions, hoarding | Fluoxetine (40 mg/d) |
| | | | | | Thioridazine (50 mg/d) |
| | | | | | Alprazolam (4 mg/d) |
| C6 | M | 16 | 37 | Intrusive aggressive images, checking behavior | Clomipramine (225 mg/d) |
| | | | | | Olanzapine (20 mg/d) |
| C7 | F | 20 | 39 | Order and symmetry, cleaning rituals, incompleteness | Clomipramine (75 mg/d) |
| C8 | M | 14 | 40 | Obsessions with dirt and grease, order and symmetry, checking, washing, cleaning, repeating, incompleteness | Venlafaxine (300 mg/d) |
| C9 | M | 12 | 24 | Obsessions about inadvertently harming others, checking, mental compulsions | Clomipramine (100 mg/d) |
| | | | | | Risperidone (4 mg/d) |
| C10 | F | 9 | 29 | Obsessions of causing harm to relatives by having wrong thoughts, compulsive "undoing," compulsive praying, repeating sentences | None |
| C11 | F | 16 | 56 | Obsessions about inadvertently harming others, checking | Clomipramine (225 mg/d) |
| | | | | | Olanzapine (10 mg/d) |
| | | | | | Chlorazepaat (40 mg/d) |
| | | | | | Nitrazepam (10 mg/d) |

implantation. Baseline evaluation included a full psychiatric assessment, a semi-structured interview, and rating scales.

Eleven patients (six female, five male), age 24 to 56 years, were enrolled between 1998 and 2005 (Table 26.1). Mean age at onset was 15 (range 9–24). Mean Y-BOCS score for severity of OCD symptoms before surgery, was

34/40 (range 30–38). Seven of eleven patients were clinically depressed at the time of inclusion. Mean baseline depression score, measured by the Hamilton depression score (17 items) was 23.8 (range 16–43). Two other patients had suffered from a depressive episode in the preceding year. Mean baseline global assessment of functioning (GAF) score was 33 (range 25–40). Mean DBS follow-up time for these patients was 38 months (rang 7–90).

## Neurosurgical Device Implantation

Neurosurgical intervention in all patients was performed by the same neurosurgeon (Bart Nuttin) as fully described elsewhere *(29–31)*. In all patients, quadripolar electrodes Model 3887 Pisces Quad Compact (1.27 mm in diameter, 4 mm contact spacing, 3 mm contact length, Medtronic Inc., Minneapolis, MN) were stereotactically implanted into the anterior limb of the internal capsule bilaterally (Figure 26.1). The four electrode contacts are numbered from 0 (most distal) to 3 (most proximal).

The implantation procedure was done using stereotaxy based on MRI and MR-angiogram to avoid passing unnecessarily through other important functional areas and blood vessels. Prophylactic antibiotics were given. Operations were performed with the patient awake under local anesthesia.

In the first several treated patients, stimulation targets in the internal capsule were similar to those used in anterior capsulotomy *(14, 24)*. The electrode was extended ventrally to the most inferior capsular fibers. Contact 0 was

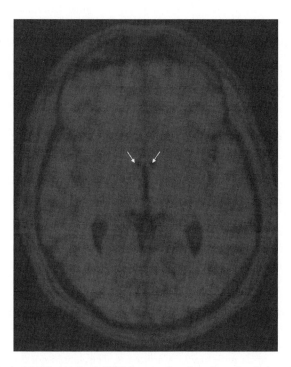

**Figure 26.1** Axial T1-weighted MRI image showing the stimulating electrodes in the anterior limbs of the internal capsules at the level of the anterior commissure. The arrows point to the electrode tract

very near to or in the nucleus accumbens, contacts 1 and 2 were situated in the internal capsule, and contact 3 was sited dorsally to the internal capsule. Bilateral electrodes were placed symmetrically via precoronal burr holes. In the coronal plane contact 0 entered the gray matter at the bottom of the internal capsule. After the third patient showed exceptional improvement *(30)*, the electrode location used in this patient was used as the target for the following patients. The target was somewhat more posterior and medial compared to the published capsulotomy target. Surgery was performed in two stages: after an episode of 2 weeks of initial testing with externalized leads and external programming devices, the electrodes were connected to two implanted pulse generators (IPGs: Itrell II, SynergyTM or KinetraTM, Medtronic Inc.) with subcutaneously tunnelled connecting wires. Depending on the type of implanted IPG, the case of the IPG can be used as the anode. These IPGs were subcutaneously implanted in the subclavicular or abdominal region, in accordance with the patient's preference. Immediate postoperative care included standard medical and surgical considerations used following any stereotactic neurosurgical procedure. Special attention was paid to signs or symptoms of potential surgical complications such as infection, haemorrhage, seizures, or altered mental status. Postoperative CT or MRI was obtained and matched to the pre-operative stereotactic MRI to document the placement of the electrodes.

## Description of Acute Effects

The quadripolar electrodes Model 3887 Pisces Quad Compact allow a multitude of options for contact combinations. Multiple, often transient, acute effects are observed with systematic exploration of various contact combinations, either unilaterally or bilaterally. Some of these have been described previously *(32)*. The exploration of these effects is a very time consuming activity. Frequent consecutive alterations in stimulation parameters induced weariness in all patients. Fatigue and sighing were often observed but it was unclear whether these effects were induced by stimulation using certain contact combinations or weariness due to the prolonged testing session Paresthesias, experienced as a warm feeling in certain body parts or the entire body, sometimes combined with perspiration and flushing, were observed in all patients although the contact combinations and threshold levels at which they appeared differed. Abrupt abolition of stimulation frequently caused a transient hot feeling, perspiration, and flushing.

Changes in affect were most prominent with bilateral stimulation. All patients reported sudden happiness, joy and a good feeling some seconds after stimulation was switched on with particular contact combinations. They smiled and laughed, sometimes extensively. When asked why they were laughing they often could not give a reason. They just felt an inner joy. They sometimes tried to swallow their laughter but this ended in a laughing fit. In four patients unilateral stimulation (both left and right) with the deepest contacts produced transient contralateral contraction of facial muscles resulting in a typical hemi-smile with higher amplitudes. They could not counteract these muscle contractions at will. Bilateral stimulation induced the same happy feeling associated with a transient smile they could barely suppress at will.

In five patients some contact combinations led to a worsening mood, depressive feelings and greater anxiety. Switching stimulation off abolished these feelings.

Six patients were more talkative and talked in a louder voice when stimulated with specific (unilateral and bilateral) contact combinations. Transient verbal perseveration was observed with bilateral stimulation and dysarthria with unilateral stimulation.

Nausea, sudden epigastric sensations and a peculiar sensation in the throat were often although not exclusively reported with unilateral stimulation. Patients often placed hands over their stomach or throat, describing a "lump," "tension," or "queasiness." Monopolar stimulation at several levels induced prolonged but transient muscle contractions in the cheek and neck leading to cramp in three patients. In one patient, torticollis was induced using bilateral stimulation with unequal amplitudes with head turning contralateral to the side of the highest amplitude. One patient reported a transient vaginal muscle contraction with bilateral stimulation while another reported transient sexual arousal.

Both bilateral and unilateral stimulation with the deepest contacts produced a transient smell sensation in three patients. In one of these patients the same contacts at slightly higher amplitudes induced a strange, uneasy feeling in the upper chest producing a fright "as if something invisible hit him." He gave a visible start when this feeling occurred but quieted down easily. Four patients reported an itchy feeling in the back of the nose. Hyperventilation and gasping for breath occurred in 6 patients with unilateral right or bilateral stimulation.

Four patients reported transient unformed visual perceptions such as black or white specks and subtle changes in the color of the walls. Sometimes they had the impression that things moved a bit, that the walls were approaching, or that everything was hazy and deformed. These reports came mostly with unilateral stimulation. Four patients reported auditory perceptions such as "water running," "ringing," "buzzing," and "throbbing."

## Postoperative Contact Selection

To determine the most appropriate contact combination for stimulation, we used a 3-hour long, double-blind crossover protocol with three branches. This protocol was implemented in the first few weeks after surgery. After an initial screening for acute effects with many contact combinations, two contact combinations with positive impact on mood, anxiety or obsessions and compulsions were chosen, based on observations of the evaluators and subjective reports of the patient. These two contact combinations were compared to stimulation off (STIM OFF) in three consecutive randomized sessions. During these sessions, the patient was exposed to a Behavioral Avoidance Test (BAT; ref. *33*) after which he/she completed visual analogue scales (VAS) for obsessions ("To which degree do you have obsessive thoughts at this moment?") and compulsions ("How strong do you feel the urge to engage in compulsive acts at this moment?").

In the BAT, trigger situations that evoke obsessive thoughts are individually chosen and hierarchically ordered from "easy to confront" to "most difficult, certainly not feasible." Patient and evaluator agreed upon a detailed and stepwise

**Table 26.2** Parameters and triggers used in postoperative acute tests.

| | Contacts | Left/right bilateral | Freq (Hz) | PW (microsec) | Ampl (V) | Randomization | BAT: Trigger |
|---|---|---|---|---|---|---|---|
| C4 | Off | — | — | — | — | 2 | Container with chlorine tablets |
| | 1-2+ | Bilateral | 100 | 200 | 7 | 3 | |
| | 0-1-2-3+ | Bilateral | 100 | 200 | 7 | 1 | |
| C5 | Off | — | — | — | — | 1 | Towel swept through toilet |
| | 0-case+ | Bilateral | 120 | 200 | 5 | 3 | |
| | 0-1-2-3+ | Bilateral | 120 | 200 | 6 | 2 | |
| C6 | Off | — | — | — | — | 3 | Sharp scissors |
| | 0-1+ | Bilateral | 100 | 200 | 7 | 1 | |
| | 0-1-2-3+ | Bilateral | 100 | 200 | 7 | 2 | |
| C7 | Off | — | — | — | — | 2 | Turning closet content upside down |
| | 0-1+ | Right | 100 | 210 | 4 | 3 | |
| | 0-1-2-3+ | Right | 100 | 210 | 5 | 1 | |
| C8 | Off | — | — | — | — | 3 | Glass jar with butter |
| | 0-1+ | Bilateral | 120 | 210 | 3 | 1 | |
| | 0-1-2-3+ | Bilateral | 120 | 210 | 4 | 2 | |

Freq, frequency; PW, pulse width; ampl, amplitude; BAT, behavioral assessment test.

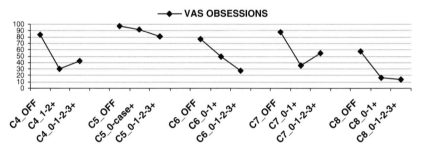

**Figure 26.2** VAS obsessions for five cases in acute tests with different contact combinations. Labeling of the *x*-axis indicates the number of the case and the contact combination used in the session

gradual exposure script. Patients were instructed to expose themselves as far as they could, without overstepping the limits of their capabilities. After completing a step, they were invited to advance to the next one, but it was made explicit that they had full freedom to renounce. Patient and evaluator gave post-hoc preferences (BEST, MEDIUM or WORST) after the third session.

Five patients (cases 4–8) participated in these behavioral, crossover tests to determine appropriate contact combinations (Table 26.2). For one patient, the behavioral assessment was done at home, since her OCD symptoms (ordering and symmetry) manifested themselves only in that location. The other patients were tested in the hospital. VAS scores after exposure at the end of BAT are shown in Figures 26.2 and 26.3.

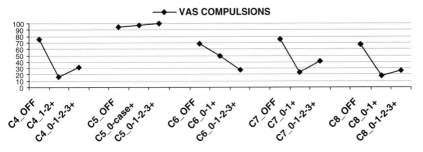

**Figure 26.3** VAS compulsions for five cases in acute tests with different contact combinations. Labeling of the *x*-axis indicates the number of the case and the contact combination used in the session

After the test sessions patient and evaluator agreed on a ranking of overall preference for each setting (STIM OFF and two contact combinations). Consequently the settings were classified as BEST, MEDIUM or WORST. The STIM OFF condition was always ranked WORST. Compared to STIM OFF, mean VAS obsessions decreased by 36% in the MEDIUM session and 53% in the BEST condition, while mean VAS compulsions dropped by 38% in the MEDIUM session and 49% in the BEST session compared to STIM OFF.

## Randomized Double-Blind Crossover

The main objective of this research was to evaluate the effects of capsular stimulation on the severity of OCD symptoms. To differentiate a placebo effect from therapeutic benefit, patients entered a randomized double blind crossover trial with two branches: stimulation on (CROSSOVER-ON) and stimulation off (CROSSOVER-OFF) or vice versa in random order, as determined by an independent person tossing coins. Patients and evaluators were blinded for the stimulation. The protocol of the crossover trial was planned for two episodes of 3 months each, but a safety procedure allowed for abbreviation of an episode if the state of the patient deteriorated beyond baseline condition or if the patient became suicidal. This crossover branch was then shortened and switched to the other condition, without unblinding the patient or evaluators.

Medication was kept at a constant level and no psychotherapy that focuses on OCD (e.g., ERP, flooding) was given until the end of the double blind crossover trial. Patients were allowed and even urged to continue supportive counseling.

Patients were considered responders if they experienced a drop in Y-BOCS of 35% during stimulation, compared to the stimulation "off" branch and if their clinical global impressions (CGI-I) score demonstrated an improvement of at least "much improved."

The electrode implantation in one patient was complicated by an intracerebral hemorrhage around the left electrode, which disturbed the target region. This patient experienced partial improvement of OCD symptoms after surgery without stimulation, probably due to a partial capsulotomy effect, but stimulation induced additional therapeutic benefit over subclinical levels. Because of the combined effect of lesion and stimulation, we excluded this patient from the crossover analysis.

Ten patients served as their own control in this trial with stimulation on (CROSSOVER-ON) and stimulation off (CROSSOVER-OFF). The stimulation parameters used for the crossover were chosen based on assessments and reports of changes in obsessive thoughts and compulsive behavior in daily life.

Contact combinations during the crossover trial were: bilateral 0-1-2-3-case+ ($n = 1$), bilateral 0-1-2-3+ ($n = 2$), bilateral 0-1-2+ ($n = 1$), bilateral 1-2+ ($n = 1$), bilateral 0+1-2+ ($n = 1$), bilateral 0-1+ ($n = 2$), unilateral right 0-1+ ($n = 1$), bilateral 0-case+ ($n = 1$); frequencies were 100 ($n = 7$) or 130 ($n = 3$) Hz; pulse widths were 210 ($n = 5$), 330 ($n = 1$), or 450 ($n = 4$) microseconds, mean amplitude was 6.8 V (range 3.5–10.5 V).

Only four of 10 patients completed the full length of the CROSSOVER-OFF episode. After 2 weeks (four patients), 3 weeks (one patient), and 5 weeks (one patient) dramatic worsening of symptoms induced a premature end of one crossover branch. This implementation of the safety procedure always took place in the CROSSOVER-OFF branch.

The mean Y-BOCS ($n = 10$) at baseline was 33.8 (SD = 3.1). It decreased by 54% from 29.5 (SD = 9.5) during CROSSOVER-OFF to 14.0 (SD = 9.3) during CROSSOVER-ON (Mean difference = 15.5; 95% $CI_{diff}$ = 6.0 to 25.0). Mean HAM-D at baseline was 23.6 (SD = 7.9). It dropped by 61% from 24.5 (SD = 5.6) during CROSSOVER-OFF to 10.2 (SD = 7.2) during CROSSOVER-ON (mean difference = 14.3; 95% $CI_{diff}$ = 5.8 to 21.0).

At the end of CROSSOVER-OFF, CGI scores for Improvement (CGI-I), compared to baseline before surgery were "much worse" ($n = 1$), "slightly worse" ($n = 2$), "the same" ($n = 5$), and "slightly improved" ($n = 1$). At the end of CROSSOVER-ON, CGI-I was "slightly improved" ($n = 2$), "much improved" ($n = 3$), and "very much improved ($n = 5$) compared to baseline. Eight of 10 patients fulfilled criteria for responders.

## Long-Term Follow-Up

After the first year of DBS, we continued to evaluate the long-term outcome of capsular stimulation. Standard visits were scheduled at 1, 3, 6, 9, and 12 months in the first year. Thereafter, they were evaluated at least once yearly. Patients could ask for supplementary visits if they felt the need. If necessary, in the opinion of a member of the multidisciplinary team, additional visits were scheduled as well. Separate qualitative information was gathered from close significant others, especially during the first years of stimulation, to complete data on current functioning and behavioral changes.

The mean number of visits for psychiatric evaluation after surgery was 11 (range 6–15) in the first year, 5 (range 4–9) in the second year, and 4 (range 1–7) in the following follow-up years 3 to 7. Multiple visits for adjustment of parameters were required: 14 (range 6–24) in the first year; 9 (range 4–15) in the second year; and 7 (range 1–14) in the following follow-up years 3 to 7. Two patients had their devices (electrodes, extension wires, and IPGs) removed, after 15 and 40 months respectively and opted for a subsequent capsulotomy. For the follow-up analysis in Figure 26.4, only the YBOCS scores of the patients who continue on DBS are included.

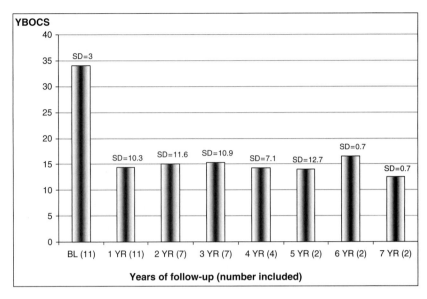

**Figure 26.4** YBOCS scores during follow-up for DBS. *x*-axis indicates years of follow-up with the number of patients included in this follow-up provided in brackets. BL, baseline

At their last psychiatric evaluation, with a follow-up time of between 12 and 84 months, mean YBOCS for the 11 patients (nine DBS, two capsulotomy) dropped by 65% from 34 (SD = 3.0) at baseline to 12 (SD = 10.3). At the most recent evaluation, of the nine patients who continue to receive capsular stimulation, five have subclinical OCD symptoms (YBOCS score between 1 and 7), three have mild OCD symptoms (YBOCS score between 8 and 15), and one has moderate symptoms (YBOCS score between 16 and 23). On the CGI, one patient has only very mild symptoms, four patients have mild symptoms without functional impairment, three patients have mild symptoms with mild impairment in daily functioning, and one patient has moderate symptoms. As long as patients are stimulated no worsening of symptoms compared to baseline has been observed. It is only when stimulation fails or is switched off that symptoms have deteriorated to baseline levels (eight patients) or become worse than at baseline (one patient).

## Complications and Adverse Effects

Side effects are a major potential concern with capsular stimulation. Surgically related adverse effects were observed in four patients. In one patient an intracranial haemorrhage around the left electrode track was detected the day after surgery. Although it gradually resolved on CT in the week following implantation, it caused profound apathy that gradually resolved over 3 months. One patient had more than usual swelling of the face for four days after surgery. This was prophylactically treated with antibiotics for 1 week even though cultures of aspirated subcutaneous fluid remained sterile. One patient had a subcutaneous hematoma around both eyes, which resolved without special care.

One patient complained of major pain after implantation of the IPGs and needed pain medications for 5 days after surgery. Sensations in the region of the burr holes or the extension wires in the neck region varied from numbness (two patients) and tingling (four patients) to a transient stinging sensation when patients moved their head (five patients).

**Acute Adverse Effects of Stimulation**

Transient acute effects were often experienced immediately after starting capsular stimulation. If side effects persisted stimulation amplitude was lowered or stimulation with the contact combination that induced them was aborted. Subjective feelings of joy and happiness or sadness, anxiety and nervousness or relief of anxiety, somatic sensations (smell, vision, hearing, muscular, throat, epigastric, warmth, tingling, vaginal contraction), sleepiness and dizziness and sudden peculiar thoughts (out of context, with sexual content) were reported on several occasions. Objective signs of laughing, crying, dysarthria, verbal perseveration, yawning, sighing, hyperventilation, dyskinesias, muscle contractions of face and neck, and flushing were observed.

**Adverse Effects Linked to Battery Life or IPGs Switched Off**

Due to the high current densities required in some patients to obtain optimal therapeutic benefit, battery life was restricted (between 5 and 18 months). The battery is an integral part of the IPG and the entire IPG unit requires replacement when batteries run down. This requires a minor surgical procedure under local anesthesia. Since OCD symptoms return with former intensity and patients abruptly become severely depressed within hours to days after battery failure, they require urgent replacement. Cognitive distortions may prevent them from identifying the cause of their suffering. After experiencing improvement with DBS, they often lost or could no longer evoke mechanisms they had previously developed to cope with severe OCD symptoms. Suicidal thoughts and desperate feelings dominated and crisis intervention was necessary on several occasions.

During the CROSSOVER-OFF period, one patient made a suicide attempt by overdosing with sertraline. Another patient experienced a severe worsening of mood with acute suicidal ideation immediately after starting the CROSSOVER-OFF branch and when batteries ran out for the first time.

After battery replacement and reinstitution of the original parameters, we witnessed amplitude-dependent behavioral disinhibition in four patients. They felt very happy and euphoric but made tactless remarks and sometimes recklessly acted on impulse. They were hyperactive but failed to plan and exhibited little concern about their illness or future. They lacked empathy and showed less concern for feelings of others. There was a lack of social restraint and an undue familiarity with strangers. Despite these marked behavioral alterations, they had no neuropsychological deficits and language and memory skills remained intact.

This abnormal behavior pattern subsided spontaneously after several days, but on one occasion, it continued for 2 weeks and normalized only after reduction of the stimulus amplitude. When questioned about this period the patient remembered the hyperactivity and happiness but denied disinhibition, recklessness, or aggression.

## Adverse Effects With Chronic Stimulation

After 1 year, weight increased in six patients (6 to 16 kg) and decreased in two patients (7 and 12 kg). Two patients each had two transient episodes of urinary incontinence that lasted for several weeks. Daytime incontinence was controlled with oxybutynin. An episode of nocturnal urinary incontinence disappeared after discontinuing trazodone. Three patients reported changes in sleeping patterns. One patient became active and energetic during daytime, but sleep need increased after 4 hours. She sleeps 12 hours nightly but requires a daytime nap. One patient experienced transient excessive fatigue during a 1-month episode following 5 hyperactive days occurring after battery replacement. He slept 10 to 12 hours a night and took daily naps before surgery, mostly to let time pass more quickly. His sleep need remained essentially unchanged but after surgery he did not wish to waste time in bed any longer. One patient had very vivid dreams and nightmares during the first few months of stimulation.

Patients and family members sometimes reported changes in behavior during stimulation. According to his partner, one patient became detached and maintained more of a distance while the patient denied being less emotionally involved. Nervousness, increased irritability leading to conflicts and verbal aggression, overconfidence, inaccurate risk assessment, and clumsiness were reported on several occasions. If complaints were persistent and intrusive, stimulation parameters were adjusted and were all reversible.

It is important to appreciate that all patients had suffered from suicidal ideations at some point in the course of their illness before considering neurosurgical treatment, although at the time of surgery, suicidality was not prominent. One patient expressed suicidal thoughts after 57 months in the trial and took a small overdose of trazodone (three 100-mg tablets) together with alcohol. She was admitted to hospital for crisis intervention. She stated that she did not want to kill herself but marital conflicts were excessive and she needed rest. After 8 months in the trial another patient sent an e-mail threatening to commit suicide because his girlfriend left him. Crisis intervention and a course of interpersonal therapy prevented further harm. One patient complained of memory problems for some time after surgery but neuropsychological tests could not objectify this. Five patients reported an increase in sexual thoughts and fantasies, without increased frequency of sexual activity and one patient had a minor decrease in sexual interest.

## Adverse Effects Linked to Hardware Failure

One patient required replacement of a malfunctioning electrode 45 months after surgery. She experienced a sudden, moderate increase in obsessions and compulsions, an increase in general anxiety and a severe worsening of mood, which prompted crisis hospitalization. X-ray documented an interruption in the left electrode just beneath the cranium. Traction on the electrode caused by a short extension wire was postulated as the cause. The electrode was replaced and the extension wire was substituted with a longer one. In one patient a contact of the left electrode malfunctioned soon after implantation. As a result, not all contact combinations could be implemented and tested. This resulted in asymmetric stimulation parameters. Moreover, 17 months after surgery, a failure in the left extension wire caused complete abortion of left-sided stimulation. Both extension wires were substituted with longer wires.

## Conclusion

Research regarding electrical stimulation in the anterior limb of the internal capsule for treatment refractory OCD overcomes two major and reasonable objections against the use of stereotactic neurosurgical lesioning procedures in psychiatric disorders. Electrical stimulation is reversible and prospective double blind randomised controlled trials can be implemented to demonstrate efficacy.

In the multidisciplinary study reported here, eleven patients with severe, treatment refractory OCD were studied. We demonstrated in a double-blind, randomized crossover protocol that electrical stimulation in the anterior limb of the internal capsule produces clinically significant therapeutic benefit in patients with severe, treatment refractory OCD. Other groups, in smaller case series, have also demonstrated symptomatic improvement following capsular or nucleus accumbens DBS for OCD *(34, 35)*. Capsular stimulation not only leads to a substantial decrease in the severity of OCD symptoms, it also has a beneficial impact on the patient's mood scores. Although frequently observed, side effects are acceptable compared to capsulotomy. Some side effects, especially overconfidence and disinhibition, are amplitude-dependent, reversible and appear to be linked to the therapeutic benefits.

With continuous capsular stimulation, improvement in everyday quality of life is apparent but not always proportional to therapeutic effects on OCD symptoms. Issues not directly affected by symptom reduction may concomitantly influence improvement of psychosocial state, role functioning and social and economic status. A structured program of psychiatric aftercare and extensive psycho-education, both for patients and responsible caregivers are indispensable in this context.

Treatment of OCD patients with capsular stimulation remains investigational and is not considered standard therapy. It necessitates considerable commitment by a multidisciplinary team and motivated patients. To this end, we have participated in the formation of the "DBS-OCD collaborative group" *(36)*. This multidisciplinary, multicenter group was established in an effort to combine expertise and limit indiscriminate and widespread application of electrical brain stimulation before adequate long-term safety data are available and to ensure adequate human subject protection while providing access to this treatment.

## References

1. Rasmussen SA, Eisen JL (1992) The epidemiology and clinical features of obsessive-compulsive disorder. Psychiatr Clin North Am 15:743–758.
2. Rasmussen SA, Tsuang MT (1984) The epidemiology of obsessive-compulsive disorder. J Clin Psychiatry 45:450–457.
3. Zitterl W, Demai U, Aigner M, et al (2000) Naturalistic course of obsessive compulsive disorder and co-morbid depression. Psychopathology 33:75–80.
4. Steketee G, Foa EB, Grayson JB (1982) Recent advances in the behavioral treatment of obsessive-compulsives. Arch Gen Psychiatry 39:1365–1371.
5. Eisen JL, Goodman WK, Keller MB, et al (1999) Patterns of remission and relapse in obsessive-compulsive disorder: a 2-year prospective study. J Clin Psychiatry 60:346–352.

6. McDougle CJ, Epperson CN, Pelton GH, et al (2000) A double blind, placebo-controlled study of risperidone addition in serotonin reuptake inhibitor-refractory obsessive-compulsive disorder. Arch Gen Psychiatry 57:794–801.
7. Francobandiera G (2001) Olanzapine augmentation of serotonin uptake inhibitors in obsessive-compulsive disorder: an open study. Can J Psychiatry 46:356–358.
8. Foa EB, Kozak MJ (1996) Obsessive-compulsive disorder: long-term outcome of psychological treatment. In Mavissakalian, Prien, eds. Long-term Treatments of Anxiety Disorders. Washington, DC: American Psychiatric Press, pp. 285–309.
9. Mindus P (1993) Present-Day indications for Capsulotomy. Acta Neurochir 58(suppl):29–33.
10. Mindus P (1991) Capsulotomy in anxiety disorders. A multidisciplinary study. Thesis-monograph. Kongl Carolinska Medico Chirurgiska Institutet. Stockholm, Sweden: Caslon Press.
11. Jenike MA (1998) Neurosurgical treatment of obsessive-compulsive disorder. Br J Psychiatry 173(Suppl 35):79–90.
12. Meyerson BA (1998) Neurosurgical treatment of mental disorders. Introduction and indications. In: Gildenberg PL, Tasker RR, eds. Tekstbook of stereotactic and functional neurosurgery. New York: McGraw-Hill, pp. 1955–1964.
13. Mindus P, Meyerson B (1995) Anterior capsulotomy for intractable anxiety disorders. In: Schmidek H, Sweet W, eds. Operative Neurosurgical Techniques, Indications, Methods and Results, third edition. Philadelphia: W.B. Saunders Company, pp. 1413–1421.
14. Lippitz B, Mindus P, Meyerson B, Kihlström L, Lindquist CH (1999) Lesion topography and outcome after thermocapsulotomy and gamma knife capsulotomie for obsessive-compulsive disorder: relevance of the right hemisphere. Neurosurgery 44:452–460.
15. Rappaport ZH (1992) Psychosurgery in the modern era. Therapeutic and ethical aspects. Med Law 11:449–453.
16. Stagno SJ, Smith ML, Hassenbusch SJ (1994) Reconsidering "psychosurgery": issues of informed consent and physician responsibility. J Clin Ethics 5:217–223.
17. Tan E, Marks IM, Marset P (1971) Bi-medial leukotomy in obsessive-compulsive neurosis: a controlled serial enquiry. Br J Psychiatry 118:155–164.
18. Kullberg G (1977) Differences in effect of capsulotomy and cingulotomy. In: Sweet WH, Obrador S, Martin-Rodriguez JG, eds. Neurosurgical treatment in psychiatry, pain, and epilepsy. Baltimore: University Park Press, pp. 301–308.
19. Hay P, Sachdev P, Cumming S, et al (1993) Treatment of obsessive-compulsive disorder by psychosurgery. Acta Psychiatr Scand 87:197–207.
20. Sachdev P, Hay P (1995) Does neurosurgery for obsessive-compulsive disorder produce personality change? J Nerv Ment Dis 183:408–413.
21. Irle E, Exner C, Thielen K, et al (1998) Obsessive-compulsive disorder and ventromedial frontal lesions: clinical and neuropsychological findings. Am J Psychiatry 155:255–263.
22. Albucher R, Curtis G, Pitts K (1999) Neurosurgery for obsessive-compulsive disorder: problem with co-morbidity. Letter Am J Psychiatry 156:495–496.
23. American Psychiatric Association (1994) Diagnostic and statistical manual of mental disorders, fourth ed. Washington, DC: American Psychiatric Association Press.
24. Cosyns P, Caemaert J, Haaijman W, et al (1994) Functional stereotactic neurosurgery for psychiatric disorders: an experience in Belgium and The Netherlands. In: Symons L et al., ed. Advances and Technical Standards in Neurosurgery. Wien-New York: Springer Verlag, pp. 242–279.
25. Gybels J, Cosyns P (2000) Cerebral lesions for psychiatric disorders and pain. In: Schmidek H, Sweet WH, eds. Operative Neurosurgical Techniques, fourth ed. Pennsylvania: WB Saunders Science Company, pp. 1660–1669.

26. Goodman WK, Price LH, Rasmussen SA, et al (1989) The Yale-Brown Obsessive Compulsive scale; I. Development, use and reliability. Arch Gen Psychiatry 46:1006–1011.
27. Goodman WK, Price LH, Rasmussen SA, et al (1989) The Yale-Brown Obsessive Compulsive scale; II. Validity. Arch Gen Psychiatry 46:1012–1016.
28. First MB, Gibbon MSW, Spitzer RL, Williams JBW, Smith BL (1997) User's guide for the structured clinical interview for DSM-IV axis II personality disorders. Washington, DC: American Psychiatric Press.
29. Gabriëls L, Cosyns P, Nuttin B, et al (2003) Deep brain stimulation for treatment-refractory obsessive-compulsive disorder: psychopathological and neuropsychological outcome in 3 cases. Acta Psychiatr Scand 107:1–8.
30. Nuttin B, Cosyns P, Demeulemeester H, et al (1999) Electrical stimulation in anterior limbs of internal capsules in patients with obsessive-compulsive disorder. Lancet 354:1526.
31. Nuttin B, Gabriëls LA, Cosyns PR, et al (2003) Long-term electrical capsular stimulation in patients with obsessive-compulsive disorder. Neurosurgery 52(6):1263–1274.
32. Nuttin BJ, Gabriëls L, van Kuyck K, Cosyns P (2003) Electrical stimulation of the anterior limbs of the internal capsules in patients with severe obsessive-compulsive disorder: anecdotical reports. Neurosurg Clin N Am 14:267–274.
33. Steketee G, Chambless DL, Tran GQ, Worden H, Gillis MM (1996) Behavioral avoidance test for obsessive-compulsive disorder. Behav Res Ther 34:73–83.
34. Greenberg BD, Malone DA, Friehs GM, et al (2006) Three-year outcomes in deep brain stimulation for highly resistant obsessive-compulsive disorder. Neuropsychopharmacology 31(11):2384–2393.
35. Abelson JL, Curtis GC, Sagher O et al (2005) Deep brain stimulation for refractory obsessive-compulsive disorder. Biol Psychiatry 57(5):510–516.
36. Nuttin BJ, Gybels J, Cosyns PR, et al (2002) The OCD-DBS Collaborative Group: Deep brain stimulation for psychiatric disorders. Neurosurgery 51(2):519.

# 27

# Deep Brain Stimulation for Medically Intractable Cluster Headache

Philip A. Starr and Andrew Ahn

## Abstract

Cluster headache (CH) is the most severe of the primary headache disorders. It affects approximately 1 in 1000 persons, and 20% of patients are significantly disabled in spite of optimal medical therapy *(1)*. Peripheral nerve ablation procedures have been performed for CH, with little benefit. Positron emission tomography (PET) using $H_2^{15}O$ as the tracer has shown a focal increase in cerebral blood flow in the ipsilateral posterior hypothalamic region during a CH attack *(2, 3)*. Based on this finding, in 2000 a promising new surgical procedure for severe CH was introduced in Milan, Italy: chronic deep brain stimulation (DBS) of the posterior hypothalamic region *(4)*. Three open-label case series have been published, two from European centers and a third from our own *(5–7)*. Additional scattered case reports are beginning to emerge *(8, 9)*. In the three case series, most patients received major benefit, but approximately 25% of patients were nonresponders.

Many aspects of this novel therapy remain to be elucidated, including the actual proportion of patients who respond favorably, the degree and duration of response, presurgical predictors of outcome, the mechanism of action, the time course of onset and washout of the therapeutic effect, optimal programming parameters, and the the safety of the procedure. Currently, no commercial DBS device has U.S. or European regulatory approval for this emerging indication. This chapter reviews the relevant features of CH, surgical indications for DBS, surgical techniques, clinical outcomes, and possible mechanism of action.

**Keywords:** cluster headache, deep brain stimulation, hypothalamus, stereotactic neurosurgery

## Overview of Cluster Headache

CH is a primary headache disorder characterized by recurrent attacks of excruciating unilateral periorbital pain, usually with evidence of disturbed ipsilateral cranial autonomic activity, including lacrimation, conjunctival injection, ptosis, or meiosis *(10)*. Attacks may occur from once every other day to eight times a day and last 15 to 180 minutes. Attacks tend to occur at regular times of the day. The prevalence of CH is approximately 0.2% *(1)*. In the episodic form of CH, affecting 80 to 90% of patients, attacks occur seasonally, with periods of complete remission. In the chronic form, affecting 10 to 20% of patients, remissions do not occur or last less than 1 month *(11)*. During the active period of headache attacks, a CH attack may be triggered by sublingual nitroglycerin, which has also been used to experimentally trigger attacks *(12)*. Alcohol consumption is also a common trigger and this history is considered useful diagnostically.

Prophylactic medical therapy of CH includes verapamil, ergot derivatives such as methysergide, lithium carbonate, divalproic acid, melatonin, and corticosteriods *(11)*. Abortive medical therapy includes the use of 100% oxygen, injectable sumatriptan, ergotomines, indomethacin, intranasal lidocaine or capsaicin, corticosteroids and opiate medications *(11)*. Among those patients who fail medical therapy, the chronic form is disproportionately represented, and those who have had chronic CH for at least 1 year are unlikely to have a spontaneous remission in the following year *(13)*.

Prior to 2000, surgical therapy for CH was directed at interruption of the trigeminal nerve by chemical ablation, balloon compression, partial or complete surgical sectioning of the trigeminal root *(14)*, or radiosurgical ablation of the trigeminal dorsal root entry zone *(15)*. The results of these procedures have been disappointing, with a low rate of persistent headache relief and a high rate of facial anesthesia. In addition, there are case reports of patients with CH who had no relief of pain with complete interruption of the trigeminal nerve, despite having complete facial anesthesia, indicating that peripheral nociception is not necessary to the experience of pain in CH *(16, 17)*.

## Evidence for Hypothalamic Involvement in CH

The striking seasonal and circadian pattern of cluster attacks suggests involvement of hypothalamic centers. Recently, both structural and functional imaging have provided evidence for specific abnormalities in the hypothalamic area in CH. Voxel-based MRI morphometry has shown an increase in the size of the ipsilateral posterior hypothalamic grey matter in 25 patients with CH, compared with 29 healthy controls *(18)*. Positron Emission Tomography (PET) using $H_2^{15}O$ has shown increased regional cerebral blood flow (rCBF) in the ipsilateral posterior hypothalamus/periventricular gray area in nine CH patients during nitroglycerin-induced CH attacks, in comparison with eight control CH patients who were not having headache *(2, 3)*. Significant increases in rCBF in this region have also been shown in an individual CH patient during a spontaneous headache, in comparison with the same individual without headache *(19)*. The results of SPECT imaging in CH have been inconsistent *(20)*. Functional MRI (fMRI) has been used to study isolated cases of headache disorders closely related to CH, included under the broader heading of trigeminal autonomic cephalgia *(21–23)*. fMRI has shown blood oxygen level dependent (BOLD) contrast changes in the ipsilateral hypothalamic area during spontaneous pain attacks in these disorders.

## Indications for DBS

The European group who developed this procedure has published guidelines for surgical treatment *(24)*. These criteria emphasize the need for the accurate diagnosis of the disorder, failure of standard medical therapy at maximally tolerated doses, and the exclusion of those in whom the natural course of spontaneous or episodic remissions would be mistaken for a DBS treatment response. Our own criteria, modified and expanded from the published guidelines, are as follows.

### Inclusion Criteria

1. Patients must meet the International Headache Society (IHS) diagnostic criteria for CH *(10)*.
2. At least six debilitating headaches per week, which should be rated by the patient at least 6 on a visual analog scale of 1 to 10.
3. Inadequate relief from prophylactic therapy, to include: verapamil, lithium, divalproex sodium, methysergide, topiramate, gabapentin, nonsteroidal anti-inflammatory agents including indomethacin, and short-term use of corticosteroids.
4. Inadequate relief from abortive therapy, to include: oxygen, sumatriptan, opiates.
5. Chronic form of CH for at least 2 years, with headache always lateralizing to the same side.
6. Successful completion of daily headache diaries over a 1-month period prior to surgery, to measure preoperative headache characteristics.

### Exclusion Criteria

1. Serious untreated psychiatric co-morbidity.
2. Any medical condition that increases the risk of stereotactic neurosurgery, including untreated hypertension, coagulopathy, severe diabetes, serious cardiac or pulmonary disease, or medical need for chronic anticoagulation with coumadin.
3. Any medical condition that greatly limits the life expectancy of the patient.
4. A concomitant headache disorder distinct from CH, such as migraine, which affects the patient greater than twice per month.
5. Any other serious chronic neurologic disorder (such as epilepsy, multiple sclerosis, degenerative brain disease).
6. Inability to undergo screening brain MRI.
7. Screening MRI showing a brain mass, prior stroke, brain atrophy out of proportion to age, small vessel ischemic disease, or ectatic blood vessels near the stereotactic target.
8. Age less than 18 or more than 75.
9. Pregnancy.

## Pre- and Postoperative Evaluation

Our patients undergo a screening visit with a headache neurologist as well as the neurosurgeon to examine inclusion and exclusion criteria for surgical therapy. Prior to surgery, patients are required to complete headache diaries daily for four consecutive weeks in the month prior to surgery, during the first 3 months after surgery, and during the 6th and 12th month following surgery. Patients were carefully instructed on how to score their daily headache diary: the time of day each headache episode occurred; the duration of the headache; the intensity of headache on a visual-analog scale of 1 to 10 (1, slight pain; 10, worst imaginable pain); and the use of abortive and prophylactic medications. Patients were also instructed to make note of headaches that were not characteristic of their usual cluster attacks, in order to screen for the presence of other concurrent primary headache disorders. Headache characteristics are averaged from headache diaries over a one month period. In our practice, patients are considered "responders" to DBS therapy if at the 1-year time point, there is a more than 50% reduction in headache frequency, intensity, or both, compared to the pre-operative baseline.

## Surgical Technique

The surgical technique is similar to that used for placement of DBS electrodes into the basal ganglia for treatment of movement disorders: MRI based stereotaxy, microelectrode recording in the region of the MRI-defined target, and intraoperative test stimulation using an external pulse generator to define voltage thresholds for stimulation-induced adverse effects (25). Intravenous sedation is used during the initial surgical exposure. Sedation is not normally used for microelectrode recording or test stimulation.

### Defining the Brain Target by Brain Atlas and by MRI

Following placement of the stereotactic headframe (Leksell series G, Elekta, Inc.), MRI is performed on a 1.5T scanner (Phillips Intera, Best, the Netherlands). Two MR image sets are obtained: a volumetric gadolinium-enhanced gradient echo (3D-GRE) MRI covering the whole brain in 1.5 mm axial slices, which is mainly for trajectory planning and visualization of the anterior and posterior commissures (parameters: TR = 20, TE = 2.9, matrix = 256×192, flip angle = 3, NEX = 1); a T2-weighted fast spin echo (T2FSE) sequence, limited to the diencephalon and midbrain, in the axial plane at 2-mm slice thickness. The T2FSE scan is mainly for visualizing structural detail in the immediate vicinity of the brain target, the mammillothalamic tract (MTT) and the red nucleus. (parameters: TR = 3000, TE = 90, matrix = 268x512, NEX = 6, bandwidth = 183 Hz/pixel, interleaved). Both image sets are imported into a stereotactic surgical planning software package (Framelink version 4.1, Medtronic-SNT, Boulder, CO), computationally fused, and reformatted to produce images orthogonal to the anterior commissure-posterior commissure (AC-PC) line and midsagittal planes.

As reported by the Milan group (26), the anatomic target in commissural coordinates is 2 mm lateral to the midline, 5 mm inferior to the axial plane containing anterior and posterior commissures, and 3 mm posterior to the midcommissural point. This target was selected to correspond to the brain region that showed increased rCBF on $H_2^{15}O$ PET during CH attacks in the study of May et al (3). The target is plotted in Figure 27.1 with respect to the appropriate axial slice from the Schaltenbrand and Warren human brain atlas (27). This brain slice (which is slightly oblique with respect to

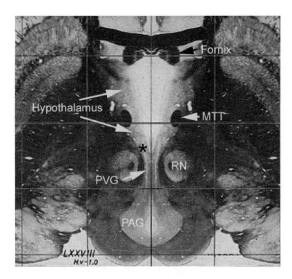

**Figure 27.1** Anatomy of the hypothalamus, periventricular gray (PVG) and periaqueductal gray (PAG), from the Schaltenbrand and Warren human brain atlas *(27)*. MTT, mammillothalamic tract; RN, red nucleus. The asterisk marks the target point for DBS in cluster headache, based on the work of Franzini et al. *(26)*. Reprinted from ref. 7 with permission

the commissural plane) shows the continuous rim of grey matter lining the inferior wall of the third ventricle and the upper Sylvian aqueduct. This continuum includes the hypothalamus proper, the periventricular grey (PVG) and the periaqueductal grey. The asterisk in Figure 27.1 indicates the Milan DBS target, which has been the surgical target in all published series. Some anatomists consider the MTT as the posterior border of the hypothalamus *(27, 28)*, but some human brain atlases depict the hypothalamus as extending several mm posterior to the MTT *(29)*. There is no consensus among anatomists regarding the precise border between the hypothalamus and the PVG *(28)*. Therefore, the "hypothalamic" DBS target published by the Milan group could be considered to be either in the posterior hypothalamus or the anterior PVG.

To account for possible variations in diencephalic anatomy that may affect target coordinates as measured from the commissures, we utilize the T2FSE sequence to confirm that the intended target point is located 3 to 5 mm posterior to the MTT and is medial to the anterior border of the red nucleus, on the axial plane 5 mm inferior to the intercommissural line. The AC-PC based coordinates are modified, if needed, to ensure that the anatomic target lies in a consistent relationship to the MTT and red nucleus.

A "default" trajectory through the brain is set at 60° from the AC-PC line in the sagittal projection and 10° lateral from the vertical in the coronal projection. This trajectory is visualized on the Gadolinium-enhanced volumetric MRI. Small adjustments in the arc and ring angles are then made to avoid traversing sulci, lateral ventricle, cortical veins, and dural venous lakes.

### 27.6.2 Single Unit Recording

A single microelectrode penetration is made to the steretotactic target, whose primary purpose is to provide physiological confirmation of the appropriate trajectory and depth of the DBS electrode. Examples of spontaneous single unit discharge in the target region are shown in Figure 27.2. In our limited series, the target area is characterized by sparse, low amplitude, wide action potentials in a regular pattern at frequency less than 20 Hz and often less than 5 Hz. The inferior boundary of the target is marked either by the interpeduncular cistern or the red nucleus, depending on the angulation of the lead and the patient's individual anatomy. If the most distal segment of the recording shows electrical silence (characteristic of cisternal entry) or dense neuronal units with narrow action potentials and high frequency discharge 30 to 50 Hz (characteristic of the red nucleus), the recording is stopped and the lead depth accordingly adjusted slightly more superiorly. Continued advancement of a microelectrode into a region of electrical silence beyond the target is not recommended due to proximity to the basilar artery bifurcation and associated perforating branches.

**Lead Placement and Intra-operative Test Stimulation**

Following confirmation of target depth with microelectrode recording, the permanent lead is placed. We have used the Medtronic model 3387 lead (contacts spaced over 10.5 mm) while others have used the smaller model 3389 lead (contacts spaced over 7.5 mm). Test stimulation is performed in bipolar mode using contacts 0-, 3+, 185 Hz, and 60 μs pulse width (model 3625 external tester, Medtronic, Inc., Minneapolis, MN). After cautioning the patient about potential stimulation induced sensations (double vision, dizziness, vertigo, mood changes) voltage is increased at 0.5 V/sec up to 6 V, during continuous

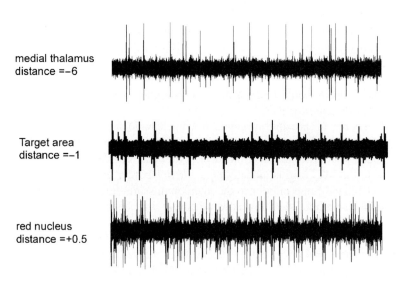

**Figure 27.2** Two second segment of single unit microelectrode recordings 6 mm dorsal, 1 mm dorsal, and 0.5 mm beyond the stereotactic target

examination of the patient's cranial nerve function. Voltage threshold for oculomotor disturbance or subjective phenomena such as mood change are noted. The patient's blood pressure and pulse are carefully monitored during test stimulation, although no changes in vital signs have been noted during our preliminary studies. A threshold for oculomotor disturbance (typically gaze paralysis, skew deviation, nystagmus or subjective double vision) of 2 to 6 V is consistent with lead placement at the intended target. Some patients experience dysphoria at more than 3 V.

**Lead Anchoring and IPG Placement**

Leads are anchored to the skull with a lead anchoring device (Stim-lock, Medtronic Inc.). After scalp closure and headframe removal, general anesthesia is induced for placement of the lead extender and pulse generator (Soletra, Medtronic Inc., Minneapolis, MN).

## Documentation of Electrode Locations

Postoperative MRI to demonstrate the location of the electrode tip is performed in all cases, according to the published safety guidelines for performing brain MRI in patients with implanted DBS systems *(30, 31)*. Figure 27.3 shows the typical location of the electrode tip on axial MRI, 5 mm inferior to the intercommissural line, from our series. In this axial plane, the mean (+/− standard deviation) distance of the lead posterior to the MTT is 4.8 +/− 0.9 mm (*N* = 7 cases).

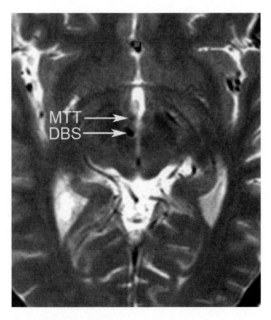

**Figure 27.3** DBS electrode location on postoperative MRI (axial T2-weighted fast spin echo). The white arrows indicate the locations of the mammillothalamic tract (MTT) and the tip of the DBS electrode. Reprinted from ref. *7* with permission

## Device Programming

Programming parameters in our patients were based on the two previously published case series (6, 26): Monopolar stimulation, pulse width of 60 μsec, frequency 185 Hz, voltage 1 to 3 V (stopping short of the threshold for acute persistent stimulation-induced adverse effects). Devices were kept activated at all times postoperatively. Our detailed postoperative programming protocol is given in Table 27.1.

## Clinical Outcomes

The short-term clinical outcomes of DBS for CH appear promising in many but not all patients. The most recent publication from the Milan series includes 16 patients with a mean follow-up time of 23 months (5). Patients were not followed using headache diaries, quality of life measures, or other standardized tools. Ten patients were reported to be pain free, three more "almost pain free" while the remaining three are "improved." Formal blinded trials with DBS on and off were not performed. However, several patients had inadvertent

**Table 27.1** Protocol for stimulator programming (Medtronic Soletra).

| Programming visit | Programming algorithm |
|---|---|
| Week 0 (1 week post-surgery) | 1. Activate the device in monopolar mode using pw = 60 μsec, frequency = 185 Hz. Record voltage threshold for stimulation-induced adverse effects (typically dizziness or visual disturbance), at all contacts in monopolar mode. |
| | 2. Review postoperative MRI to determine which contact is closest to the intended target (usually contact 0 or 1), and select this contact. Slowly increase the voltage up to 2.0 V, or to 0.1 V less than the threshold for persistent side effects, whichever is higher. |
| | 3. Verify normal impedances and battery life using the programmer. |
| Weeks 4, 8, 12, 26 | 1. Review headache diaries. If debilitating headaches have persisted in the prior month, increase voltage by 0.5 V, or to 0.1 V less than the threshold for persistent side effects whichever is greater. |
| | 2. If the patient has reached 3.0 V without headache relief, switch contact choice to the next most superior contact. Slowly increase the voltage up to 3.0 V, or to 0.1 V less than the threshold for persistent side effects, whichever is greater. |
| | 3. Verify normal impedances and battery life using the programmer. |

Abbreviations: PW, pulse width; V, voltage.

inactivation of the device (due to electrical malfunction of the device) with recurrence of attacks, indicating that the benefit of stimulation was unlikely to be due to placebo. A detailed 4-year follow up on their initial patient cohort was recently published, showing that the headache attacks have been consistently eliminated with the stimulator on *(17)*.

A group in Liege, Belgium reported on four of their six implanted patients with a mean clinical follow-up of 14.5 months *(6)*. Two of the four are free of headache attacks; a third had the frequency of attacks reduced to less than three per month, while the fourth has had only transient benefit with each reprogramming session.

Our own series includes seven patients, with follow-up presently available on the first five (Table 27.2). Patients were followed using headache diaries in which the frequency, intensity, and duration of headaches were recorded daily for 1 month prior to surgery and for 1 month at the 6- and 12-month follow-up times. The length of follow-up is 12 months for the first four patients and 6 months for the final patient. Three of five patients (cases 1, 2, and 5) may be considered "responders" based on a more than 50% reduction in headache frequency, intensity, or both. One of the three responders (case 2) had been using sumatripitan injections to reduce the intensity and duration of each headache, and has not required any abortive therapy postoperatively due to the much lower intensity. Case 3 had transient complete suppression of headaches for 1 to 2 weeks following each re-programming session, but no persistent benefit in headaches, or reduction in abortive therapy, in the intervals between programming changes. He no longer uses the device. Case 4 has had a 30% reduction in headache intensity, which failed to meet the 50% threshold to be considered a "responder."

In sum, these open-label series indicate that 50 to 75% of CH patients have substantial relief of headache symptoms 1 to 2 years postoperatively.

**Table 27.2** Outcome of hypothalamic DBS for CH in five patients. The percentage change in headache parameters compared to the baseline preoperative status is given in parentheses. Headache intensity is rated on a 1 to 10 visual analog scale with 10 equal to the most severe possible pain, and 1 equal to the mildest perceivable pain. The mean values are averaged from all headaches in a 1-week period as reported on headache diaries completed daily at home. Cases 1, 2, and 5 are considered "responders" to DBS based on a more than 50% reduction in headache intensity or frequency.

| | | PRE-OPERATIVE | | MOST RECENT F/U | |
|---|---|---|---|---|---|
| Case no. | Length of f/u (months) | # HA in week | Mean HA intensity (VAS 1–10) | # HA in week | Mean HA intensity (VAS 1–10) |
| 1 | 12 | 13 | 6.7 | 12 (−8%) | 2.6 (−61%) |
| 2 | 12 | 22 | 4.9 | 4 (−82%) | 2.5 (−49%) |
| 3 | 12 | 16 | 7.5 | 16 (0%) | 7.5 (0%) |
| 4 | 12 | 51 | 6.4 | 56 (+10%) | 4.0 (−37.5%) |
| 5 | 6 | 6 | 7.8 | 1 (−83%) | 6.5 (−17%) |

Abbreviations: f/u, follow-up; HA, headache; VAS, visual analog scale

In those who benefit, headache episodes remain present but are decreased in intensity and frequency. Prophylactic and abortive medications are reduced in many cases. These early findings should be confirmed with controlled blinded studies. Since a proportion of patients with CH appear to not benefit in a significant way from DBS, a method of prospectively predicting response to therapy is needed.

## Time Course for Stimulation-Induced Relief

The time course for wash-in and wash-out of the stimulation induced relief has been studied in detail in only one published case *(17)*. This patient had the unusual occurrence of bilateral attacks and was thus implanted bilaterally. The devices were turned off several times over four years, and only turned on again when headaches recurred. The mean time for onset of headache suppression following DBS activation was 16 days (range 2–46 days) and the mean time for headache recurrence following DBS inactivation was 73 days (range 2–290 days). The longest time for headache recurrence, 290 days, occurred on the side of the head where headaches were episodic, not chronic, and thus may reflect a temporary spontaneous remission on that side rather than a true prolonged washout time. Other patients in the Milan series, as well as those in the UCSF and Liege series were also noted to require days to weeks for onset of benefit, but the exact time course was not quantified.

## Complications

### Peri-operative Complications

The authors of the Milan series of 16 patients reported one asymptomatic third ventricular hemorrhage. In the Liege series, there were surgical complications in two of the six patients: one died of a large intracerebral and intraventricular hemorrhage several hours after surgery, and one could not complete the implantation due to a panic attack during physiological mapping of the target site. In our series of seven patients, there was a single surgical complication: an intra-operative transient ischemic attack (TIA) in the first case. This occurred immediately following intra-operative test stimulation using the deepest contact at 60 μsec, 185 Hz, up to 10 V. The patient was noted to be drowsy and hemiplegic on the side ipsilateral to the implant, which resolved completely in 5 minutes. Pulse and blood pressure were unchanged during the episode. Emergent head CT scan showed no hemorrhage. However, the DBS tip was noted to be slightly deep to the target, having exited the floor of the third ventricle, in the interpeduncular cistern at the midline. It is possible that test stimulation in the setting of the interpeduncular tip placement may have induced spasm of a contralateral thalamoperforating vessel, resulting in transient capsular ischemia and ipsilateral motor deficit. Contact 0 was not used in subsequent programming. TIAs did not recur in this patient and did not occur in the subsequent six patients.

### Stimulation-Induced Adverse Events

In all three series, voltage-limiting stimulation-induced adverse effects were reported to be oculomotor disturbance or dizziness above 1.5 to 3 V. One patient developed stimulation-induced bradycardia at therapeutic stimulation parameters requiring temporary cessation of therapy *(17)*. Long-term stimulation-induced adverse effects of unilateral implantation have been minor: In the Milan series, detailed blood pressure measurements showed that chronically stimulated patients developed asymptomatic orthostatic hypotension *(32)*. Persistent mood changes have not been observed. In the Milan series, most patients experienced mild weight loss which was attributed to cessation of corticosteroids *(5)*.

## Potential Mechanism of Action

The anatomy of the target region immediately posterior to the MTT is complex. This area harbors cells containing melatonin as well as a variety of opiate peptides *(28)*. The median forebrain bundle, which contains fiber tracts involved in all major ascending catecholaminergic systems, as well as hypothalamic efferent projections to brainstem and spinal cord, traverses this area. The fasciculus retroflexus, a pathway connecting the habenular nucleus with the serotonergic interpeduncular nucleus, also travels within the target region.

Although this complex anatomy raises many possible mechanisms, several physiologic studies have narrowed the possibilities. In the four implanted patients in the Liege series *(6)*, chronic DBS had no effect on urinary excretion of cortisol or melatonin, and no effect on plasma levels of oxytocin and vasopressin. There was no long-term effect on pressure pain thresholds in the supraorbital area, indicating that a general analgesic effect could not explain the headache benefit. Ten of the patients implanted in Milan have undergone PET imaging during acute activation and deactivation of the DBS device *(33)*. Acute activation was associated with increased activity in the ipsilateral hypothalamus, ipsilateral thalamus, somatosensory cortex and precuneous, anterior cingulate cortex, and trigeminal nucleus. There was deactivation in the posterior cingulate and contralateral insula. Major structures of the descending anti-nociceptive system, including periaqueductal gray and rostral ventromedial medulla, were not affected, suggesting that the effect is not mediated through these descending systems in spite of their extensive hypothalamic connections. This PET study only examined acute effects of DBS (within minutes of activation). These acute DBS-induced changes may not reflect chronic changes underlying the HA suppression, given that the time course for onset of the anti-headache effect appears to be days to weeks.

Although the treatment of CH with DBS of the posterior hypothalamic region is a new approach, nearby brain targets have been previously explored for the treatment of other chronic pain disorders. A number of investigators, working mainly between 1975 and 1990, reported deep brain stimulation of the PVG for neuropathic pain syndromes. Young et al. *(34)* reported the PVG target to be 10 mm posterior to the midcommissural point and 3 to 4 mm lateral to the midline. This target is 8.5 mm superior and posterior to the Milan CH target. An autopsy study of seven patients who had undergone DBS for neuropathic pain confirmed that effective electrodes were located near the posterior commissure, well posterior to the CH target *(35)*. Based on anatomic considerations, the Milan procedure is in a brain region that is distinct from prior attempts at neuromodulation for other chronic pain conditions. Likewise, previously explored targets for ablative surgeries for pain were not identical to the CH target. Sano et al. *(36)* utilized hypothalamotomy for chronic neuropathic pain, but his target was immediately lateral to the MTT and thus 3 to 5 mm anterior to the CH target. The thalamic centromedian and parafascicular nuclei have also been lesioned for pain treatment, but this target is 6 to 8 mm superior and lateral to the CH target *(37–39)*.

## Summary

CH is the most severe primary headache disorder known. Ten to 20% of cases are medically intractable. DBS of the posterior hypothalamic area has shown effectiveness for alleviation of CH in many but not all of the 20 reported cases from two European centers and the five cases studied at UCSF. This surgical strategy was based on the finding of increased blood flow in the posterior hypothalamic area on $H_2^{15}O$ PET scanning during spontaneous and nitroglycerin-induced CH attacks. The target point used, 4 to 5 mm posterior to the mamillothalamic tract, is in the border zone between posterior hypothalamus and anterior periventricular gray matter. Important questions remain to be answered, including a determination of the proportion of patients who respond to this therapy in blinded studies, measurement of wash-in and wash-out times, pre-operative predictors of clinical success, risks of hemorrhage and stimulation-induced adverse effects, optimal location of the active contact, and mechanism of action. Further characterization of this stimulation procedure in humans and in experimental systems may also yield important physiological insights into the pathogenesis of this primary headache disorder.

## References

1. Russell MB (2004) Epidemiology and genetics of cluster headaches. Lancet Neurol 3:279–283.
2. May A, Bahra A, Buchel C, Frackowiak RS, Goadsby PJ (1998) Hypothalamic activation in cluster headache attacks. Lancet 352(9124):275–278.
3. May A, Bahra A, Buchel C, Frackowiak RS, Goadsby PJ (2000) PET and MRA findings in cluster headache and MRA in experimental pain. Neurology 55:1328–1335.
4. Leone M, Franzini A, Bussone G (2001) Stereotactic stimulation of posterior hypothalamic gray matter in a patient with intractable cluster headache. N Engl J Med 345:1428–1429.
5. Leone M, Franzini A, Broggi G, Bussone G (2006) Hypothalamic stimulation for intractable cluster headache: long-term experience. Neurology 67(1):150–152.
6. Schoenen J, DiClemente L, Vandenheede M, Fumal A, Pasqua VD, Mouchamps M, Remacle JM, Noordhout AMD (2005) Hypothalamic stimulation in chronic cluster headache: a pilot study of efficacy and mode of action. Brain 128:940–947.
7. Starr PA, Barbaro N, Raskin N, Ostrem JL (in press) Chronic stimulation of the posterior hypothalamic region for cluster headache: technique and one-year results in four patients. J Neurosurg.
8. Wilkinson SB, Dafer R, Overman J (2004) Posterior hypothalamic stimulation benefits intractable cluster headaches. In: American Society for Stereotactic and Functional Neurosurgery, Cleveland, OH.
9. Rasche D, Foethke D, Gliemroth J, Tronnier VM (2006) Deep brain stimulation in the posterior hypothalamus for chronic cluster headache Case report and review of the literature. Schmerz.

10. The International Headache Society (2004) The international classification of headache disorders. Cephalalgia 24(Suppl 1):44–46.
11. May A, Leone M (2003) Update on cluster headache. Curr Opin Neurol 16:333–340.
12. May A (2005) Cluster headache: pathogenesis, diagnosis, and management. Lancet 366(9488):843–855.
13. Manzoni GC, Micieli G, Granella F, Tassorelli C, Zanferrari C, Cavallini A (1991) Cluster headache–course over ten years in 189 patients. Cephalalgia 11(4):169–174.
14. Jarrar RG, Black DF, Dodick DW, Davis DH (2003) Outcome of trigeminal nerve section in the treatment of chronic cluster headache. Neurology 60:1360–1362.
15. Donnet A, Valade D, Regis J (2005) Gamma knife treatment for refractory cluster headache: prospective open trial. J Neurol Neurosurg Psychiatry 76:218–221.
16. Matharu MS, Goadsby PJ (2002) Persistence of attacks of cluster headache after trigeminal nerve root section. Brain 125:976–984.
17. Leone M, Franzini A, Broggi G, May A, Bussone G (2004) Long-term follow-up of bilateral hypothalamic stimulation for intractable cluster headache. Brain 127:2259–2264.
18. May A, Ashburner J, Buchel C, McGonigle DJ, Friston KJ, Frackowiak RS, Goadsby PJ (1999) Correlation between structural and functional changes in brain in an idiopathic headache syndrome. Nature Med 5:836–838.
19. Sprenger T, Boecker H, Tolle TR, Bussone G, May A, Leone M (2004) Specific hypothalamic activation during a spontaneous cluster headache attack. Neurology 62(3):516–517.
20. May A (2003) Headache: lessons learned from functional imaging. Brit Med Bull 65:223–234.
21. May A, Bahra A, Buchel C, Turner R, Goadsby PJ (1999) Functional magnetic resonance imaging in spontaneous attacks of SUNCT: short-lasting neuralgiform headache with conjunctival injection and tearing. Ann Neurol 46(5):791–794.
22. Sprenger T, Valet M, Platzer S, Pfaffenrath V, Steude U, Tolle TR (2005) SUNCT: bilateral hypothalamic activation during headache attacks and resolving of symptoms after trigeminal decompression. Pain 113(3):422–426.
23. Sprenger T, Valet M, Hammes M, Erhard P, Berthele A, Conrad B, Tolle TR (2004) Hypothalamic activation in trigeminal autonomic cephalgia: functional imaging of an atypical case. Cephalalgia 24(9):753–757.
24. Leone M, May A, Franzini A, Broggi G, Dodick D, Rapoport A, Goadsby PJ, Schoenen J, Bonavita V, Bussone G (2004) Deep brain stimulation for intractable chronic cluster headache: proposals for patient selection. Cephalalgia 24(11):934–937.
25. Starr PA (2003) Placement of deep brain stimulators into the subthalamic nucleus or globus pallidus internus: technical approach. Stereotact Funct Neurosurg 79:118–145.
26. Franzini A, Ferroli P, Leone M, Broggi G (2003) Stimulation of the posterior hypothalamus for treatment of chronic intractable cluster headaches: First reported series. Neurosurgery 52:1095–1101.
27. Schaltenbrand G, Wahren W (1977) Introduction to stereotaxis with an atlas of the human brain. Stuttgart: Georg Thieme.
28. Swaab DF (2003) The human hypothalamus: basic and clinical aspects, Part I. Amsterdam: Elsevier.
29. Talairach J, Tournoux P (1988) Co-planar stereotaxic atlas of the human brain. Stuttgart: Thieme.
30. Available at: www.medtronic.com/neuro/parkinsons/techmanuals.html.
31. Rezai AR, Phillips M, Baker KB, Sharan AD, Nyenhuis J, Tkach J, Henderson J, Shellock FG (2004) Neurostimulation system used for deep brain stimulation (DBS): MR safety issues and implications of failing to follow safety recommendations. Invest Radiol 39(5):300–303.

32. Franzini A, Ferroli P, Leone M, Bussone G, Broggi G (2004) Hypothalamic deep brain stimulation for the treatment of chronic cluster headaches: A series report. Neuromodulation 7:1–8.
33. May A, Leone M, Boecker H, Sprenger T, Juergens T, Bussone G, Tolle TR (2006) Hypothalamic deep brain stimulation in positron emission tomography. J Neurosci 26(13):3589–3593.
34. Young RF, Kroening R, Fulton W (1985) Electrical stimulation of the brain in treatment of chronic pain. J Neurosurg 47:178–194.
35. Baskin DS, Mehler WR, Hosobuchi Y, Richardson DE, Adams JE, Flitter MA (1986) Autopsy analysis of the safety, efficacy and cartography of electrical stimulation of the central gray in humans. Brain Res 371(2):231–236.
36. Sano K, Sekino H, Hashimoto I, Amano K, Sugiyama H (1975) Posteromedial Hypothalamotomy in the treatment of intractable pain. Confin Neurol 37(1–3):285–290.
37. Whittle IR, Jenkinson JL (1995) CT-guided stereotactic antero-medial pulvinotomy and centromedian-parafascicular thalamotomy for intractable malignant pain. Br J Neurosurg 9:195–200.
38. Jeanmonod D, Magnin M, Morel A (1993) Thalamus and neurogenic pain: physiological, anatomical and clinical data. Neuroreport 4:475–478.
39. Young RF, Jacques DS, Rand RW, Copcutt BC, Vermeulen SS, Posewitz AF (1995) Technique of stereotactic medial thalamotomy with the Leksell Gamma Knife for treatment of chronic pain. Neurol Res 17:59–65.

# 28
# Deep Brain Stimulation in Epilepsy

William J. Marks, Jr.

## Abstract

Epilepsy describes a variety of disorders in which the brain produces recurrent seizures—events characterized by abnormal, hypersynchronous neuronal activity. Although numerous etiologies underlie epilepsy, ranging from genetic susceptibility to acquired lesions of the brain, the net result is a paroxysmal disruption of cerebral electrical activity. It therefore seems appealing to apply electrical stimulation to combat the storms of electricity that erupt in the epileptic brain. Indeed, neurostimulation has been applied to epilepsy in a variety of ways, both in animal models and in humans with various forms of epilepsy. Approaches have included stimulation of cranial nerves, particularly the vagus nerve (the only Food and Drug Administration [FDA]-approved neurostimulation therapy for epilepsy at the present time), and direct stimulation of cortical epileptogenic regions. This chapter focuses on the application of stimulation to deep brain structures in an effort to treat epileptic disorders.

**Keywords:** deep brain stimulation, DBS, epilepsy, seizure disorder

## Overview of Epilepsy and its Treatment

To assess the application of deep brain stimulation (DBS) to epilepsy, an extremely heterogeneous group of disorders, it is useful to understand the syndromic classification of epilepsy *(1)*. From the standpoint of brain stimulation strategies, the most important means of epilepsy classification pertains to the extent of brain involvement at seizure onset. In the *generalized epilepsies*, the electrical disturbance appears to arise diffusely throughout the cerebral cortex. Associated seizure types include *absence seizures* (producing momentary staring and disruption of awareness), *myoclonic seizures* (producing brief, lightning-like jerks of the body), *tonic seizures* (producing stiffening of the limbs and body), *clonic seizures* (producing repetitive jerking of the body), *tonic-clonic seizures* (alternating tonic and clonic activity), and *atonic seizures* (in which there is abrupt loss of muscle tone usually resulting in the patient's falling to the ground). In the *localization-related epilepsies* (also called partial or focal epilepsies), the initial zone of electrical abnormality is confined to a specific, focal region or regions of the brain. The most common brain region implicated in localization-related epilepsy is the temporal lobe, but any neocortical or medial temporal (hippocampus, amygdala) region can serve as the nidus for seizure initiation. Seizure types include *simple partial seizures* (clinical events in which patients experience stereotyped symptoms, such as somatosensory changes, muscle twitching, or experiential phenomena, but in which conscious awareness remains fully preserved) and *complex partial seizures* (in which conscious awareness is impaired and often associated with behavioral arrest and automatic motor movements). Patients with localization-related epilepsy may also experience *secondarily generalized seizures*, in which abnormal electrical activity in the brain begins focally but then spreads diffusely throughout the cerebral cortex, typically resulting in a tonic-clonic seizure with loss of consciousness.

First-line treatment of epilepsy is pharmacological in nature. Today, a large number of effective anti-epileptic medications are available and the majority of patients with epilepsy are able to achieve complete seizure control by taking one or more medications. A substantial number of patients, perhaps 30% or more, fail to achieve adequate control of seizures or are unable to tolerate the adverse effects produced by multiple medications *(2)*. Patients with pharmaco-resistant epilepsy desperately need other treatments that are effective in controlling seizures, produce reliable and durable seizure control, and are free from intolerable adverse effects. For some of these medically refractory patients, surgical resection of the epileptogenic brain tissue can fully control seizures or reduce their frequency and intensity. However, not all patients are appropriate candidates for resective surgery and, for those who are, the likelihood of achieving a long-lived seizure-free outcome varies from 95% for some syndromes to only 50% for others. Additionally, surgical resection entails irreversible removal of brain tissue, sometimes resulting in cognitive or other neurological deficits. For these reasons, availability of an effective and well tolerated non-destructive, non-pharmacological approach is urgently needed to more effectively control seizures and improve quality of life. Neurostimulation strategies, including DBS, have therefore been pursued in an attempt to satisfy this large unmet medical need.

## Approaches to DBS for Epilepsy

In applying DBS to the treatment of epilepsy, a number of different tactics and paradigms are available for consideration. Variables include location of the stimulating electrodes, configuration of the stimulating electrodes, stimulation protocols, and stimulation parameters.

Two general approaches to electrode location have been employed. One approach, which is applicable to localization-related epilepsies, seeks to locate the stimulating electrode(s) within or near the confirmed or suspected focus or foci that are generating seizures. The goal is to use local electrical stimulation to disrupt the ability of the epileptogenic neuronal network to initiate seizures or to limit spread of seizure activity beyond the confines of the site of origination. This strategy is best suited in cases where there is a discrete, readily identifiable, and accessible seizure focus. In the case of a neocortical focus, cortical stimulation using electrodes placed in a subdural or epidural location might be undertaken, whereas with a hippocampal or amygdala focus, the approach would involve DBS using electrodes implanted into the parenchyma of the seizure focus. Other deep foci, such as the insular cortex, might also be accessed via a DBS approach. Stimulation located at the seizure focus becomes less practical, however, when the epileptogenic zone is widespread in its distribution; when multiple discrete epileptogenic foci are at play; when it is difficult to ascertain the localization or extent of the epileptogenic region; or potentially, depending on stimulation parameters needed to suppress seizures and their effects on normal brain function, when seizures arise from eloquent brain areas.

Another approach to electrode location utilizes stimulation sites implicated in the genesis or propagation of seizures but remote from the actual seizure focus or foci. This strategy would obviously be applicable to the generalized epilepsies in which no discrete seizure focus exists. It also has applicability to the localization-related epilepsies, where DBS of a central target might have anti-epileptogenic effects to mitigate the occurrence of seizures or might interfere with seizure propagation within one or both cerebral hemispheres. Brain target candidates for this approach include various nuclei of the thalamus due to the widespread connectivity of the thalamus and its role in the entrainment of thalamocortical brain rhythms that have been implicated in at least some forms of epilepsy. Presuming that a location for stimulation has been chosen, the arrangement of anode and cathode configuration is likely to play a large role in the effects that are achieved and the morphology of the waveform used to deliver stimulation.

In brain stimulation for epilepsy, three general stimulation paradigms may be applied. These are continuous, cyclical, or seizure-initiated stimulation. Continuous stimulation, in which repetitive stimulation is administered around the clock, is the paradigm used for DBS in movement disorders. Continuous stimulation might also be useful in treating epilepsy in order to provide ongoing anti-epileptic effects at a seizure focus or within epileptogenic networks. Cyclical stimulation delivers repetitive stimulation for a specified epoch of time, interposed with periods free from stimulation. Modern neurostimulation devices typically offer the user the ability to program a wide range of on- and off-stimulation times. Such duty cycles can alternate rapidly (e.g., 1 second on stimulation, 1 second off stimulation) or less frequently (e.g., 5 minutes on stimulation, 5 minutes off stimulation). Duration of on- and off-stimulation times need not be identical. Cyclical stimulation could also be delivered with reference to the time of day so that a patient with nocturnal seizures might have stimulation initiated at night. Finally, a more sophisticated approach to the paradigm of stimulation is to deliver stimulation around the time of a seizure *(3–5)*. Presuming that stimulation at a brain target could promptly and reliably terminate a seizure soon after its onset, seizure-initiated stimulation would deliver therapy on demand. This paradigm relies on the ability to accurately and rapidly detect the onset of a seizure or to predict in advance when a seizure is likely to occur *(6)*. Coupling of a detection algorithm and delivery of contingent stimulation is sometimes referred to as closed-loop stimulation. A system delivering closed-loop stimulation could have the stimulation electrodes also serve as sensing electrodes or could have sensing electrodes at one site and stimulation electrodes at another.

## Deep Brain Targets for Epilepsy

Animal and human studies that have evaluated DBS to treat epilepsy at various targets are summarized here.

**Anterior Nucleus of the Thalamus**

Thalamic nuclei are attractive targets for stimulation given their extensive connectivity with cerebral cortex and their potential ability to broadly modulate cortical physiological activity through stimulation of a discrete thalamic target. Animal models demonstrate frequency-dependent effects of thalamic stimulation on cortical synchronization, with higher frequency stimulation being capable of desynchronizing cortical activity *(7, 8)*, a useful attribute when attempting to disrupt the hypersynchronous epileptic state.

The anterior nucleus of the thalamus has generated particular attention as a candidate region for anti-epileptic stimulation for several reasons. First, based on metabolic mapping studies in animal models, this region appears to be involved in generalized seizures *(9)*. Second, by virtue of its role in the circuit of Papez, its anatomic connectivity seems highly relevant in seizure generation *(10)*. Third, high-frequency stimulation of the anterior nucleus inhibits generalized seizures in a chemo-convulsant model in the rat *(11)*. These and other encouraging observations have led to investigation of anterior thalamic stimulation in humans with epilepsy.

One small-scale study in five patients, some with generalized epilepsy and others with localization-related or multi-focal epilepsy, found a 54% mean reduction in seizure frequency after mean follow-up duration of 15 months *(12)*. Long-term follow-up (mean duration 5 years) of these subjects plus one additional patient, during which multiple changes in stimulation parameters and paradigms were made, demonstrated at least 50% seizure reduction *(13)*. In some cases seizure reduction occurred following implantation of the DBS leads, but before activation, suggesting a possible "microlesion" effect. In addition, benefit was seemingly delayed by 5 to 6 years in two patients, so that medication manipulation may have been at least partially responsible for improved seizure control. A separate study of five patients with intractable localization-related epilepsy treated with bilateral stimulation of the anterior thalamic nucleus using cyclical stimulation (1 minute on, 10 minutes off) documented improved severity of seizures in four patients and statistically significant reduction in total seizure frequency in another *(14)*. In a multi-center pilot study of bilateral anterior thalamic nucleus stimulation to treat 14 patients with pharmaco-resistant localization-related epilepsy or, in several cases, symptomatic generalized epilepsy, mean reduction in seizure frequency was 64% 3 months following stimulator activation *(15)*. Eight of the 14 patients experienced a 50% or greater rate of seizure reduction. These findings persisted at 6 and 12 months of follow-up. In this study, sub-group analysis suggested that patients with temporal and/or frontal lobe localization experienced the most robust level of seizure suppression.

Based on this preliminary work, a prospective multi-center, randomized, controlled study investigating stimulation of the anterior nucleus of the thalamus for epilepsy (the SANTE study) has commenced *(16)*. In this study, patients with intractable localization-related epilepsy are receiving surgical implantation of DBS leads into the anterior thalamic nuclei and are then randomized in a double-blind manner to receive an initial period of active stimulation versus no stimulation. When results of this study become available, they will provide valuable information concerning the efficacy of anterior thalamic stimulation and on a variety of other issues related to this approach to the treatment of epilepsy.

### Centromedian Nucleus of the Thalamus

Physiologic studies in humans suggest a role for the centromedian nucleus of the thalamus in influencing reticulo-thalamic cortical neurons implicated in the genesis or propagation of generalized seizures *(17)*. Several open-label studies from one research group have investigated stimulation of the centromedian nucleus in patients with various types of epilepsy *(18–23)*. Reported outcomes have been generally favorable, ranging from 50 to 100% reduction in various seizure types across the various studies. A report of 49 patients followed over 6 months to 15 years concluded that stimulation of the centromedian nucleus was effective in reducing generalized tonic-clonic, atypical absence, and tonic seizures but did not control complex partial seizures *(18)*. An additional study, using a double-blind, cross-over design in seven patients, demonstrated a mean reduction in tonic-clonic seizure frequency of 30% with stimulation compared to an 8% reduction during the off-stimulation period, a suggestive but statistically insignificant difference *(24)*. During the open-label follow-up phase of this study, three of six patients had a 50% or greater reduction in generalized seizures.

### Caudate Nucleus

Stimulation of the caudate nucleus in various animal models of epilepsy has been reported to decrease interictal and ictal epileptiform activity *(25, 26)*. One study suggested a frequency-dependent effect, with lower frequency (<100 Hz) stimulation reducing seizure occurrence and higher frequency stimulation increasing seizure activity *(26)*. No controlled human studies of caudate nucleus stimulation have been conducted, but an open-label study showed reduction of epileptiform activity in some patients *(27)*.

### Cerebellar Nuclei

Uncontrolled early studies cited considerable efficacy of cerebellar stimulation in treating seizures *(28)*. A double-blind, randomized, controlled trial investigated stimulation of the superomedial surface of the cerebellum in five patients with symptomatic generalized epilepsy syndromes. They found a significant reduction in seizure frequency during periods when patients were receiving stimulation but not during non-stimulation control periods. Other controlled studies, however, have failed to demonstrate significant seizure reduction with stimulation of the cerebellum *(29, 30)*.

### Hippocampus and Amygdala

Medial temporal (amygdalohippocampal) stimulation has been shown to suppress epileptiform discharges in animal models, human slice preparations, and in humans with epilepsy *(31–33)*. In a short-term study, continuous electrical stimulation within the hippocampus prevented seizure occurrence and reduced the number of interictal epileptiform transients *(34)*. An open-label study of chronic bilateral hippocampal region stimulation in three patients with medial temporal lobe epilepsy found reduction of complex partial seizure rates ranging from 50 to 97% at 4 to 6 months of follow-up *(35)*. No stimulation-induced adverse effects were identified. However, a double-blind, crossover design trial of unilateral hippocampal stimulation in four patients with refractory left medial temporal lobe epilepsy demonstrated only modest (mean 15%) reduction of seizures during stimulation *(31)*. Also noted was an apparent carry-over effect in seizure suppression following cessation of stimulation and a long-term (4-year) benefit in one patient.

**Locus Coeruleus**

Two published case reports discuss the effects of locus coeruleus stimulation in humans with epilepsy. In a report of a single patient, stimulation was found to suppress generalized epileptiform activity *(36)*. In a report of two patients, one experienced a 75% reduction in seizure frequency while the other experienced prolongation in the time between onset of simple partial seizure activity and conversion to a more disabling seizure type *(37)*.

**Subthalamic Nucleus (STN)**

Experimental data have led to the theory of an endogenous control system that modulates cortical excitability and exerts an anti-seizure effect. Components of this system include the substantia nigra pars reticulata and its GABA-ergic inhibitory effects on the so-called dorsal midbrain anticonvulsant zone (DMAZ), a region ventral to the superior colliculi *(38)*. Stimulation of the STN is postulated to exert an anti-epileptic effect through activation of the DMAZ. In a rat model of generalized epilepsy, high frequency stimulation of the STN aborted spontaneous seizures *(39)*. A study of kainic acid-induced seizures in rats found that STN stimulation shortened the duration of generalized seizures but prolonged the duration of partial seizures *(40)*. Physiological studies in humans demonstrate that interictal epileptiform spikes and epileptic seizures (captured on simultaneously recorded scalp EEG) can be recorded from the STN *(41)*. In human patients with epilepsy, several case reports have suggested an anti-epileptic effect of STN stimulation. Subthalamic stimulation in a child with epilepsy caused by centroparietal focal cortical dysplasia documented an 80% reduction in seizure frequency that continued to endure 30 months later *(42)*. Another report described three patients with symptomatic localization-related epilepsy and one patient with myoclonic epilepsy who received substantial benefit (up to 80% reduction in seizure frequency) following subthalamic stimulation, although one patient with a genetic frontal lobe epilepsy syndrome failed to respond *(43)*. In another study, two patients with cryptogenic frontal lobe epilepsy, one followed for 6 months and the other for 18 months, had greater than 80% reduction in seizure frequency with chronic STN DBS *(44)*.

# Conclusions and Future Directions

Intriguing observations and data from animal and human studies appear to provide a compelling rationale for further study of DBS for the treatment of epilepsy. To date, however, most human studies have been very small in scale, uncontrolled and unblinded, have included patients with heterogeneous epilepsy syndromes, have targeted a variety of anatomic sites, and have lacked a systematic approach to choice of electrode polarity, stimulation parameters, and treatment paradigms. Thus, it is extraordinarily difficult to discern which targets of stimulation are likely to be successful, and for which epilepsy syndromes. The SANTE study discussed above will be the first rigorously conducted large-scale study of DBS for epilepsy and is expected to yield data that should provide greater insight into the promising but to date unrealized application of DBS to patients with epilepsy.

## References

1. Commission on Classification and Terminology of the International League Against Epilepsy (1989) Proposal for revised classification of epilepsies and epileptic syndromes. Epilepsia 30:389–399.
2. Brodie MJ (2005) Diagnosing and predicting refractory epilepsy. Acta Neurol Scand Suppl 181:36–39.
3. Osorio I, Frei MG, Manly BF, et al (2001) An introduction to contingent (closed-loop) brain electrical stimulation for seizure blockage, to ultra-short-term clinical trials, and to multidimensional statistical analysis of therapeutic efficacy. J Clin Neurophysiol 18:533–544.
4. Osorio I, Frei MG, Sunderam S, et al (2005) Automated seizure abatement in humans using electrical stimulation. Ann Neurol 57:258–268.
5. Fountas KN, Smith JR, Murro AM, et al (2005) Implantation of a closed-loop stimulation in the management of medically refractory focal epilepsy: a technical note. Stereotact Funct Neurosurg 83:153–158.
6. Litt B, Echauz J (2002) Prediction of epileptic seizures. Lancet Neurol 1:22–30.
7. Dempsey EW, Morrison RS (1942) The production of rhythmically recurrent cortical potentials after localized thalamic stimulation. Am J Physiol 135:293–300.
8. Monnier M, Kalberer M, Krupp P (1960) Functional antagonism between diffuse reticular and intralaminary recruiting projections in the medial thalamus. Exp Neurol 2:271–289.
9. Mirski MA, Ferrendelli JA (1986) Anterior thalamic mediation of generalized pentylenetetrazol seizures. Brain Res 399:212–223.
10. Theodore W, Fisher RS (2004) Brain stimulation for epilepsy. Lancet Neurol 3:111–118.
11. Mirski MA, Rossell LA, Terry JB, Fisher RS (1997) Anticonvulsant effect of anterior thalamic high frequency electrical stimulation in the rat. Epilepsy Res 28:89–100.
12. Hodaie M, Wennberg RA, Dostrovsky JO, Lozano AM (2002) Chronic anterior thalamus stimulation for intractable epilepsy. Epilepsia 43:603–608.
13. Andrade DM, Zumsteg D, Hamani C, et al (2006) Long-term follow-up of patients with thalamic deep brain stimulation for epilepsy. Neurology 66:1571–1573.
14. Kerrigan JF, Litt B, Fisher RS, et al (2004) Electrical stimulation of the anterior nucleus of the thalamus for the treatment of intractable epilepsy. Epilepsia 45:346–354.
15. Graves NM, Fisher RS (2005) Neurostimulation for epilepsy, including a pilot study of anterior nucleus stimulation. Clin Neurosurg 52:127–134.
16. Fisher RS, SANTE Study Group (2006) SANTE (Stimulation of the anterior nucleus of thalamus for epilepsy) interim report. Abstract 4.122, presented December 4, 2006 at the Annual Meeting of the American Epilepsy Society.
17. Velasco F, Velasco M, Marquez I, Velasco G (1993) Role of the centromedian nucleus in the genesis, propagation, and arrest of epileptic activity: an electrophysiological study in man. Acta Neurochir Suppl (Wien) 58:201–204.

18. Velasco F, Velasco M, Jimenez F, Velasco AL, Marquez I (2001) Stimulation of the central median thalamic nucleus for epilepsy. Stereotact Funct Neurosurg 77:228–232.
19. Velasco F, Velasco M, Velasco AL, Jimenez F (1993) Effect of chronic electrical stimulation of the centromedian thalamic nuclei on various intractable seizure patterns: I. Clinical seizures and paroxysmal EEG activity. Epilepsia 34:1052–1064.
20. Velasco F, Velasco M, Velasco AL, et al (1995) Electrical stimulation of the centromedian thalamic nucleus in control of seizures: long-term studies. Epilepsia 36:63–71.
21. Velasco M, Velasco F, Alcal H, Davila G, Diaz-de-Leon AE (1991) Epileptiform EEG activity of the centromedian thalamic nuclei in children with intractable generalized seizures of the Lennox-Gastaut syndrome. Epilepsia 32:310–321.
22. Velasco M, Velasco F, Velasco AL, et al (2000) Acute and chronic electrical stimulation of the centromedian thalamic nucleus: modulation of reticulo-cortical systems and predictor factors for generalized seizure control. Arch Med Res 31:304–315.
23. Velasco M, Velasco F, Velasco AL, Lujan M, Vazquez del Mercado J (1989) Epileptiform EEG activities of the centromedian thalamic nuclei in patients with intractable partial motor, complex partial, and generalized epilepsies. Epilepsia 30:295–306.
24. Fisher RS, Uematsu S, Krauss GL, et al (1992) Placebo-controlled pilot study of centomedian thalamic stimulation in treatment of intractable seizures. Epilepsia 33:841–851.
25. La Grutta, Sabatino M, Gravante G, et al (1988) A study of caudate inhibition on an epileptic focus in the cat hippocampus. Arch Int Physiol Biochim 96:113–120.
26. Oakley JC, Ojemann GA (1982) Effects of chronic stimulation of the caudate nucleus on a preexisting alumina seizure focus. Exp Neurol 75:360–367.
27. Chkhenkeli SA, Chkhenkeli IS (1997) Effects of therapeutic stimulation of nucleus caudatus on epileptic electrical activity of brain in patients with intractable epilepsy. Stereotact Funct Neurosurg 69:221–224.
28. Cooper IS, Amin I, Riklan M, Waltz JM, Poon TP (1976) Chronic cerebellar stimulation in epilepsy. Clinical and anatomical studies. Arch Neurol 33:559–570.
29. Van Buren JM, Wood JH, Oakley J, Hambrecht F (1978) Preliminary evaluation of cerebellar stimulation by double-blind stimulation and biological criteria in the treatment of epilepsy. J Neurosurg 48:407–416.
30. Wright GD, McLellan DL, Brice JG (1984) A double-blind trial of chronic cerebellar stimulation in twelve patients with severe epilepsy. J Neurol Neurosurg Psychiatr 47:769–774.
31. Tellez-Zenteno JF, McLachlan RS, Parrent A, Kubu CS, Wiebe S (2006) Hippocampal electrical stimulation in mesial temporal lobe epilepsy. Neurology 66:1490–1494.
32. Yamamoto J, Ikeda A, Satow T, et al (2002) Low-frequency electric cortical stimulation has an inhibitory effect on epileptic focus in mesial temporal lobe epilepsy. Epilepsia 43:491–495.
33. Chkhenkeli SA, Sramka M, Lortkipanidze GS, et al (2004) Electrophysiological effects and clinical results of direct brain stimulation for intractable epilepsy. Clin Neurol Neurosurg 106:318–329.
34. Velasco M, Velasco F, Velasco AL, et al (2000) Subacute electrical stimulation of the hippocampus blocks intractable temporal lobe seizures and paroxysmal EEG activities. Epilepsia 41:158–169.
35. Vonck K, Boon P, Achten E, De Reuck J, Caemaert J (2002) Long-term amygdalohippocampal stimulation for refractory temporal lobe epilepsy. Ann Neurol 52:556–565.
36. Faber J, Vladyka V (1983) Anti-epileptic effect of electric stimulation of the locus coeruleus in man. Act Nerv Super (Praha) 25:304–308.
37. Feinstein B, Gleason CA, Libet B (1989) Stimulation of locus coeruleus in man. Preliminary trials for spasticity and epilepsy. Stereotact Funct Neurosurg 52:26–41.

38. Loddenkemper T, Pan A, Neme S, et al (2001) Deep brain stimulation in epilepsy. J Clin Neurophysiol 18:514–532.
39. Vercueil L, Benazzouz A, Deransart C, et al (1998) High-frequency stimulation of the subthalamic nucleus suppresses absence seizures in the rat: comparison with neurotoxic lesions. Epilepsy Res 31:39–46.
40. Usui N, Maesawa S, Kajita Y, et al (2005) Suppression of secondary generalization of limbic seizures by stimulation of subthalamic nucleus in rats. J Neurosurg 102:1122–1129.
41. Dinner DS, Neme S, Nair D, et al (2002) EEG and evoked potential recording from the subthalamic nucleus for deep brain stimulation of intractable epilepsy. Clin Neurophysiol 113:1391–1402.
42. Benabid AL, Minotti L, Koudsié A, de Saint Martin A, Hirsch E (2002) Antiepileptic effect of high-frequency stimulation of the subthalamic nucleus (corpus luysi) in a case of medically intractable epilepsy caused by focal dysplasia: a 30-month follow-up technical case report. Neurosurgery 50:1385–1392.
43. Chabardes S, Kahane P, Minotti L, et al (2003) Deep brain stimulation in epilepsy with particular reference to the subthalamic nucleus. Epileptic Disord 4:83–93.
44. Shon YM, Lee KJ, Kim HJ (2005) Effect of chronic deep brain stimulation of the subthalamic nucleus for frontal lobe epilepsy: subtraction SPECT analysis. Stereotact Funct Neurosurg 83:84–90.

# 29
# The Future of Deep Brain Stimulation

Julie G. Pilitsis and Roy A.E. Bakay

## Abstract

The success of deep brain stimulation (DBS) in movement disorders has prompted evaluation of its efficacy in the treatment of a number of other disease processes. To truly assess the efficacy of DBS in these emerging applications, an understanding of the neurophysiology of DBS is mandated. Device optimization is also necessary to both adequately treat these diseases and to allow younger patients who may have the devices for decades to function relatively normally. Ultimately, these systems may be augmented with other available technologies to further growth in the fields of neuroprosthesis, cellular, and gene therapy. This chapter reviews the current uses of DBS, the understanding of underlying neurophysiology, and of devices. This discussion is followed by emerging applications, progress in device optimization, and the future of functional neurosurgery.

**Keywords:** deep brain stimulation, future, psychosurgery, technology, device optimization

## Introduction

Over the last 10 years, DBS has emerged as a mainstay in the surgical treatment of movement disorders. In fact, a recent prospective randomized-pairs trial has shown DBS to be significantly more effective than medical management of patients with Parkinson's disease (PD) at 6-month follow-up *(1)*. The success of DBS in the treatment of movement disorders has prompted evaluation of its efficacy in the treatment of a number of other disease processes, such as obsessive–compulsive disorder (OCD), depression, epilepsy, pain, eating disorders, and minimally conscious states *(2)*.

To evaluate the success of DBS on these emerging applications, work must first be directed to understanding the effects of DBS on neural tissues and the optimal targets for each disease process. With the current somewhat limited insight into the effects of DBS *in vivo*, it will be difficult to accurately determine the efficacy of the devices, as the treated disease processes expand outside the realm of movement disorders. Furthermore, a better understanding of the neurophysiology of DBS and the electrical properties needed to provide efficacious treatment will lead to optimization of the devices and improved outcomes for each treated disorder. The next logical step is the augmentation of these devices with other available technologies to further the growth of the fields of neuroprosthesis, cellular, and gene therapy. Because of the already widespread success and use of DBS as an empiric therapy, it is impossible to have "a bench to bedside" approach to such issues. Instead, research occurring in the laboratory and in the clinical setting will need to occur simultaneously and will hopefully complement other-ongoing research. Furthermore, the aforementioned areas of research will occur concurrently. This chapter first reviews the current uses of DBS, then turnstotle understanding of neurophysiology, and devices used. We will finally focus on the emerging applications and future of device optimization and functional neurosurgery.

## History of DBS

The first report of human cortical stimulation was published in 1874 following Fritz and Hitzig's demonstration of localized electrical excitability of the cortex *(3)*. However, it was over a century later before it was appreciated that chronic brain stimulation resulted in clinical benefits similar to those achieved with surgical lesioning, but were reversible *(4)*. In the 1990s, Benabid et al. combined implantable pacemaker technology with other technical advances which enabled placement of chronically implanted deep brain electrodes and followed this observation with the first reports of successful DBS *(4, 5)*. Since that time, DBS has become increasingly used in the treatment of movement disorders. The first widespread use of DBS in the United States and Europe was for the treatment of tremor *(4, 5)*. Thalamic targets were the first to be assessed followed by stimulation of the globus pallidus internus (GPi), which was based on previous pallidotomy studies. Introduction of the subthalamic nucleus (STN) as a target was based on primate research *(6, 7)*, which, previous to stimulation, had been considered a potentially dangerous location due to neurological side effects associated with surgical procedures in this site such as hemiballismus.

A controlled comparison of GPi DBS vs STN DBS *(8)* confirmed the comparable clinical benefits from stimulation at either site. Other small, randomized comparative trials have also produced similar data *(9, 10)*; however, definitive comparisons of safety and efficacy awaits randomized trials organized by the National Institutes of Health and the Veterans Administration. The first randomized controlled study comparing DBS to medical management was recently published and revealed a significant benefit of bilateral STN DBS over best medical therapy for the treatment of PD *(1)*. The success of DBS in treating drug-induced dyskinesia and dystonia associated with PD led to assessments of its efficacy in dystonia. With the success of pallidotomy for generalized dystonia the globus pallidus became the primary target for primary dystonia, but thalamic and STN targets have also been used *(11–15)*. In a recent controlled trial of pallidal DBS in 22 patients with primary generalized dystonia, there was a mean decrease of 51% in Burke–Fahn–Marsden dystonia scores at 1-year follow-up as compared to pre-operative scores *(16)*.

Gait disturbance and postural instability associated with PD, especially when poorly responsive to L-dopa, was only moderately improved with STN or GPi stimulation, leading researchers to investigate other targets for treatment of these symptoms. Experimental stimulation of the pedunculopontine nucleus in animals increases locomotor activity *(17, 18)*. Interestingly, it is low-frequency stimulation (i.e., less than 10 Hz) in parkinsonian monkeys that leads to increased motor activity *(19)*. Two patients who underwent placement of bilateral DBS electrodes in the pedunculopontine nucleus had significant improvement in gait and postural instability at low frequencies (20–25 Hz; ref. *20*).

Target selection for DBS in the treatment of movement disorders has been based primarily on results that previously occurred with lesioning, animal research, and lessons learned while treating other movement disorders. This trial and error methodology has for the most part been successful, although it has left clinicians and scientists wondering whether other more ideal targets may exist. This work has not always resulted in a clear consensus as to which target was best and whether different targets should be advocated for different symptoms. The use of trial and error methodology will be more problematic as DBS leaves the arena of movement disorders, since psychiatric and behavioral disorders are even less well understood than movement disorders. Furthermore, lack of adherence to the scientific method in psychosurgery performed in the 1930s and 1940s resulted in public outcries that led to virtually a complete collapse of the field for the past 60 years.

## Psychosurgery

The term psychosurgery was first used by Moniz, a neurologist at the University of Lisbon. He worked with the neurosurgeon Almeida Lima to perform the first surgery to disrupt afferent and efferent pathways from the frontal lobe, results of which were published in 1936 *(21, 22)*. This work resulted in the award of the Nobel Prize in 1949. In 1937, the neurologist Walter Freeman and neurosurgeon James Watts modified the European procedure of prefrontal ablation in the hope of producing more consistent results; in their procedure white matter tracts were transected by inserting a leukotome in a 1-cm burr-hole along the coronal suture superior to the zygomatic arch *(23)*. Freeman then began performing transorbital frontal lobotomy (without a neurosurgeon present) by inserting the instrument into the orbital roof and sweeping it across the prefrontal cortex. *(24)*.

It is important to note that at that time over half the hospital beds were taken up by psychiatric patients and, by the 1940s, $1.5 billion was required to treat mental illness *(25)*. It was estimated that this procedure would save Americans $1 million per day in taxes to fund psychiatric institutions *(26)*. The procedure soon was increasingly used by physicians without surgical training *(27, 28)*. Once some of the abuses and adverse long-term effects of these procedures on patients were appreciated, a congressional commission investigated the procedures. However opponents successfully frightened and even misled the public into being so appalled by the concept of psychosurgery that even the finding of usefulness of the procedure and recommendation for its continued use by the commission could not prevent the procedure from falling out of favor *(29)*. Beginning in the late 1950s, public outcry in combination with the advent of antipsychotic medications caused the field of psychosurgery to be largely abandoned.

However, a few neurosurgeons at a handful of centers continued the practice. The most commonly treated psychiatric conditions were medical failures such as OCD. They were treated using a variety of procedures which selectively lesioned portions of the limbic system. Anterior cingulotomy, subcaudate tractomy, and anterior capsulotomy were all attempted. Therefore, the greatest experience neurosurgeons had with psychiatric disease was in the treatment of OCD, which has therefore been the logical starting point for the functional neurosurgeon's venture into the realm of DBS treatment of psychiatric disease.

The anterior limb of the internal capsule near the ventral striatum was chosen as the initial site for DBS placement based on the previous success with capsulotomy *(30)*.

Small-scale controlled *(31–34)* and open studies *(30, 35–37)* have suggested that DBS of the internal capsule and/or the adjacent ventral striatal region improved symptoms in severely affected OCD patients who have failed other therapies. Based on long-term follow-up studies of Nuttin et al. *(32)*, multicenter studies have utilized the capsular target adjacent to the ventral striatum. Greenberg et al. recently published their 3-year follow-up on eight patients using the Yale-Brown Obsessive Compulsive Scale (YBOCS) (38). Fifty percent of patients continued to have greater than 35% improvement in YBOCS at follow-up. These patients also had significant improvement in depression and anxiety measures at 3 years. Because of previous greater success with anterior cingulotomy as compared to anterior capsulotomy in the treatment of depression *(39)*, together with PET studies suggesting abnormalities in metabolism in this area the subgenual cingulate, white matter was chosen as a target for DBS for depression *(40)*. In a small open-label study, improved mood was reported in four of six patients with treatment-resistant depression *(40)*.

## Lessons Learned From Psychosurgery

Although DBS is obviously a far cry from the use of ice picks by non-surgeons to sever white matter tracts, many lessons can be learned from the history of psychosurgery. Most crucially, it is important to carefully select the patients that may benefit from these procedures and to monitor them closely in both the peri-operative period and during the long term. It is essential to have a scientific basis for the choice of targets and alterations in methodology. It is also crucial not to let social pressures dictate the decisions to treat patients and to be able to defend choices of surgical intervention in appropriate cases.

The success of DBS in the treatment of patients with movement disorders is due in no small part to the multidisciplinary approach that has been used in the peri-operative management of these patients. The collaboration of the neurosurgeon and neurologist has developed over a long time with combined endeavors, not only to treat movement disorders, but also epilepsy, stroke, tumor, and other conditions. Relationships between neurosurgeons and psychiatrists are not as familiar and currently few centers have a well-developed collaboration between the two specialties. Collegiality is essential for the successful development of a functional psychosurgery program. Additionally, while the initial U.S. experience with DBS in movement disorders was restricted to a limited number of centers with well-developed teams especially trained to deal with patients, the pending FDA limited approval of DBS for OCD will likely impact the development of multidisciplinary psychiatric teams even in established movement disorder centers. Such a team must be established before DBS can be responsibly offered as a treatment option in order to assure proper patient selection and programming. Pre-operative testing and intensive initial programming are very time consuming and cannot be done independently by a neurosurgeon with a busy practice. Acute disruption of stimulation may lead to severe psychiatric effects *(41)*. Furthermore, these patients have very complex issues and needs that necessitate the involvement of not only a general psychiatrist, but also a psychiatrist specializing in OCD.

The appreciation that depressive symptoms have improved in OCD patients following DBS has led to clinical trials assessing the efficacy of DBS in major depression. These case series and their effects are too small to adequately determine whether these improvements are epiphenomena, and very few of the emerging applications have the underpinnings of relevant animal models. Much like DBS in the treatment of movement disorders, a trial and error progression of target selection is occurring, based on past successes and observed clinical effects. Functional imaging has also played and will continue to play an important role in the refinement of targets for psychiatric disease. For example, Mayberg et al. *(42)* chose to target the cingulate region in their study of DBS for depression because of increased fluorodeoxyglucose (FDG) uptake in this area in some patients with depression.

While such a method of target selection in the treatment of movement disorders has been relatively safe, this modality must be used carefully as we tread into the realm of psychosurgery. Our current understanding of psychiatric disorders is limited and greater appreciation of the neurobiology of emotion, addiction, and cognition is necessary before selecting precise targets. As cognitive and emotional processing become better understood, the role of DBS in these diseases will likely increase. Most effects of DBS are reversible and the device can be turned off, removed, or repositioned in a more appropriate target as the field progresses. However, the potential for microlesioning and important long-term sequelae may also exist. The potential for cognitive and unpredicted neuropsychological sequelae is probably greater than in movement disorders surgery because the limbic system is being directly altered. DBS will likely be a useful tool in the treatment of some psychiatric conditions, but should be approached scientifically and cautiously.

A role for DBS in the treatment of addiction and eating disorders has also been suggested, although little published data is yet available in these fields. There is preliminary evidence in rodents that hypothalamic stimulation may lead to a reduction in weight gain *(43)*. The social implication of the use of DBS in these fields is far-reaching, as two of the leading current health crises in the United States are obesity and tobacco addiction. Consider the recent explosion in the frequency of gastric bypass operations. Gastric bypass surgery had been performed for years with strict patient selection and peri-operative management with reasonable success. However, the "quick fix" of gastric bypass surgery over the last decade without careful peri-operative management has led to a number of surgical failures *(44)*. Likewise, if DBS becomes a treatment option for addiction and eating disorders and is used to treat large numbers of patients, poor peri-operative management will likely lead to its eventual failure, when indeed it might turn out to be efficacious if used in properly selected and carefully managed patients.

## Other Emerging Applications

### Epilepsy

Open-loop stimulation systems (i.e., those in which no feedback is present to alter stimulation parameters) were first introduced for the treatment of epilepsy in the late 1970s *(45)*. Cerebellar hemispheric stimulation was used first *(45)*. The advent of DBS led to investigation of a number of targets for the treatment of epilepsy. In animal models stimulation of the STN, anterior thalamus, and substantia nigra has been found to inhibit limbic seizures *(46–48)*.

In humans, stimulation of the STN, caudate, hippocampus and thalamic nuclei have all been attempted for the treatment of epilepsy. In the first nine patients who underwent STN stimulation in uncontrolled studies, two-thirds had up to an 80% reduction in seizure frequency *(49)*. In another series of patients, ventral stimulation of the caudate nucleus led to a reduction of epileptic discharges and electrical spread *(50)*. In a third uncontrolled series, three patients with complex partial seizures had DBS electrodes implanted in the amygdalo-hippocampal region and all had a greater than 50% reduction in seizure frequency *(51)*.

Stimulation of thalamic nuclei for the treatment of epilepsy has become an area of active investigation. An open series of 49 treated patients showed subjective beneficial stimulation effects in those receiving centromedian-nucleus (CM) stimulation for various types of intractable seizures *(52)*. However, an earlier, small placebo-controlled study of CM stimulation showed no significant benefit *(53)*. Bilateral DBS of the anterior nucleus (AN) in epilepsy has been promising in open-label studies. In a recently published follow-up of patients treated with bilateral AN DBS, five of six patients had more than 50% seizure reduction at 1-year follow-up and no changes in AEDs were necessary for the first 2 years *(54)*. From years 3 to 5, one patient remained stable, three had one medication added, and two had multiple medication changes. A multicenter study to assess efficacy of AN DBS is currently in progress.

### Other Clinical Applications

Other potential applications of DBS are even more foreign to the general neurosurgeon. These applications are less well studied and often for diseases which have been refractory to medical treatment. The potential role of DBS in Tourette's syndrome (TS), cluster headaches, and minimally conscious states has been investigated. Unfortunately, there are no reliable animal models for these disorders and the underlying neuronal circuitries and pathophysiology are poorly understood. Importantly, however, the targets for DBS in TS and cluster headache have been selected as a result of functional imaging findings *(55–59)*.

There have been several recent reports of DBS for TS *(60, 61)*. The centromedian-parafascicular complex of the thalamus has been targeted bilaterally in the majority of cases *(62, 63)*, but the GPi *(60, 62)* and the anterior limb of the internal capsule *(64)* also have been targeted. Because of the small number of patients who have undergone surgery, the ideal target has not been defined, although short-term follow-up reveals that most patients have experienced some degree of tic reduction.

The DBS target selected for the treatment of cluster headache has been the posterior hypothalamus and the results of treatment in as many as 22 patients have been published *(65–68)*. DBS of the posterior inferior hypothalamus was successful in the majority of these cases although one death did occur. A case series summarizing 21 patients examined the role of DBS in the minimally conscious state with 10 years of follow-up *(69)*. In 19 of these cases, the thalamic centromedian parafascicular (CM-pf) complex was targeted and eight of 21 patients reportedly emerged from their minimally conscious state and were able to obey commands *(69)*.

Although these case series represent potential uses of DBS in very different conditions and the efficacy of these treatments has not yet been well-defined, the alternative treatment options which exist for all of these diseases is very limited and conservative therapies have failed in a significant number of patients. In addition to further research toward establishing a precise target, multidisciplinary teams should be established before initiating treatment of patients with these disorders. Depending on the disorder being treated, team members should include a neurologist, pain management specialist, and rehabilitation specialist.

## Future Technical Considerations

As applications for DBS continue to expand, the number of patients with implantable devices will grow exponentially. Although the need to replace DBS electrodes due to infection and other hardware complications has become less common with improvements in securing the devices and other technical advances, one estimate of the complication rate per electrode per year is 8.4% *(70)*. Thus, the revision rates following DBS surgeries remain significantly higher than in other neurosurgical procedures and widespread use of these devices will mandate optimization of these devices to minimize re-operation rates and the overall cost of implantation.

With the advent of the Stimloc™ (Medtronic IGN, Minneapolis, MN) and a lower profile connector (Medtronic Model 7482), the frequency of lead migration and lead erosion has decreased. The connector should ideally be placed at the parieto-occipital junction 4 cm posterior to the pinna and therefore above the mastoid to minimize the risk of lead fracture *(70, 71)*. We have noted a further decrease in erosion by covering the Stimloc with pericranium and the connector with temporalis muscle/fascia and have not experienced an erosion in the last 300 leads placed (unpublished observations). Further technological advances will be mandated as DBS becomes increasingly used. Simple additions may aid in resolving the most common problems. Because of the potentially devastating effect of infection, antibiotic coating of the plastic may decrease the potential for infection. Because of the frequency of fractures at the distal end of the lead, a rescue option of additional contacts on the proximal end of the lead could save the need to replace the lead.

## Device Optimization

### Daily Living

The Medtronic Soletra™ Model 7426 Neurostimulator (Medtronic, Inc.) is currently the most commonly used IPG and consists of a lithium-thionyl chloride battery, with a median lifespan of approximately 45 months *(72)*. In general, PD patients will require a battery change every 3 to 5 years. However, pulse generators used in patients with higher energy consumptions, such as essential tremor and dystonia patients, have a significantly reduced life span *(72, 73)*. While the rate of battery replacement has not been high in patients with PD, more frequent battery changes in patients with dystonia or ET would mean a minimum of 10 battery changes in a 30 year old with an average lifespan. In children with dystonia requiring a repeated change in hardware, the wisdom of DBS vs a lesion can be questioned *(73)*.

The Medtronic Kinetra Model 7428 Neurostimulator, introduced in 2003, is a silver lithium vanadium oxide battery in a titanium case capable of accepting bilateral DBS through two quadripolar leads which connect into one pulse generator allowing for independent programming. It is FDA-approved for PD but the reimbursement is less, it is bulky, and has had some manufacturing problems so that it has not been used as frequently in the United States as in Europe. Vesper et al. have described the special programming features of the Kinetra system *(74)*. The dual-channel Kinetra is more useful for dystonia because power consumption is linear and battery life is longer in the higher voltage range. However, it is not FDA-approved for use in dystonia at this time *(75)*.

Research toward creating an implantable pulse generator (IPG) with a longer life span will no doubt continue, much as cardiac pacemaker technology has advanced from mercury-zinc batteries to nuclear to rechargeable lithium batteries *(76)*. Although the demands on a cardiac pacemaker battery are different than those for an IPG, the ideal IPG will no doubt also have a high energy density and low internal resistance. Pacemakers also have memory, which allows for data storage and processing as well as remote telemetry. IPGs of the future ideally will be equipped with similar features.

Another major issue with current IPGs is the effect of electromagnetic interference (EMI) encountered during daily life and during medical care for other diseases. The magnetic switch of the IPG may be activated by a number of household items. Notorious culprits are refrigerator doors with magnetic locks that may turn the IPG on or off. Other household devices that may interfere include small motors, stereo speakers, some cordless telephones, and radios. Metal detection devices in airports or shopping malls can also affect the IPG. The Kinetra can shield the on/off switch from these external sources of electromagnetic interference (EMI) but the Soletra cannot.

These are all inconveniences but the real problem is from MRI exposure (www.medtronic.com /physician/activa/downloadablefiles/ M925038A_a_001.pdf). It is clearly necessary to protect patients with implanted DBS systems from MR EMI because of the risk of heating the intracerebral electrode, which may cause brain injury. Henderson et al. *(77)* recently published a case report of a PD patient with bilateral STN DBS electrodes who underwent MRI of the lumbar spine and developed hemiplegia immediately after, presumably secondary to heating of the stimulating electrode. MR related heat generation is due to a multitude of factors including the electronic characteristics of the general DBS system and the schematics of each individual DBS, the relationship of the DBS lead to the radiofrequency coil, and the field strength and amount of radiofrequency (SAR) delivered by specific MR equipment *(78–82)*. It is crucial to realize that the SAR varies with MR model and software packages employed and thus may vary from scanner to scanner *(80)*.

Body MRI is currently not advised in patients implanted with DBS and cranial MRI should only be performed in MR scanners configured to safety specifications determined by the manufacturer. Functional neuroimaging is potentially a very important asset for researchers to have in order to assess the effects of DBS and help select more precise targets for DBS in various disease processes. However, currently patients with implanted DBS systems have a limited ability to undergo functional MRI (fMRI) or high resolution MRI scans. The majority of functional imaging studies concerning the effects of DBS to date have used PET *(83–88)*. The employment of fMRI, which has a higher resolution than PET, would be extremely useful. As more patients are implanted with DBS devices and other neuromodulatory devices, both MR technology and DBS systems will need to be adapted so these procedures can be performed safely and routinely, even in smaller hospitals or MR centers. For more details regarding MRI safety see the chapter by Baker and Phillips in this volume.

While difficulties among DBS patients concerning MRI will most commonly be encountered by the neurosurgeon, these patients may also have difficulty undergoing other medical procedures. A patient implanted with DBS who underwent diathermy for pain control after dental work entered a vegetative state due to electrode heating *(89)*. The safety of cardioversion in the DBS patient has also been questioned. One case report documents that cardioversion in an ET patient with unilateral DBS resulted in a thalamotomy lesion *(90)*. However, cardioversion has been performed safely in a patient with bilateral STN DBS *(91)* and there have been case series of patients who have been safely implanted with both DBS systems and pacemakers *(92, 93)*. However, great care must be taken in the implantation and programming of these patients as safety specifications have not been published and the potential for adverse interactions of these devices continues to exist.

The device specifications published by Medtronic, Inc. also warn concerning the use of gamma radiation and high output ultrasonic aspirators such as those used for lithotripsy, electrocautery, and electroconvulsive therapy in patients with implanted DBS systems. The safety of DBS patients undergoing transcranial magnetic stimulation, which can be used to better define human neurophysiology in both normal and disease processes is also undetermined. Although it would be difficult, if not impossible, to design a DBS system which would not interact with any of these systems, bioengineers need to take into account that as the applications of DBS expand and implanted patients become younger, these devices must be compatible with other frequently encountered medical technologies.

**Lead Technology**

The electrode lead and the means by which it delivers current will also be adapted over time as the principles of electrical stimulation are better understood.

The current electrodes used are the Medtronic 3389 and 3387 models, which are quadripolar. Each contact is made of cylindrical platinum/iridium alloy that is 1.5 mm long and 1.27 mm in diameter. Electrodes are available with individual contacts spaced 1.5 mm apart, typically used for Vim or GPi DBS (Medtronic Model 3387) or contacts spaced 0.5 mm apart which are often used for STN DBS (Medtronic model 3389). The proximal portion of the electrode consists of four nickel conductor wires insulated with a polytetraflouroethylene jacket (94). Our understanding of the effects of these electrodes on surrounding brain parenchyma and of the impact of stimulation parameters on neuronal response is currently limited.

Most studies examining the impact of the electrodes on surrounding brain tissue have been post-mortem case reports. Autopsy data exists for 12 patients with electrodes with PD (95–99), one patient with ET (100) and one with chorea-acanthocytosis (101). These reports have shown very limited neuropathological damage induced by chronic DBS implantation and stimulation. However one study which examined explanted DBS electrodes using electron microscopy, showed a foreign body multinucleated giant cell-type reaction, which occurred after 3 months of implantation (102). The researchers hypothesized that this reaction may have been due to the polyurethane component of the electrodes' surface coat and that by altering tissue impedance or distorting current distribution, the resultant reaction and local gliosis may be responsible for the tolerance that may develop following chronic stimulation (102). However, to date this report is unique and other researchers have not documented foreign body giant cell reactions (97–100). The material sciences may develop improved leads that are more durable, less inflammatory, and would provide satisfactory stimulation but resist EMI. As our understanding of electrode properties on brain parenchyma increases, lead technology will be adapted accordingly. Medtronic, as part of a post-market surveillance program, is conducting a "Brain Autopsy Research program."

Future lead characteristics are likely to change. When DBS technology was first invented, neural engineering design tools were limited (101). Another potential area of development is the alteration of electrode geometries in order to more precisely deliver targeted stimulation. Finite element models (FEM) have been used to assess the effects of varying the height and radius of the contacts on electrodes on the volume of tissue activated (VTA) at stimulation parameters used in clinical settings (103). Compared to the dimensions of contacts in standard 3387 or 3389 electrodes, increases in contact height led to an increase in VTA, while increasing the radius led to a decrease in VTA (103). The shape of the VTA was also affected. FEM, in combination with a three-dimensional representation of Vim have also demonstrated that relatively minor modifications in contact height and diameter, within manufacturing limitations of the current electrode tubing, could result in increased VTA by 28% without spread of stimulation to surrounding areas (103). In addition to altering contact dimensions, customizing the spacing and number of contacts can offer additional improvements in stimulation (103). With the use of computer modeling techniques, lead technology may be customized based on targets in the near future.

Multiple leads can also be coordinated to optimize beneficial effects. There has been some success using dual-lead technology in controlling tremor in patients, by passing electrode current between both electrodes (104). In one report, the electrodes were inserted in parallel and connected to a dual receiver (Mattrix, model 3272, Medtronic, Inc). The most effective stimulation parameter used contact 1 on the second electrode as the cathode and contact 1 on the first electrode as the anode *(104)*. The authors noted that the development of a Y-shaped extension cable with two active connections, would make dual lead technology possible with pulse generators that are currently used *(104)*.

Other potential modifications involve altering the current itself. Available leads are circumferential and the spread of current is reasonably symmetrical. In the future, by bisecting or quartering the lead current, it could be distributed toward areas of optimal effect and away from areas that induce side effects. Directing a side arm could have the same effect. Microelectrode arrays could potentially more effectively stimulate targets. In general, increasing sources of competition in the field of DBS technology should help improve the safety and efficacy of these devices.

**Stimulation Technology**

The electrical field generated by DBS affects the surrounding neural processes in a variable fashion related to the distribution of extracellular potentials and depolarization/hyperpolarization *(105–109)*. The result may be activation or inhibition depending on the neuronal subtype, the neuronal process being stimulated, and the nucleus involved *(109)*. These questions are impossible to answer through the use of historical experimental models and will likely be resolved only through well-developed neural modeling systems. Some preliminary data has been collected by combining physiological data obtained from diffusion tensor imaging combined with finite element models *(109, 110)*. If DBS technology can be developed which enables targeted activation of specific nuclei, cellular subtypes, and neuronal processes by altering electrode geometries, a great number of alterations and potential clinical benefits are possible *(111)*.

Improving our understanding of the effects of stimulation parameters on specific neural activity will also greatly alter the field of DBS and expand potential applications. The current stimulation parameters which are usually employed (monopolar or bipolar stimulation; 1 to 5 V stimulus amplitude; 60 to 200 5s stimulus pulse duration; 120 to 180 Hz stimulus frequency), much like target selection, are the result of trial and error *(112–115)*. Past successes of this methodology were effective because of the immediate responses of the diseases being treated, such as tremor control in PD or essential tremor, but may not be possible in emerging applications in which clinical benefit may occur over longer periods of time. A better understanding of the mechanisms of stimulation and its effects on neural activity will require multi-modality research techniques including histochemical analyses, electrophysiological recordings, functional imaging and neural modeling. The potential exists that DBS hardware and stimulation parameters will no longer be generic and will be customized for disease processes, affected nuclei, and ultimately perhaps even individual patients *(109)*.

It may also turn out that constant stimulation may not be the best therapeutic mode. Currently DBS is an open-loop system, in which no feedback is present to alter stimulation parameters as needed. Development of sensor technology in the DBS system could improve the efficacy of DBS in the treatment of diseases such as epilepsy or possibly TS, where seizures or tics occur intermittently. Currently, another form of neuromodulation, the Neuropace system (RNS, NeuroPace, Inc., Mountain View, CA), is being investigated in a multi-center study. This device consists of an IPG, one or two quadripolar subdural strip or depth leads, and a programmer. It is capable of analyzing the patient's electrocortigram and then triggering electrical stimulation when specific electrocortigram characteristics programmed by the clinician as ictal events occur. An initial small open label study reported that seven of eight patients using this system had greater than 45% reduction in seizures *(116)*. However, specific and sensitive algorithms will need to be developed which optimally detect ictal activity before true efficacy can be determined. As discussed earlier, there has been initial success in open label studies with chronic DBS of the anterior nucleus of the thalamus for epilepsy in an open-loop system *(54, 117)*. The employment of this target in a remote closed-loop system resulted in a 40% seizure reduction in a small number of treated patients *(118)*.

Technology enabling DBS to be used as part of closed-loop systems is available, although the details and practical aspects remain to be refined. For example, stimulation for movement disorders could potentially be controlled by feedback concerning ongoing motor activity. Further beyond the horizon may be the employment of DBS technology in the augmentation of brain–computer interface systems (BCI). Some existing BCIs use invasive electrode techniques *(119–125)* to obtain recordings from populations of individual neurons. The ability of these electrodes to stimulate as well as record may have some benefit in facilitating learning and rehabilitation. Preliminary studies have shown that electrical stimulation of the cortex may improve motor outcome in impaired individuals *(126–128)*. Although much work is needed to optimize microelectrodes for BCI and ultimately to develop BCIs which are capable of three-dimensional control, it is possible that eventually a combination of BCI technology with high-frequency stimulation may lead to further advances in neurorehabilitation.

## Combination of DBS With Alternative Technologies

In the more immediate future, clinicians will have the ability to combine DBS systems with delivery systems technology, much as endovascular technologies have advanced with the advent of drug eluting stents *(129, 130)*. Several potential types of adjuvant therapies may be possible including drug infusions, gene therapies, and stem cell implantations. Microdialysis work in models of DBS have demonstrated that increases in extracellular glutamate are induced by STN DBS at frequencies up to 60 Hz and that progressive GABA increases which parallel frequency amplitudes also occur *(131)*. Microinjections of muscimol, a GABAa agonist, administered intra-operatively in 10 patients undergoing DBS demonstrated tremor suppression in two patients *(132)*. Thus, the potential exists for drug infusions used as adjunctive therapies that could selectively activate specific neurotransmitter receptors or neurotrophic factors. Work in gene therapy has included gene transfer of tyrosine hydroxylase and aromatic acid decarboxylase (AADC), two enzymes involved in dopamine synthesis, as well as co-regulators of the process such as GTP cyclohydrolase and vesicular monoamine transporters in animal models *(133–144)*. Possibly the most promising thus far is the transfer of the aromatic acid decarboxylase (AADC) gene which resulted in increased striatal dopamine levels in response to systemic L-dopa in primate models of parkinsonism *(145)*. The introduction of growth factors has also shown promise. The infusion of glial-derived neurotrophic factor (GDNF) into the putamen of five patients with PD resulted in significant motor improvement *(146)*. A phase II trial was initiated and at 6-month follow-up, the GDNF-treated patients failed to show significant changes in their off medication UPDRS III scores. However, methodological differences between this study and previous open label studies may have led to some of the discrepancy *(147)*. The results with fetal neural transplantation for PD to date have not been well received because of lack of efficacy compared with results of sham surgery and the appearance of intractable dyskinesias *(148)*. Work with neural transplantation is ongoing utilizing stem cells, retinal pigment epithelial cells, and auto-transplanted dopaminergic cells *(149–151)*. Closed-loop low-frequency stimulation of transplanted cell populations could augment the effectiveness of these therapies. As advances are made in these therapies, the potential exists to use them in combination with DBS both because DBS systems of the future may offer a delivery mechanism, and because stimulation itself may result in more responsive cellular milieu *(152, 153)*.

## Conclusions

The future of DBS has enormous possibilities. The question is which areas will offer the greatest clinical benefit. The future success of DBS is dependent on refinement of target and patient selection and the development of multidisciplinary teams specific to the diseases being treated. Much work will be directed at device optimization to enable customized stimulation delivery and developing systems that will be more compatible with activities of daily living in the real world environment. The potential for adjuncts to DBS are limitless and will no doubt be a major focus of research for years to come. Although DBS has the potential to become a basis for treatment of a number of disease processes, great caution, due diligence, and basic and preclinical research will be needed to truly assess the efficacy of implant stimulation in a scientific fashion.

## References

1. Deuschl G, Schade-Brittinger C, Krack P, et al (2006) A randomized trial of deep-brain stimulation for Parkinson's disease. N Engl J Med 355:896–908.
2. Benabid AL, Chabardes S, Seigneuret E, Pollak P, Fraix V, Krack P, Lebas JF, Grand S, Piallat B (2005) Functional neurosurgery: past, present, and future. Clin Neurosurg 52:265–70.
3. Bartholow R (1874) Experimental investigations into the functions of the human brain. Am J Med Sci 67:305–313.
4. Benabid AL, Pollak P, Gervason C, Hoffmann D, Gao DM (1991) Long-term suppression of tremor by chronic stimulation of the ventral intermediate thalamic nucleus. Lancet 337:403–406.
5. Benabid AL, Pollak P, Gao D, Hoffmann D, Limousin P (1996) Chronic electrical stimulation of the ventralis intermedius nucleus of the thalamus as a treatment of movement disorders. J Neurosurg 84:203–214.
6. Bergman H, Wichmann T, DeLong MR (1990) Reversal of experimental parkinsonism by lesions of the subthalamic nucleus. Science 249:1436–1438.

7. Aziz TZ, Peggs D, Sambrook MA, Crossman AR (1991) Lesion of the subthalamic nucleus for the alleviation of 1-methyl-4-phenyl-1,2,3,6-tetrahydropyridine (MPTP)-induced parkinsonism in the primate. Mov Disord 6:288–292.
8. Anderson VC, Burchiel KJ, Hogarth P, Favre J, Hammerstad JP (2005) Pallidal vs subthalamic nucleus deep brain stimulation in Parkinson disease. Arch Neurol 62:554–560.
9. Burchiel KJ, Anderson VC, Favre J, Hammerstad JP (1999) Comparison of pallidal and subthalamic nucleus deep brain stimulation for advanced Parkinson's disease: results of a randomized, blinded pilot study. Neurosurgery 45:1375–1382.
10. Katayama Y, Kasai M, Oshima H, Fukaya C, Yamamoto T, Mizutani T (2000) Double blinded evaluation of the effects of pallidal and subthalamic nucleus stimulation on daytime activity in advanced Parkinson's disease. Parkinsonism Relat Disord 7:35–40.
11. Eltahawy HA, Saint-Cyr J, Giladi N, Lang AE, Lozano AM (2004) Primary dystonia is more responsive than secondary dystonia to pallidal interventions: outcome after pallidotomy or pallidal deep brain stimulation. Neurosurgery 54:613–619.
12. Lozano AM, Kumar R, Gross RE, Giladi N, Hutchison WD (1997) Globus pallidus internus pallidotomy for generalized dystonia. Mov Disord 12:865–870.
13. Vitek JL, Zhang J, Evatt M, Mewes K, DeLong MR (1998) GPi pallidotomy for dystonia: clinical outcome and neuronal activity. Adv Neurol 78:211–219.
14. Yoshor D, Hamilton WJ, Ondo W, Jankovic J, Grossman RG (2001) Comparison of thalamotomy and pallidotomy for the treatment of dystonia. Neurosurgery 48:818–824.
15. Detante O, Vercueil L, Krack P, Chabardes S, Benabid AL, Pollak P (2004) Off-period dystonia in Parkinson's disease but not generalized dystonia is improved by high-frequency stimulation of the subthalamic nucleus. Adv Neurol 94:309–314.
16. Vidailhet M, Vercueil L, Houeto JL, Krystkowiak P, Benabid AL (2005) Bilateral deep-brain stimulation of the globus pallidus in primary generalized dystonia. N Engl J Med 352:459–467.
17. Brudzynski SM, Houghton PE, Brownlee RD, Mogensen GJ (1986) Involvement of neuronal cell bodies of the mesencephalic locomtor region in the initiation of locomotor activity of freely behaving rats. Brain Res Bull 16:377–381.
18. Milner KL, Mogensen GJ (1988) Electrical and chemical activation of the mesenchephalic and subthalamic locomotor regions in freely moving rats. Brain Res 452:273–285.
19. Jenkinson N, Nandi D, Miall RC, Stein JF, Aziz TZ (2004) Pedunculopontine nucleus stimulation improves akinesia in a Parkinsonian monkey. Neuroreport 15:2621–2624.
20. Plaha P, Gill SS (2005) Bilateral deep brain stimulation of the pedunculopontine nucleus for Parkinson's disease. Neuroreport 16:1883–1887.
21. Moniz E (1936) Essai d'un traitement chirugical de certaine psychoses. Bull Acad Med 115:385–393.
22. Moniz E (1937) Prefrontal leucotomy in the treatment of mental disorders, Am. J. Psychiatry 93:1379–1385.
23. Freeman W, Watts JW (1937) Prefrontal leucotomy in the treatment of mental disorders, South Med J 30:23–31.
24. Freeman W (1948) Transorbital leucotomy. Lancet 2:371–373.
25. Deutsch A (1937) The Mentally Ill in America. New York: Doubleday.
26. Fulton JF (1948) The Frontal Lobes: Research Publication for the Association for Research in Nervous and Mental Disease. Baltimore: Williams & Wilkins.
27. Rodgers JE (1992) Psychosurgery: Damaging the Brain to Save the Mind. New York: Harper-Collins.
28. Valenstein ES (1986) Great and Desperate Cures. New York: Basic Books.

29. Mashour GA, Walker EE, Martuza RL (2005) Psychosurgery: past, present, and future. Brain Res Review 48:409–419.
30. Anderson D, Ahmed A (2003) Treatment of patients with intractable obsessive–compulsive disorder with anterior capsular stimulation. Case report. J Neurosurg 98:1104–1108.
31. Nuttin B, Cosyns P, Demeulemeester H, Gybels J, Meyerson B (1999) Electrical stimulation in anterior limbs of internal capsules in patients with obsessive–compulsive disorder. Lancet 354:1526.
32. Nuttin BJ, Gabriels LA, Cosyns PR, Meyerson BA, Andreewitch S, Sunaert SG (2003) Long-term electrical capsular stimulation in patients with obsessive–compulsive disorder. Neurosurgery 52:1263–1272.
33. Gabriels L, Cosyns P, Nuttin B, Demeulemeester H, Gybels J (2003) Deep brain stimulation for treatment-refractory obsessive–compulsive disorder: psychopathological and neuropsychological outcome in three cases. Acta Psychiatr Scand 107:275–282.
34. Abelson JL, Curtis GC, Sagher O, Albucher RC, Harrigan M, Taylor SF (2005) Deep brain stimulation for refractory obsessive–compulsive disorder. Biol Psychiatry 57:510–516.
35. Sturm V, Lenartz D, Koulousakis A, Treuer H, Herholz K, Klein JC (2003) The nucleus accumbens: a target for deep brain stimulation in obsessive–compulsive- and anxiety-disorders. J Chem Neuroanat 26:293–299.
36. Aouizerate B, Cuny E, Martin-Guehl C, Guehl D, Amieva H, Benazzouz A (2004) Deep brain stimulation of the ventral caudate nucleus in the treatment of obsessive–compulsive disorder and major depression. Case report. J Neurosurg 101:682–686.
37. Aouizerate B, Martin-Guehl C, Cuny E, Guehl D, Amieva H, Benazzouz A (2005) Deep brain stimulation for OCD and major depression. Am J Psychiatry 162:2192.
38. Greenberg BD, Malone DA, Friehs GM, et al (2006) Three-year outcomes in deep brain stimulation for highly resistant obsessive-compulsive disorder. Neuropsychopharmacology.
39. Matthews K, Eljamel M, Christmas D, MacVicar R (2005) Neurosurgical treatments for Chronic Refractory Depression: Controlled comparison of anterior capsulotomy, anterior cingulotomy, and vagus nerve stimulation. Neurosurg 57:426 (Abstr.).
40. Mayberg HS, Lozano AM, Voon V, McNeely HE, Seminowicz D (2005) Deep brain stimulation for treatment-resistant depression. Neuron 45:651–660.
41. Abelson JL, Curtis GC, Sagher O, Albucher RC, Harrigan M, Taylor SF, Martis B, Giordani B (2005) Deep brain stimulation for refractory obsessive-compulsive disorder. Biol Psychiatry 57:510–516.
42. Mayberg HS, Brannan SK, Mahurin RK, Jerabek PA, Brickman JS, Tekell JL, Silva JA, McGinnis S, Glass TG, Martin CC, Fox PT (1997) Cingulate function in depression: a potential predictor of treatment response. Neuroreport 8:1057–1061.
43. Sani SB, Jobe KW, Kordower J, Bakay RAE (2006) Deep brain stimulation for the treatment of obesity in the rat. J Neurosurg 102:783(Abstr).
44. Foust RF, Burke R, Gordon N (2006) Best practice for obesity and weight management: finding success through linking effective gastric bypass surgery policy and health management. Dis Manag 9:182–188.
45. Van Buren JM, Wood JH, Oakley J, Hambrecht F (1978) Preliminary evaluation of cerebellar stimulation by double-blind stimulation and biological criteria in the treatment of epilepsy. J Neurosurg 48:407–416.
46. Mirski MA, Rossell LA, Terry JB, Fisher RS (1997) Anticonvulsant effect of anterior thalamic high frequency electrical stimulation in the rat. Epilepsy Res 28:89–100(Abstr.).

47. Velisek L, Veliskova J, Moshe SL (2002) Electrical stimulation of substantia nigra pars reticulata is anticonvulsant in adult and young male rats. Exp Neurol 173:145–152.
48. Vercueil L, Benazzouz A, Deransart C (1998) High-frequency stimulation of the subthalamic nucleus suppresses absence seizures in the rat: comparison with neurotoxic lesions, Epilepsy Res 31:39–46.
49. Theodore WH, Fisher RS (2004) Brain stimulation for epilepsy. Lancet Neurol 3:111–118.
50. Chkhenkeli SA, Chkhenkeli IS (1997) Effects of therapeutic stimulation of nucleus caudatus on epileptic electrical activity of brain in patients with intractable epilepsy, Stereotact Funct Neurosurg 69:221–224.
51. Vonck K, Boon P, Achten E, De Reuck J, Caemaert J (2002) Long-term amygdalohippocampal stimulation for refractory temporal lobe epilepsy. Ann Neurol 52:556–565.
52. Velasco F, Velasco M, Jimenez F, Velasco AL and Marquez I (2002) Stimulation of the central median thalamic nucleus for epilepsy. Stereotact Funct Neurosurg 77:228–232.
53. Fisher RS, Uematsu S, Krauss GL (1992) Placebo-controlled pilot study of centromedian thalamic stimulation in treatment of intractable seizures. Epilepsia 33:841–851.
54. Andrade DM, Zumsteg D, Hamani C, Hodaie M, Sarkissian S, Lozano AM, Wennberg RA (2006) Long-term follow-up of patients with thalamic deep brain stimulation for epilepsy. Neurology 66:1571–1573.
55. Braun AR, Stoetter B, Randolph C, et al. (1993) The functional anatomy of Tourette's syndrome: an FDG-PET study. I. Regional changes in cerebral glucose metabolism differentiating patients and controls. Neuropsychopharmacology 9:277–291.
56. Braun AR, Randolph C, Stoetter B, et al (1995) The functional anatomy of Tourette's syndrome: an FDG-PET study. II. Relationships between regional cerebral metabolism and associated behavioral and cognitive features of the illness. Neuropsychopharmacology 13:151–168.
57. Peterson BS, Skudlarski P, Anderson AW, Zhang H, Gatenby JC, Lacadie CM, Leckman JF, Gore JC (1998) A functional magnetic resonance imaging study of tic suppression in Tourette syndrome. Arch Gen Psychiatry 55:326–333.
58. May A, Bahra A, Buchel C, Frackowiak RS, Goadsby PJ (1998) Hypothalamic activation in cluster headache attacks. Lancet 352:275–278.
59. Sprenger T, Boecker H, Toelle TR, Bussone G, May A, Leone M (2004) Specific hypothalamic activation during a spontaneous cluster headache attack. Neurology 3:516–517.
60. Diederich NJ, Kalteis K, Stamenkovic M, Pieri V, Alesch F (2005) Efficient internal pallidal stimulation in Gilles de la Tourette syndrome: a case report. Mov Disord 20:1496–1499.
61. Temel Y, Visser-Vandewalle V (2005) Surgery in Tourette syndrome. Mov Disord 19:3–14.
62. Houeto JL, Karachi C, Mallet L, Pillon B, Yelnik J (2005) Tourette's syndrome and deep brain stimulation. J Neurol Neurosurg Psych 76:992–995.
63. Visser-Vandewalle V, Temel Y, Boon P, Vreeling F, Colle H (2003) Chronic bilateral thalamic stimulation: a new therapeutic approach in intractable Tourette syndrome. J Neurosurg 99:1094–1100.
64. Flaherty AW, Williams ZM, Amirnovin R, Kasper E, Rauch SL, Cosgrove GR, Eskandar EN (2005) Deep brain stimulation of the anterior internal capsule for the treatment of Tourette syndrome: technical case report. Neurosurg 57:E403.
65. Leone M, Franzini A, Broggi G, May A, Bussone G (2004) Long-term follow-up of bilateral hypothalamic stimulation for intractable cluster headache. Brain 127:2259–2264.

66. Leone M, Franzini A, D'Amico D, Grazzi L, Mea E, Curone M, Tullo V, Broggi G, D'Andrea G, Bussone G (2004) Strategies for the treatment of autonomic trigeminal cephalalgias. Neurol Sci 25:S167–S170.
67. Leone M, May A, Franzini A, Broggi G, MD, Dodick D, Rapoport A, Goadsby PJ, Schoenen J, Bonavita V, Bussone G (2004) Deep brain stimulation for intractable chronic cluster headache: proposals for patient selection. Cephalgia 24:934–937.
68. Schoenen J, Di Clemente L, Vandenheede M Fumal A, De Pasqua V, Mouchamps M, Remacle JM, de Noordhout AM (2005) Hypothalmic stimulation in chronic cluster headache: a pilot study of efficacy and mode of action. Brain 128:940–947.
69. Yamamoto T, Katayama Y (2005) Deep brain stimulation therapy for the vegetative state. Neuropsychol Rehabil 15:406–413.
70. Oh MY, Abosch A, Kim SH, et al (2002) Long-term hardware-related complications of deep brain stimulation. Neurosurgery 50:1268–1274.
71. Starr PA (2002) Placement of deep brain stimulators into the subthalamic nucleus or Globus pallidus internus: technical approach. Stereotact Funct Neurosurg 79:118–145.
72. Bin-Mahfoodh M, Hamani C, Sime E, Lozano AM (2003) Longevity of batteries in internal pulse generators used for deep brain stimulation. Stereotact Funct Neurosurg 80:56–60.
73. Okun MS, Vitek JL (2004) Lesion therapy for Parkinson's disease and other movement disorders: update and controversies. Mov Disord 19:375–389.
74. Vesper J, Chabardes S, Fraix V, Sunde N, Ostergaard K; Kinetra Study Group (2002) Dual channel deep brain stimulation system (Kinetra) for Parkinson's disease and essential tremor: a prospective multicentre open label clinical study. J Neurol Neurosurg Psychiatry 73:275–280.
75. Krauss JK, Yianni J, Loher TJ, Aziz TZ (2004) Deep brain stimulation for dystonia. J Clin Neurophysiol 21:18–30.
76. Mallela VS, Ilankumaran V, Rao NS (2004) Trends in cardiac pacemaker batteries. Indian Pacing Electrophysiol J 4:201–212.
77. Henderson JM, Tkach J, Phillips M, Baker K, Shellock FG, Rezai AR (2005) Permanent neurological deficit related to magnetic resonance imaging in a patient with implanted deep brain stimulation electrodes for Parkinson's disease: case report. Neurosurgery 57:E1063.
78. Finelli DA, Rezai AR, Ruggieri P, Tkach J, Nyenhuis JA, Hrdlicka G, Sharan A, Gonzalez-Martinez J, Stypulkowski PH, Shellock FG (2002) MR-related heating of deep brain stimulation electrodes: An in vitro study of clinical imaging sequences. AJNR Am J Neuroradiol 23:1795–1802.
79. Rezai AR, Finelli DA, Nyenhuis JA, Hrdlicka G, Tkach J, Sharan A, Ruggieri P, Stypulkowski PH, Shellock FG (2002) Neurostimulation systems for deep brain stimulation: In vitro evaluation of magnetic resonance imaging-related heating at 1.5 tesla. J Magn Reson Imaging 15:241–250.
80. Rezai AR, Phillips M, Baker K, Sharan A, Nyenhuis JA, Tkach J, Henderson JM, Shellock FG (2004) Neurostimulation systems used for deep brain stimulation (DBS): MR safety issues and implications for failing to follow guidelines. Invest Radiol 39:300–303.
81. Shellock FG (2005) Reference Manual for Magnetic Resonance Safety, Implants, and Devices: 2005 Edition. Los Angeles: Biomedical Research Publishing Group.
82. Tronnier VM, Stauber A, Hanhnel S, Sarem-Aslani A (1999) Magnetic resonance imaging with implanted neurostimulation systems: An in vitro and in vivo study. Neurosurgery 44:118–125.
83. Ceballos-Baumann AO, Boecker H, Bartensetin P, von Falkenhayn I, Riescher H (2001) A positron emission tomographic study of subthalamic nucleus stimulation in Parkinson's disease: enhanced movement-related activity of motor-association cortex and decreased motor cortex resting activity. Neurology 56:1347–1354.

84. Davis KD, Taub E, Houle S, Lang AE, Dostrovsky JO, Tasker RR, Lozano AM (1997) Globus pallidus stimulation activates the cortical motor system during alleviation of parkinsonian symptoms. Nat Med 3:671–674.
85. Fukuda M, Mentis MJ, Ma Y, Dhawan V, Antonini A (2001) Networks mediating the clinical effects of pallidal brain stimulation for Parkinson's disease: a PET study of resting-state glucose metabolism. Brain 124:1601–1609.
86. Haslinger B, Boecker H, Buchel C, Vesper J, Tronnier VM, Pfister R, Alesch F, Moringlane JR, Krauss JK, Conrad B, Schwaiger M, Ceballos-Baumann AO (2003) Differential modulation of subcortical target and cortex during deep brain stimulation. Neuroimage 18:517–524.
87. Hilker R, Voges J, Thiel A, Ghaemi M, Herholz K (2002) Deep brain stimulation of the subthalamic nucleus versus levodopa challenge in Parkinson's disease: measuring the on- and off-conditions with FDG-PET. J Neural Transm 109:1257–1264.
88. Perlmutter JS, Mink JW, Bastian AJ, Zackowski K, Hershey T, Miyawaki E, Koller W, Videen TO (2002) Blood flow responses to deep brain stimulation of thalamus. Neurology 58:1388–1394.
89. Nutt JG, Anderson VC, Peacock JH, Hammerstad JP, Burchiel KJ (2001) DBS and diathermy interaction induces severe CNS damage. Neurology 56:1384–1386.
90. Yamamoto T, Katayama Y, Fukaya C, Kurihara J, Oshima H, Kasai M (2000) Thalamotomy caused by cardioversion in a patient treated with deep brain stimulation. Stereotact Funct Neurosurg 74:73–82.
91. Rosenow JM, Tarkin H, Zias E, Sorbera C, Mogilner A. Simultaneous use of bilateral subthalamic nucleus stimulators and an implantable cardiac defibrillator. Case report. J Neurosurg 99:167–169.
92. Capelle HH, Simpson RK Jr, Kronenbuerger M, Michaelsen J, Tronnier V, Krauss JK (2005) Long-term deep brain stimulation in elderly patients with cardiac pacemakers. J Neurosurg 102:53–59.
93. Senatus PB, McClelland S 3rd, Ferris AD, et al (2004) Implantation of bilateral deep brain stimulators in patients with Parkinson disease and preexisting cardiac pacemakers. Report of two cases. J Neurosurg 101:1073–1077.
94. Yelnik J, Damier P, Demeret S, Gervais D, Bardinet E, Bejjani BP, Francois C, Houeto JL, Arnule I, Dormont D, Galanaud D, Pidoux B, Cornu P, Agid Y (2003) Localization of stimulating electrodes in patients with Parkinson disease by using a three-dimensional atlas-magnetic resonance imaging coregistration method. J Neurosurg 99:89–99.
95. Caparros-Lefebvre D, Ruchoux MM, Blond S, Petit H, Percheron G (1994) Long-term thalamic stimulation in Parkinson's disease: postmortem anatomo-clinical study. Neurology 44:1856–1860.
96. Haberler C, Alesch F, Mazal PR, Pilz P, Jellinger K, Pinter MM, Hainfellner JA, Budka H (2000) No tissue damage by chronic deep brain stimulation in Parkinson's disease. Ann Neurol 48:372–376.
97. Henderson JM, O'Sullivan DJ, Pell M, Fung VS, Hely MA, Morris JG, Halliday GM (2001) Lesion of thalamic centromedian—parafascicular complex after chronic deep brain stimulation. Neurology 56:1576–1579.
98. Henderson JM, Pell M, O'Sullivan DJ, McCusker EA, Fung VS, Hedges P, Halliday GM (2002) Postmortem analysis of bilateral subthalamic electrode implants in Parkinson's disease. Mov Disord 17:133–137.
99. Jarraya B, Bonnet AM, Duyckaerts C, Houeto JL, Cornu P, Hauw JJ, Agid Y (2003) Parkinson's disease, subthalamic stimulation, and selection of candidates: a pathological study. Mov Disord 18:1517–1520.
100. Boockvar JA, Telfeian A, Baltuch GH, Skolnick B, Simuni T, Stern M, Schmidt ML, Trojanowski JQ (2000) Long-term deep brain stimulation in a patient with essential tremor: clinical response and postmortem correlation with stimulator termination sites in ventral thalamus. Case report. J Neurosurg 93:140–144.

101. Burbaud P, Vital A, Rougier A, Bouillot S, Guehl D, Cuny E, Ferrer X, Lagueny A, Bioulac B (2002) Minimal tissue damage after stimulation of the motor thalamus in a case of chorea-acanthocytosis. Neurology 59:1982–1984.
102. Moss J, Ryder T, Aziz TZ, Graeber MB, Bain PG (2004) Electron microscopy of tissue adherent to explanted electrodes in dystonia and Parkinson's disease. Brain 127:2755–2763.
103. Butson CR, McIntyre CC (2006) Role of electrode design on the volume of tissue activated during deep brain stimuliaton. J Neural Eng 3:1–8.
104. Yamamoto T, Katayama Y, Fukaya C, Oshima H, Kasai M, Kobayashi K (2001) New method of deep brain stimulation therapy with two electrodes implanted in parallel and side by side. J Neurosurg 95:1075–1078.
105. McIntyre CC, Mori S, Sherman DL, Thakor NV, Vitek JL (2004) Electric field and stimulating influence generated by deep brain stimulation of the subthalamic nucleus. Clin Neurophysiol 115:589–595.
106. McNeal DR (1976) Analysis of a model for excitation of myelinated nerve. IEEE Trans Biomed Eng 23:329–337.
107. Lee DC, McIntyre CC, Grill WM (2003) Extracellular electrical stimulation of central neurons: quantitative studies. In: Finn WE, Lopresti PG, eds. Handbook of Neuroprosthetic Methods. Boca Raton, FL: CRC Press.
108. Rattay F (1999) The basic mechanism for the electrical stimulation of the nervous system. Neuroscience 89:335–346.
109. McIntyre CC, Grill WM (2002) Extracellular stimulation of central neurons: influence of stimulus waveform and frequency on neuronal output. J Neurophysiol 88:1592–1604.
110. Tuch DS, Wedeen VJ, Dale AM, George JS, Belliveau JW (2001) Conductivity tensor mapping of the human brain using diffusion tensor MRI. Proc Natl Acad Sci 98:11,697–11,701.
111. McIntyre CC, Grill WM (2000) Selective microstimulation of central nervous system neurons. Ann Biomed Eng 28:219–233.
112. Moro E, Esselink RJ, Xie J, Hommel M, Benabid AL, Pollak P (2002) The impact on Parkinson's disease of electrical parameter settings in STN stimulation. Neurology 59:706–713.
113. O'Suilleabhain PE, Frawley W, Giller C, Dewey RB Jr (2003) Tremor response to polarity, voltage, pulse width and frequency of thalamic stimulation. Neurology 60:786–790.
114. Rizzone M, Lanotte M, Bergamasco B, Tavella A, Torre E, Faccani G, Melcarne A, Lopiano L (2001) Deep brain stimulation of the subthalamic nucleus in Parkinson's disease: effects of variation in stimulation parameters. J Neurol Neurosurg Psychiatry 71:215–219.
115. Volkmann J, Herzog J, Kopper F, Deuschl G (2002) Introduction to the programming of deep brain stimulators. Mov Disord 17:181–187.
116. Fountas KN, Smith JR, Murro AM, Politsky J, Park YD, Jenkins PD (2005) Implantation of a closed-loop stimulation in the management of medically refractory focal epilepsy: a technical note. Stereotact Funct Neurosurg 83:153–158.
117. Kerrigan JF, Litt B, Fisher RS, Cranstoun S, French JA, Blum DE, Dichter M, Shetter A, Baltuch G, Jaggi J, Krone S, Brodie M, Rise M, Graves N (2004) Electrical stimulation of the anterior nucleus of the thalamus for the treatment of intractable epilepsy. Epilepsia 45:346–354.
118. Osorio I, Frei MG, Sunderam S, Giftakis J, Bhavaraju NC, Schaffner SF, Wilkinson SB (2005) Automated seizure abatement in humans using electrical stimulation. Ann Neurol 57:258–268.
119. Serruya MD, Hatsopoulos NG, Paninski L, Fellows MR, Donoghue J (2002) Instant neural control of a movement signal. Nature 416:141–142.
120. Taylor DM, Tillery SIH, Schwartz AB (2002) Direct cortical control of 3D neuroprosthetic devices. Science 296:1829–1832.

121. Carmena JM, Lebedev MA, Crist RE, O'Doherty JE, Santucci DM, Dimitrov DF, Patil PG, Henriquez CS, Nicolelis MA (2003) Learning to control a brain-machine interface for reaching and grasping by primates. PLoS Biol 1:E42.
122. Musallam S, Corneil BD, Greger B, Scherberger H, Andersen RA (2004) Cognitive control signals for neural prosthetics. Science 305:258–262.
123. Kennedy PR, Bakay RA, Moore MM, Adams K, Goldwaithe J (2000) Direct control of a computer from the human central nervous system. IEEE Trans Rehabil Eng 8:198–202.
124. Hochberg LR, Serruya MD, Friehs GM, Mukand JA, Saleh M, Caplan AH, Branner A, Chen D, Penn RD, Donoghue JP (2006) Neuronal ensemble control of prosthetic devices by a human with tetraplegia. Nature 442:164–171.
125. Patil PG, Carmena JM, Nicolelis MA, Turner DA (2004) Ensemble recordings of human subcortical neurons as a source of motor control signals for a brain-machine interface. Neurosurgery 55:27–38.
126. Hummel FC, Cohen LG (2006) Non-invasive brain stimulation: a new strategy to improve neurorehabilitation after stroke? Lancet Neurol 5:708–712.
127. Levy RM, Ruth A, Huang ME, Harvery RL, Ruland S, Dafer S, Lowry D, Weinand ME (2006) Cortical stimulation for motor recovery after stroke: impact on Neuropsychological performance and functional imaging. Neurosurg 59:480.
128. Brown JA, Lutsep HL, Weinand M, Cramer SC (2006) Motor cortex stimulation for the enhancement of recovery from stroke: a prospective, multicenter safety study. Neurosurgery 58:464–473.
129. Eisenberg MJ, Konnyu KJ (2006) Review of randomized clinical trials of drug-eluting stents for the prevention of in-stent restenosis. Am J Cardiol 98:375–382.
130. Gupta R, Al-Ali F, Thomas AJ, et al (2006) Safety, feasibility, and short-term follow-up of drug-eluting stent placement in the intracranial and extracranial circulation. Stroke 37:2562–2566.
131. Windels F, Bruet N, Poupard A, Feuerstein C, Bertrand A, Savasta M (2003) Influence of the frequency parameter on extracellular glutamate and gamma-aminobutyric acid in substantia nigra and globus pallidus during electrical stimulation of subthalamic nucleus in rats. J Neurosci Res 2:259–267.
132. Levy R, Lang AE, Dostrovsky JO, et al (2001) Lidocaine and muscimol microinjections in subthalamic nucleus reverse Parkinsonian symptoms. Brain 124:2105–2118.
133. Ozawa K, Fan DS, Shen Y, et al (2000) Gene therapy of Parkinson's disease using adeno-associated virus (AAV) vectors. J Neural Transm Suppl 58:181–191.
134. Kordower JH, Bloch J, Ma SY, et al (1999) Lentiviral gene transfer to the nonhuman primate brain. Exp Neurol 160:1–16.
135. During MJ, Naegele JR, O'Malley KL, Geller AI (1994) Long-term behavioral recovery in parkinsonian rats by an HSV vector expressing tyrosine hydroxylase. Science 266:1399–1403.
136. Azzouz M, Martin-Rendon E, Barber RD, et al (2002) Multicistronic lentiviral vector-mediated striatal gene transfer of aromatic L-amino acid decarboxylase, tyrosine hydroxylase, and GTP cyclohydrolase I induces sustained transgene expression, dopamine production, and functional improvement in a rat model of Parkinson's disease. J Neurosci 22:10,302–10,312.
137. Shen Y, Muramatsu SI, Ikeguchi K, et al (2000) Triple transduction with adeno-associated virus vectors expressing tyrosine hydroxylase, aromatic-L-amino-acid decarboxylase, and GTP cyclohydrolase I for gene therapy of Parkinson's disease. Hum Gene Ther 11:1509–1519.
138. Fan D, Shen Y, Kang D, et al (2001) Adeno-associated virus vector-mediated triple gene transfer of dopamine synthetic enzymes. Chin Med J (Engl) 114:1276–1279.
139. Leff SE, Spratt SK, Snyder RO, Mandel RJ (1999) Long-term restoration of striatal L-aromatic amino acid decarboxylase activity using recombinant adeno-

associated viral vector gene transfer in a rodent model of Parkinson's disease. Neuroscience 92:185–196.
140. Muramatsu S, Fujimoto K, Ikeguchi K, et al (2002) Behavioral recovery in a primate model of Parkinson's disease by triple transduction of striatal cells with adeno-associated viral vectors expressing dopamine-synthesizing enzymes. Hum Gene Ther 13:345–354.
141. During MJ, Samulski RJ, Elsworth JD, et al (1998) In vivo expression of therapeutic human genes for dopamine production in the caudates of MPTP-treated monkeys using an AAV vector. Gene Ther 5:820–827.
142. Muramatsu S, Fujimoto K, Ikeguchi K, et al (2002) Behavioral recovery in a primate model of Parkinson's disease by triple transduction of striatal cells with adeno-associated viral vectors expressing dopamine-synthesizing enzymes. Hum Gene Ther 13:345–354.
143. Lee WY, Chang JW, Nemeth NL, Kang UJ (1999) Vesicular monoamine transporter-2 and aromatic L-amino acid decarboxylase enhance dopamine delivery after L-3,4-dihydroxyphenylalanine administration in Parkinsonian rats. J Neurosci 19:3266–3274.
144. Sanchez-Pernaute R, Harvey-White J, Cunningham J, Bankiewicz KS (2001) Functional effect of adeno-associated virus mediated gene transfer of aromatic L-amino acid decarboxylase into the striatum of 6-OHDA-lesioned rats. Mol Ther 4:324–330.
145. Bankiewicz KS, Eberling JL, Kohutnicka M, et al (2000) Convection-enhanced delivery of AAV vector in parkinsonian monkeys; in vivo detection of gene expression and restoration of dopaminergic function using pro-drug approach. Exp Neurol 164:2–14.
146. Gill SS, Patel NK, Hotton GR, et al (2003) Direct brain infusion of glial cell line-derived neurotrophic factor in Parkinson disease. Nat Med 9:589–595.
147. Lang AE, Gill SS, Patel NK, et al (2006) Randomized controlled trial of intraputamenal glial cell line-derived neurotrophic factor infusion in Parkinson disease. Ann Neurol 59:459–466.
148. Freed CR, Greene PE, Breeze RE, et al (2001) Transplantation of embryonic dopamine neurons for severe Parkinson's disease. N Engl J Med 344:710–719.
149. Watts RL, Raiser CD, Stover NP, et al (2003) Stereotaxic intrastriatal implantation of human retinal pigment epithelial (hPRE) cells attached to gelatin microcarriers: a potential new cell therapy for Parkinson's disease. J Neural Transm Suppl 65:215–227.
150. Yoshizaki T, Inaji M, Kouike H, et al (2004) Isolation and transplantation of dopaminergic neurons generated from mouse embryonic stem cells. Neurosci Lett 363:33–37.
151. Zhao M, Momma S, Delfani K, et al (2003) Evidence for neurogenesis in the adult mammalian substantia nigra. Proc Natl Acad Sci USA 100:7925–7930.
152. Lee PY, Chesnoy S, Huang L (2004) Electroporatic delivery of TGF-beta1 gene works synergistically with electric therapy to enhance diabetic wound healing in db/db mice. J Invest Dermatol 123:791–798.
153. Iida Y, Oda Y, Nakamori S, Tsunoda S, Kishida T, Gojo S, Shin-Ya M, Asada H, Imanishi J, Yoshikawa T, Matsubara H, Mazda O (2006) Transthoracic direct current shock facilitates intramyocardial transfection of naked plasmid DNA infused via coronary vessels in canines. Gene Ther 13:906–916.

# Index

**A**
Activities-specific balance confidence (ABC) scale, 335
Air embolism, after DBS, 139–140
Alzheimer's disease, 292
Anterior cingulate cortex (ACC), 44, 50
Anterior commissure (AC), 100
Aripiprazole, 327
Aspiny striatal neurons, 6
Attention deficit hyperactivity disorder (ADHD), 322
Atypical parkinsonism (AP), DBS in
   diagnosis of MSA, 293–299
   diagnosis of the syndrome, 292–293
   features suggestive of an AP disorder, 292
   future targets for, 299–300
   subthalamic nucleus (STN) DBS, 299
Axonal spikes, 113

**B**
Bartholow, Roberts, 65
Basal ganglia (BG)
   integration across Cortico-BG circuits, 43
   pallidal complex and SN, SNr, 38–40
   pathways of the GP/SNr, 46
   role of, in parallel circuit and integrative network, 49–50
   SN, SNc and VTA, 41–43
   STN, 40–41
   striato-nigro-striatal network, 46–48
   striatum, 35–38
      functional organization of frontal cortical striatal projections, 43–46
   structures and connectivity, 34–35
   thalamo-cortico-thalamic interface, 48–49
Basal ganglia–thalamocortical network
   consequences of abnormalities
      dystonia, 17
      effects of lesions, 15
      hemiballism, 17
      Parkinson's disease or parkinsonism, 15–16
   between cortical neurons, 5
   dopamine receptors (D1-D5) in, 12
   effect of DBS, 169–170
   general structure, 4–5
   inputs to basal ganglia
      cortico-and thalamo-subthalamic projections, 10
      sensorimotor corticostriatal projections, 7–8
      thalamostriatal projections, 8–10
   intrinsic connections
      direct and indirect pathways, 10–11
      dopaminergic projections, 11–13
   intrinsic neuronal organization of nuclei
      GABAergic projection neurons, 7
      SNc neurons, 7
      SNr neurons, 7
      striatum, 5–7
   output projections
      nigrofugal pathways, 13
      pallidofugal pathways, 13–14
   role in motor control, 14–15
   segregation, anatomic concept of, 5
   sensorimotor portion of, 5
Beck Depression Inventory, 87
Behr's syndrome, 224
Ben-Gun method, 117
Biochemical studies, of DBS mechanisms, 154
Bipolar stimulations, 479
Bipolar testing, 481
Blood oxygenation level-dependent (BOLD)-fMRI, 180
Botulinum toxin injection, 322
Burke–Fahn–Marsden (BFM) scale, 306

# Index

## C
Calbindin (CaBP), 41
Center of gravity (CoG) sway, 336
Centromedian-parafascicular complex (CM-Pf), 323, 325
Cholinergic interneurons, 12
Clinical applications, of DBS, 576–577
Clonazepam, 322
Clonidine, 322, 327–328
Clozapine, 327
Cognitive testing tools, 88
Complications and management, in DBS
  air embolism, 139–140
  damage to lead or lead extender due to patient manipulation of the IPG, 145–146
  electrolysis and gas production, 145
  inadvertent thermal lesioning, 145
  infections, 140–141
  long-term hardware-related, 143–145
  misplaced electrodes, 142
  postoperative cognitive decline in patients with Parkinson's disease (PD), 146
  reasons for failure of device, 146–147
  sterile clear fluid collections, 141–142
  stroke, 135–139
Computer modeling, of DBS mechanisms, 154–155
Cortex-basal ganglia-thalamic-cortical circuits, 4
Cortico-subthalamic projection, 10

## D
Deep brain stimulation (DBS), 3, 50. *See also* Microelectrode recordings
  affective effects of depth electrode stimulation, 518–519
  CAPSIT criteria, 84
  case histories, 490–493
  circuit, 475–480
  combination with alternative technologies, 582–583
  commonly used tools for cognitive testing, 88
  complications and management
    air embolism, 139–140
    damage to lead or lead extender due to patient manipulation of the IPG, 145–146
    electrolysis and gas production, 145
    inadvertent thermal lesioning, 145
    infections, 140–141
    long-term hardware-related, 143–145
    misplaced electrodes, 142
    postoperative cognitive decline in patients with Parkinson's disease (PD), 146
    reasons for failure of device, 146–147
    sterile clear fluid collections, 141–142
    stroke, 135–139
  components and materials used, 455–456
  cost effectiveness of, 503
  in depression
    adverse effects, 516
    background, 513–514
    mechanisms, 515–516
    simulation technique, 515
    technical aspects, 514–515
  devices
    daily living, 578–579
    lead technology, 579–581
    simulation technology, 581–582
  dystonia
    clinical results, 306
    complications of therapy, 312
    dystonia-plus syndromes and other exceptional cases, 310
    evaluation of the efficacy of treatment, 306
    focal and segmental, 309–310
    generalized, 307–309
    management and practical issues, 313–314
    neuropsychological performance and mood, 312
    patient selection, 313
    safety, 312
    secondary, 310–311
    stimulation arrest and safety, 313
  emerging applications
    clinical applications, 576–577
    epilepsy, 576
  for epilepsy, 73
    approaches to, 562–563
    deep brain targets for, 564–566
  globus pallidus (GPi)
    adverse events, 285
    clinical results of patients treated for PD, 280, 282
    effect against cardinal features of PD and "off" disability, 281–284
    effect in the "On" medication state, 284–285
    functional imaging, 192–194
    treatment for PD, 244–250
  hardwares, 466
  history of, 70, 572–573
  importance of multidisciplinary assessment prior to, 83
  invasive testing, 486–488
  issues and recommendations, 522–524
  mechanisms of
    biochemical studies, 154
    computer modeling, 154–155
    effect on neuronal activity, 155–167
    effect on the network, 169–170
    imaging, 154
    methodologies, 153–155
    neural recordings, 153–154
    therapeutic, 167–168

Deep brain stimulation (DBS) (*Continued*)
  medically intractable cluster headache
    clinical outcomes, 554–556
    complications, 556–557
    device programming, 554
    documentation of electrode locations, 553
    indications for, 549
    mechanisms, 557–558
    pre-and postoperative evaluation, 549–550
    surgical technique, 550–553
    time course for stimulation-induced relief, 556
  neuropsychological issues in
    areas of functioning assessed, 405–411
    depression, neurobehavioral outcomes in, 428–429
    dystonia, neurobehavioral outcomes in, 426–427
    epilepsy, neurobehavioral outcomes in, 427–428
    ET, neurobehavioral outcomes in, 425–426
    evaluation of patients, 401–411
    interpretative and practical challenges for the neuropsychologist, 411–413
    methods of neuropsychological evaluation for, 404–405
    MS, neurobehavioral outcomes in, 428
    OCD, neurobehavioral outcomes in, 429
    other conditions, neurobehavioral outcomes in, 430
    overview, 400–401
    PD, neurobehavioral outcomes in, 413–425
    purposes of neuropsychological evaluation for, 403–404
    TS, neurobehavioral outcomes in, 430
  noninvasive active testing, 482–486
  noninvasive testing, 480–482
  obsessive–compulsive behavior (OCB)
    capsular, 532–535
    complications and adverse effects, 541–543
    description of acute effects, 536–537
    long-term follow-up, 540–541
    neurosurgical intervention, 535–536
    postoperative contact selection, 537–539
    randomized double blind crossover, 539–540
  for OCD, 73–74, 516–518
  for pain, 65
  patient selection
    in dystonia, 90–91
    in essential tremor (ET), 91–92
    in neuropsychiatric disorders, 92
    in PD, 84–89
  possible complications, 89
  potential interactions, 456–460
  for primary depressive illness, 520–522
  programming for movement disorders
    amplitude, 363–364
    basic approach to, 367–375
    electrode configuration, 366–367
    frequency, 365–366
    future directions, 390
    issues related to GPi, 387–390
    issues related to STN, 379–387
    issues related to targets, 376–379
    pulse width, 364–365
    stimulation parameters, 362–363
  published and reported adverse events, 466–467
  responsiveness of PD Symptoms with, 86
  risk factors
    age, 89
    imaging, 89–90
    medical co-morbidities, 90
    patients with prior ablative surgery, 90
  subthalamic nucleus (STN)
    adverse events, 285
    aspects of gait, 261
    balance, 260–261
    bladder functions, 264
    clinical results of patients treated for PD, 279
    cognitive effects, 262
    dysarthria/hypophonia and weight gain effects, 267
    dyskinesias, 259, 267
    effect against cardinal features of PD and "off" disability, 281–284
    effect in the "On" medication state, 284–285
    effects on motor aspects, 256–262
    effects on nonmotor aspects, 262–264
    group of behaviors, 262–264
    indications and contraindications, 254–256
    motor fluctuations, 259–260
    postural instability, 268
    psychiatric complications, 266–267
    quality of life, 264–265
    rationale, 253–254
    sexual functions, 264
    side effects and complications, 265–268
    sleep, 264
    subthalamotomy *vs.*, 268–269
  system, 474–475
  technical alternatives in implantation procedure
    interventional MRI, 107–110
    localization using peri-operative and intra-operative imaging, 105–107
    Medtronic NexFrame, 101–103
    StarFix micro Targeting Platform, 104–105
    surgical navigation systems, 100–101
  testing methodology, 488–490
  of thalamus, 205–211
    general experience of VL DBS for MS, 216–224
    head tremor, 209–210
    "Off-label" *vs.* "Experimental" use of DBS and insurance coverage, 224–225
    selected studies of, 206–208, 210–211

Deep brain stimulation (DBS) (*Continued*)
  surgical issues unique to non-ET and non-PD tremor, 224
  as "symptomatic," 225
  thalamotomy *vs.*, 211–213
  for treatment of Parkinson's disease (PD) tremor, 230–236
  for tremors other than MS, 224
  unilateral *vs.* bilateral stimulation, 209
  voice tremor, 210–211
 Tourette's syndrome (TS)
  clinical and surgical evaluation, 327–328
  neuroanatomical basis for, 325–327
  other considerations, 329
  reports on deep brain stimulation in patients, 330
 treatment of postural stability and gait disorders in PD
  clinical assessments and quantitative measures, 334–337
  effect on PPN, 352–353
  effects, 338–352
  long-term effects of STN and GPi DBS on, 353
 for tremor, 71
 types of motor fluctuations, 84–85
 *vs.* psychosurgery, 573–576
Dementia with Lewy bodies, 292
Depression
 background, 511–512
 deep brain stimulation (DBS)
  adverse effects, 516
  background, 513–514
  mechanisms, 515–516
  simulation technique, 515
  technical aspects, 514–515
 pathophysiology, 513
 phenomenology, 512–513
 treatment resistance, 512
Depression, neurocircuitry of, 50–51
Diagnostic and Statistical Manual of Mental Disorders (DSM-IV TR), 322
Diagnostic Confidence Index (DCI), 327
Direct and indirect striatofugal projections, 10
Dopamine (DA)
 cells in striatum, 46–47
 functional correlates of the cells, 43
 neurons, 37, 42
 receptors, 37
 transporter (DAT), 42
Dopaminergic projections, 11–13
Dorsal pallidal segments, 39
Dorsolateral prefrontal cortex (DLPFC), 44–45
Dyskinesias, 259
Dystonia, 3, 17, 73, 388–389
 DBS in, 305–314
 neurobehavioral outcomes after DBS, 426–427

 quality of life, GPi DBS effects, 501
DYT1 gene, 73

E
Electricity, therapeutic use on brain development
 modern era of DBS, 70–74
 stimulation between 1700–1900, 64–65
 stimulation between 1900–1987, 65–70
 stimulation up to 1700, 63–64
 use by ancient Greeks, 63
Electroconvulsive therapy (ECT), 402
Electromyography (EMG) software, 482
Enkephalin (ENK), 37
Entopeduncular nucleus (EPN), 4
Epilepsy
 DBS
  anterior nucleus of the thalamus, effects of, 565
  approaches to, 562–563
  caudate nucleus, effects of, 565
  centromedian nucleus of thalamus, effects of, 565
  cerebellar nuclei, effects of, 565
  deep brain targets for, 564–566
  hippocampus and amygdala, effects of, 565–566
  locus coeruleus stimulation in humans, effects of, 566
  neurobehavioral outcomes after DBS, 427–428
  stimulation of the STN, effects of, 566
 overview, 561–562
 treatment approaches, 561–562
Essential tremor (ET), 91–92
 thalamic DBS effects on quality of life, 500–501
Extended Disability Status Scale (EDSS) scale, 216
External globus pallidus (GPe), 4, 124–125
Extracellular recordings. *See* Microelectrode recordings

F
Faradic current, 65
Fibers, 39, 51
 GPi, 40
FLASQ-PD, 85
[$^{18}$F] Fluorodeoxyglucose (FDG)-PET technique, 180
Focal and segmental dystonia, 309–310
FOG, DBS effects on, 351–352
Functional imaging, of DBS
 globus pallidus (GPi)
  for generalized dystonia, 193–194
  for PD, 192–193
 subthalamic nucleus (STN )
  acute, in a resting state visualized by, 181–185
  L-dopa effects, 188–189
  motor tasks, 185–188
 use and purpose of, 180
 ventral intermediate nucleus (VIM)
  of essential tremor, 190–191
  of Parkinsonian tremor, 191–192

## G

GABAergic neurons, 4–5, 7, 38, 45
Gait disorder, DBS effects
  act of sit-to-stand, 345
  initiation, 345–346
  long-term effects, 353
  treatment of PPN, 352–353
  walking, 346–351
Galen, 64
Galvani, Luigi, 64
Generalized dystonia, 307–309
Gilbert, William, 63
Globus pallidus (GPi)
  altered sensory feedback, effect of DBS, 341
  anatomy, 387–388
  DBS, functional imaging
    for generalized dystonia, 193–194
    for PD, 192–193
  DBS treatment for Parkinson's disease (PD) patients
    ADL scores off medication/on stimulation, 248
    adverse events, 249
    clinical results of patients treated, 280, 282
    effect against cardinal features of PD and "off" disability, 281–284
    effect in the "On" medication state, 284–285
    impact on quality of life, 248–249
    status of, 249–250
    unilateral vs. bilateral stimulation, 244–247
  dystonia, 388–389
  external perturbations, effect of DBS, 341
  medical adjustments, 389
  optimal contact selection, 388
  quality of life and DBS, 499
  during quiet stance, effect of DBS, 341
  rationale for targeting, 326
  stimulantion-related adverse events, 389–390
GP/SNr pathways, 46

## H

Haloperidol, 322, 327
Hamilton Anxiety Rating Scale, 87–88
Hamilton Depression Rating Scale, 87
Head tremor DBS, 209–210
Heath, Robert, 68
Hemiballism, 17
Huntington's disease, 7

## I

Imaging, of DBS mechanisms, 154
Implantable pulse generator (IPG), 475
IMRI technique, 108
Infection, after DBS, 140–141
Internal globus pallidus (GPi), 4, 72, 90
  microelectrode recording, 124–127

Intra-operative microelectrode recording
  anesthesia, 118
  setup and procedure, 116–117
  single- vs. multitrajectory recording, 117
  stimulation, 117–118
Intrinsic neuronal organization, of nuclei
  GABAergic projection neurons, 7
  SNc neurons, 7
  SNr neurons, 7
  striatum, 5–7
Invasive testing, 486–488

## L

Largus, Scribbonius, 64
Lateral habenular nucleus, 4
Levodopa, 16, 68, 84, 324
Levodopa Equivalent Dose (LDED), 256–259
Lormetazepam, 328

## M

Mattis Dementia Rating Scale (MDRS), 87
Medically intractable cluster headache
  DBS
    clinical outcomes, 554–556
    complications, 556–557
    device programming, 554
    documentation of electrode locations, 553
    indications for, 549
    mechanisms, 557–558
    pre-and postoperative evaluation, 549–550
    surgical technique, 550–553
    time course for stimulation-induced relief, 556
  evidence for hypothalamic involvement in, 548
  overview, 547–548
Medium spiny neurons (MSNs), 37
Medtronic Kinetra Model 7428 Neurostimulator, 578
Medtronic Soletra™ Model 7426 Neurostimulator, 578
Meige syndrome, 91
Methylphenidate, 322
MPTP-induced toxicity, 42
Microelectrode recordings
  benefits and risks, 127–130
  methods
    electronic equipment, 115–116
    intra-operative procedure, 116–118
    microelectrodes, 114–115
  physiology, 112–113
  target specific strategies
    internal globus pallidus (GPi), 124–127
    nucleus ventrointermedius thalami (VIM), 123–124
    subthalamic nucleus (STN), 119–123
    tetrodes, use of, 114–115
Micro Targeting Platform (MTP), 104
Mini Mental State Exam (MMSE), 87

Monopolar impedances and currents, 481–482
Monopolar stimulations, 479
Montgomery Asberg Depression Rating Scale, 87
Montreal procedure, 65
Motor fluctuations, 259–260
Movement disorders, 3
  affective changes after DBS, 519–520
MP35N, 475
MRI environment, 460–461
  potential interactions
    artifacts, 465–466
    gradient-induced currents, 462
    RF field, 462–465
    static field interactions, 461–462
MSN. *See* Medium spiny neurons (MSNs)
Multiple sclerosis (MS), 501–502
Multiple system atrophy (MSA), 255, 292
  globus pallidus DBS, 298–299
  published case reports of, 294–295
  STN DBS in
    with features of PD, 293–297
    with typical MSA, 298

N
Neural recordings, examining DBS mechanisms, 153–154
Neuronal activity, effect of DBS
  computer models, 165–167
  neurochemical and gene expression studies, 161–165
  recordings in downstream nuclei, 157–161
  recordings in the stimulated nucleus, 156–157
Neurostimulation, 64–65
NexFrame™, 101–103, 107–108
Nigro-collicular fibers, 13
Nigrofugal pathways, 13
Nigro-tegmental projections, 13
Nitric oxide synthase (NOS), 38
Noninvasive active testing, 482–486
Noninvasive testing, 480–482

O
Obsessive–compulsive behavior (OCB), 322
  capsulotomy for, 532
  deep brain stimulation (DBS), 516–518
    capsular, 532–535
    complications and adverse effects, 541–543
    description of acute effects, 536–537
    long-term follow-up, 540–541
    neurosurgical intervention, 535–536
    postoperative contact selection, 537–539
    randomized double blind crossover, 539–540
  neurobehavioral outcomes after DBS, 429
  treatment options, 532

Obsessive–compulsive Disorder (OCD), neurocircuitry of, 50–51
[$^{15}$O]H$_2$O PET, 180
Olanzapine, 327
Orbital frontal cortex (OFC), 44–45, 50

P
Pallidal complex, 38–40
Pallidofugal pathways, 13–14
PAN. *See* Phasically active neurons (PANs)
Pantothenate kinase associated neurodegeneration (PANK2), 310–311
Parkinsonism-plus syndromes. *See* Atypical parkinsonism (AP), DBS in
Parkinson's disease, 3, 15–16, 40, 50, 68
  DBS treatment of globus pallidus (GPi)
    ADL scores off medication/on stimulation, 248
    adverse events, 249
    impact on quality of life, 248–249
    status of, 249–250
    unilateral *vs.* bilateral stimulation, 244–247
  DBS treatment of subthalamic nucleus (STN)
    aspects of gait, 261
    balance, 260–261
    bladder functions, 264
    cognitive effects, 262
    dysarthria/hypophonia and weight gain effects, 267
    dyskinesias, 259, 267
    effects on motor aspects, 256–262
    effects on nonmotor aspects, 262–264
    group of behaviors, 262–264
    indications and contraindications, 254–256
    motor fluctuations, 259–260
    postural instability, 268
    psychiatric complications, 266–267
    quality of life, 264–265
    rationale, 253–254
    sexual functions, 264
    side effects and complications, 265–268
    sleep, 264
    subthalamotomy *vs.*, 268–269
  idiopathic, 300
  neurobehavioral outcomes after DBS, 413–425
  quality of life
    GPi DBS effects, 499
    predictive indicators, 499–500
    STN DBS effects, 496–499
    thalamic DBS effects, 499
  thalamic deep brain stimulation
    adverse effects, 235–236
    background, 230–231
    importance, 232–233
    patient selection, 231–232
    problem of progressive parkinsonism after, 232
    results, 233–234

treatment of postural stability and gait disorders of
 clinical assessments and quantitative measures,
 334–337
  effect DBS on the PPN, 352–353
  effect of DBS, 338–352
  long-term effects of STN and GPi DBS on, 353
Pars compacta (SNc), 41–43
Pars reticulata (SNr), 38–40, 120, 156
Parvicellular reticular formation, 4
Patient selection, for DBS
 role of neurologist, 84–86
 role of neuropsychologist, 86–87
 role of neurosurgeon, 88
 role of psychiatrist, 87–88
PD. *See* Parkinson's disease
Pedunculopontine nucleus (PPN), 4, 10, 16
Pergolide, 327
Peri-operative and intra-operative imaging, in DBS, 105–107
Pharmacologic dopamine replacement therapy, 16
Phasically active neurons (PANs), 37
1.5T Philips Intera MRI, 107
Pimozide, 327
Pool, J. Lawrence, 66
Posterior commissure (PC), 100, 326, 550, 557
Postural stability
 clinical assessments, 334–335
 effect of DBS
  instability in PD, 338–342
  long-term effects, 353
  long-term or adaptive changes, 343
  treatment of PPN, 352–353
  underlying pathophysiology and theories, 343–344
 effect of medication, 339–341
 quantitative measures of
  kinematics-3-D motion analysis, 337
  posturography, 335–336
  voluntary movement, 336–337
Posturography, 335–336
Primary depressive illness, 520–522
Progressive supranuclear palsy, 292
Propofol Target Controlled Infusion, 328
Psychostimulants, 322
Psychosurgery, 573–574

## Q

Quality of life
 DBS effect on multiple sclerosis (MS), 501–502
 dystonia, GPi DBS effects on, 501
 GPi DBS effects in PD, 499
 predictive indicators in PD, 499–500
 STN DBS effects in PD, 496–499
 subthalamic nucleus (STN), 264–265
 thalamic DBS effects in PD, 499

## R

RCBF SPECT, 180
Repetitive transcranial magnetic stimulation (rTMS), 402–403
Risperidone, 327

## S

Self-injurious behavior (SIB), 322
Sensorimotor corticostriatal projections, 7–8
SF-36 scale, 307, 309
SN. *See* Substantia nigra (SN)
SNc. *See* Pars compacta (SNc)
SNc neurons, 7
SNc-v neurons, 11
SNr. *See* Pars reticulata (SNr)
SNr neurons, 7
Spiegel, Ernest, 67
Spiegel-Wycis device, 67
StarFix™ micro Targeting® Platform, 101, 104–105
Static electricity, 63
Status dystonicus, 310
StealthStation®, 100
Sterile clear fluid collection, after DBS, 141–142
STN. *See* Subthalamic nucleus (STN)
Striato-nigro-striatal network, 46–48
Striatum, 5–7
 afferent connections, 35–37
 dorsolateral, 33
 functional organization of frontal cortical striatal projections, 43–46
 intrinsic cells of, 37–38
 ventral, 38
Stroke, after DBS, 135–137
 avoidance, 137–139
 management of, 139
Stryker® Navigation System, 100
Substance P (SP), 37
Substantia nigra (SN), 38–43
Subthalamic nucleus (STN), 4, 40–41, 72–73, 107
 altered sensory feedback, effect of DBS, 341
 anatomy, 379
 DBS
  with features of PD, 293–297
  in other forms of AP, 299
  with typical MSA, 298
 DBS, functional imaging
  acute, in a resting state visualized by, 181–185
  chronic state, 184–185
  L-dopa effects, 188–189
  local and distant effects of, 183
  motion-related fMRI activity, effects on, 185–186
  motion-related rCBF, effects on, 187–188
  motor tasks, 185–186
  motor tasks, in PET and SPECT, 186–188
  rCBF in cognitive tasks, effects on, 188

Subthalamic nucleus (STN), (*Continued*)
  DBS treatment for atypical parkinsonism, 299
  DBS treatment for PD
    aspects of gait, 261
    balance, 260–261
    bladder functions, 264
    clinical results of patients, 279
    cognitive effects, 262
    dysarthria/hypophonia and weight gain effects, 267
    dyskinesias, 259, 267
    effect against cardinal features of PD and "off" disability, 281–284
    effect in the "On" medication state, 284–285
    effects on motor aspects, 256–262
    effects on nonmotor aspects, 262–264
    group of behaviors, 262–264
    indications and contraindications, 254–256
    motor fluctuations, 259–260
    postural instability, 268
    psychiatric complications, 266–267
    quality of life, 264–265
    rationale, 253–254
    sexual functions, 264
    side effects and complications, 265–268
    sleep, 264
    subthalamotomy *vs.*, 268–269
  electrophysiologic mapping, 119–123
  external perturbations, effect of DBS, 341
  medication adjustments, 381–383
  optimal contact selection, 379–381
  quality of life and DBS, 496–499
  during quiet stance, effect of DBS, 341
  stimulation-related adverse events, 383
  target-related adverse events, 383–387
  therapeutic mechanisms, of DBS, 167–168
Subthalamotomy, 268–269
Sulpiride, 327
Superior colliculus, 4

**T**
TANS. *See* Tonically active neurons (TANS)
Tetrabenazine, 322
Thalamic deep brain stimulation
  general experience of VL DBS for MS, 216–224
  head tremor, 209–210
  "Off-label" *vs.* "Experimental" use of DBS and insurance coverage, 224–225
  and quality of life, 499–501
  rationale for targeting the medial portion, 325–326
  selected studies of, 206–208, 210–211
  surgical issues unique to non-ET and non-PD tremor, 224
  as "symptomatic," 225

  thalamotomy *vs.*, 211–213
  for the treatment of Parkinson's disease (PD) tremor
    adverse effects, 235–236
    background, 230–231
    importance, 232–233
    patient selection, 231–232
    problem of progressive parkinsonism after, 232
    results, 233–234
  for tremors other than MS, 224
  unilateral *vs.* bilateral stimulation, 209
  voice tremor, 210–211
Thalamo-cortico-thalamic interface, 48–49
Thalamostriatal projections, 8–10
Thalamotomy
  Pahwa and coworkers experiments, 212
  Schuurman and colleagues experiments, 212
  Tasker and colleagues experiments, 212
Theory of animal electricity, 64
Therapeutic mechanisms, of DBS, 167–168
Tics, 321–322
Tonically active neurons (TANS), 38
Toronto Western Spasmodic Torticollis Rating Scale (TWSTRS), 90, 306, 310
Tourette's syndrome (TS)
  clinical characteristics and prevalence, 321–322
  DBS
    clinical and surgical evaluation, 327–328
    neuroanatomical basis for, 325–327
    other considerations, 329
    reports on deep brain stimulation in patients, 330
  neurobehavioral outcomes after DBS, 430
  targets, 324–325
  treatment of, 322–323
    neurosurgical, 323–324
Tremor Activities of Daily Living Scale (TADLS), 500
Tyrosine hydroxylase-immunoreactive interneurons, 7

**U**
Unified Parkinson's Disease Rating Scale (UPDRS), 71–72, 84–85, 118, 254–256, 268, 335, 343
Unilateral *vs.* bilateral stimulation, 209

**V**
Vascular pathology, 292
VectorVision®, 100
Ventral intermediate nucleus (VIM)
  adverse effect of DBS, 235–236
  DBS for treatment of PD tremor, 233–234
  DBS, functional imaging
    of essential tremor, 190–191
    of Parkinsonian tremor, 191–192
  microelectrode recording of, 123–124
  stimulation, for PD, 70, 72

*vs.* thalamotomy, 236–237
Ventral motor thalamic nuclei, 4
Ventral pallidum (VP), 39
Ventral tegmental area (VTA), 34, 41–43
Ventrolateral nucleus of the thalamus (VL) DBS
  conundrum, 221–222
  general experience, for MS, 216–219
  long-term efficacy, for MS, 219–221
  published literature on the efficacy of, 217–218
  unique pre-operative and postoperative issues related to non-ET and non-PD tremor, 222–224
Voice tremor DBS, 210–211
Volta, Allesandro, 64
Volta's pile, 64
Von Musschebroek, Pieter, 64

**W**
Weinhold, Karl, 65
Wilson's disease, 91
Wycis, Henry, 67

**X**
X-linked progressive dystonia-parkinsonism, 6

**Y**
Yale Global Tic Severity Scale (YGTSS), 328
Young Mania Scale, 87

Printed in the United States of America